SLEEP APNEA

LUNG BIOLOGY IN HEALTH AND DISEASE

Executive Editor

Claude Lenfant
Director, National Heart, Lung and Blood Institute
National Institutes of Health
Bethesda, Maryland

1. Immunologic and Infectious Reactions in the Lung, *edited by C. H. Kirkpatrick and H. Y. Reynolds*
2. The Biochemical Basis of Pulmonary Function, *edited by R. G. Crystal*
3. Bioengineering Aspects of the Lung, *edited by J. B. West*
4. Metabolic Functions of the Lung, *edited by Y. S. Bakhle and J. R. Vane*
5. Respiratory Defense Mechanisms (in two parts), *edited by J. D. Brain, D. F. Proctor, and L. M. Reid*
6. Development of the Lung, *edited by W. A. Hodson*
7. Lung Water and Solute Exchange, *edited by N. C. Staub*
8. Extrapulmonary Manifestations of Respiratory Disease, *edited by E. D. Robin*
9. Chronic Obstructive Pulmonary Disease, *edited by T. L. Petty*
10. Pathogenesis and Therapy of Lung Cancer, *edited by C. C. Harris*
11. Genetic Determinants of Pulmonary Disease, *edited by S. D. Litwin*
12. The Lung in the Transition Between Health and Disease, *edited by P. T. Macklem and S. Permutt*
13. Evolution of Respiratory Processes: A Comparative Approach, *edited by S. C. Wood and C. Lenfant*
14. Pulmonary Vascular Diseases, *edited by K. M. Moser*
15. Physiology and Pharmacology of the Airways, *edited by J. A. Nadel*
16. Diagnostic Techniques in Pulmonary Disease (in two parts), *edited by M. A. Sackner*
17. Regulation of Breathing (in two parts), *edited by T. F. Hornbein*
18. Occupational Lung Diseases: Research Approaches and Methods, *edited by H. Weill and M. Turner-Warwick*
19. Immunopharmacology of the Lung, *edited by H. H. Newball*
20. Sarcoidosis and Other Granulomatous Diseases of the Lung, *edited by B. L. Fanburg*
21. Sleep and Breathing, *edited by N. A. Saunders and C. E. Sullivan*
22. *Pneumocystis carinii* Pneumonia: Pathogenesis, Diagnosis, and Treatment, *edited by L. S. Young*
23. Pulmonary Nuclear Medicine: Techniques in Diagnosis of Lung Disease, *edited by H. L. Atkins*
24. Acute Respiratory Failure, *edited by W. M. Zapol and K. J. Falke*
25. Gas Mixing and Distribution in the Lung, *edited by L. A. Engel and M. Paiva*

26. High-Frequency Ventilation in Intensive Care and During Surgery, *edited by G. Carlon and W. S. Howland*
27. Pulmonary Development: Transition from Intrauterine to Extrauterine Life, *edited by G. H. Nelson*
28. Chronic Obstructive Pulmonary Disease: Second Edition, *edited by T. L. Petty*
29. The Thorax (in two parts), *edited by C. Roussos and P. T. Macklem*
30. The Pleura in Health and Disease, *edited by J. Chrétien, J. Bignon, and A. Hirsch*
31. Drug Therapy for Asthma: Research and Clinical Practice, *edited by J. W. Jenne and S. Murphy*
32. Pulmonary Endothelium in Health and Disease, *edited by U. S. Ryan*
33. The Airways: Neural Control in Health and Disease, *edited by M. A. Kaliner and P. J. Barnes*
34. Pathophysiology and Treatment of Inhalation Injuries, *edited by J. Loke*
35. Respiratory Function of the Upper Airway, *edited by O. P. Mathew and G. Sant'Ambrogio*
36. Chronic Obstructive Pulmonary Disease: A Behavioral Perspective, *edited by A. J. McSweeny and I. Grant*
37. Biology of Lung Cancer: Diagnosis and Treatment, *edited by S. T. Rosen, J. L. Mulshine, F. Cuttitta, and P. G. Abrams*
38. Pulmonary Vascular Physiology and Pathophysiology, *edited by E. K. Weir and J. T. Reeves*
39. Comparative Pulmonary Physiology: Current Concepts, *edited by S. C. Wood*
40. Respiratory Physiology: An Analytical Approach, *edited by H. K. Chang and M. Paiva*
41. Lung Cell Biology, *edited by D. Massaro*
42. Heart–Lung Interactions in Health and Disease, *edited by S. M. Scharf and S. S. Cassidy*
43. Clinical Epidemiology of Chronic Obstructive Pulmonary Disease, *edited by M. J. Hensley and N. A. Saunders*
44. Surgical Pathology of Lung Neoplasms, *edited by A. M. Marchevsky*
45. The Lung in Rheumatic Diseases, *edited by G. W. Cannon and G. A. Zimmerman*
46. Diagnostic Imaging of the Lung, *edited by C. E. Putman*
47. Models of Lung Disease: Microscopy and Structural Methods, *edited by J. Gil*
48. Electron Microscopy of the Lung, *edited by D. E. Schraufnagel*
49. Asthma: Its Pathology and Treatment, *edited by M. A. Kaliner, P. J. Barnes, and C. G. A. Persson*
50. Acute Respiratory Failure: Second Edition, *edited by W. M. Zapol and F. Lemaire*
51. Lung Disease in the Tropics, *edited by O. P. Sharma*
52. Exercise: Pulmonary Physiology and Pathophysiology, *edited by B. J. Whipp and K. Wasserman*
53. Developmental Neurobiology of Breathing, *edited by G. G. Haddad and J. P. Farber*
54. Mediators of Pulmonary Inflammation, *edited by M. A. Bray and W. H. Anderson*
55. The Airway Epithelium, *edited by S. G. Farmer and D. Hay*

56. Physiological Adaptations in Vertebrates: Respiration, Circulation, and Metabolism, *edited by S. C. Wood, R. E. Weber, A. R. Hargens, and R. W. Millard*
57. The Bronchial Circulation, *edited by J. Butler*
58. Lung Cancer Differentiation: Implications for Diagnosis and Treatment, *edited by S. D. Bernal and P. J. Hesketh*
59. Pulmonary Complications of Systemic Disease, *edited by J. F. Murray*
60. Lung Vascular Injury: Molecular and Cellular Response, *edited by A. Johnson and T. J. Ferro*
61. Cytokines of the Lung, *edited by J. Kelley*
62. The Mast Cell in Health and Disease, *edited by M. A. Kaliner and D. D. Metcalfe*
63. Pulmonary Disease in the Elderly Patient, *edited by D. A. Mahler*
64. Cystic Fibrosis, *edited by P. B. Davis*
65. Signal Transduction in Lung Cells, *edited by J. S. Brody, D. M. Center, and V. A. Tkachuk*
66. Tuberculosis: A Comprehensive International Approach, *edited by L. B. Reichman and E. S. Hershfield*
67. Pharmacology of the Respiratory Tract: Experimental and Clinical Research, *edited by K. F. Chung and P. J. Barnes*
68. Prevention of Respiratory Diseases, *edited by A. Hirsch, M. Goldberg, J.-P. Martin, and R. Masse*
69. *Pneumocystis carinii* Pneumonia: Second Edition, *edited by P. D. Walzer*
70. Fluid and Solute Transport in the Airspaces of the Lungs, *edited by R. M. Effros and H. K. Chang*
71. Sleep and Breathing: Second Edition, *edited by N. A. Saunders and C. E. Sullivan*
72. Airway Secretion: Physiological Bases for the Control of Mucous Hypersecretion, *edited by T. Takishima and S. Shimura*
73. Sarcoidosis and Other Granulomatous Disorders, *edited by D. G. James*
74. Epidemiology of Lung Cancer, *edited by J. M. Samet*
75. Pulmonary Embolism, *edited by M. Morpurgo*
76. Sports and Exercise Medicine, *edited by S. C. Wood and R. C. Roach*
77. Endotoxin and the Lungs, *edited by K. L. Brigham*
78. The Mesothelial Cell and Mesothelioma, *edited by M.-C. Jaurand and J. Bignon*
79. Regulation of Breathing: Second Edition, *edited by J. A. Dempsey and A. I. Pack*
80. Pulmonary Fibrosis, *edited by S. Hin. Phan and R. S. Thrall*
81. Long-Term Oxygen Therapy: Scientific Basis and Clinical Application, *edited by W. J. O'Donohue, Jr.*
82. Ventral Brainstem Mechanisms and Control of Respiration and Blood Pressure, *edited by C. O. Trouth, R. M. Millis, H. F. Kiwull-Schöne, and M. E. Schläfke*
83. A History of Breathing Physiology, *edited by D. F. Proctor*
84. Surfactant Therapy for Lung Disease, *edited by B. Robertson and H. W. Taeusch*
85. The Thorax: Second Edition, Revised and Expanded (in three parts), *edited by C. Roussos*

86. Severe Asthma: Pathogenesis and Clinical Management, *edited by S. J. Szefler and D. Y. M. Leung*
87. *Mycobacterium avium*–Complex Infection: Progress in Research and Treatment, *edited by J. A. Korvick and C. A. Benson*
88. Alpha 1–Antitrypsin Deficiency: Biology • Pathogenesis • Clinical Manifestations • Therapy, *edited by R. G. Crystal*
89. Adhesion Molecules and the Lung, *edited by P. A. Ward and J. C. Fantone*
90. Respiratory Sensation, *edited by L. Adams and A. Guz*
91. Pulmonary Rehabilitation, *edited by A. P. Fishman*
92. Acute Respiratory Failure in Chronic Obstructive Pulmonary Disease, *edited by J.-P. Derenne, W. A. Whitelaw, and T. Similowski*
93. Environmental Impact on the Airways: From Injury to Repair, *edited by J. Chrétien and D. Dusser*
94. Inhalation Aerosols: Physical and Biological Basis for Therapy, *edited by A. J. Hickey*
95. Tissue Oxygen Deprivation: From Molecular to Integrated Function, *edited by G. G. Haddad and G. Lister*
96. The Genetics of Asthma, *edited by S. B. Liggett and D. A. Meyers*
97. Inhaled Glucocorticoids in Asthma: Mechanisms and Clinical Actions, *edited by R. P. Schleimer, W. W. Busse, and P. M. O'Byrne*
98. Nitric Oxide and the Lung, *edited by W. M. Zapol and K. D. Bloch*
99. Primary Pulmonary Hypertension, *edited by L. J. Rubin and S. Rich*
100. Lung Growth and Development, *edited by J. A. McDonald*
101. Parasitic Lung Diseases, *edited by A. A. F. Mahmoud*
102. Lung Macrophages and Dendritic Cells in Health and Disease, *edited by M. F. Lipscomb and S. W. Russell*
103. Pulmonary and Cardiac Imaging, *edited by C. Chiles and C. E. Putman*
104. Gene Therapy for Diseases of the Lung, *edited by K. L. Brigham*
105. Oxygen, Gene Expression, and Cellular Function, *edited by L. Biadasz Clerch and D. J. Massaro*
106. Beta$_2$-Agonists in Asthma Treatment, *edited by R. Pauwels and P. M. O'Byrne*
107. Inhalation Delivery of Therapeutic Peptides and Proteins, *edited by A. L. Adjei and P. K. Gupta*
108. Asthma in the Elderly, *edited by R. A. Barbee and J. W. Bloom*
109. Treatment of the Hospitalized Cystic Fibrosis Patient, *edited by D. M. Orenstein and R. C. Stern*
110. Asthma and Immunological Diseases in Pregnancy and Early Infancy, *edited by M. Schatz, R. S. Zeiger, and H. N. Claman*
111. Dyspnea, *edited by D. A. Mahler*
112. Proinflammatory and Antiinflammatory Peptides, *edited by S. I. Said*
113. Self-Management of Asthma, *edited by H. Kotses and A. Harver*
114. Eicosanoids, Aspirin, and Asthma, *edited by A. Szczeklik, R. J. Gryglewski, and J. R. Vane*
115. Fatal Asthma, *edited by A. L. Sheffer*
116. Pulmonary Edema, *edited by M. A. Matthay and D. H. Ingbar*
117. Inflammatory Mechanisms in Asthma, *edited by S. T. Holgate and W. W. Busse*
118. Physiological Basis of Ventilatory Support, *edited by J. J. Marini and A. S. Slutsky*

119. Human Immunodeficiency Virus and the Lung, *edited by M. J. Rosen and J. M. Beck*
120. Five-Lipoxygenase Products in Asthma, *edited by J. M. Drazen, S.-E. Dahlén, and T. H. Lee*
121. Complexity in Structure and Function of the Lung, *edited by M. P. Hlastala and H. T. Robertson*
122. Biology of Lung Cancer, *edited by M. A. Kane and P. A. Bunn, Jr.*
123. Rhinitis: Mechanisms and Management, *edited by R. M. Naclerio, S. R. Durham, and N. Mygind*
124. Lung Tumors: Fundamental Biology and Clinical Management, *edited by C. Brambilla and E. Brambilla*
125. Interleukin-5: From Molecule to Drug Target for Asthma, *edited by C. J. Sanderson*
126. Pediatric Asthma, *edited by S. Murphy and H. W. Kelly*
127. Viral Infections of the Respiratory Tract, *edited by R. Dolin and P. F. Wright*
128. Air Pollutants and the Respiratory Tract, *edited by D. L. Swift and W. M. Foster*
129. Gastroesophageal Reflux Disease and Airway Disease, *edited by M. R. Stein*
130. Exercise-Induced Asthma, *edited by E. R. McFadden, Jr.*
131. LAM and Other Diseases Characterized by Smooth Muscle Proliferation, *edited by J. Moss*
132. The Lung at Depth, *edited by C. E. G. Lundgren and J. N. Miller*
133. Regulation of Sleep and Circadian Rhythms, *edited by F. W. Turek and P. C. Zee*
134. Anticholinergic Agents in the Upper and Lower Airways, *edited by S. L. Spector*
135. Control of Breathing in Health and Disease, *edited by M. D. Altose and Y. Kawakami*
136. Immunotherapy in Asthma, *edited by J. Bousquet and H. Yssel*
137. Chronic Lung Disease in Early Infancy, *edited by R. D. Bland and J. J. Coalson*
138. Asthma's Impact on Society: The Social and Economic Burden, *edited by K. B. Weiss, A. S. Buist, and S. D. Sullivan*
139. New and Exploratory Therapeutic Agents for Asthma, *edited by M. Yeadon and Z. Diamant*
140. Multimodality Treatment of Lung Cancer, *edited by A. T. Skarin*
141. Cytokines in Pulmonary Disease: Infection and Inflammation, *edited by S. Nelson and T. R. Martin*
142. Diagnostic Pulmonary Pathology, *edited by P. T. Cagle*
143. Particle–Lung Interactions, *edited by P. Gehr and J. Heyder*
144. Tuberculosis: A Comprehensive International Approach, Second Edition, Revised and Expanded, *edited by L. B. Reichman and E. S. Hershfield*
145. Combination Therapy for Asthma and Chronic Obstructive Pulmonary Disease, *edited by R. J. Martin and M. Kraft*
146. Sleep Apnea: Implications in Cardiovascular and Cerebrovascular Disease, *edited by T. D. Bradley and J. S. Floras*
147. Sleep and Breathing in Children: A Developmental Approach, *edited by G. M. Loughlin, J. L. Carroll, and C. L. Marcus*

148. Pulmonary and Peripheral Gas Exchange in Health and Disease, *edited by J. Roca, R. Rodriguez-Roisen, and P. D. Wagner*
149. Lung Surfactants: Basic Science and Clinical Applications, *R. H. Notter*
150. Nosocomial Pneumonia, *edited by W. R. Jarvis*
151. Fetal Origins of Cardiovascular and Lung Disease, *edited by David J. P. Barker*
152. Long-Term Mechanical Ventilation, *edited by N. S. Hill*
153. Environmental Asthma, *edited by R. K. Bush*
154. Asthma and Respiratory Infections, *edited by D. P. Skoner*
155. Airway Remodeling, *edited by P. H. Howarth, J. W. Wilson, J. Bousquet, S. Rak, and R. A. Pauwels*
156. Genetic Models in Cardiorespiratory Biology, *edited by G. G. Haddad and T. Xu*
157. Respiratory-Circulatory Interactions in Health and Disease, *edited by S. M. Scharf, M. R. Pinsky, and S. Magder*
158. Ventilator Management Strategies for Critical Care, *edited by N. S. Hill and M. M. Levy*
159. Severe Asthma: Pathogenesis and Clinical Management, Second Edition, Revised and Expanded, *edited by S. J. Szefler and D. Y. M. Leung*
160. Gravity and the Lung: Lessons from Microgravity, *edited by G. K. Prisk, M. Paiva, and J. B. West*
161. High Altitude: An Exploration of Human Adaptation, *edited by T. F. Hornbein and R. B. Schoene*
162. Drug Delivery to the Lung, *edited by H. Bisgaard, C. O'Callaghan, and G. C. Smaldone*
163. Inhaled Steroids in Asthma: Optimizing Effects in the Airways, *edited by R. P. Schleimer, P. M. O'Byrne, S. J. Szefler, and R. Brattsand*
164. IgE and Anti-IgE Therapy in Asthma and Allergic Disease, *edited by R. B. Fick, Jr., and P. M. Jardieu*
165. Clinical Management of Chronic Obstructive Pulmonary Disease, *edited by T. Similowski, W. A. Whitelaw, and J.-P. Derenne*
166. Sleep Apnea: Pathogenesis, Diagnosis, and Treatment, *edited by A. I. Pack*

ADDITIONAL VOLUMES IN PREPARATION

Biotherapeutic Approaches to Asthma, *edited by J. Agostl and A. L. Sheffer*

Proteoglycans in Lung Disease, *edited by H. G. Garg, P. J. Roughley, and C. A. Hales*

Disease Markers in Exhaled Breath, *edited by N. Marczin, S. Kharitonov, M. Yacoub, and P. J. Barnes*

Gene Therapy in Lung Disease, *edited by S. M. Albelda*

SLEEP APNEA

Pathogenesis, Diagnosis, and Treatment

Edited by

Allan I. Pack

University of Pennsylvania
Philadelphia, Pennsylvania, U.S.A.

MARCEL DEKKER

MARCEL DEKKER, INC. NEW YORK • BASEL

ISBN: 0-8247-0312-X

This book is printed on acid-free paper.

Headquarters
Marcel Dekker, Inc.
270 Madison Avenue, New York, NY 10016
tel: 212-696-9000; fax: 212-685-4540

Eastern Hemisphere Distribution
Marcel Dekker AG
Hutgasse 4, Postfach 812, CH-4001 Basel, Switzerland
tel: 41-61-261-8482; fax: 41-61-261-8896

World Wide Web
http://www.dekker.com

The publisher offers discounts on this book when ordered in bulk quantities. For more information, write to Special Sales/Professional Marketing at the headquarters address above.

Current printing (last digit):
10 9 8 7 6 5 4 3 2

PRINTED IN THE UNITED STATES OF AMERICA

To my father,
Sidney Edward Pack,
who was a great friend and counselor

INTRODUCTION

The study of apnea is no small challenge, nor is it a new one. Yet, the definition is quite simple; it is "cessation of respiration"—temporary cessation, of course!

Around 1870, I. Rosenthal introduced the name apnea to designate the lack of breathing that follows hyperventilation. Eventually, posthyperventilation apnea became the object of intensive physiological investigations, all aiming to understand the chemical and neural control of breathing. This subject attracted some of the most brilliant physiologists of the latter part of the 19th century and through the 20th century.

Toward the end of the 20th century, apnea was recognized as a disorder, a pathological manifestation with major systemic consequences. This awareness was coupled with the dawning recognition that sleep disorders are a significant public health problem.

Research on sleep and sleep disorders, as well as debates about the importance of sleep and lack thereof, have greatly intensified. An article entitled "Mortality Associated with Sleep Duration and Insomnia" and a companion editorial, "Can Sleep Be Bad for You? Can Insomnia Be Good?", published in the *Archives of General Psychiatry*, illustrate the controversy. These publications provide evidence and support the need for more investigation. We already know much about sleep, but we must endeavor to disseminate and apply this knowledge.

In 1984, the Lung Biology in Health and Disease series of monographs reported on sleep and breathing in Volume 21. Since then, it has remained at the cutting edge of the field by adding new publications focusing on many aspects of the biology of sleep in addition to many others on the control of breathing in health and disease, a field intimately related to sleep.

The series is currently presenting to its readership *Sleep Apnea: Pathogenesis, Diagnosis, and Treatment.* This volume's 21 chapters bring the reader up to date on this vibrant field of research and clinical application. The editor, Dr. Allan I. Pack, has been not only a faithful and generous contributor to the series, but also a career-long pioneer in the field of sleep research. For the development of this book, Dr. Pack assembled a group of experts who have made many premier contributions. As Executive Editor, I welcome this new volume to the series, and express my gratitude to Dr. Pack and his ''team'' for the opportunity to publish it.

Claude Lenfant, M.D.
Bethesda, Maryland

PREFACE

This book represents another step forward in the study of a common disorder, obstructive sleep apnea. Since the original description of the disorder by Gastout et al. in 1965 (1), much has been learned. We have recognized how common the disorder is based on landmark studies such as that by Young et al. from the Wisconsin Sleep Cohort (2). We have learned a lot about the consequences of obstructive sleep apnea and there is growing interest in its role as a risk factor for cardiovascular disease (3).

Chapters in this book indicate our growing knowledge about the biomechanics of the upper airway, upper airway structures, and the complex neurobiology that underlie the sleep-related decrements in the activity of the relevant upper airway muscles (4) and the neurobiology of arousal. Moreover, we are beginning to study the genetics of the disorder and finding evidence of family aggregation (5).

Fortunately, with growing awareness of the high prevalence of this disorder and its important consequences, new treatments have become available. Foremost among these is the use of nasal continuous positive airway pressure (6). However, none of the currently available treatments is ideal, and the search continues for new treatment approaches, some of which are modifications of those currently available, while others are more forward-looking but not yet attainable. All of these issues are covered in chapters in this book.

Our constantly improving knowledge generated by science has firmly established obstructive sleep apnea as a major common disorder (7) and is overcoming the skepticism of our colleagues in other areas of medicine.

The research and conclusions presented in this volume would not have been possible without the leadership of the National Heart, Lung and Blood Institute (NHLBI) at the National Institutes of Health. In 1988, at a time when skepticism about this disorder was high, the Institute took the bold step of establishing the Special Centers of Research in Cardiopulmonary Disorders of Sleep. The Institute has continued its strong support of sleep research and, with the establishment of the National Center for Sleep Disorders Research (NCSDR), has continued to facilitate new scientific developments in this field.

Thus this book owes a great debt of gratitude to Dr. Claude Lenfant, Director of NHLBI; Dr. James Kiley, founding Director of NCSDR; and Dr. William Dement, whose leadership of the National Commission on Sleep Disorders Research (8) facilitated the establishment of the NCSDR. Their contributions have been invaluable to the millions of patients who have obstructive sleep apnea.

At a more local level, I wish to thank my longtime Administrative Assistant, Daniel C. Barrett, whose great efforts made publication of this book possible. I also thank my wonderful colleagues in the Center for Sleep and Respiratory Neurobiology at the University of Pennsylvania. We have had great fun conducting our research together as a collegial group of scholars. Many of them—Richard O. Davies, David F. Dinges, Warren B. Gefter, Andrew Goldberg, Joan C. Hendricks, Leszek Kubin, Richard J. Schwab, Sigrid C. Veasey, and Terri E. Weaver—have contributed chapters to this volume, as have Basil Petrof and Richard Horner, investigators who spent time training with us at the University of Pennsylvania. Finally, I want to thank my understanding wife (Frances), children (the 4 A's), and now grandchildren, who have endured with my workaholic habits.

Allan I. Pack

References

1. Gastaut H, Tassinari CA, Duron B. Etude polygraphique des manifestations épisodiques (hypniques et respiratoires), diurnes et nocturnes, du syndrome de Pickwick. Rev Neurol 1965; 115:456.
2. Young T, Palta M, Dempsey J, Skatrud J, Weber S, Badr S. The occurrence of sleep-disordered breathing among middle-aged adults. N Engl J Med 1993; 328:1230–1235.
3. Shahar E, Whitney CW, Redline S, Lee ET, Newman AB, Nieto JF, O'Connor GT, Boland LL, Schwartz JE, Samet JM. Sleep-disordered breathing and cardiovascular disease. Am J Respir Crit Care Med 2001; 163:19–25.
4. Kubin L, Davies RO, Pack AI. Control of upper airway motoneurons during REM sleep. News Physiol Sci 1998; 13:91–97.
5. Redline S, Tishler PV, Tosteson TD, Williamson J, Kump K, Browner I, Ferrette V, Krejci P. The familial aggregation of obstructive sleep apnea. Am J Respir Crit Care Med 1995; 151:682–687.

6. Sullivan CE, Berthon-Jones M, Issa FG, Eves L. Reversal of obstructive sleep apnoea by continuous positive airway pressure applied through the nares. Lancet 1981; i:862–865.
7. Phillipson EA. Sleep apnea—a major public health problem. N Engl J Med 1993; 328: 1271–1273.
8. Wake Up America: A National Sleep Alert. Bethesda, MD: National Commission on Sleep Disorders Research, 1993.

CONTRIBUTORS

T. Douglas Bradley, M.D. Professor of Medicine and Director of the Centre for Sleep and Chronobiology, University of Toronto, Toronto, Ontario, Canada

Dina Brooks, Ph.D., M.Sc. Assistant Professor, Department of Physical Therapy, University of Toronto, Toronto, Ontario, Canada

Gregory G. Brown, Ph.D. University of California, San Diego, and VA San Diego Healthcare System, San Diego, California

Monte S. Buchsbaum, M.D. Professor, Department of Psychiatry, Mount Sinai School of Medicine, New York, New York

William E. Bunney, Jr., M.D. Distinguished Professor, Department of Psychiatry and Human Behavior, University of California College of Medicine, Irvine, California

Deepak K. Chugh, M.B.B.S., M.D. Department of Neurology, MCP Hahnemann University Hospital, Philadelphia, Pennsylvania

Camellia P. Clark, M.D. Assistant Adjunct Professor, Department of Psychiatry, University of California, San Diego, and VA San Diego Healthcare System, San Diego, California

Richard O. Davies, D.V.M., Ph.D. Professor, Department of Animal Biology, School of Veterinary Medicine, University of Pennsylvania, Philadelphia, Pennsylvania

Robert J. O. Davies, M.B., B.S., D.M. Senior Lecturer in Medicine, University of Oxford; Consultant Physician, Oxford Centre for Respiratory Medicine, Churchill Hospital, Oxford, England

Jerome A. Dempsey, Ph.D. John Robert Sutton Professor of Health Sciences, University of Wisconsin, Madison, Wisconsin

David F. Dinges, Ph.D. Professor and Chief, Division of Sleep and Chronobiology, Department of Psychiatry, University of Pennsylvania School of Medicine, Philadelphia, Pennsylvania

Sean P. A. Drummond, Ph.D. Department of Psychiatry, University of California, San Diego, and VA San Diego Healthcare System, San Diego, California

Peter R. Eastwood, Ph.D. Department of Pulmonary Physiology, Sir Charles Gairdner Hospital, and University of Western Australia, Perth, Western Australia, Australia

Eugene C. Fletcher, M.D. Professor and Director, Division of Respiratory and Critical Care Medicine, Department of Medicine, University of Louisville, Louisville, Kentucky

Warren B. Gefter, M.D. Professor of Radiology and Chief, Chest Radiology Division, University of Pennsylvania Medical Center, Philadelphia, Pennsylvania

J. Christian Gillin, M.D. Professor, Department of Psychiatry, University of California, San Diego, and VA San Diego Healthcare System, San Diego, California

Andrew N. Goldberg, M.D., F.A.C.S. Department of Otolaryngology–Head and Neck Surgery, University of California, San Francisco, San Francisco, California

Louis A. Gottschalk, M.D., Ph.D. Professor Emeritus, Department of Psychiatry and Human Behavior, University of California College of Medicine, Irvine, California

Ronald R. Grunstein, M.B., B.S., M.D., Ph.D., F.R.A.C.P. Associate Professor and Head, Centre for Respiratory Failure and Sleep Disorders, Royal Prince Alfred Hospital, Sydney, New South Wales, Australia

Joan C. Hendricks, V.M.D., Ph.D. Professor, Center for Sleep and Respiratory Control, School of Veterinary Medicine; Center for Sleep and Respiratory Neurobiology, University of Pennsylvania, Philadelphia, Pennsylvania

Charles Hong, M.D., Ph.D. Johns Hopkins University School of Medicine, Baltimore, Maryland

Richard L. Horner, Ph.D. Assistant Professor, Departments of Medicine and Physiology, University of Toronto, Toronto, Ontario, Canada

Michael C. K. Khoo, Ph.D. Professor, Department of Biomedical Engineering, University of Southern California, Los Angeles, California

Leszek Kubin, Ph.D. Research Associate Professor, Department of Animal Biology, School of Veterinary Medicine, University of Pennsylvania, Philadelphia, Pennsylvania

Geraldo Lorenzi-Filho Centre for Sleep and Chronobiology, University of Toronto, Toronto, Ontario, Canada

Alan A. Lowe, D.M.D., Ph.D., F.R.C.D. (C), F.A.C.D., F.C.D.S. (BC) Professor and Chair, Division of Orthodontics, Department of Oral Health Sciences, Faculty of Dentistry, University of British Columbia, Vancouver, British Columbia, Canada

Mark R. Opp, Ph.D. Associate Professor, Department of Anesthesiology, University of Michigan, Ann Arbor, Michigan

Basil J. Petrof, M.D., F.R.C.P.(C) Associate Professor, Respiratory Division, McGill University Health Centre, Montreal, Quebec, Canada

Eliot A. Phillipson, M.D., F.R.C.P.(C) Professor and Chair, Department of Medicine, University of Toronto, Toronto, Ontario, Canada

Susan Redline, M.D., M.P.H. Professor, Department of Pediatrics, Rainbow Babies and Children's Hospital, and Case Western Reserve University, Cleveland, Ohio

Mark H. Sanders, M.D., F.C.C.P., A.B.S.M. Professor and Chief, Pulmonary Sleep Disorders Program, Montefiore University Hospital, and University of Pittsburgh School of Medicine, Pittsburgh, Pennsylvania

Wolfgang W. Schmidt-Nowara, M.D. Associate Professor Emeritus, University of New Mexico, Albuquerque, New Mexico, and Sleep Medicine Institute, Dallas, Texas

Richard J. Schwab, M.D. Associate Professor, Pulmonary, Allergy, and Critical Care Division, University of Pennsylvania Medical Center, Philadelphia, Pennsylvania

Alan R. Schwartz, M.D. Associate Professor, Pulmonary and Critical Care Division, Department of Medicine, Johns Hopkins University School of Medicine, Baltimore, Maryland

Frederic Sériès, M.D. Department of Medicine, Laval University, and Director, Sleep Laboratory, Laval Hospital, Sainte-Foy, Quebec, Canada

Aaron E. Sher, M.D. Capital Region Otolaryngology–Head and Neck Surgery Group; Medical Director, Capital Region Sleep Wake Disorders Center; and Associate Clinical Professor, Albany Medical College, Albany, New York

Curtis A. Smith, Ph.D. Department of Population Health Sciences, University of Wisconsin, Madison, Wisconsin

Philip L. Smith, M.D. Professor, Department of Medicine, Johns Hopkins University School of Medicine, Baltimore, Maryland

Virend K. Somers, M.D., Ph.D. Cardiovascular Division, Department of Internal Medicine, The University of Iowa, Iowa City, Iowa

John R. Stradling, M.D., F.R.C.P.(UK) Professor, Oxford Center for Respiratory Medicine, Churchill Hospital, Oxford, England

Kingman P. Strohl, M.D. Professor, Department of Medicine, Case Western Reserve University, Cleveland, Ohio

Peter V. Tishler, M.D. Associate Professor, Department of Medicine, VA Boston Healthcare System and Harvard Medical School, Boston, Massachusetts

Sigrid C. Veasey, M.D. Assistant Professor, Department of Medicine, University of Pennsylvania, Philadelphia, Pennsylvania

Terri E. Weaver, Ph.D., R.N., C.S., F.A.A.N. Associate Professor, University of Pennsylvania School of Nursing, Philadelphia, Pennsylvania

David P. White, M.D. Division of Sleep Medicine, Brigham and Women's Hospital, and Harvard Medical School, Boston, Massachusetts

Christine R. Wilson, Ph.D. Assistant Professor, Department of Physical Therapy, Northeastern University, Boston, Massachusetts

Joseph Wu, M.D. Associate Professor, Department of Psychiatry, University of California College of Medicine, Irvine, California

CONTENTS

1

Anatomical Factors
Insights from Imaging Studies

RICHARD J. SCHWAB and WARREN B. GEFTER

University of Pennsylvania Medical Center
Philadelphia, Pennsylvania

Although obstructive sleep apnea is a major public health problem affecting at least 2–4% of the middle-aged population, the pathogenesis of this disorder is poorly understood. Upper airway imaging studies have provided insights into the biomechanical basis for obstructive sleep apnea and the mechanisms underlying the efficacy of various therapeutic interventions for this disorder [i.e., continuous positive airway pressure (CPAP), weight loss, oral appliances, and surgery]. High-resolution anatomical information can be obtained on static and dynamic changes in upper airway dimensions and surrounding soft tissue structures with magnetic resonance imaging (MRI) and computed tomography (CT). Magnetic resonance volumetric three-dimensional reconstructions of the airway and surrounding soft tissue structures are being utilized to accurately quantify anatomical structural risk factors in patients with obstructive sleep apnea. Such imaging studies have allowed us to study the effects of obesity and gender on upper airway structure and function. Upper airway imaging studies have highlighted the singular importance of thickening of the lateral pharyngeal walls in mediating upper airway narrowing during wakefulness and sleep in normals and patients with sleep apnea. Although obstructive sleep apnea involves both an anatomical and neurological component (discussed in other chapters in this volume), we will primarily focus on the anatomical component in this chapter.

I. Upper Airway Anatomy

The upper airway is an extremely complicated structure that performs several different physiological functions including deglutition, vocalization, and respiration. The dynamic biomechanical relationships among the upper airway muscles (over 24 have been described) that allow these functions to occur are not well understood (1). Nonetheless, the upper airway has been categorized into three anatomical regions: (1) nasopharynx (the nasal turbinates to the hard palate); (2) oropharynx, which is subdivided into the retropalatal (the caudal margin of the hard palate to the caudal margin of the soft palate) and retroglossal (the caudal margin of the soft palate to the base of the epiglottis) regions; and (3) hypopharynx (the base of the tongue to the cervical esophagus) (2–4) (see Fig. 1). Upper airway closure in the majority of patients with obstructive sleep apnea occurs in the retropalatal and retroglossal regions (5–7). Therefore, we will focus predominantly on the oropharyngeal region in the remainder of this chapter.

The oropharynx can be further delineated by examining the structures that form its anterior, posterior, and lateral walls. The soft palate and tongue form the

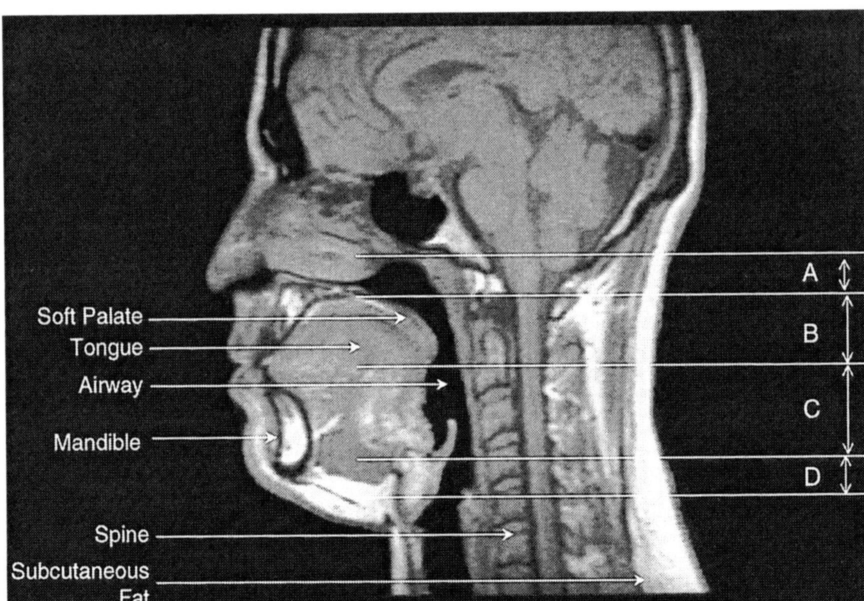

Figure 1 Midsagittal magnetic resonance image in a normal subject demonstrating the upper airway regions: (A) nasopharynx—from the nasal turbinates to the hard palate; (B) retropalatal—from the level of the hard palate to the caudal margin of the soft palate; (C) retroglossal—from the caudal margin of the soft palate to the base of the epiglottis; and (D) hypopharynx—from the base of the epiglottis to the larynx.

majority of the anterior wall of the oropharynx (4,8). The posterior wall of the oropharynx is formed primarily by the superior, middle, and inferior constrictor muscles (these muscles also make up a portion of the lateral wall). Structures lateral to the airway include the mandibular rami, pharyngeal tonsils, parapharyngeal fat pads, and lateral pharyngeal walls. In the retropalatal region, the lateral pharyngeal walls are defined as the tissue between the lateral edge of the airway and the medial edge of the parapharyngeal fat pads (see Fig. 2). In the retroglossal region, since the parapharyngeal fat pads disappear, the lateral walls are defined as the tissue between the lateral edge of the airway and the mandible (see Fig. 3). These lateral walls are formed by lymphoid tissue (palatine tonsils) and several muscles. These muscles include the pharyngeal constrictors (superior, middle, and inferior) and the hyoglossus, styloglossus, stylohyoid, stylopharyngeus, palatoglossus, and palatopharyngeus

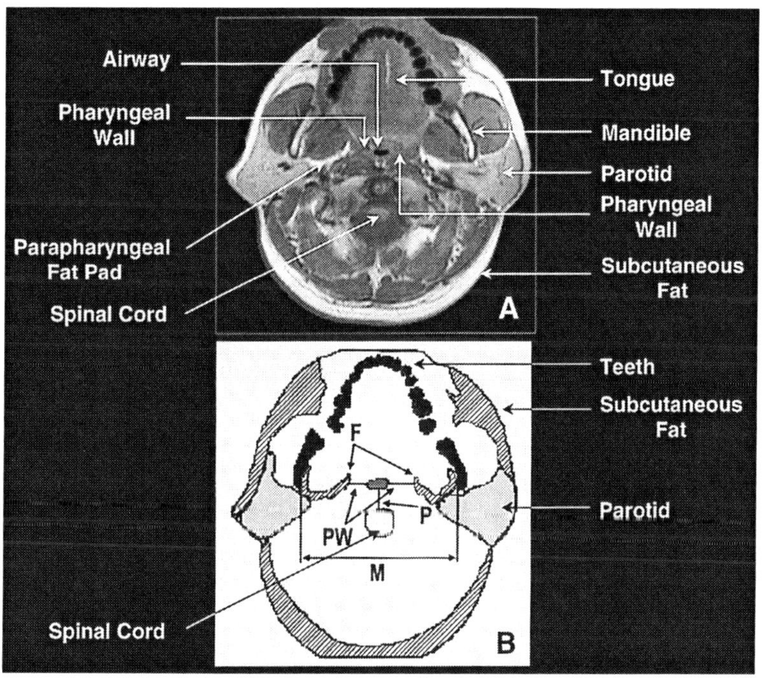

Figure 2 (A) Axial magnetic resonance image in a normal subject at the retropalatal region. Note the location of the lateral parapharyngeal walls, parapharyngeal fat pads, mandibular rami, parotids, and spinal cord. The lateral pharyngeal walls are defined as the muscles between the airway and the medial edge of the lateral parapharyngeal fat pads. Fat is white on MR scans. (B) Diagram of axial MR anatomy at the retropalatal level demonstrating the important soft tissue structures surrounding the upper airway. Soft tissue measurements displayed include: PW, lateral pharyngeal wall thickness; M, distance between the rami of the mandible; F, distance between the fat pads; and P, posterior airway wall thickness.

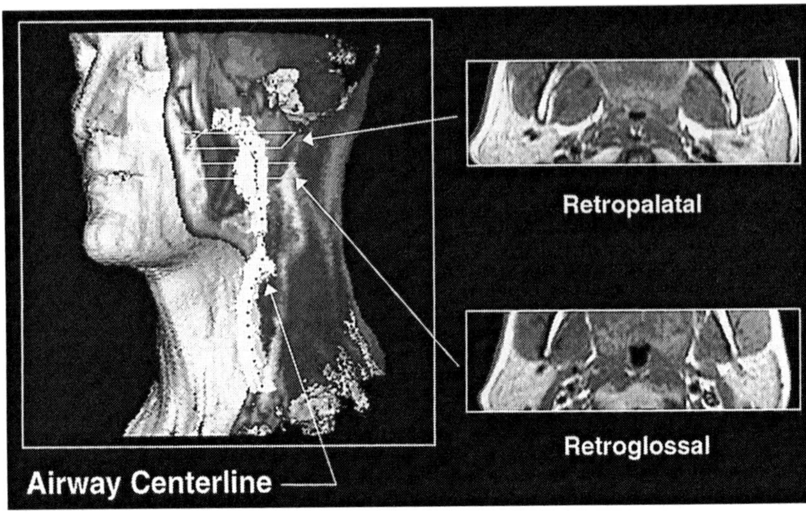

Figure 3 Three-dimensional volume rendering of the head with an extracted upper airway (white) and a three-dimensional centerline (represented by the black dots within the white airway). Two oblique images locally perpendicular to the airway are displayed at the retropalatal and retroglossal regions.

(3,6,9). The biomechanical relationships between these muscles and how they modulate movement of lateral walls are not well understood. Moreover, the interaction between the muscles that form the lateral walls and the tongue, soft palate, parapharyngeal fat pads, and mandible are also not well understood. Although the tongue, soft palate, and mandible are thought to be important in the pathogenesis of sleep apnea, the lateral pharyngeal walls may turn out to be the principal structure mediating upper airway caliber and closure in patients with sleep apnea. However, it is likely that all of these structures and intrinsic muscles closely interact to modulate upper airway caliber. For instance, movement of the soft palate may directly affect the size and configuration of the lateral walls since fascicles of the palatopharyngeus muscle, which arise from the soft palate and insert on the thyroid cartilage, form part of the lateral pharyngeal walls. In order to fully understand the biomechanics of the upper airway, we will need to carefully define in three dimensions the complex relationships between the upper airway soft tissue and craniofacial structures.

II. Upper Airway Anatomy and Its Relationship to Obstructive Sleep Apnea

The majority of CT and MR imaging studies (3,5,10–27), although not all (21,23), indicate that during wakefulness the upper airway of apneics is smaller than normals. In general, the upper airway is smallest in the retropalatal region in both normal subjects and patients with sleep apnea (3,16,18,26). These studies (3,5,10–27) lead to a fundamental question: Why is the upper airway smaller in patients with sleep apnea compared to normal subjects during wakefulness? The answer is likely to be related to alterations in the soft tissue and craniofacial structures that surround the upper airway. Multiple craniofacial abnormalities have, in fact, been demonstrated with cephalometric studies of patients with sleep apnea, including reductions in mandibular body length (retrognathia/micrognathia), inferiorly positioned hyoid bone, and retroposition of the maxilla (15,28–36). Mandibular body length in particular, or the distance between the most posterior and inferior points on the convexity of the mandible, has been demonstrated in a clinical meta-analysis to be significantly associated with obstructive sleep apnea (37). In addition to these craniofacial risk factors for sleep apnea, increases in the size of the upper airway soft tissue structures have been associated with obstructive sleep apnea. Increases in the cross-sectional area and volume of the soft palate, tongue, parapharyngeal fat pads and lateral pharyngeal walls have been demonstrated with CT and MR imaging in patients with sleep apnea (3,18,21,38,39). Figure 4 demonstrates enlargement of the soft palate and tongue in a patient with sleep apnea compared to a normal subject on a midsagittal MR image. Figure 5 (an axial MR image in the retropalatal region) highlights the thickening of the lateral pharyngeal walls in patients with sleep apnea. Three-

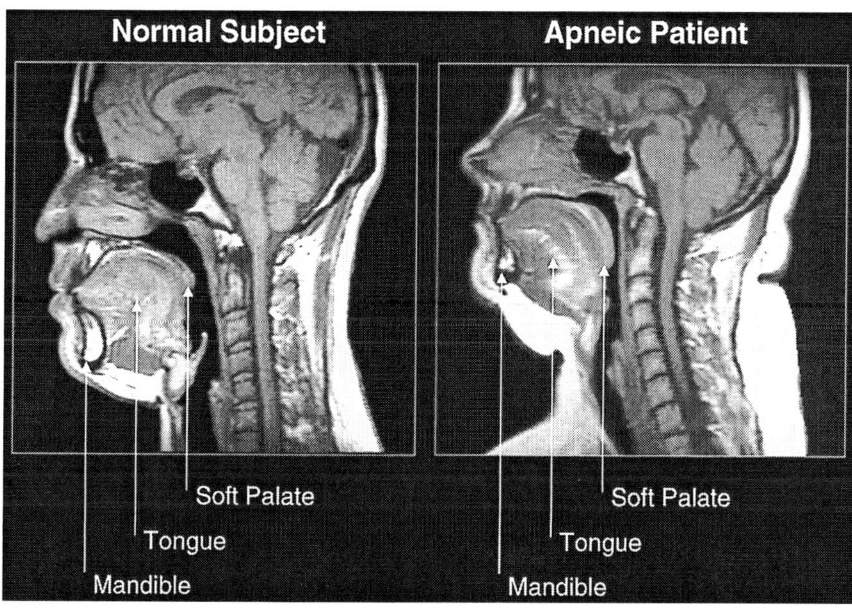

Figure 4 Comparison of a midsagittal MR image of a normal subject and patient with sleep apnea. Airway caliber is smaller in the apneic. Soft palate and tongue area are larger in the apneic.

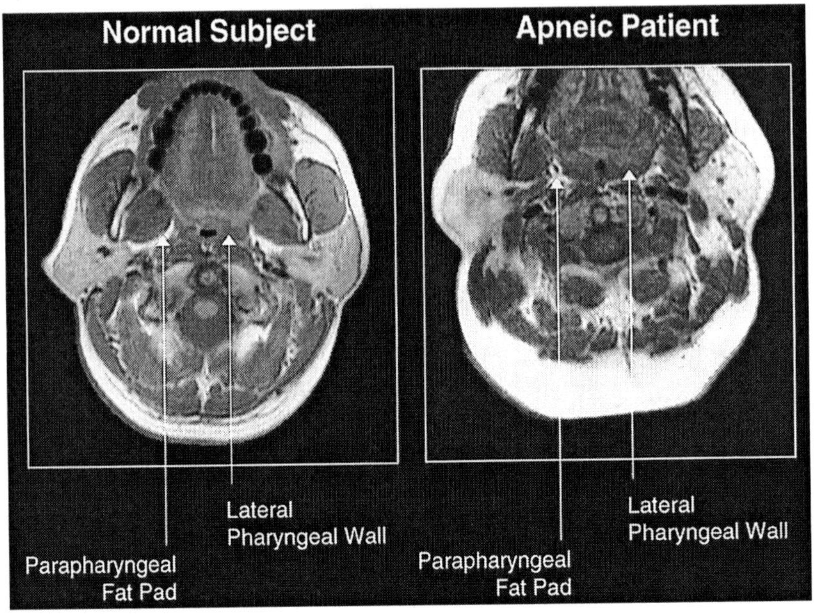

Figure 5 Comparison of an axial MR image in the retropalatal region of a normal subject and a patient with sleep apnea. The patient with sleep apnea has a smaller airway area and width and a larger lateral pharyngeal wall. However, the size of the parapharyngeal fat pads is similar between the normal subject and the patient with sleep apnea.

dimensional MR reconstructions (see Fig. 6) can also be utilized to demonstrate volumetric increases in the size of the upper airway soft tissue structures (tongue, soft palate, lateral parapharyngeal fat pads and lateral/posterior pharyngeal walls) in patients with sleep apnea.

A. Craniofacial Structure

In order to learn more about the pathogenesis of sleep apnea, we need to understand why the size of these upper airway structures are increased (soft tissue structures) or decreased (craniofacial structures) in patients with sleep apnea. The craniofacial abnormalities (reduced mandibular body length, inferiorly positioned hyoid bone, and retroposition of the maxilla) are likely to be genetically determined, although gender and race may play a role. Studies using cephalometrics suggest that craniofacial abnormalities are inherited in patients with obstructive sleep apnea (30,40). Guilleminault et al. performed a study on first-degree relatives of probands with sleep apnea and demonstrated that family members had a significantly smaller SNB [angle measurement from sella (S) to nasion (N) to point B (supramentale—deepest point on the outer mandibular contour between the mandibular incisor and pogonion—most anterior median point on the mandible)], longer MPH (distance from

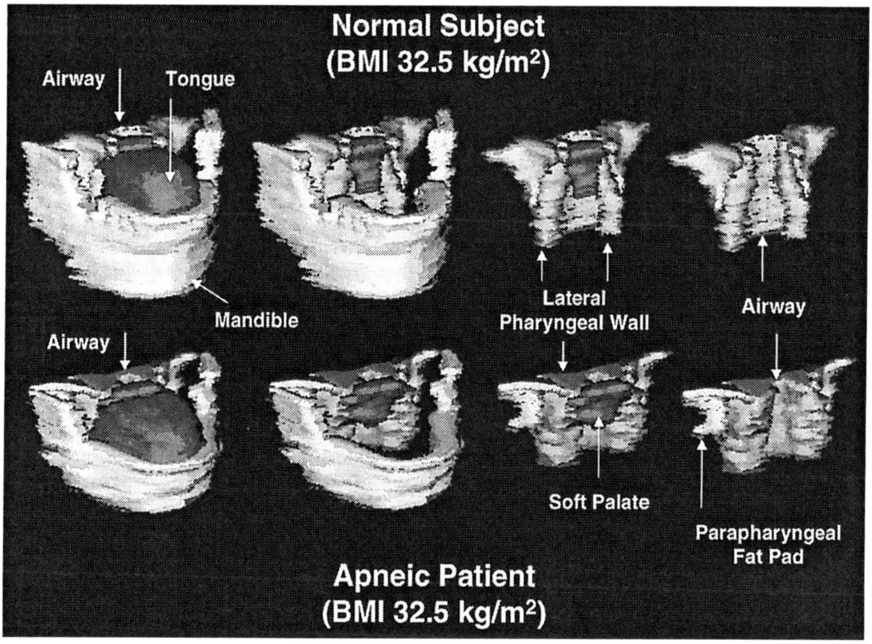

Figure 6 Volumetric reconstructions from a series of 3 mm contiguous axial MR images of the mandible, tongue, soft palate, lateral parapharyngeal fat pads, and lateral/posterior pharyngeal walls in a weight-matched normal and patient with sleep apnea, both with an elevated body mass index (32.5 kg/m^2). Note that the airway is larger in the normal than the apneic. The volume of the tongue, parapharyngeal fat pads, and lateral pharyngeal walls are larger in the apneic.

mandibular plane to hyoid), and decreased PAS (posterior airway space) (30). These data indicated that first degree relatives of patients with sleep apnea had retroposed mandibles and inferiorly placed hyoid bones. In addition, first-degree relatives of the probands with sleep apnea had an odds ratio of 10.9 for the presence of a high narrow hard palate. Mathur and Douglas (41) also noted cephalometric differences in the first-degree relatives of nonobese patients with sleep apnea compared to age-, sex-, height-, and weight-matched controls. The relatives of patients with sleep apnea demonstrated retroposed maxillae and mandibles, shorter mandibles, longer soft palates, and wider uvulas than the matched controls. In addition, differences in craniofacial form have been demonstrated in different ethnic groups (40). In this study (40), African-Americans demonstrated statistically significant bimaxillary prognathism compared to Hispanics and Caucasians. Hispanics, however, demonstrated statistically significant bimaxillary retrognathism compared to the other ethnic groups. In another cephalometric investigation (42) statistically significant differences were demonstrated in (1) sella-nasion-subspinale angle (SNA) between black men and both Caucasian and Hispanic men and (2) sella-nasion-supramentale angle (SNB) between black men and Caucasian men. The data from all these studies suggest that elements of craniofacial structure in patients with sleep apnea are likely to be inherited and may depend on ethnicity. Differences in craniofacial morphology may also be related to gender (42). Differences have been demonstrated in cephalometric measurements of posterior airway space, posterior nasal spine to the soft palate, and mandibular plane to hyoid distance in Caucasian men and women (42). Specific craniofacial morphometric features of women with mild sleep apnea have also been demonstrated (43). These features include a triangular chin, overjet, a narrow hard palate, and class II malocclusion (43). These and other craniofacial morphometric characteristics of men and women need to be studied further since such information may be useful in understanding gender-related differences in the pathogenesis of sleep-disordered breathing.

B. Soft Tissue Structure

As discussed above, imaging studies have demonstrated enlargement of the soft palate, tongue, parapharyngeal fat pads, and lateral pharyngeal walls in patients with obstructive sleep apnea (3,18,21,38,39). Increases in the size of these soft tissue structures will, in turn, narrow the upper airway and predispose to airway closure during sleep. Why are these soft tissue structures enlarged in apneics? The underlying pathogenesis of the increase in size of these soft tissue structures surrounding the upper airway remains unknown, but possible etiological mechanisms include: (1) edema from negative pressure generated in the upper airway during sleep; (2) weight gain/obesity; (3) primary muscle disorder/injury; and (4) genetic/gender factors. We will discuss each of these factors separately.

Upper airway edema is considered to be an important contributor to enlargement of these soft tissue structures, and continuous positive airway pressure (CPAP) is thought to reduce this edema (39). This may be especially important for the soft palate, which can be tugged caudally and constricted during apneic events. We recently performed a study (44) examining T_2 relaxation times of the lingual musculature in normals and patients with sleep apnea with quantitative magnetic resonance mapping. The T_2 relaxation time is a physical property that varies with changes in tissue structure. Short T_2 relaxation times are typically associated with fibrosis, while long T_2 relaxation times are often associated with tissue edema or increased fat content (44). Our results demonstrate that the mean T_2 relaxation times of apneic lingual muscles are significantly longer than those of the control group. These data are compatible with increased edema or possibly increased fat content of the tongue muscles in patients with sleep-disordered breathing.

Obesity is thought to be an important reason why the upper airway soft tissue structures are enlarged in patients with obstructive sleep apnea. Obesity is a major structural risk factor for obstructive sleep apnea in adults, and obesity has reached epidemic proportions in the United States, with approximately one-third of the population considered to be at least mildly obese (21,45). Clinic-based and epidemiological studies have confirmed that obesity is an important risk factor for obstructive sleep apnea (46,47). Obesity was the strongest predictor of sleep-disordered breathing in a study of 720 individuals (48). In addition, weight loss has been demonstrated in over 15 clinical studies to decrease the severity of obstructive sleep apnea (47,49–51) and results in decreased collapsibility of the airway (as measured by increased Pcrit) (22) (for further discussion on Pcrit, see Chap. 2). In the Wisconsin Sleep Cohort Study (52) an increase in body mass index by one standard deviation tripled the prevalence of sleep apnea. Neck size was the strongest predictor of sleep-disordered breathing among all anthropomorphic variables studied in this cohort (52). Increased neck size has been demonstrated in other population studies to be the best predictor of the presence of sleep apnea (53–55). That neck circumference is the strongest predictor of sleep-disordered breathing indicates that upper body obesity (fat deposition around the upper airway), rather than a more generalized distribution of body fat, is important for the development of sleep apnea.

Therefore, it has been hypothesized (24,25) that increased adipose tissue, specifically deposited in the lateral parapharyngeal fat pads (see Figs. 2, 5), results in airway compression, which ultimately induces apneic events during sleep. Indeed, upper airway imaging studies have found that the area and volume of the lateral parapharyngeal fat pads are enlarged in obese patients with apnea (5,24,25,56). Furthermore, animal studies have also shown that enlargement of the lateral pharyngeal fat pads results in airway narrowing (57). There is, moreover, a correlation between the respiratory disturbance index and the volume of adipose tissue surrounding the apneic upper airway (25). Increased adipose tissue surrounding the upper airway has been demonstrated not only in obese but importantly also in nonobese patients with sleep apnea (58). Upper airway MR imaging studies (3,25,57) have confirmed that the total volume of fat in the lateral parapharyngeal fat pads is greater in apneics than normals. While we hypothesize that fat deposition in the lateral pharyngeal fat pads is a primary risk factor for sleep apnea, there are other possible anatomical sites in which upper airway fat deposition can lead to increased neck size and obstructive sleep apnea. For instance, fat deposited under the mandible, within the tongue or soft palate, may be important in the pathogenesis of sleep apnea. Increased fat has also been demonstrated histologically in the uvula of patients with sleep apnea (59). An excess of fatty infiltration was found in the surgically resected distal soft palate of patients with sleep apnea in comparison to normal subjects (59). Alternatively, the total amount of fat deposited around the upper airway rather than fat in a particular location may be important. Shelton and coworkers have argued (24) that fat deposited in the space bounded by the mandibles leads to an increase in tissue pressure and hence compression of the airway.

Obesity may also directly alter the biomechanical properties of the upper airway soft tissue structures. Rather than obesity predisposing to sleep apnea on the basis of increased fat deposition, weight gain may directly affect the muscular tissue surrounding the upper airway. Weight gain is known to increase muscle mass in addition to fat (60,61). Fat-free tissue accounts for approximately 25–30% of the increased weight in obese patients (61,62). An increased percentage of muscle has been demonstrated in the uvula of patients with sleep apnea compared to normals (23,59). Such studies lead to the hypothesis that obesity may predispose to sleep apnea by increasing the size of the upper airway soft tissue structures (tongue, soft palate, lateral pharyngeal walls) rather than by the direct deposition of fat in the parapharyngeal fat pads or by compression of the lateral airway walls by these fat pads. Studies in normal women (19,63) support this hypothesis by demonstrating that the lateral pharyngeal walls (as well as the parapharyngeal fat pads) decrease in size with weight loss (see Fig. 7). In these studies tongue and soft palate size did not change significantly with weight loss. It is possible that weight loss has a differential effect on upper airway muscular soft tissue structures, i.e., affecting the lateral walls more than the tongue and soft palate. Moreover, weight gain/loss may also change upper airway compliance and the mechanical actions of the upper airway muscles (47). Unfortunately the mechanism whereby obesity predisposes to sleep apnea remains controversial. However, imaging studies should increase our understanding of the relationship between obesity and the size of the upper airway structures by allowing us to: (1) assess the entire three-dimensional configuration of upper airway adipose tissue; (2) examine volumetric anatomical changes in upper airway

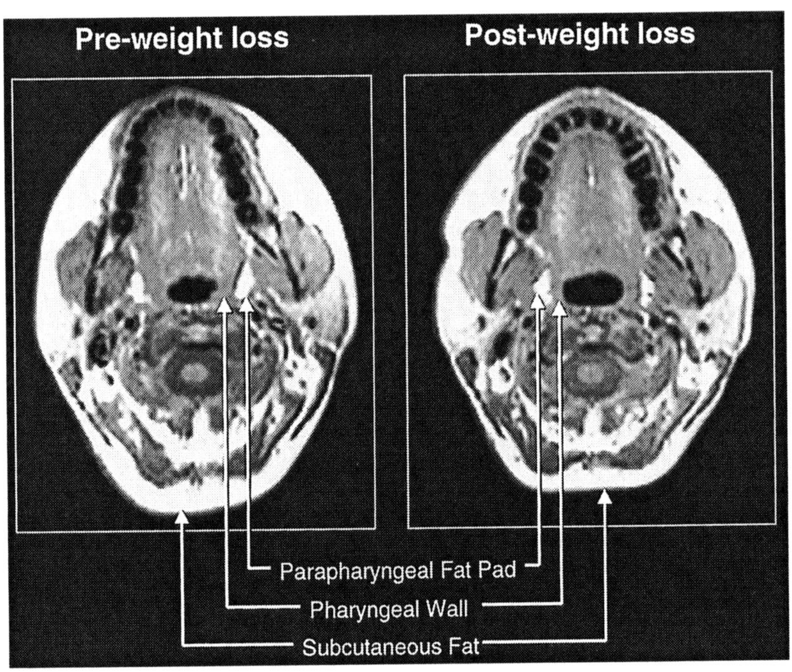

Figure 7 Axial MR images in a normal subject at the retropalatal region, pre– and post–weight loss during wakefulness. Note lateral airway enlargement and thinning of lateral pharyngeal walls with weight loss.

soft tissue structures (tongue, soft palate, lateral pharyngeal walls, parapharyngeal fat pads) with weight loss/gain; and (3) evaluate three-dimensional biomechanical interrelationships between the tongue, soft palate, lateral pharyngeal walls, parapharyngeal fat pads, and mandible with weight loss/gain.

In addition to the effects of obesity on the upper airway soft tissue structures, patients with obstructive sleep apnea are thought to have altered muscle properties based on histological findings. Several studies have demonstrated increased type II fast twitch fibers in the genioglossus of patients with sleep apnea compared to controls (23,64–66). Similar findings have been demonstrated in the sternohyoid muscle of the English bulldog (67). Type II fibers are known to be less resistant to fatigue than type I fibers. These investigators (23,64–66) believe that remodeling of the upper airway muscles that occurs in patients with sleep apnea is a secondary phenomenon rather than a cause of sleep apnea. Friberg and colleagues (65) performed biopsies on palatopharyngeal muscle in 21 snorers/apneics and 10 nonsnoring controls. They (65) also found increased type II muscle fibers in the palatopharyngeal muscle and an increase in morphological abnormalities, including signs characteristic of neurogenic lesions in patients with sleep-disordered breathing. These investigators (65) hypothesized that the local neurogenic lesions (i.e., denervated regions) were secondary to tissue vibration produced by snoring. Carrera and coworkers (64) investigated the structure and function of the genioglossus muscle in 16 apneics and 11 normals. They also found increased type II fibers in the genioglossus muscle and demonstrated that the muscle had a greater susceptibility to fatigue. These functional and structural changes were reversed by CPAP. The fact that the changes were reversed by CPAP indicates that the abnormalities in genioglossus structure and function are a consequence of the sleep apnea and not the cause of the disease. Nonetheless, these investigations (23,64–66) demonstrate that patients with sleep apnea manifest muscle changes, including injury, which may alter the size and configuration of the upper airway muscles (see Chap. 7).

Genetic factors may also be important in mediating the size of the upper airway soft tissue structures (68). There are several reasons that obstructive sleep apnea is thought to have a genetic basis (see also Chap. 8): (1) there is a high prevalence of sleep apnea in patients with a number of disorders with single gene or chromosomal defects, e.g., Treacher Collins syndrome, Down syndrome, Apert syndrome (45); (2) obstructive sleep apnea has been reported to cluster in families (68–71); and (3) studies comparing family members of patients with sleep apnea with relatives of randomly selected neighbors (72) and controls (41) demonstrate that a first-degree relative of a patient with sleep-disordered breathing has approximately twice the risk of having sleep apnea (72). Moreover, the relative risk increases if there are more family members with sleep apnea (72). Several studies have also demonstrated family aggregation of craniofacial morphology in patients with sleep apnea (30,41), and these studies provide evidence for a genetic basis to the skeletal risk factors for sleep apnea. Thus, there is compelling evidence that sleep apnea has a genetic component. However, the genetics or development of the upper airway soft tissue structures have not been well studied. Macroglossia is a known risk factor for sleep apnea in children with trisomy 21 (73), but otherwise there is very little information on the genetic determinants of upper airway soft tissue structures. Nonetheless, the size of the tongue, soft palate, and lateral pharyngeal walls may all be genetically determined. Future studies are needed to determine if enlargement of the upper airway soft tissue structures demonstrate family aggregation in normals and patients with sleep apnea. Such studies could be performed with MR imaging since it provides an ideal tool to accurately quantify the structural risk factors in patients with obstructive sleep apnea. MR imaging can examine in three dimensions craniofacial structure, upper airway soft tissue morphology, and fat deposition in the neck (see Fig. 6), all potentially important risk factors for sleep apnea.

Gender may also play an important role in the size of upper airway soft tissue structures. In order to examine gender-related differences in upper airway caliber and the surrounding soft tissue structures, Whittle and colleagues (74) studied age- and weight-matched normal men and women with magnetic resonance imaging. There were no significant differences in the minimum cross-sectional area between men and women in this investigation (74). Although mean cross-sectional area was similar between men and women in the palatal region, it was significantly greater in men in the subpalatal region (74). These data (74) indicate that at least in certain anatomical regions upper airway area is similar between men and women; however, volumetric differences (which may be a more definitive measurement than upper airway area) were not determined in this investigation. Further studies are needed to determine if there are gender-related differences in upper airway volume or regional volumes (retropalatal and retroglossal).

In addition to upper airway caliber, Whittle and colleagues (74) also studied gender-related differences in the soft tissue structures surrounding the upper airway. Women are known to have a smaller neck size than men, so it would be reasonable to hypothesize that the size of the critical upper airway soft tissue structures (tongue, soft palate, lateral pharyngeal walls, lateral parapharyngeal fat pads) should be smaller in women than men. In addition, fat distribution is known to be different in men than in women (75,76). Fat distribution in women is primarily in the lower body and extremities, whereas in men it is distributed primarily in the upper body and trunk (75,76). Therefore, it would be reasonable to hypothesize that adipose tissue deposited around the upper airway and specifically the size of the lateral parapharyngeal fat pads would be greater in men than women. However, the data from Whittle and colleagues (74) did not support such a hypothesis. In their study, there was no significant difference in the volume of upper airway fat (assessed by MRI) between normal men and women. Although there were no differences in upper airway fat deposition, they found that total neck soft tissue volume was significantly greater in men than in women (74).

The increased tissue volume in men compared to women in Whittle et al.'s investigation (74) was related to enlargement of other upper airway soft tissue structures. The mean cross-sectional area of the tongue and soft palate was larger in men than women (74). Unfortunately, the lateral pharyngeal walls were not evaluated in this investigation (74). The lateral walls, if measured, may have also contributed to the increased upper airway tissue in men. In order to definitively determine if gender-related differences exist in upper airway soft tissue structures volumetric measurements of the tongue, soft palate, and lateral walls will need to be compared in men and women both in normals and apneics. Nonetheless Whittle et al.'s data (74) indicate that there are gender-related differences in the upper airway soft tissue structures that they assessed.

III. Importance of the Lateral Pharyngeal Walls

Changes in the size of the tongue, soft palate, mandible, parapharyngeal fat pads and lateral pharyngeal walls have all been implicated in the pathogenesis of obstructive sleep apnea, but we do not know which of these structures are most important in mediating upper airway narrowing (18,77). It is likely that all these structures may interact to narrow the upper airway. Soft palate and tongue size have been shown to be increased in patients with sleep apnea (38,39). Several studies (3,6,16–21,45,77–83) have suggested that the lateral pharyngeal walls are the critical structure controlling upper airway caliber in normals and apneics. Data from upper airway imaging studies and investigations evaluating anatomical risk factors for sleep apnea support this assertion (3,6,16–21,45,77–83). We also performed a careful oropharyngeal examination in a cohort of 420 patients to identify the upper airway craniofacial and soft tissue structural abnormalities that were associated with an increased risk for obstructive sleep apnea (78). In this study (78) we hypothesized that anatomical abnormalities of the oropharynx, particularly narrowing of the airway by the lateral pharyngeal walls, tonsils, and tongue, would be associated with an increased risk for obstructive apnea. The association between individual variables in the clinical model and sleep apnea as defined by a respiratory disturbance index (RDI) greater than or equal to 15 was compared using odds ratios (OR). Multivariable logistic regression was used to estimate the independent contribution of each variable in predicting sleep apnea and to identify the minimal subset of variables necessary to predict sleep apnea using a backward stepwise algorithm. The backward stepwise analysis was also performed with neck circumference and body-mass index (BMI) forced into the model. In the backward regression model, lateral airway narrowing had the highest association with sleep apnea (OR 2.4) followed by tonsillar enlargement (OR 2.0), enlargement of the uvula (OR 1.9), and tongue enlargement (OR 1.8). Low-lying palate, retrognathia, and overjet were not found to be significantly associated with sleep apnea in this study. When BMI and neck circumference were forced into the model, only lateral narrowing was significant in both models (OR of 2.4 and 2.0, respectively). These data demonstrate that lateral narrowing of the airway during wakefulness is associated with an increased risk for sleep apnea.

Upper airway imaging studies (3,6,16–21,25,26,45,77,79,80) have allowed us to investigate the mechanism of this lateral narrowing. These studies have provided strong evidence for the importance of the lateral pharyngeal walls in addition to the tongue and soft palate in mediating upper airway caliber. If increases in the size of the soft palate and tongue played the major role in compromising airway caliber in apneics, then the majority of airway narrowing should be in the anterior-posterior (AP) direction. But the apneic airway narrows primarily in the lateral dimension. Studies have demonstrated that the major axis of the normal airway is horizontal, whereas in the apneic airway it is in anterior-posterior dimension (16,84) (see Fig. 8). This airway configuration in apneics may adversely affect upper airway muscle activity, which in turn could predispose the airway to closure during sleep (85). But what mediates this lateral narrowing? The lateral pharyngeal walls and lateral parapharyngeal fat pads are the two primary soft tissue structures lateral to the upper airway (see Figs. 2, 5). Although both of these structures have been proposed to be important in compromising upper airway caliber, imaging studies conducted by us have demonstrated that increased thickness of the lateral pharyngeal muscular walls rather than enlargement of the parapharyngeal fat pads was the predominant anatomical factor causing airway narrowing in apneics (3–5). Figure 5 is a comparison of an axial image in the retropalatal region of a normal subject and a patient with sleep apnea and highlights the findings from this investigation (3). In Figure 5 the retropalatal airway area and width are smaller and the thickness of the lateral pharyngeal wall is larger in the patient with sleep apnea. If the airway was compromised by fat in the parapharyngeal fat pads, then the fat pads would be expected to be closer together, i.e., the distance between the lateral dimension would be smaller. We did not find this to be so. In addition, our study demonstrated that the dimensions of the soft tissue structure, which most correlated with airway size in all subject groups (normals, snorers and apneics), was the thickness of the lateral pharyngeal

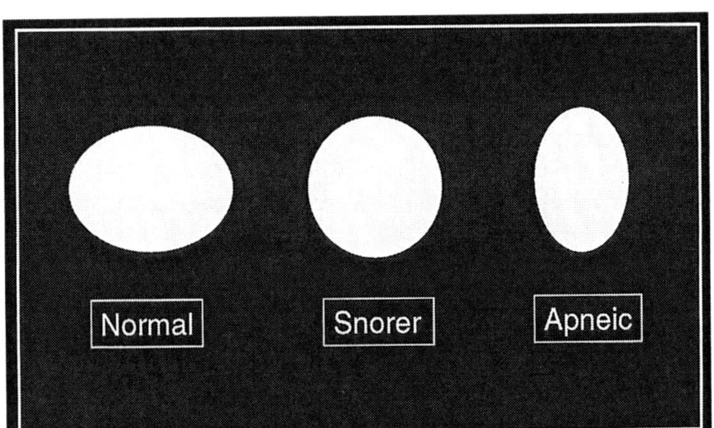

Figure 8 Diagram of the differences in upper airway geometry in a normal, snorer, and apneic. Note that the longest axis of the apneic airway is anterior-posterior dimension, whereas the longest axis of the normal airway is lateral dimension.

walls (3). These data indicate that the lateral pharyngeal walls are important structures mediating changes in airway caliber in normals and apneics.

Why are the lateral walls thickened in patients with sleep apnea? Unfortunately, we currently do not know the answer to this question. However, all the mechanisms discussed above that might explain increased size of upper airway soft tissue structures could play a role: (1) edema from negative pressure generated in the upper airway during sleep; (2) weight gain/obesity; (3) primary muscle disorder/injury; (4) changes in blood flow and capillary volume; and (5) genetic/gender factors. In addition to these mechanisms, the lateral walls may be thickened secondary to a reduced tracheal tug (tethering of these walls by the negative pleural pressure on the trachea) since obesity raises the diaphragm and reduces functional residual capacity (77,82). Alternatively, changes in the configuration of the surrounding tissues (hyoid bone, mandible, soft palate, and tongue) may be important in mediating the size of the lateral walls by altering the mechanical action of key upper airway muscles. Understanding the mechanisms that control the dimensions of the lateral walls is likely to be fundamental to our understanding of the pathogenesis of sleep apnea. Stimulation of the lateral walls with simultaneous upper airway imaging may allow us to understand the control mechanisms of these walls. Such studies could be performed in animals.

If the lateral pharyngeal walls are the critical structures controlling the upper airway, then treatment of patients with sleep apnea might be directed at these lateral walls. In fact, the effects of CPAP, the treatment of choice in patients with sleep apnea, are mediated, at least in part, through the lateral pharyngeal walls. CPAP results in significant thinning of the lateral walls as the airway expands with the application of positive airway pressure (Figs. 9–11). Initially it was proposed that the beneficial effects of CPAP were due to anterior displacement of the tongue and

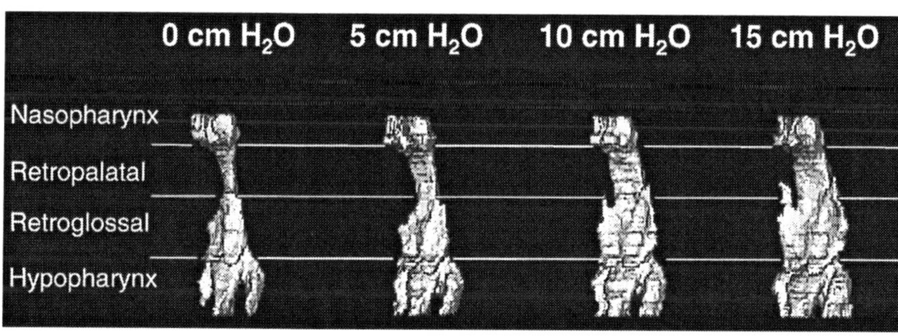

Figure 9 Three-dimensional surface renderings of the upper airway in a normal subject demonstrating the enlargement in upper airway volume with progressive increases in CPAP (0–15 cmH_2O). CPAP significantly increases airway volume primarily in the retropalatal and retroglossal regions. Note that the airway widens predominantly in the lateral dimension.

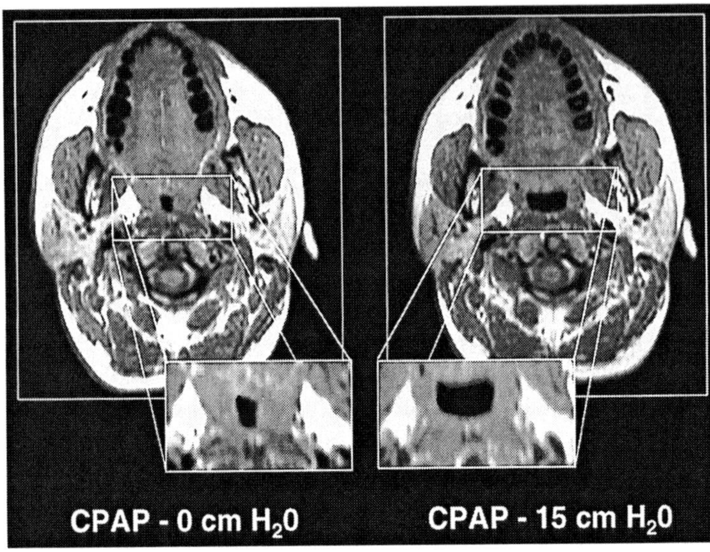

Figure 10 Axial MR image at the retropalatal region in a normal subject with 0 cmH_2O and CPAP of 15 cmH_2O. Airway enlargement is demonstrated predominantly in the lateral dimension with the application of 15 cmH_2O of CPAP. The anterior-posterior airway dimension is not significantly changed with CPAP at 15 cmH_2O.

soft palate. However, Kuna and colleagues, using CT scanning, demonstrated that upper airway dilatation with CPAP was greatest in the lateral dimension (14). A recent study (80) with MRI confirmed Kuna's findings and showed that progressive increases in CPAP (up to 15 cmH_2O), at least in normals, increased airway volume, area, and lateral airway dimensions in the retropalatal and retroglossal regions (Figs. 9–11). The lateral airway dimensional changes with CPAP were significantly greater than the anterior-posterior changes (80). CPAP resulted in significant thinning of the lateral walls as the airway expanded with positive airway pressure (Figs. 10, 11). There was an inverse relationship between CPAP level and thickness of the lateral pharyngeal walls. Thus, increases in CPAP predominantly affect structures lateral to the upper airway rather than the tongue and soft palate. These data also suggest that the lateral pharyngeal walls are a more ''compliant'' structure than the tongue or soft palate.

In addition to CPAP, other treatment options for sleep apnea (weight loss, oral appliances, and uvulopalatopharyngoplasty) also have an effect on the dimensions of the lateral pharyngeal walls. Weight loss, as discussed above, decreases the size of the lateral walls and parapharyngeal fat pads more than the tongue and soft palate at least in normal, somewhat obese women (19,63). There are currently very few data on the effect of upper airway surgery on the lateral pharyngeal walls; prelimi-

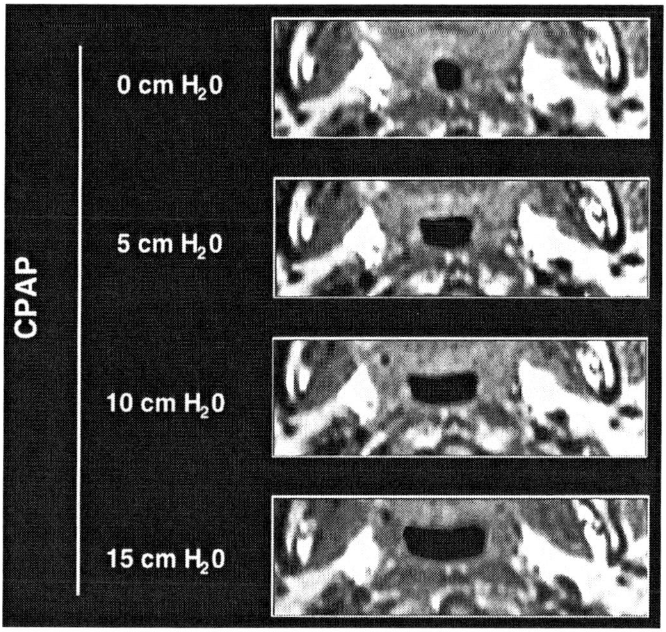

Figure 11 Axial MR images in a normal subject (same subject as in Fig. 10) at the retropalatal region with CPAP ranging from 0 to 15 cmH_2O. Progressive increases in CPAP result in airway enlargement and thinning of the lateral pharyngeal wall. The distance between the lateral pharyngeal fat pads does not change with incremental increases in CPAP.

nary data from imaging studies (83) in patients pre- and postuvulopalatopharyngoplasty demonstrate that following this surgery the lateral walls may thin (see Fig. 12). Several studies (45,86–88) have demonstrated that mandibular repositioning devices are an effective treatment for patients with mild to moderate sleep apnea (45). Although cephalometric studies have demonstrated that mandibular repositioning devices advance and rotate the mandible (87), the specific biomechanical changes that underlie the effectiveness of these devices are unknown. Airway enlargement has been proposed to occur in the AP dimension with mandibular repositioning devices since these appliances advance the mandible and increase the posterior airway space. However, recent data (20) indicate that airway caliber increases in the lateral dimension with oral appliances, adding support to the concept that structures lateral to the airway are important in understanding the mechanisms whereby oral appliances increase upper airway caliber. Preliminary studies using a SnoreGuard mandibular repositioning device in fact demonstrate that not only does airway caliber increase but the lateral walls also thin (20) (see Fig. 13). It is conceivable that advancing the mandible may put traction on the lateral walls, resulting in

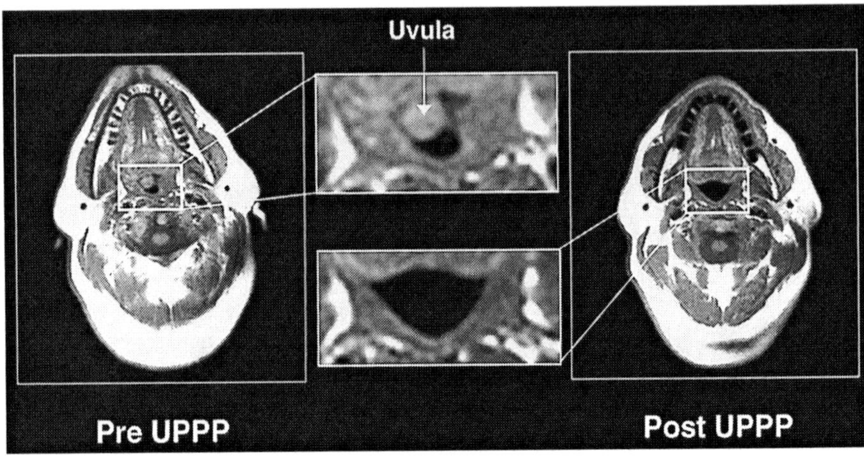

Figure 12 Axial MR images in a patient with sleep apnea at the retropalatal region before and after uvulopalatopharyngoplasty (UPPP) during wakefulness. Note the large lateral increase in airway size and decrease in the thickness of the lateral pharyngeal walls after surgery.

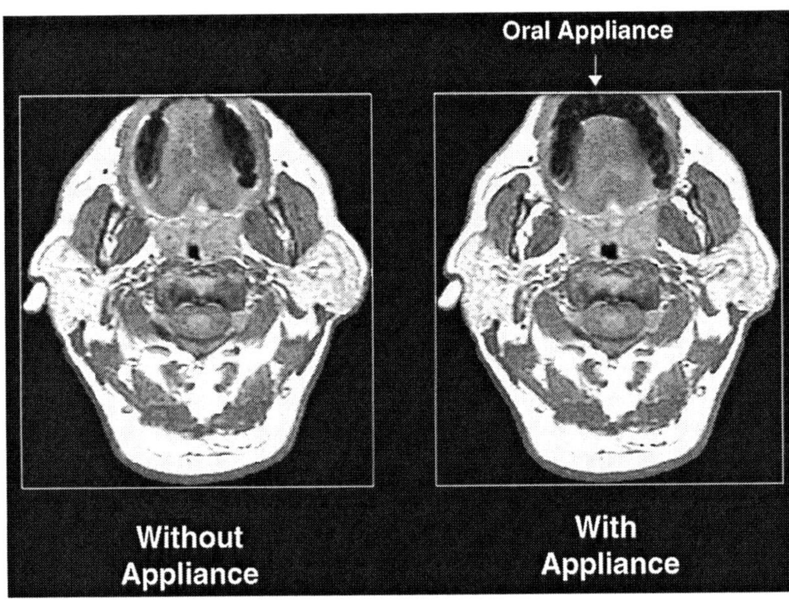

Figure 13 Axial MR images in a patient with sleep apnea at the retropalatal region before and after a mandibular repositioning device (SnoreGuard) during wakefulness. The oral appliance appears as a black band around the teeth on MRI. Note the lateral increase in airway size and decrease in the thickness of the lateral pharyngeal walls with the oral appliance.

thinning of these walls. Upper airway imaging studies with and without oral appliances may help in allowing us to understand the complicated biomechanical interactions between the mandible, tongue, soft palate, and lateral walls. Such information may lead to new insights into the pathogenesis of sleep apnea.

IV. State-Dependent Upper Airway Imaging

In order to fully understand the pathogenesis of sleep apnea, we need to understand how and where the upper airway closes during sleep. Imaging studies during sleep are particularly relevant because they can demonstrate state-dependent changes in upper airway caliber and the surrounding soft tissue structures. Such studies have demonstrated that airway narrowing during sleep occurs in both the retropalatal and retroglossal region with the retropalatal region being the more common site of closure (5,7,81,89). The upper airway is thought to narrow as a tube during sleep. Trudo and coworkers performed a study examining state-dependent changes in airway caliber and surrounding soft tissue structures in normal subjects using spin echo magnetic resonance imaging and found that the narrowest portion of the airway was in the retropalatal region in the majority of subjects (81). This study demonstrated that in normal subjects the volume of the retropalatal airway was reduced by 19% during sleep; in contrast, airway volume in the retroglossal region was not significantly reduced during sleep (81). These data indicate that the upper airway does not act as a homogeneous tube. The retropalatal (RP) region appears to be more likely to collapse than the RG region during sleep, at least in normal individuals.

The study of Trudo et al. (81) also directly addressed the fundamental question of which soft tissue structures (tongue, soft palate, or lateral pharyngeal walls) mediate upper airway narrowing during sleep (81). The RP airway area changes in this investigation were due to a reduction in both AP and lateral airway dimensions. The reduction in the lateral airway diameter during sleep was associated with thickening of the lateral pharyngeal walls, whereas the AP narrowing was primarily related to posterior movement of the soft palate. These data indicate that thickening of the lateral pharyngeal walls and posterior movement of the soft palate are likely to be important in the biomechanics of airway narrowing in both normal subjects and, potentially, in patients with sleep apnea (21) (Fig. 14). Other investigators have demonstrated AP and lateral narrowing during sleep in normals and apneics (5,7,89–91). Utilizing conventional CT imaging in apneics, Homer et al. (5) demonstrated that airway obstruction during sleep was due to posterior displacement of the soft palate and tongue, as well as lateral displacement of the pharyngeal walls. Suto and colleagues (7) also demonstrated retropalatal airway closure in both normals and apneics during sleep utilizing sagittal ultrafast MR imaging. The state-dependent retropalatal narrowing resulted from reductions in both the AP and lateral airway dimensions (7). Morrell and colleagues (91) performed nasopharyngoscopy in eight apneics during sleep. These investigators examined dynamic flow volume relationships in inspiration and expiration over four breaths preceding apneas. They found

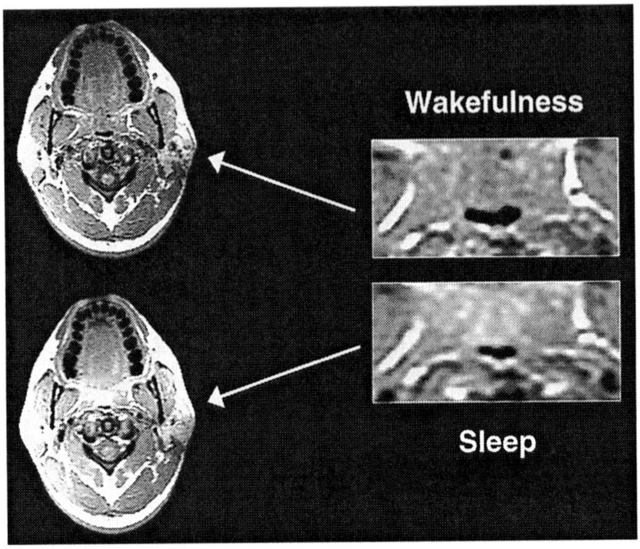

Figure 14 Axial MR images in a normal subject at the retropalatal region during wakefulness and sleep. Anterior-posterior and lateral airway narrowing is demonstrated during sleep. Thickening of the lateral pharyngeal walls occurs during sleep, reducing airway cross-sectional area.

a progressive reduction in end-expiratory cross-sectional area in each successive breath prior to the obstructive apnea. Airway closure was demonstrated in the AP and lateral dimension. All of these studies indicate that airway narrowing during sleep occurs in both the lateral and AP dimensions. In the lateral dimension the narrowing is associated with thickening of the lateral pharyngeal walls.

Why do these walls thicken during sleep, and what controls their motion? We do not know the answer to these questions, but possible mechanisms causing the lateral walls to thicken during sleep include: (1) reduction in muscle tone with concomitant shortening and thickening of these muscles; (2) a decreased lung volume, which would be expected to reduce tracheal tug and potentially allow an increase in the size of the lateral walls; and (3) changes in the configuration/conformation of the hyoid, mandible, tongue, and soft palate altering muscle action and hence the pull on the lateral wall. It is likely that complex three-dimensional state-dependent biomechanical interactions exist between the tongue, soft palate, mandible, and lateral pharyngeal walls. Dynamic and volumetric imaging studies will be necessary in order to develop a biomechanical model of the state-dependent changes in these upper airway soft tissue structures. Developing such knowledge is essential in order to fully understand the mechanism of state-dependent airway narrowing and the relative role of the different upper airway soft tissue structures.

V. Dynamic Upper Airway Imaging

In order to fully understand the pathogenesis of sleep apnea, we need to understand mechanisms involved in upper airway narrowing or closure. Examination of the upper airway during sleep provides such information. Another paradigm to examine airway narrowing is to evaluate the dynamic behavior of the upper airway during respiration or during a Müller maneuver. Significant changes in upper airway caliber and the surrounding soft tissue structures occur during the respiratory cycle and in conjunction with the negative pressure induced by a Müller maneuver. Examination of these physiological processes will allow us to determine if airway narrowing occurs laterally or in the AP dimension.

Respiratory-related dynamic upper airway imaging has been performed with nasopharyngoscopy, CT, and MR. The respiratory-related changes that take place in upper airway geometry during wakefulness in normal subjects and patients with sleep apnea have been carefully studied with electron beam CT (16,17). From these studies four distinct phases of the respiratory cycle emerge (16,17) (Fig. 15). At the onset of inspiration (phase 1), there is a small increase in upper airway area, presumably reflecting increased activity of the upper airway dilator muscles. However, during most of the duration of inspiration (phase 2 → 3), the airway area remains relatively constant. This suggests a balance between upper airway dilator muscle action and negative intraluminal pressure. In early expiration (phase 3 → 4), the

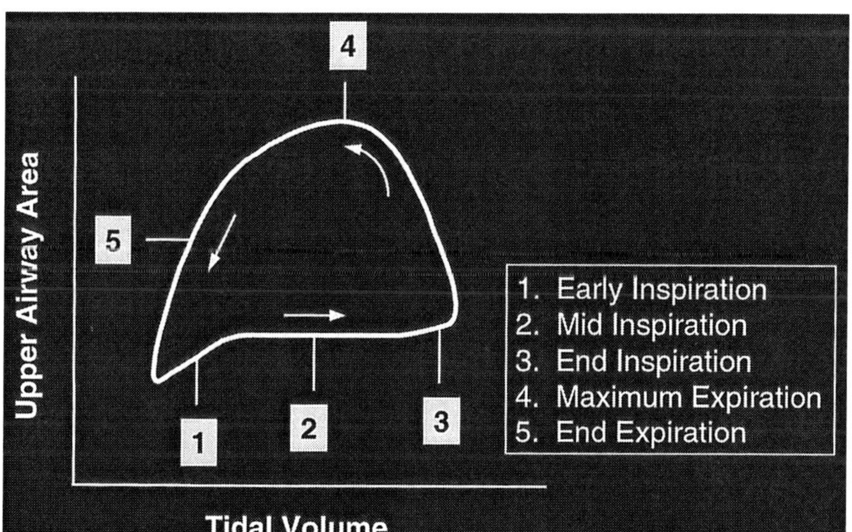

Figure 15 Diagram of the changes in upper airway area as a function of tidal volume during the respiratory cycle in an apneic.

upper airway enlarges, presumably secondary to positive intraluminal pressure. It is during this phase of respiration that airway caliber is largest. At the end of expiration (phase 5), there is a large reduction in upper airway size. Airway caliber is smallest at the end of expiration when it is no longer maintained open by the phasic action of the upper airway dilator muscles (phases 1 → 3, during inspiration) or positive intraluminal pressure (phase 3 → 4, early expiration). These data suggest that the upper airway may be particularly susceptible to collapse or narrowing at the end of expiration.

Other imaging studies (27,91,92) have also demonstrated that airway caliber is smallest at the end of expiration. Morrell and coworkers (91) demonstrated progressive end-expiratory upper airway narrowing in apneic subjects with nasopharyngoscopy during sleep. The observation that airway narrowing occurs during expiration may have important implications with respect to the timing of upper airway closure during apneas. It was originally proposed that airway closure during an apnea occurred during inspiration secondary to negative intraluminal pressure generated by chest wall contraction (93). However, studies by Sanders and colleagues (94,95) have suggested that airway occlusion in apneics occurs during expiration, not during inspiration. Moreover, other studies (96) have found that closing pressure (Pcrit) is greater than atmospheric pressure in patients with sleep apnea. Such data suggest that airway closure occurs during expiration (positive atmospheric pressure) before the generation of negative pressure during inspiration. Thus, these studies indicate that the end of expiration may be important in the genesis of apneas. This, in turn, suggests that the delivery of positive airway pressure near the end of expiration may help prevent apneas (16,21,45,79).

In addition to the understanding the timing of airway closure, it is important to understand the mechanism of airway narrowing during the respiratory cycle. The respiratory-related changes in upper airway caliber demonstrated in the CT studies (16,17) were predominantly in the lateral dimension, suggesting that the lateral walls have an important role in modulating airway caliber. A study utilizing cine (ultrafast) MRI confirmed these CT findings by demonstrating an inverse relationship between airway caliber and the size of the lateral pharyngeal walls (79,82). The size of the lateral pharyngeal walls was relatively unchanged during inspiration, thinned in early expiration, and thickened towards the end of expiration (82). These data indicated that changes in the dimensions of the lateral walls were more important than the tongue and soft plate in mediating respiratory-related dynamic changes in upper airway area (82). These studies again highlight the importance of the lateral walls in modulating airway narrowing.

Similar findings have been demonstrated with nasopharyngoscopy during a Müller maneuver (97). Nasopharyngoscopy is ideally suited to examine and quantify dynamic intraluminal changes in upper airway caliber. The Müller maneuver, a forced inspiratory effort with the mouth closed and nose occluded, is thought to simulate an apneic event (45,97). Changes in upper airway caliber during a Müller maneuver are directly related to changes in intraluminal pressure, which are effort-dependent. Therefore, simultaneous objective measurements of changes in airway caliber and negative intraluminal pressure are necessary to accurately interpret upper airway narrowing during a Müller maneuver.

In order to investigate the mechanism of airway closure, Ritter and colleagues, performed a study to quantitatively examine changes in upper airway caliber of normal subjects during maximal effort Müller maneuvers and at graded negative intraluminal pressures (−10, −20, −30, and −40 cmH_2O) generated by Müller maneuvers (97). This study (97) also examined positional (supine vs. sitting) and regional (retropalatal or retroglossal) differences in upper airway caliber and dimensions during the Müller maneuver. Cross-sectional area may be narrowed primarily in the lateral (movement of the lateral pharyngeal walls) or anterior-posterior (A-P) dimension (movement of the soft palate and tongue) during a Müller maneuver. There were several important findings from this investigation (97): (1) upper airway area was progressively reduced in the retropalatal region as intraluminal pressure

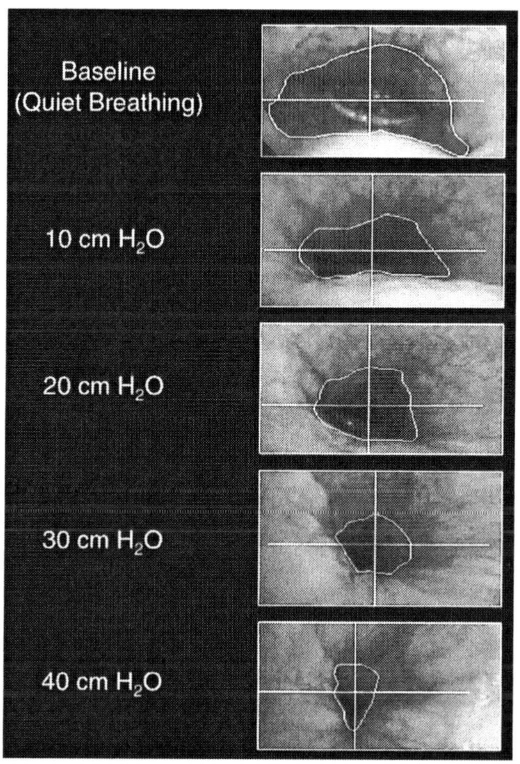

Figure 16 Representative images of the upper airway in a normal subject in the retropalatal region at baseline and during submaximal Müller maneuvers of increasing negative pressure (−10 to −40 cmH_2O). This figure demonstrates the predominant lateral narrowing and minor anterior-posterior narrowing during the Müller maneuvers.

became more negative from −10 to −40 cmH_2O during the Müller maneuver (see Fig. 16); (2) retropalatal narrowing was significantly greater than the retroglossal narrowing at all pressure levels; (3) retroglossal area did not change significantly with the Müller maneuver but demonstrated an alteration in airway configuration that consisted of lateral narrowing and an increase in the A-P airway; (4) lateral airway narrowing was significantly greater than A-P narrowing at all pressure levels; and (5) changes in body position (sitting vs. supine) did not result in significant differences in airway caliber or dimensions. These data indicate that in normals changes in airway caliber during a Müller maneuver are mediated primarily through changes in the lateral pharyngeal walls and that the retropalatal and retroglossal regions of the upper airway respond differently to forced negative intraluminal pressure. The latter finding indicates that the upper airway does not collapse as a homogeneous tube when exposed to negative intraluminal pressure. Analogous upper airway findings have been demonstrated during sleep (state-dependent changes in upper airway caliber do not occur uniformly in the retropalatal and retroglossal regions; see Sec. IV). Preliminary studies (98) examining nasopharyngoscopy with the Müller maneuver in patients with sleep apnea have demonstrated similar findings. However, reductions in airway area in the apneics with graded and maximal Müller maneuvers were greater than in the normals at all pressure levels suggesting that the apneic airway is more compliant than the normal airway (98). These studies add support to the concept that the lateral pharyngeal walls are an important structure in mediating airway collapse and are intimately involved in the pathogenesis of dynamic airway closure.

VI. Conclusions

Upper airway imaging is a powerful technique to study the mechanisms underlying the pathogenesis and biomechanics of obstructive sleep apnea. Imaging studies have provided important insights into the static and dynamic structure and function of the upper airway and surrounding soft tissue structures during wakefulness and sleep. Volumetric three-dimensional reconstructions of the airway and surrounding soft tissue structures accurately quantify anatomic structural differences between normals and apneics. Such imaging studies have highlighted the singular importance of the lateral pharyngeal walls, in addition to the tongue and soft palate, in mediating upper airway caliber. Upper airway imaging has provided the framework to allow us to begin to examine the pathogenesis of obstructive apneas, which, in time, may lead to newer, more effective approaches to the treatment of sleep apnea.

Acknowledgments

This chapter was supported by the National Institutes of Health Grants HL-57843, HL-03124, and HL-42236.

References

1. Fleetham JA. Upper airway imaging in relation to obstructive sleep apnea. Clin Chest Med 1992; 13:399–416.
2. Hudgel DW. The role of upper airway anatomy and physiology in obstructive sleep apnea. Clin Chest Med 1992; 13:383–398.
3. Schwab RJ, Gupta KB, Gefter WB, Hoffman EA, Pack AI. Upper airway soft tissue anatomy in normals and patients with sleep disordered breathing. Significance of the lateral pharyngeal walls. Am J Respir Crit Care Med 1995; 152:1673–1689.
4. Van Lunteren E. Muscles of the pharynx: structural and contractile properties. ENT J 1993; 72:27–29.
5. Horner RL, Shea SA, McIvor J, Guz A. Pharyngeal size and shape during wakefulness and sleep in patients with obstructive sleep apnoea. Q J Med 1989; 72:719–735.
6. Schwab RJ. Radiographic imaging in the diagnostic evaluation of sleep apnea. In: Weinberger SE, ed. UpToDate (4.3) in Pulmonary and Critical Care Medicine.electronic media, 1996.
7. Suto Y, Matsuo T, Kato T, Hori I, Inoue Y, Ogawa S, Suzuki T, Yamada M, Ohta Y. Evaluation of the pharyngeal airway in patients in sleep apnea: Value of ultrafast MR imaging. Am J Roentgenol 1993; 160:311–314.
8. Van Lunteren E, Strohl KP. The muscles of the upper airway. Clin Chest Med 1986; 7:171–188.
9. Kuna ST, Smickley JS, Vanoye CR. Respiratory-related pharyngeal constrictor muscle activity in normal human adults. Am Rev Respir Dis 1997; 155:1991–1999.
10. Bohlman ME, Haponik EF, Smith PL, Allen RP, Bleecker ER, Goldman SM. CT demonstration of pharyngeal narrowing in adult obstructive sleep apnea. Am J Roentgenol 1983; 140:543–548.
11. Brown IG, Zamel N, Hoffstein V. Pharyngeal cross-sectional area in normal men and women. J Appl Physiol 1986; 61:890–895.
12. Ell SR, Jolles H, Galvin JR. Cine CT demonstration of nonfixed upper airway obstruction. Am J Roentgenol 1986; 146:669–677.
13. Hoffstein V, Zamel N, Phillipson EA. Lung volume dependence of pharyngeal cross-sectional area in patients with obstructive sleep apnea. Am Rev Respir Dis 1984; 130: 175–178.
14. Kuna ST, Bedi DG, Ryckman C. Effect of nasal airway positive pressure on upper airway size and configuration. Am Rev Respir Dis 1988; 138:969–975.
15. Rivlin J, Hoffstein V, Kalbfleisch J, McNicholas W, Zamel N, Bryan AC. Upper airway morphology in patients with idiopathic obstructive sleep apnea. Am Rev Respir Dis 1984; 129:355–360.
16. Schwab RJ, Gefter WB, Hoffman EA, Gupta KB, Pack AI. Dynamic upper airway imaging during respiration in normal subjects and patients with sleep disordered breathing. Am Rev Respir Dis 1993; 148:1385–1400.
17. Schwab RJ, Gefter WB, Pack AI, Hoffman EA. Dynamic imaging of the upper airway during respiration in normal subjects. J Appl Physiol 1993; 74:1504–1514.
18. Schwab RJ, Goldberg AN. Upper airway assessment—radiographic and other imaging techniques. Otolaryngol Clin North Am 1998; 31:931–968.
19. Schwab RJ, Gupta KB, Metzger LJ, Pack AI, Gefter WB. Weight related changes in

upper airway size and surrounding soft tissue structures in normals. Am J Respir Crit Care Med 1995; 151:A372.

20. Schwab RJ, Gupta KB, Doung G, Schmidt-Nowara WW, Pack AI, Gefter WB. Upper airway soft tissue structural changes with a dental appliance in apneics. Am J Respir Crit Care Med 1996; 153:A719.
21. Goldberg AN, Schwab RJ. Identifying the patient with sleep apnea: upper airway assessment and physical examination. Otolaryngol Clin North Am 1998; 31:919–930.
22. Schwartz AR, Gold AR, Schubert N, Stryzak A, Wise RA, Permutt S, Smith PL. Effect of weight loss on upper airway collapsibility in obstructive sleep apnea. Am Rev Respir Dis 1991; 144:494–498.
23. Series F, Cote C, Simoneau JA, Gelinas Y, St Pierre S, Leclerc J, Ferland R, Marc I. Physiologic, metabolic, and muscle fiber type characteristics of musculus uvulae in sleep apnea hypopnea syndrome and in snorers. J Clin Invest 1995; 95:20–25.
24. Shelton KE, Gay SB, Hollowell DE, Woodson H, Surratt PM. Mandible enclosure of upper airway and weight in obstructive sleep apnea. Am Rev Respir Dis 1993; 148: 195–200.
25. Shelton KE, Gay SB, Woodson H, Surratt PM. Pharyngeal fat in obstructive sleep apnea. Am Rev Respir Dis 1993; 148:462–466.
26. Shepard JW Jr, Thawley SE. Evaluation of the upper airway by computerized tomography in patients undergoing uvulopalatopharyngoplasty for obstructive sleep apnea. Am Rev Respir Dis 1989; 140:711–716.
27. Shepard JW, Stanson AW, Sheedy PF, Westbrook PR. Fast-CT evaluation of the upper airway during wakefulness in patients with obstructive sleep apnea. In: Suratt PM, Remmers J, eds. Proceedings of the First International Symposium on Sleep and Respiration. New York: Alan R Liss, Inc., 1990:273–282.
28. Bacon WH, Turlot JC, Krieger J, Stierle J-L. Cephalometric evaluation of pharyngeal obstructive factors in patients with sleep apnea syndrome. Angle Orthod 1990; 60:115–122.
29. Deberry-Borowiecki B, Kukwa A, Blanks RH. Cephalometric analysis for diagnosis and treatment of obstructive sleep apnea. Laryngoscope 1988; 98:226–234.
30. Guilleminault C, Partinen M, Hollman K, Powell N, Stoohs R. Familial aggregates in obstructive sleep apnea syndrome. Chest 1995; 107:1545–1551.
31. Lowe AA, Fleetham JA, Adachi S, Ryan CF. Cephalometric and computed tomographic predictors of obstructive sleep apnea severity. Am J Orthod Dentofac Orthoped 1995; 107:589–595.
32. Lyberg T, Krogstad O, Djupesland G. Cephalometric analysis in patients with obstructive sleep apnoea syndrome. Skeletal morphology. J Laryngol Otol 1989; 103:287–292.
33. Lyberg T, Krogstad O, Djupesland G. Cephalometric analysis in patients with obstructive sleep apnoea syndrome: II. Soft tissue morphology. J Laryngol Otol 1989; 103: 293–297.
34. Partinen M, Guilleminault C, Quera-Salva M, Jamieson A. Obstructive sleep apnea and cephalometric roentgenograms. The role of anatomic upper airway abnormalities in the definition of abnormal breathing during sleep. Chest 1988; 93:1199–1205.
35. Pracharktam N, Hans MG, Strohl KP, Redline S. Upright and supine cephalometric evaluation of obstructive sleep apnea syndrome and snoring subjects. Angle Orthod 1994; 64:63–73.
36. Riley R, Guilleminault C, Herran J, Powell N. Cephalometric analysis and flow-volume loops in obstructive sleep apnea patients. Sleep 1983; 6:303–311.

37. Miles PG, Vig PS, Weyant RJ, Forrest TD, Rockette HE. Craniofacial structure and obstructive sleep apnea syndrome—a qualitative analysis and meta-analysis of the literature. Am J Orthod Dentofac Orthop 1996; 109:163–172.
38. Lowe AA, Gionhaku N, Takeuchi K, Fleetham JA. Three-dimensional CT reconstructions of tongue and airway in adult subjects with obstructive sleep apnea. Am J Orthod Dentofac Orthop 1986; 90:364–374.
39. Ryan CF, Lowe AA, Li D, Fleetham JA. Three-dimensional upper airway computed tomography in obstructive sleep apnea. Am Rev Respir Dis 1991; 144:428–432.
40. Will MJ, Ester MS, Ramirez SG, Tiner BD, McAnear JT, Epstein L. Comparison of cephalometric analysis with ethnicity in obstructive sleep apnea syndrome. Sleep 1995; 18:873–875.
41. Mathur R, Douglas NJ. Family studies in patients with the sleep apnea-hypopnea syndrome. Ann Intern Med 1995; 122:174–178.
42. Lee JJ, Ramirez SG, Will MJ. Gender and racial variations in cephalometric analysis. Otolaryngol Head Neck Surg 1997; 117:326–329.
43. Guilleminault C, Stoohs R, Kim YD, Chervin R. Black J. Clerk A. Upper airway sleep-disordered breathing in women. Ann Intern Med 1995; 122:493–501.
44. Schotland HM, Insko EK, Schwab RJ. Alterations of the lingual musculature in obstructive sleep apnea with quantitative magnetic resonance imaging. Sleep 1999; 22:605–613.
45. Schwab RJ, Goldberg AN, Pack AI. Sleep apnea syndromes. In: Fishman AP, ed. Pulmonary Diseases and Disorders, 3d ed. New York: McGraw-Hill, Inc., 1998:1617–1637.
46. Bliwise D, Feldman D, Bliwise N, Carskadon M, Kraemer H, North C, et al. Risk factors for sleep disordered breathing in heterogeneous geriatric populations. J Am Geriatr Soc 1987; 35:132–141.
47. Strobel RJ, Rosen RC. Obesity and weight loss in obstructive sleep apnea: a critical review. Sleep 1996; 19:104–115.
48. Burger CD, Stanson AW, Sheedy PF, Sheedy, PF, Shepard JW. Fast-computed tomography evaluation of age-related changes in upper airway structure and function in normal men. Am Rev Respir Dis 1992; 145:846–852.
49. Loube MI, Loube AA, Mitler MM. Weight loss for obstructive sleep apnea: the optimal therapy for obese patients. J Am Diet Assoc 1994; 94:1291–1295.
50. Smith PL, Gold AR, Meyers DA, Haponik EF, Bleecker ER. Weight loss in mildly to moderately obese patients with obstructive sleep apnea. Ann Intern Med 1985; 103: 850–855.
51. Wittels EH, Thompson S. Obstructive sleep apnea and obesity. Otolaryngol Clin North Am 1990; 23:751–760.
52. Young T, Palta M, Dempsey J, Skatrud J, Weber S, Badr S. The occurrence of sleep-disordered breathing among middle-aged adults. N Engl J Med 1993; 328:1230–1235.
53. Zohar Y, Sabo R, Strauss M, Schwartz A, Gal R, Oksenberg A. Oropharyngeal fatty infiltration in obstructive sleep apnea patients: a histologic study. Ann Otol Rhinol Laryngol 1998; 107:170–174.
54. Davies RJ, Ali NJ, Stradling JR. Neck circumference and other clinical features in the diagnosis of the obstructive sleep apnoea syndrome. Thorax 1992; 47:101–105.
55. Davies RJ, Stradling JR. The relationship between neck circumference, radiographic pharyngeal anatomy, and the obstructive sleep apnoea syndrome. Eur Respir J 1990; 3:509–514.

56. Horner RL, Mohiaddin RH, Lowell DG, Shea SA, Burman ED, Longmore B, Guz A. Sites and sizes of fat deposits around the pharynx in obese patients with obstructive sleep apnoea and weight matched controls. Eur Respir J 1989; 2:613–622.
57. Winter WC, Gampper T, Gay SB, Suratt PM. Enlargement of the lateral pharyngeal fat pad space in pigs increases upper airway resistance. J Appl Physiol 1995; 79:726–731.
58. Mortimore IL, Marshall I, Wraith PK, et al. Neck and total body fat deposition in non-obese and obese patients with sleep apnea compared with that in control subjects. Am J Respir Crit Care Med 1998; 157:280–283.
59. Stauffer JL, Buick MK, Bixler EO, Sharkey FE, Abt AB, Manders EK, Kales A, Cadieux RJ, Barry JD, Zwillich CW. Morphology of the uvula in obstructive sleep apnea. Am Rev Respir Dis 1989; 140:724–728.
60. Hill JO, Sparling PB, Shields TW, Heller PA. Effects of exercise and food restriction on body composition and metabolic rate in obese women. Am J Clin Nutr 1987; 46: 622–630.
61. Wadden TA, Foster GD, Letizia KA, Mullen JL. Long-term effects of dieting on resting metabolic rate in obese outpatients. JAMA 1990; 264:707–711.
62. Foster GD, Wadden TA, Mullen JL, Stunkard AJ, Wang J, Feurer ID, Pierson RN, Yang MU, Presta E, Van Itallie TB, Lemberg PS, Gold J. Resting energy expenditure, body composition and excess weight in the obese. Metabolism 1988; 37:467–472.
63. Welch KC, Schellenberg JB, Ritter CT, Foster GD, Wadden TA, Maislin G, Schwab RJ. A novel volumetric magnetic resonance imaging paradigm to study upper airway anatomy. Sleep (submitted).
64. Carrera M, Barbe F, Sauleda J, Tomas M, Gomez C, Agusti AG. Patients with obstructive sleep apnea exhibit genioglossus dysfunction that is normalized after treatment with continuous positive airway pressure. Am J Respir Crit Care Med 1999; 159:1960–1966.
65. Friberg D, Ansved T, Borg K, Carlsson-Nordlander B, Larsson H, Svanborg E. Histological indications of a progressive snorers disease in an upper airway muscle. Am J Respir Crit Care Med 1998; 157:586–593.
66. Petrof BJ, Hendricks JC, Pack AI. Does upper airway muscle injury trigger a vicious cycle in obstructive sleep apnea? A hypothesis. Sleep 1996; 19:465–471.
67. Petrof BJ, Pack AI, Kelly AM, Eby J, Hendricks JC. Pharyngeal myopathy of loaded upper airway in dogs with sleep apnea. J Appl Physiol 1994; 76:1746–1752.
68. Redline S, Tishler PV. The genetics of sleep apnea. Sleep Med Rev 2000; 4:583–602.
69. Bayadi SE, Millman RP, Tishler PV, Rosenberg C, Saliski W, Boucher MA, Redline S. A family study of sleep apnea. Anatomic and physiologic interactions. Chest 1990; 98:554–559.
70. Douglas NJ, Luke M, Mathur R. Is the sleep apnoea/hypopnoea syndrome inherited? Thorax 1993; 48:719–721.
71. Redline S, Tishler PV, Tosteson TD, Williamson J, Kump K, Browner I, Ferrette V, Kregci P. The familial aggregation of obstructive sleep apnea. Am J Respir Crit Care Med 1995; 151:682–687.
72. Redline S, Tosteson T, Tishler PV, Carskadon MA, Millman RP. Studies in the genetics of obstructive sleep apnea. Familial aggregation of symptoms associated with sleep-related breathing disturbances. Am Rev Respir Dis 1992; 145:440–444.
73. Marcus CL, Keens TG, Bautista DB, von Pechmann WS, Davidson Ward SL. Obstructive sleep apnea in children with Down syndrome. Pediatrics 1991; 88:132–139.
74. Whittle AT, Marshall I, Mortimore IL, Wraith PK, Sellar RJ, Douglas NJ. Neck soft

tissue and fat distribution: comparison between normal men and women by magnetic resonance imaging Thorax 1999; 54:323–328.
75. Legato MJ. Gender-specific aspects of obesity. Int J Fertil 1997; 42:184–197.
76. Millman RP, Carlisle CC, McGarvey ST, et al. Body fat distribution and sleep apnea severity in women. Chest 1995; 107:362–366.
77. Schwab RJ. Upper airway imaging. Clinics Chest Med 1998; 19:33–54.
78. Schellenberg J, Maislin G, Schwab RJ. Physical findings and the risk for obstructive sleep apnea: the importance of soft tissue structures. Am J Respir Crit Care Med 2000; 162:740–748.
79. Schwab RJ. Properties of tissues surrounding the upper airway. Proceedings of the Fourth International Symposium on Sleep and Respiration. Sleep 1996; 19:S170–S174.
80. Schwab RJ, Pack AI, Gupta KB, Metzger LJ, Oh E, Getsy JE, Hoffman EA, Gefter WB. Upper airway and soft tissue structural changes induced by CPAP in normal subjects. Am J Respir Crit Care Med 1996; 154:1106–1116.
81. Trudo FJ, Gefter WB, Welch KC, Gupta KB, Maislin G, Schwab RJ. State related changes in upper airway caliber and surrounding soft tissue structures in normals. Am J Respir Crit Care Med 1998; 158:1259–1270.
82. Welch KC, Gefter WB, Ritter CT Maislin G, Schwab RJ. Dynamic respiratory related upper airway imaging during wakefulness in normal subjects and patients with sleep disordered breathing using MRI. Am J Respir Crit Care Med 1998; 157:A54.
83. Welch KC, Goldberg AN, Trudo FJ, Gefter WB, Ritter CT, Schwab RJ. Upper airway anatomic changes with magnetic resonance imaging in uvulopalatopharyngoplasty patients. Am J Respir Crit Care Med 1997; 155:A938.
84. Rodenstein DO, Dooms G, Thomas Y, Liistro G, Stanescu DC, Culee C, Aubert-Tulkins G. Pharyngeal shape and dimensions in healthy subjects, snorers, and patients with obstructive sleep apnoea. Thorax 1990; 45:722–727.
85. Leiter JC. Upper airway shape. Is it important in the pathogenesis of obstructive sleep apnea? Am J Respir Crit Care Med 1996; 153:894–898.
86. Pack AI. Obstructive sleep apnea. Adv Intern Med 1994; 49:517–567.
87. Schmidt-Nowara W, Lowe AA, Wiegand L, et al. Oral appliances for the treatment of snoring and obstructive sleep apnea: A review. Sleep 1995; 18:501–510.
88. Strollo PJ Jr, Rogers RM. Obstructive sleep apnea. N Engl J Med 1996; 334:99–104.
89. Stein MG, Gamsu G, DeGeer G, Golden JA, Crumley RL, Webb WR. Cine CT in obstructive sleep apnea. Am J Roentgenol 1987; 148:1069–1074.
90. Badr MS, Toiber F, Skatrud JB, Dempsey J. Pharyngeal narrowing/occlusion during central sleep apnea. J Appl Physiol 1995; 78:1806–1815.
91. Morrell MJ, Arabi Y, Zahn B, Badr MS. Progressive retropalatal narrowing preceding obstructive apnea. Am J Respir Crit Care Med 158:1974–1981, 1998.
92. Burger CD, Stanson AW, Daniels BK, Sheedy, PF, Shepard JW. Fast-CT evaluation of the effect of lung volume on upper airway size and function in normal men. Am Rev Respir Dis 1992; 146:335–339.
93. Suratt PM, Wilhoit SC, Cooper K. Induction of airway collapse with subatmospheric pressure in awake patients with sleep apnea. J Appl Physiol 1984; 57:140–146.
94. Sanders MH, Moore SE. Inspiratory and expiratory partitioning of airway resistance during sleep in patients with sleep apnea. Am Rev Respir Dis 1983; 127:554–558.
95. Sanders MH, Kern N. Obstructive sleep apnea treated by independently adjusted inspiratory and expiratory positive airway pressures via a nasal mask. Chest 1990; 98:317–324.

96. Gold AR, Schwartz AR. The pharyngeal critical pressure (Pcrit): the why's and how's of using nasal continuous positive airway pressure diagnostically. Chest 1996; 110: 1077–1088.
97. Ritter CT, Trudo FJ, Goldberg AN Welch KC, Maislin G, Schwab RJ. Quantitative evaluation of the upper airway during nasopharyngoscopy with Müller maneuver. Laryngoscope 1999; 109:954–963.
98. Ritter CT, Trudo FJ, Goldberg AN, Welch KC, Schwab RJ. Quantitative evaluation of upper airway changes in normals and apneics during Müller maneuver. Am J Respir Crit Care Med 1998; 157:A54.

2

Biomechanics of the Upper Airway During Sleep

PHILIP L. SMITH and ALAN R. SCHWARTZ

Johns Hopkins University School of Medicine
Baltimore, Maryland

I. Introduction

As has been outlined in Chapter 1, the major structural components of the pharyngeal airway demonstrate clear abnormalities in patients with obstructive sleep apnea compared to normal. Nevertheless, one of the more intriguing aspects of this sleep disorder is the fact that many patients with more markedly narrowed airways (e.g., acromegaly, achondroplasia) do not necessarily succumb to recurrent upper airway collapse. Moreover, our understanding of the structural aspects of the pharynx and the surrounding tissues have derived primarily from studies during wakefulness.

Varying degrees of upper airway obstruction have been observed clinically, although it has been difficult to discern consistent anatomical functional differences in the upper airway of normals, snorers, and patients with obstructive apneas and hypopneas. Thus far, clear differences have been noted among apneic patients compared to normals as demonstrated in morphometric studies examining upper airway size and tissue composition utilizing techniques such as acoustic reflection (1), CT scanning (2,3), or MRI (4–6). Furthermore, awake flow-volume curves (7,8) and pharyngeal resistance measurements (9–11) have not yielded specific physiological abnormalities among the various groups. Similarly, in neurophysiological studies in sleeping humans, no clear disturbances of neural control of the upper airway account for the variable airway obstruction among these groups.

While it might be possible to make certain statements about the pathophysiology of the upper airway prior to sleep onset, ultimately it will be necessary to elucidate the sleep-related mechanisms responsible for the collapse and occlusion that are the hallmark of this disorder. An appropriate analogy might be that our studies of exercise physiology have allowed us to predict the maximum ventilation as a function of the resting FEV_1, a relationship that could only be derived from the comparison of exercise and resting states. On the other hand, there are other physiological changes, such as gas exchange, that occur during exercise that simply cannot be predicted from rest studies; hence, the need for the study of exercise.

We have several objectives in this chapter. First, we will build on a previous published volume on sleep and breathing (12) that has extensively reviewed the airway mechanics to that point. Second, we will emphasize work on the biomechanics of the upper airway that has been performed during the sleep or sleep-like (anesthesia) state. Third, the chapter will have an expressed point of view that builds on a specific model that can begin to address the mechanical and neural factors responsible for upper airway collapse. This chapter focuses primarily on the mechanisms of airflow obstruction during sleep.

II. Site of Collapse

From the initial studies by Remmers, it has been clear that the predominant site of upper airway collapse during sleep in patients with obstructive sleep apnea resides within the pharyngeal segment between the tip of the soft palate to the glottic inlet (13). Studies by both Hudgel (14) and Shepard and Thawley (15) have further defined whether the sites for collapse are predominantly retropalatal or retroglossal in an attempt to correlate responses to specific therapeutic interventions. In general, however, these studies have tended to demonstrate that while collapse differs between various patients, it is also apparent that the site of collapse can vary within a patient. Utilizing a nasopharyngoscope in patients who were sleeping, Launois et al. have shown that approximately half the patients displayed narrowing in the nasopharynx and the other half in the oral or hypopharyngeal region (16,17). Additional studies have also demonstrated that the upper airway collapse seems to begin in the oropharynx, progressing to the hypopharynx (15). These latter, more dynamic, observations strongly suggest that regardless of the origin of the collapse, eventually the entire pharyngeal segment of the upper airway may be involved.

III. Anatomy

It is well recognized that the anatomy of the pharyngeal segment of the airway is complicated, extending caudally from the nasal choanae to the supraglottic space. Even though it is surrounded by bony structures, the caliber and function are modulated predominantly by an alteration in the pattern of neuromuscular activities of the skeletal muscles, including the intrinsic muscles of the pharyngeal wall, the tongue, and supra- and infrahyoid strap muscles. Functionally, the airway can be partitioned into a relatively collapsible nasopharyngeal segment, which is limited by the rim of the soft palate, and the oro- and hypopharyngeal segments which extend to the aryepiglottic folds.

As has been noted in Chapter 1, the airway size of patients with sleep apnea is significantly smaller than normals studied awake. Moreover, utilizing the acoustic-reflection technique, it has been possible to show that the pharyngeal cross-sectional area in awake patients with obstructive sleep apnea has a greater tendency to narrow as lung volume falls compared to controls without apnea (18,19). This linkage between the determination of airway size and state of lung inflation has been confirmed by additional animal (20,21) and human experiments.

During wakefulness, patency of the upper airway is under both volitional and nonvolitional control. However, during sleep, pharyngeal patency is almost exclusively under nonvolitional control. Even though it is clear that the airway collapses in patients with sleep apnea, the precise mechanism is unknown. Because of the complicated arrangement of the muscles as well as the varying sleep states, it has not been possible to precisely define whether the collapse is due primarily to altered neural or mechanical control, or a combination of both factors. Moreover, our ability to dissect out the relative contribution of neuromuscular activity and the contraction and/or relaxation of various muscles has been hampered by our inability to develop a biomechanical model that could determine the relative influences of the various factors causing collapse. Currently there are two theoretical models that have been put forth and are discussed below.

IV. Balance of Forces Model

Since the original physiological description of airway collapse, it has been proposed that the upper airway patency is determined by the balance between the negative intraluminal airway pressure and the dilator muscle tone (22) (Fig. 1). Remmers and others noted a demonstrable fall in phasic genioglossus activation at the onset of the apneas and suggested that an inappropriately low level of activity did not counterbalance the collapsing force exerted by the respiratory pump muscles (13) (Fig. 1). According to this model, the airway patency is dependent on the relative balance between the intraluminal pressure (airway suction) and the upper airway dilator muscle tone. Various inputs including the peripheral and central chemoreceptors as well as other factors that increase neural input to either the diaphragm (inspiratory drive) or upper airway muscles (upper airway drive) will be important in determining upper airway patency.

There are several difficulties with this model. First, it has not been possible to quantitate the forces generated by the specific dilator muscles relative to the negative intraluminal pressure. Measurements of the EMG activity, while useful in defining

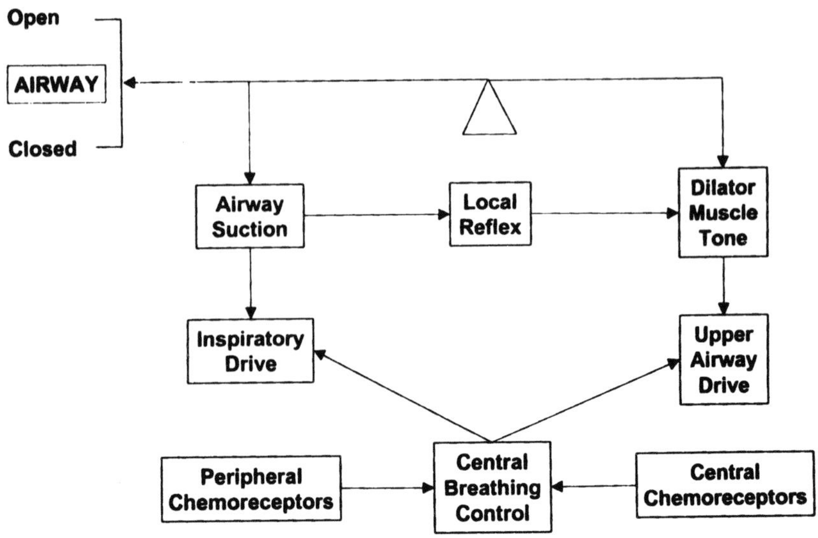

Figure 1 Balance of forces model to explain the maintenance of upper airway patency. In general, a balance between negative intraluminal airway pressure and upper airway dilator muscle tone are the primary forces that are modulated by additional factors. (From Ref. 22.)

relative change in the drive, do not necessarily translate into specific force measurements that yield to easy quantitation. Second, because of the multiple pharyngeal muscles involved in maintaining airway patency, it has not been possible to determine the constrictor and dilator muscle activity of each muscle relative to the pressure generated within the airway. Third, the inherent assumption that the negative airway suction is primarily responsible for airway closure has not been clearly demonstrated. In fact, as has been frequently observed, increasingly negative inspiratory esophageal pressure swings in a partially occluded airway is accompanied by a plateauing of flow (flow limitation) rather than occlusion of the airway.

V. Starling Resistor Model

In order to examine the effects of intraluminal pressure on flow through the upper airway, it is possible to model the behavior of the upper airway as a collapsible tube that is devoid of neural activity. In fact, the relationship between pressure and flow through collapsible biological structures has been well-defined in the pulmonary and systemic vasculature as well as the intrathoracic airway (23–26). The upper airway can be represented as a simple tube with collapsible segments bordered by two more rigid segments upstream (nasal passages) and downstream (hypopharyngeal segment) (Fig. 2). The segments upstream and downstream to the collapsible site have fixed diameters and resistances, R_{US} and R_{DS}, respectively, and the pres-

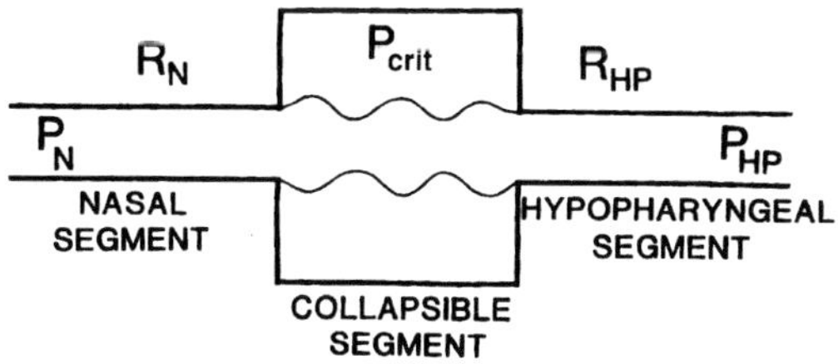

Figure 2 Starling mechanical analog of the upper airway consisting of a collapsible locus (P_{crit}) and relatively rigid segments upstream in the nose and downstream in the hypopharynx with nasal pressures P_N and hypopharyngeal (P_{HP}), and resistances, R_N and R_{HP}, respectively. (From Ref. 28.)

sures upstream and downstream are P_{US} and P_{DS}, utilizing this approach, respectively.

Several features of this model are worth emphasizing. First, as previously stated, changes in the pressure downstream do not influence the maximal flow through this system once the flow-limited condition exists. The development of inspiratory airflow limitation is illustrated for several breaths in an apneic patient as nasal pressure is increased (Fig. 3). As the hypopharyngeal pressure (P_{HP}) falls during inspiration, airflow ($\dot{V}$) remains independent of changes in the downstream pressure (Fig. 3).

In breaths with partial airflow obstruction (Fig. 3B, C), inspiratory airflow plateaus at a maximal level. Second, maximal flow in a collapsible tube is determined by the P_N, R_N, and P_{crit} as described in the following, e.g.,

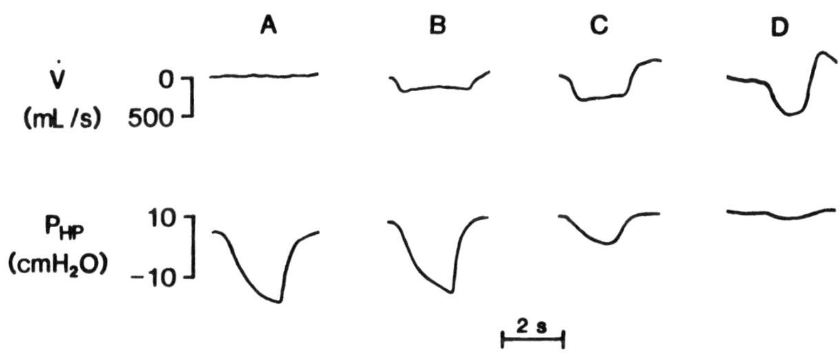

Figure 3 Single breath pressure (P_{HP}) – inspiratory flow (V) relationships in a patient with sleep apnea during stage II sleep at several levels of positive nasal pressure. (A) At a P_N of approximately 4 cmH_2O, the inspiratory flow was zero. (B) At a P_N of 6 cmH_2O, V_I plateaued at a low level and was associated with hypopneas. (C) At a P_N of 9 cmH_2O, flow limitation was observed, but no arousals or desaturations occurred. (D) At a P_N of approximately 12 cmH_2O, V was normal with no evidence of flow limitation (see text for details). (From Ref. 29.)

$$\dot{V}i_{max} = (P_N - P_{crit}) \div R_N \tag{1}$$

under conditions of flow limitation. The response in maximal flow to increases in upstream nasal pressure can be seen in Figure 3. By varying P_N, it is possible to obtain pressure-flow relationships that describe the collapsibility (pharyngeal critical pressure, P_{crit}) and nasal resistance upstream from the collapsible site (R_N) as determined by the zero-flow intercept and inverse of the slope, respectively (Fig. 4).

Third, based on this model, it is possible to describe distinct pressure-flow relationships for a range of physiological states that characterize the human upper airway (see Fig. 5). Moreover, these pressure-flow curves can describe physiological states and will serve as the basis for the remainder of the discussion. A more detailed description of the model and the specific methods employed to evaluate it are provided in a recent review (27) of several studies (28–31).

During sleep, several distinct breathing patterns have been recognized depending on the degree of upper airway obstruction. In general, individuals with a normal upper airway do not snore and have minimal episodes of periodic breathing during sleep. On the other hand, it is now recognized that individuals who snore have altered pressure-flow relationships (see below) and individuals who have apneas and hypopneas clearly have disrupted sleep characterized by alterations in oxyhemo-

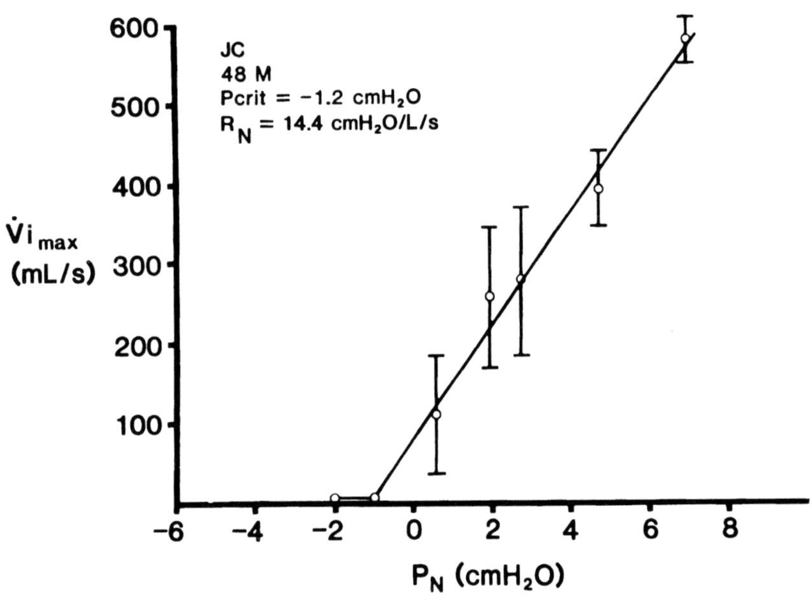

Figure 4 Maximal inspiratory airflow ($\dot{V}i_{max}$) versus nasal pressure (P_N) in a representative patient with obstructive hypopnea demonstrates a P_{crit} of -1.2 cmH_2O (defined by the nasal pressure at which airflow ceases). Each point represents the mean ± SD for breaths sampled at each level of P_N shown. (From Ref. 28.)

globin saturation and micro-arousal from sleep. As outlined below, it is possible to characterize the pressure-flow relationships for each of the various types of breathing.

VI. Normal Individuals

In normal individuals, the airway remains patent during sleep. Under these circumstances, changes in the esophageal pressure (downstream pressure) are directly related to the change in inspiratory airflow. When nasal pressure is lowered incrementally, however, a flow-limited condition ensues and a pressure-flow relationship can be obtained as previously shown in Figure 4. In studies of normal individuals, it has been found that the critical pressure is approximately -13 in adults during non-REM sleep (29) (see Fig. 5). In contrast, it has been shown that the upper airway during wakefulness demonstrates a much more markedly negative critical closing pressure of approximately -40 to -80 cmH_2O (32). Thus, with the onset of sleep, there is a dramatic change in the collapsible properties of the normal human upper airway.

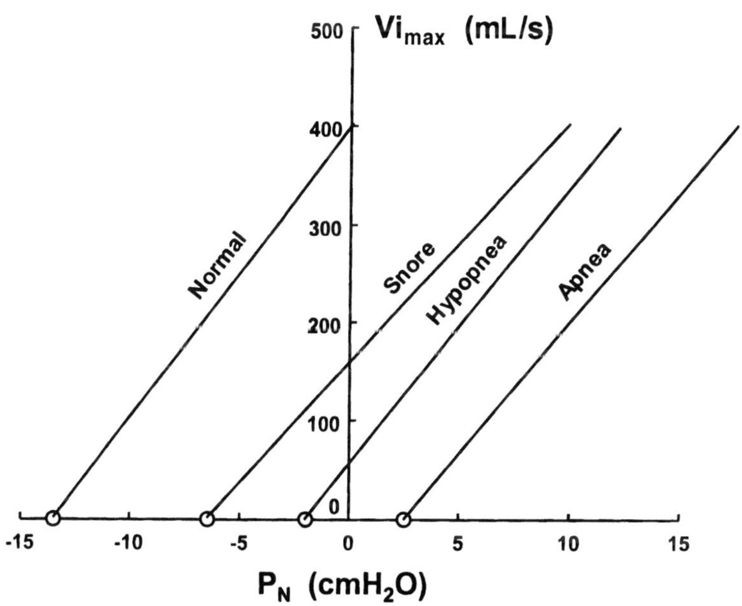

Figure 5 Characteristic upper airway pressure-flow relationships and critical pressures are represented for normals, subjects with snoring, and patients with hypopnea and apnea. The zero-flow intercept represents the various critical pressures (P_{crit}) for the different subject types. (Adapted from Refs. 28, 29.)

VII. Snorers

In normal individuals who snore, the upper airway narrows and inspiratory flow is reduced. With increasing negative downstream pressure, the inspiratory flow plateaus or "flow limits." If one plots the relationship between inspiratory flow and esophageal pressure (downstream) one would obtain the curve as seen in Figure 6. The relatively linear portion of the curve up to the point, P'_{HP}, represents the non–flow-limited condition. Beyond P'_{HP}, the flow plateaus, indicating that flow limitation has occurred. While airflow limitation can occur intermittently or continuously throughout the night, there is no evidence of desaturation or arousal from sleep if inspiratory airflow remains above 150 mL/s (28). Moreover, markedly negative pressures as much as −30 to −50 cmH_2O can be observed without evidence of disruption of sleep. As has been previously stated, the large negative pleural pressure swings do not lead to airway occlusion but rather airflow limitation, and thus the large swings in downstream pressure should be viewed as a consequence, rather than the cause, of upper airway narrowing.

Again, as in normal individuals, the P_{crit} can be determined by lowering the pressure upstream from the collapsible site until no flow is evident (28). From additional studies of individuals who snored, but did not have evidence of sleep-disor-

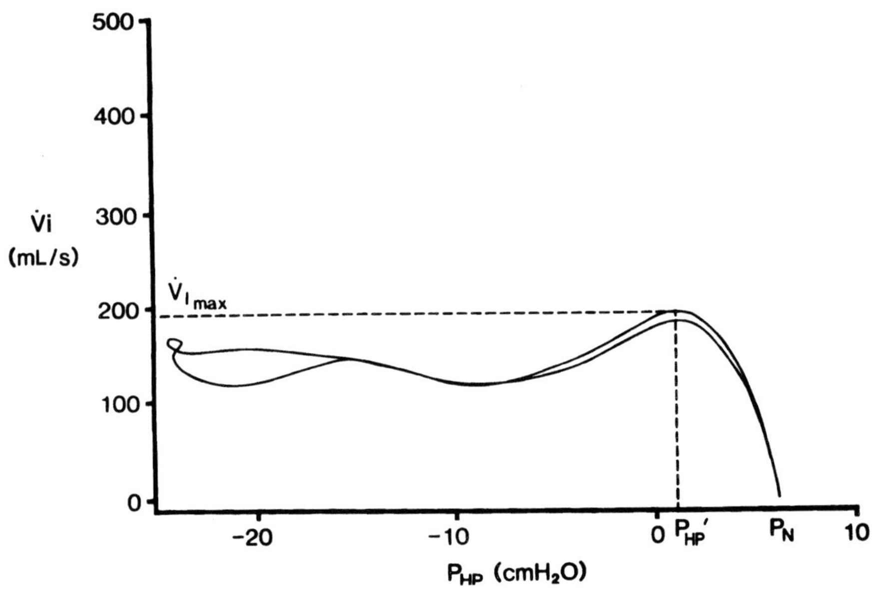

Figure 6 Maximal inspiratory flow ($\dot{V}i$) versus hypopharyngeal pressure (P_{HP}) during a single flow-limited inspiration. During early inspiration, $\dot{V}i$ increases as P_{HP} falls. When P_{HP} decreases below a specific P_{HP} (P'_{HP}), $\dot{V}_i$ becomes maximal and independent of downstream pressure. (From Ref. 20.)

dered breathing, the P_{crit} was approximately -6 cmH_2O during sleep but more positive than the normal individuals, thus indicating a more collapsible airway (see Fig. 5).

VIII. Hypopnea

In certain individuals, as the upper airway narrows further, and maximal flow is reduced below 150 mL/s (see Fig. 5), disordered breathing ensues (hypopnea) and is characterized by oscillations in oxygen saturation and/or arousal from sleep (28). The endo-esophageal pressures may be more or less negative than individuals who snore. The P_{crit} in these individuals is approximately -2 cmH_2O during sleep as derived from the pressure-flow curve described above (28). Thus, it is the critical pressure, not the relative swings in esophageal pressure, that are responsible for the progressive increase in restricted flow through the upper airway.

Recently it has been proposed that a form of sleep-disordered breathing characterized by flow limitation and recurrent arousal and/or possible minimal desaturation be classified as ''upper airway resistance syndrome'' (33). Nevertheless, the characteristic of this particular subclassification appears similar to that of hypopnea, which has been defined as a disordered breathing event characterized by reduced flow in association with either an arousal and/or desaturation. Moreover, the original description of this syndrome includes pressure and flow recordings similar to those noted with individuals with hypopnea (33). In individuals defined with upper airway resistance syndrome, it has been shown that the critical pressures are similar when compared to patients with hypopnea (34). Regardless of the types of classification, it can be seen that each of the subgroups demonstrate critical pressures that fall on a line between health (more negative critical pressures) to disease (slightly negative to positive critical pressures).

IX. Obstructive Sleep Apnea

When the upper airway occludes, no airflow can occur and an apnea ensues. In this case, the critical pressure surrounding the airway is at least atmospheric or above. Under circumstances of airway occlusion, it is necessary to raise rather than lower the upstream pressure in order to generate a pressure-flow relationship and determine the P_{crit} (28,31) (see Fig. 5). Critical pressures as high as 10–15 cmH_2O have been recorded in individuals with severe obstructive sleep apnea (31). However, in a study of patients with moderately severe obstructive sleep apnea who were matched for body mass index (BMI), the mean P_{crit} during sleep was approximately 3.0 cmH_2O (28). It has been recently noted that the frequency of apnea bears a weak relationship to the P_{crit} (35). We have also examined apnea frequency as a function of P_{crit} and found almost no relationship (Fig. 7A). Our own notion is that the periodicity of the disordered breathing events is a function of a complex interaction of multiple respiratory inputs and is discussed in more detail in Chapter 3. On the other hand,

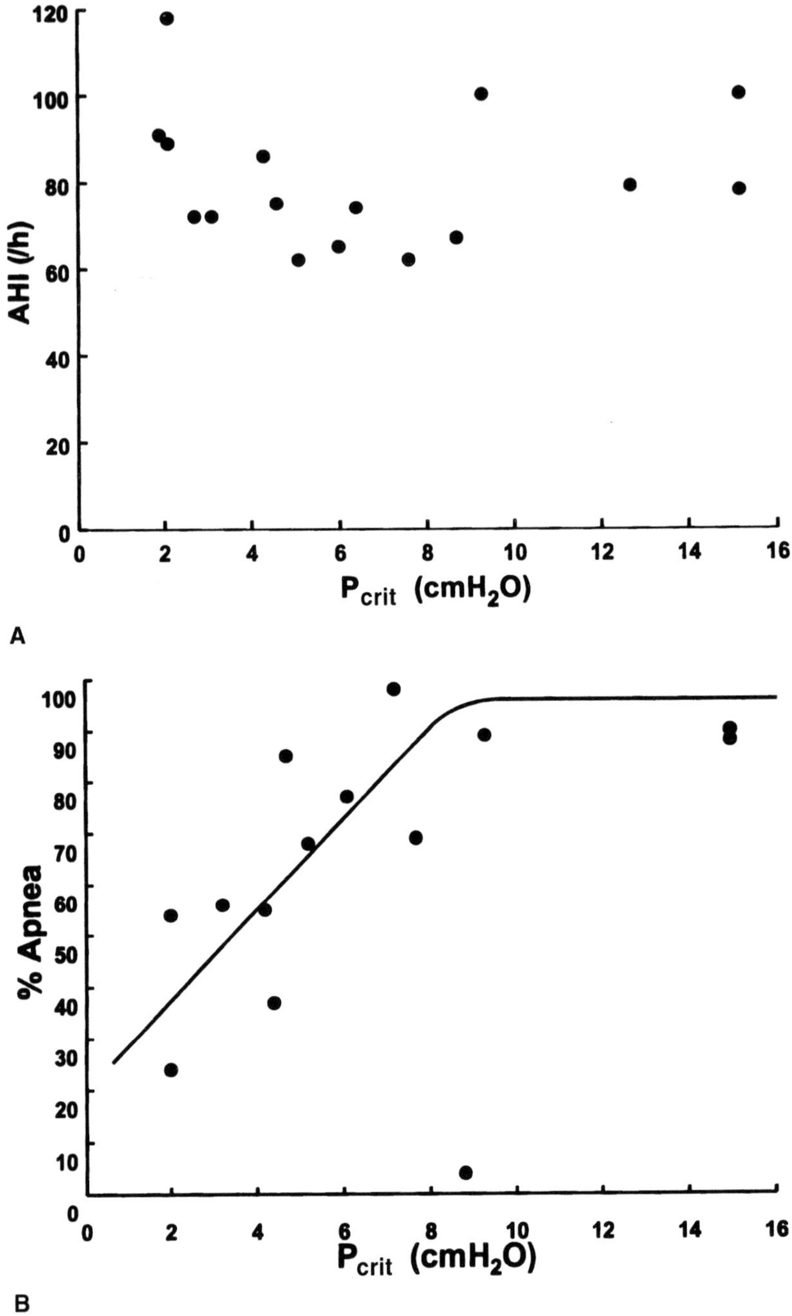

Figure 7 (A) Relationship of critical pressure to apnea-hypopnea index (see text for details). (B) Relationship of critical pressures and ratio of apnea/hypopnea expressed as a percentage (see text for details).

when P_{crit} is examined as a function of the predominant type of disordered breathing event, it is clear that a closer correlation exists (Fig. 7B).

There is an additional aspect of the model that is worth emphasizing. Since the nasal passages are exposed to atmospheric pressure, the pressure upstream from the oropharyngeal collapse remains constant and equal to zero. Thus, under conditions of flow limitation, $\dot{V}i_{max}$ is determined either by the P_{crit} or the R_{US}, as noted in Eq. (1). In addition, as shown in Figure 5, the reciprocal of the slopes of the pressure-flow curves (R_{US}) for each of the various patient groups are almost parallel to each other based on additional empirical observations (28). Thus, for practical purposes, the maximal inspiratory flow under conditions of flow limitation is primarily a function of the upper airway collapsibility.

The implications of the above relationship are severalfold. First, it has become apparent that the collapsibility of the upper airway is the major determinant of flow rather than resistive changes in the upstream segment. This may, in part, be due to the fact that the collapsible segment of the upper airway is either very limited and that the upstream segment is rather fixed in its properties due to the stiffness of the bony structures. Second, in patients with airflow limitation (snorer/hypopnea), rough estimates of the critical pressure can be derived by measuring the $\dot{V}i_{max}$ and assuming a constant range of R_{US} from previously published data (28). These estimates of critical pressure may prove useful for clinical epidemiological purposes to describe populations at risk or in transition from health to disease. Third, in cases of disease characterized by hypopnea or apnea, a knowledge of the critical pressure may provide unique insight into the probability of being able to decrease the P_{crit} into a more normal range and reestablish health (see Sec. XIII).

X. Analysis of Pressure-Flow Relationships: Assumptions

In contrast to adults, when pressure-flow curves are developed in children, there is a remarkably different slope in normal snorers compared to children with sleep apnea (36). In fact, when negative pressure is applied to children who snore, the P_{crit} is often very negative with an R_{US} that is considerably higher than adults.

When constructing the pressure-flow curves, it has been assumed that there are minimal influences of neuromuscular tone. In fact, the Starling resistor model was developed as a pure mechanical analog with the underlying premise that neural activity was absent. Nevertheless, it is well recognized that either lowering or raising upstream nasal pressure in human or animal airways leads to significant stimulation of mechanical receptors that cause activation or deactivation of neuromuscular activity (37,38). In spite of this, in adults, the slope of the pressure-flow relationship ($1/R_{US}$) is remarkably similar between the various normal individuals (normals and snorers) and the patient groups (apnea and hypopnea). Thus, it has been assumed that even if neuromuscular activity changes dynamically during the construction of the pressure-flow curves, the relationship is relatively similar. On the other hand, clear differences in these relationships between children and adults suggest that neuromuscular responses in children are altered compared to adults.

XI. Mechanical Determinants of Pharyngeal Collapsibility

Because of the empirical observations noted above and the fact that there is significant tonic and phasic neuromuscular activity during sleep, techniques that eliminate neural input have been developed to dissect out the purely mechanical properties of the upper airway. To study this issue, a decerebrate isolated upper airway preparation has been developed (39,40). In this preparation, the trachea is bisected and cannulated rostrally and caudally. Pressure-flow relationships have been generated through the upper airway segment by altering pressures systematically.

In using this preparation, it has been shown that increasing airway length, either by neck extension or caudal tracheal traction, caused a marked decrease in pharyngeal collapsibility, which led to an increase in the maximal airflow through the upper airway (40). In contrast, anterior traction on the tongue led to variable changes in collapsibility (P_{crit}) as follows: P_{crit} fell with tongue displacement only after the airway had been elongated, whereas no change in P_{crit} was observed when the trachea was in the neutral position. To account for such variability in the P_{crit} response to the tongue and tracheal displacement, the following mechanical model has been elaborated (Fig. 8).

In this model, the effect of tongue displacement is represented in panels B and D, while the effect of lengthening the upper airway can be represented in panels C and D. When the trachea is displaced caudally, decreases in P_{crit} can be attributed to increases in tension in the upper airway wall/mucosa. In contrast, the tongue is thought to exert a radial force on the pharyngeal airway (41). With outward displacement, the pressure surrounding the collapsible site decreases to a variable degree, depending on the wall tension as follows. When wall tension is low (panel A and B), outward tongue movement causes little change in surrounding pressure (P_{crit}). Under conditions of increased wall tension (panels C and D), but such outward movement results in a larger decrease in P_{crit}. Thus, it is possible in an experimental model to apportion the changes in pharyngeal collapsibility to alterations in tracheal and tongue tension in a fashion analogous to that previously described for the intrathoracic airways (42,43).

The clinical implications of this model help in understanding how different pathophysiological mechanisms might explain increases in critical pressure observed in apneic patients. For example, the scarring of the upper airway that accompanies uvulopalatopharyngoplasty may be responsible for decreases in pharyngeal collapsibility in selected patients (44). In contrast, patients failing to respond to uvulopalatopharyngoplasty may have increased levels of wall tension causing increased collapsibility due to elevated pressures surrounding the pharynx. Under these circumstances, patients might be treated with other procedures that displace surrounding structures anteriorly such as mandible repositioning or reconstruction (45–47).

To extend the animal studies and define the purely mechanical determinants of upper airway collapsibility in humans, the effect of neuromuscular hypotonia on airflow dynamics has been performed. It is known that marked reductions in pharyngeal neuromuscular activity occur during rapid eye movement sleep (48). Moreover,

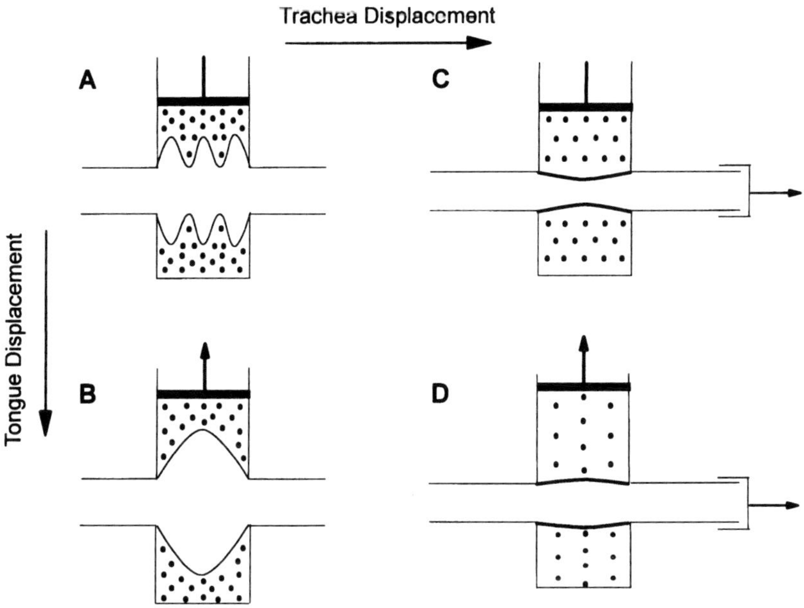

Figure 8 Model illustrating interactive effect of tongue and tracheal displacement on surrounding pressure (P_{crit}). (A–D): Starling model of airway modified to show a plunger representing tongue and dots representing P_{crit}. Static condition of upper airway after either tongue or tracheal displacement is shown. Concentration of dots within surrounding space is proportional to P_{crit}. Thick solid line = increase in airway wall longitudinal tension with tracheal displacement within flow-limiting site. (From Ref. 56.)

as has been previously noted (49,50), studies have demonstrated significant hypotonia of the pharyngeal muscles with the application of positive pressure during sleep and have shown that this hypotonia persists even after the nasal pressure is abruptly reduced. By repeatedly lowering the nasal pressure to various levels, a complete pressure-flow curve can be constructed and repeated measurements of the critical pressures and upstream resistance can be obtained over multiple breaths throughout the night.

As can be seen in Figure 9, critical pressures increased progressively for the first through the third breath after an abrupt decrease in nasal pressure in both non-REM and REM sleep, even though genioglossal electromyographic activity had increased. In addition, no significant difference was detected between non-REM and REM sleep, despite the fact that genioglossal electromyographic activity had decreased significantly when compared to baseline. Assuming that REM sleep represents the most hypotonic state of the airway, similarities in critical pressure suggest that the predominantly mechanical properties of the upper airway during non-REM sleep are represented under these circumstances. Moreover, utilizing similar tech-

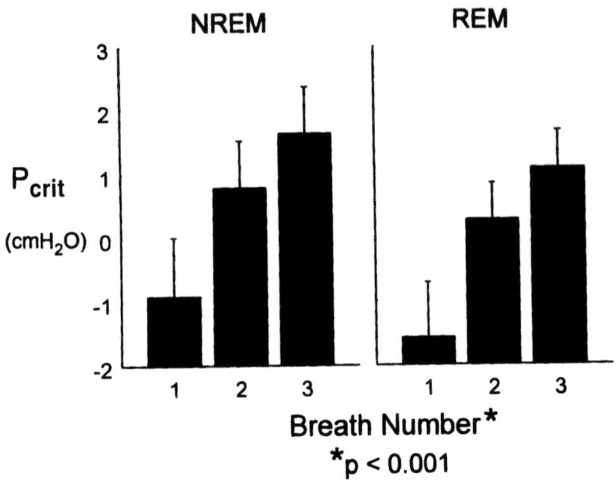

Figure 9 P_{crit} versus breath number for non-REM (left panel) and REM (right panel) sleep for three breaths after an abrupt drop in nasal pressure. P_{crit} increased ($p < 0.001$) with breath number. (From Ref. 108.)

niques in humans under general anesthesia and neuromuscular blockade, comparable critical pressures have been demonstrated in apneic patients (Fig. 10) (49,51). These findings are consistent with the notion that increases in pharyngeal collapsibility in patients with obstructive sleep apnea are due to an underlying mechanical or structural alteration.

Although the structural basis for increased pharyngeal collapsibility in humans is not known, Isono and coworkers (49,51,52) have examined the role of anatomical factors in anesthetized humans after having eliminated neuromuscular activity pharmacologically. In their work, pharyngeal cross-sectional area is measured over a range of nasal pressure encompassing the critical pressure at which the airway closes (49,52). Analyzing the pressure-area relationship, they have defined the critical pressure and compliance of the oropharyngeal and velopharyngeal segments. The critical pressures for the oropharyngeal segment are generally lower (often more negative) than those for the velopharynx, a finding that correlates with earlier observations (49). In further studies, they have determined that anterior mandibular advancement improves velopharyngeal patency (P_{crit} falls) and attributes the change to a decrease in the pressure exerted by the tongue on the ventral surface of the soft palate. It also appears that the response in the velopharyngeal P_{crit} to anterior mandibular displacement was greater in lean compared to obese individuals, suggesting that adiposity alters the response in pharyngeal collapsibility to the application of dilating forces (53,54) (Fig. 11).

There are several possible explanations for the interaction between adiposity and airway dilating forces. First, dilating forces produced by anterior tongue/man-

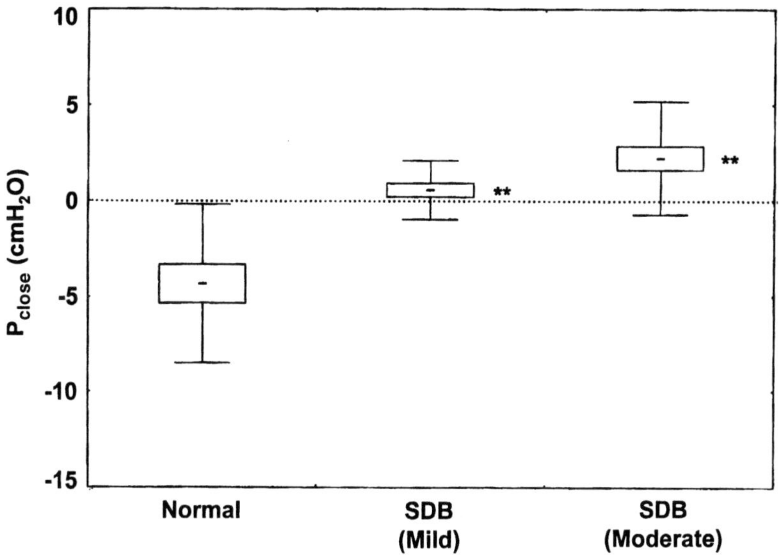

Figure 10 Box plots illustrating closing pressure (P_{close}). The magnitude of closing pressure is represented for three groups: normal, mild sleep-disordered breathing (SDB) defined as patients with oxygen desaturation under 5–20 per hour, and moderate SDB, defined as greater than 20 desaturations per hour. Mean values are indicated by horizontal bar within each box; bars above and below each box represent SE. $^{**}p < 0.01$ vs. normal group. (Adapted from Ref. 51.)

dibular displacement may have a variable effect on pressure at the ventral surface of the soft palate, depending on the level of tension within the palate and its attachments to the lateral pharyngeal mucosa and caudal structures. Second, adiposity may slacken these palatal attachments, as suggested by studies demonstrating enfolding of the lateral pharyngeal walls in obese patients with obstructive sleep apnea (6). Third, conformational changes in the lateral wall may alter the shape of the velopharyngeal lumen, thereby further diminishing the improvement in pharyngeal patency with anterior tongue and mandibular displacement (55,56). It is therefore likely that adiposity is associated with a complex array of anatomical changes, which alters the response in pharyngeal collapsibility to forces which dilate the airway.

Other lines of investigation also suggest that anatomical alterations predispose to increases in pharyngeal collapsibility in obstructive sleep apnea. Hendricks et al. in a bulldog model have shown that anatomical compromise of the pharyngeal airway is associated with histological evidence of muscle injury (57,58). Others have demonstrated physiological and metabolic changes in upper airway muscles, suggesting that pharyngeal muscles compensate for structural narrowing of the upper airway (59). (These muscle changes are discussed in more detail in Chap. 7.) Finally, it has been thought that increased activation of the genioglossal muscle during wake-

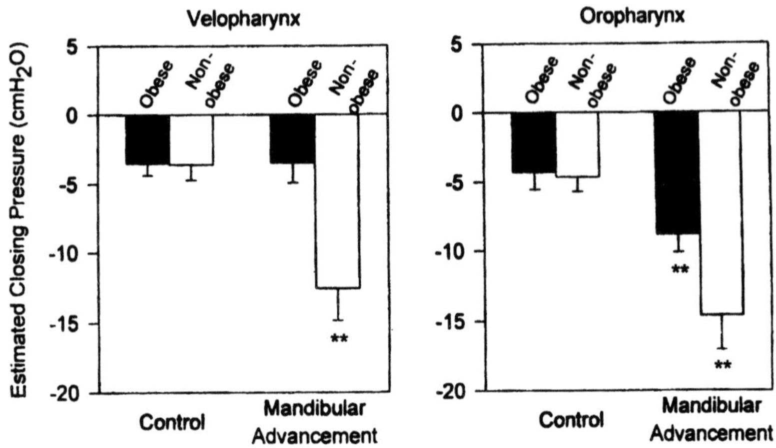

Figure 11 Effects of mandibular advancement on estimated closing pressure at the velopharynx (left panel) and oropharynx (right panel). At the level of the oropharynx, mandibular advancement significantly decreased the closing pressure in both obese and nonobese subjects, whereas only the nonobese group responded to this maneuver at the level of the velopharynx. $^{**}p < 0.01$ vs. control. Values are means ± SE. (From Ref. 54.)

fulness in apneic patients is required to compensate for an underlying anatomical defect (60).

XII. Neural Determinants of Pharyngeal Collapsibility

In addition to anatomical factors predisposing to pharyngeal collapse, it is also likely that neural factors play a role. For example, we know that the expression of the disease is quite distinct in children compared to adults since most of the children have marked tonsillar hypertrophy as a major feature of the disease (36,61). In contrast, most adults who develop sleep apnea do not have gross anatomical alterations, but rather subtle generalized changes in upper airway size that could represent decrements in neural control of the airway (11). A more detailed review of the various neural reflexes that might play a role in sleep apnea is discussed in detail in Chapter 5. In particular, previous experimental evidence has suggested specific changes due to alterations in chemoreceptors and upper airway mucosal afferents (62–71). While it is known that stimulation of these reflexes is associated with an increase in upper airway muscle activity, few studies have actually examined the relative effect of the various chemoreceptors and upper airway reflexes on airway collapsibility as defined by measurements of the pharyngeal critical pressure.

The relative effect of chemoreceptor, vagal, and mucosal afferents on upper airway function have been examined (72). In general, increasing levels of CO_2 caused an increase in maximal inspiratory airflow that was due primarily to a decrease in critical pressure, indicating that airway collapsibility had fallen. Moreover, the alterations in airflow and critical pressure were accentuated during inspiration after having stimulated phasic upper airway neuromuscular activity with CO_2 (39).

These phasic differences in airflow dynamics suggest that neural activity can play an important role in stabilizing the upper airway during inspiration. In spite of the marked response in upper airway collapsibility to CO_2, hypoxemia did not appreciably change critical pressures at any level of CO_2. It is of note that other investigators examining changes in upper airway resistance and neural muscular activity have not seen consistent changes in upper airway resistance or compliance with administration of CO_2 (73–75).

Given the graded response in pharyngeal collapsibility to CO_2, it is likely that the relationship between critical pressures and CO_2 exhibit both a threshold and slope, analogous to the ventilatory response to CO_2. The threshold to this response is suggested by the fact that when levels of CO_2 were significantly reduced, critical pressure increased to a level seen during complete neuromuscular blockade. In addition, pressure-flow relationships were generated in an isolated feline upper airway preparation to determine the critical pressure under a variety of experiment conditions. As can be seen in Figure 12, when mucosal afferents were blocked by topical anesthesia (Fig. 12, curve B), there was a minimal but definite shift in the threshold of the CO_2 response toward a slightly lower critical pressure without any change in the slope of this response. In contrast, vagal afferents had no independent effect on the critical pressure suggesting that this reflex did not influence the threshold of the CO_2 response. Rather, there was a significant interaction between the vagal afferents in the CO_2 reflex responses as demonstrated by a remarkably attenuated slope of this relationship. Thus, it appears that vagal afferents markedly depressed the sensitivity in upper airway collapsibility to CO_2. Although it is difficult to know whether similar neuromuscular control mechanisms modulate human pharyngeal collapsibility during sleep, it must be recognized that CO_2 was significantly higher in the aforementioned experimental preparation than that ordinarily seen in normal sleeping apneic and nonapneic individuals (76,77).

While it is still unclear whether a generalized disturbance in pharyngeal neuromotor tone might be a cause of sleep apnea control, it has been postulated that isolated reductions in genioglossal neuromuscular activity might be responsible for pharyngeal airflow obstruction. This notion has led several investigators to stimulate the genioglossus muscle with transcutaneous (78,79), percutaneous (80), and intraoral electrodes (81–84). Unfortunately, it has been difficult to determine the degree to which these devices activated the genioglossus muscle or whether responses in airway patency were related to arousals rather than selective genioglossal recruitment during stimulation (80). The most recent evidence, however, strongly suggests that activation of the genioglossus muscle either with fine wire electrodes or a cuff electrode placed around the hypoglossal nerve can lead to both an increase in inspiratory airflow as well as a fall in critical pressure of 5 cmH_2O during sleep (77).

In the most recent work, it has been noted that the effect on the upper airway depended on the location of the electrodes and the actual movement of the tongue

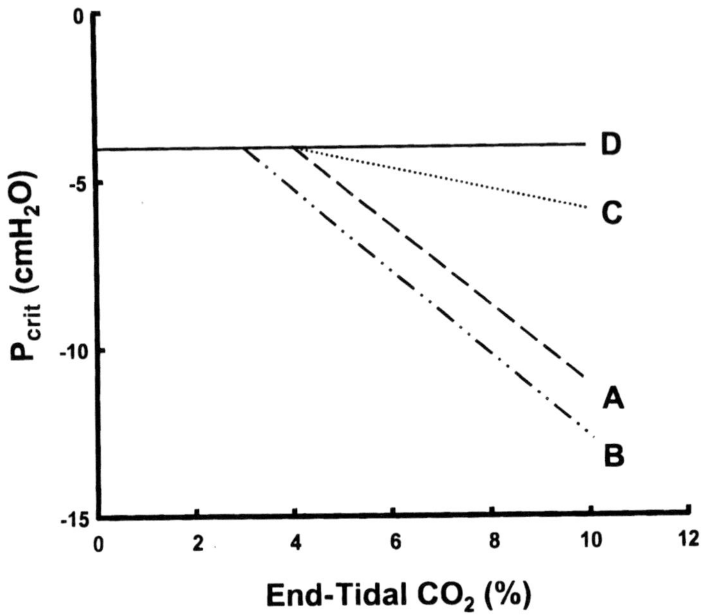

Figure 12 Schematic illustrating influence of chemoreceptor, airway mucosal receptor, and vagally mediated pulmonary reflexes on critical pressure (P_{crit}) vs. end-tidal CO_2 ($ETCO_2$). (A) Response of P_{crit} to increasing $ETCO_2$ in the absence of airway and pulmonary reflex modulation; (B) effects of airway mucosal receptor reflexes on $P_{crit}-CO_2$ relationship; (C) effects of pulmonary receptor reflexes on $P_{crit}-CO_2$ relationship; (D) P_{crit} after neuromuscular blockade. (From Ref. 72.)

(76,77,85,86). For example, when lingual retractor muscles were selectively stimulated, airflow fell significantly. In contrast, selective stimulation of the genioglossus was consistently associated with an increase in inspiratory airflow and a fall in critical pressure. Although it appears that selective recruitment of tongue retractors or protrusors has opposite effects on airway patency, recent animal data suggest that the combined action of these antagonist muscle groups enhances pharyngeal stability and reduces airflow obstruction (87,88). It is still unclear what role the lingual musculature plays in maintaining pharyngeal patency during sleep, and whether a selective or generalized defect in neuromuscular control of the pharyngeal musculature plays a primary role in the pathogenesis of obstructive sleep apnea.

XIII. A Pathophysiological Approach to Treatment

As the pathophysiology of pharyngeal airflow obstruction is better elucidated, it is now possible to delineate a general framework for considering approaches to treating obstructive sleep apnea. Initially, the site of upper airway obstruction was bypassed with a tracheostomy, the earliest treatment for this disorder. Subsequent developments, however, have now led to treatments which relieve airflow obstruction by either (1) raising the upstream nasal pressure above the pharyngeal critical pressure or by (2) decreasing the critical pressure itself (27).

Nasal CPAP is the current mainstay of treatment for obstructive sleep apnea and depends on elevating the pressure above the pharyngeal critical pressure (30,31). It should be noted that the pressure at which flow limitation ceases can be quite variable. In fact, it is often necessary to raise the upstream pressure considerably above the critical pressure (89). In part, this is due to the activation of mucosal reflexes that cause the critical pressure to rise with increased nasal pressure (29). In general, individuals with lower critical pressures tend to have somewhat lower final CPAP pressures; nevertheless, it is necessary to titrate each patient individually for optimal determination. Whether it is necessary to eliminate all evidence of flow limitation is somewhat controversial (90,91). There have been several recent modifications of CPAP devices that will adjust the pressure based on evidence of flow limitation resulting in lower mean nasal pressures of approximately 2–3 cmH_2O (89). It is unknown whether this minimal difference in nasal pressure will lead to significant improvement in patient compliance (92–95).

The second major therapeutic strategy involves lowering critical pressure. If the critical pressure is reduced to a level of -5 to -8 cmH_2O, flow limitation may still be present; however, recurrent arousals from sleep and desaturations can be eliminated (27,44,96). If critical pressure is reduced within the normal range, normal respiration would be expected. Currently, there is good evidence that a 15% reduction in body weight lowers the P_{crit} by approximately 6 cmH_2O. Depending on the baseline critical pressure, a 6 cmH_2O reduction could completely normalize the breathing pattern as in the case of patients with obstructive hypopneas. Other maneuvers that may be effective include electrical stimulation of the hypoglossal nerve (77,97) and pharmacological agents such as protriptyline (98–101), which are designed to increase pharyngeal neuromuscular activity (98). Based on present evidence, these later strategies may be associated with critical pressure changes of approximately 2–5 cmH_2O.

Although there are minimal available studies on the effect of structural changes on upper airway collapsibility, one recent study examining the effect of body position noted a reduction in P_{crit} of approximately 4–5 cmH_2O when the patient assumed an upright position compared to the supine and lateral decubitus position (102,103). In addition, dental appliances and surgical procedures that move the mandible anteriorly might possibly help to augment dilating forces on the pharynx that could result in similar falls in the critical pressure (46,104–107). Finally, it has been noted that surgical reconstruction of the upper airway—in particular uvulopalatopharyngoplasty—has been associated with a variable, yet demonstrable 4–6 cmH_2O fall in P_{crit} among those patients who respond to surgery (44).

As noted above, relief of airflow obstruction can only be achieved if the critical pressure falls to sufficiently negative levels after intervention. With both the structural and neuromuscular strategies mentioned above, improvements in obstructive sleep apnea have been relatively modest, suggesting that many of these interventions lead to only modest decreases in critical pressure. With such reductions in critical pressure, apnea is most likely to remit in those patients in whom the initial critical pressure is close to atmospheric. In patients with higher levels of critical pressure, a greater effect might be achieved if multiple interventions are combined or if specific therapeutic strategies that augment the response in critical pressure are designed.

In summary, many of the newer therapies that are being considered for sleep apnea will be very dependent on a more complete understanding of the interaction between the neural and structural properties of the upper airway. At this juncture, there are minimal data regarding the pharmacological manipulation of the airway and how this might possibly be utilized as a strategic therapy. It is also conceivable that multiple therapeutic strategies could be combined to achieve a more effective result. For example, weight loss in combination with other strategies might prove particularly effective. Regardless of the method attempted, strategies directed at quantitating the changes in the upper airway collapsibility should yield insights into newer treatment regimens that might otherwise be dismissed if the apnea/hypopnea index were the only measurement of improvement.

References

1. Bradley TD, Brown IG, Grossman RF, Zamel N, Martinez D, Phillipson EA, et al. Pharyngeal size in snorers, nonsnorers, and patients with obstructive sleep apnea. N Engl J Med 1986; 315:1327–1331.
2. Haponik EF, Smith PL, Bohlman ME, Allen RP, Goldman SM, Bleecker ER. Computerized tomography in obstructive sleep apnea: Correlation of airway size with physiology during sleep and wakefulness. Am Rev Respir Dis 1983; 127:221–226.
3. Suratt PM, Dee P, Atkinson RL, Armstrong P, Wilhoit SC. Fluoroscopic and computed tomographic features of the pharyngeal airway in obstructive sleep apnea. Am Rev Respir Dis 1983; 127:487–492.
4. Schwab RJ, Gefter WB, Hoffman EA, Gupta KB, Pack AI. Dynamic upper airway imaging during awake respiration in normal subjects and patients with sleep disordered breathing. Am Rev Respir Dis 1993; 148:1385–1400.
5. Schwab RJ, Gupta KB, Metzger LJ, Pack AI, Gefter WB. State related changes in upper airway caliber and surrounding soft tissue structures in normals and apneics. Am J Respir Crit Care Med 1995; 151:A667.
6. Schwab RJ, Gupta KB, Gefter WB, Metzger LJ, Hoffman EA, Pack AI. Upper airway and soft tissue anatomy in normal subjects and patients with sleep-disordered breathing. Am J Respir Crit Care Med 1995; 152:1673–1689.
7. Haponik EF, Allen RP, Smith PL, Kaplan J, Bleecker ER. Flow volume curves and obstructive sleep apnea: serial changes. Am Rev Respir Dis 1981; 123:94.
8. Sanders MH, Martin RJ, Pennock BE, Rogers RM. The detection of sleep apnea in the awake patient. The 'saw-tooth' sign. JAMA 1981; 245:2414–2418.

9. Gleeson K, Zwillich CW, Bendrick TW, White DP. Effect of inspiratory nasal loading on pharyngeal resistance. J Appl Physiol 1986; 60:1882–1886.
10. Stauffer JL, Zwillich CW, Cadieux RJ, Bixler EO, Kales A, Varano LA, et al. Pharyngeal size and resistance in obstructive sleep apnea. Am Rev Respir Dis 1987; 136: 623–627.
11. White DP, Lombard RM, Cadieux RJ, Zwillich CW. Pharyngeal resistance in normal humans: influence of gender, age, and obesity. J Appl Physiol 1985; 58:365–371.
12. Sullivan CE. Sleep and Breathing. 2d ed. New York: Marcel Dekker, Inc., 1994.
13. Remmers JE, deGroot WJ, Sauerland EK, Anch AM. Pathogenesis of upper airway occlusion during sleep. J Appl Physiol 1978; 44:931–938.
14. Hudgel DW. Variable site of airway narrowing among obstructive sleep apnea patients. J Appl Physiol 1986; 61:1403–1409.
15. Shepard JW, Thawley SE. Localization of upper airway collapse during sleep in patients with obstructive sleep apnea. Am Rev Respir Dis 1990; 141:1350–1355.
16. Launois SH, Feroah TR, Campbell WN, Whitelaw WA, Remmers JE. Site of obstruction in obstructive sleep apnea: Influence on the outcome of uvulopalatopharyngoplasty. Am Rev Respir Dis 1990; 141:A861.
17. Launois SH, Feroah TR, Campbell WN, Issa FG, Morrison D, Whitelaw WA, et al. Site of pharyngeal narrowing predicts outcome of surgery for obstructive sleep apnea. Am Rev Respir Dis 1993; 147:182–189.
18. Bradley TD, Brown IG, Grossman RF, Zamel N, Martinez D, Phillipson EA, et al. Pharyngeal size on snorers, non-snorers, and patients with obstructive sleep apnea. N Engl J Med 1986; 315:1327–1331.
19. Hoffstein V, Zamel N, Phillipson EA. Lung volume dependence of pharyngeal cross-sectional area in patients with obstructive sleep apnea. Am Rev Respir Dis 1984; 130: 175–178.
20. Van de Graaff WB. Thoracic influence on upper airway patency. J Appl Physiol 1988; 65:2124–2131.
21. Van de Graaff WB. Thoracic traction on the trachea: mechanisms and magnitude. J Appl Physiol 1991; 70:1328–1336.
22. Cistulli PA, Sullivan CE. Pathophysiology of Sleep Apnea. In: Saunders NA, Sullivan CE, eds. Sleep and Breathing. Lung Biology in Health and Disease. 2d ed. New York: Marcel Dekker, 1994:405–448.
23. Permutt S, Bromberger-Barnea B, Bane HN. Alveolar pressure, pulmonary venous pressure, and the vascular waterfall. Med Thorac 1962; 19:239–260.
24. Permutt S, Riley RL. Hemodynamics of collapsible vessels with tone: the vascular waterfall. J Appl Physiol 1963; 18:924–932.
25. Sylvester JT, Brower RG, Permutt S. Effects of hypoxic vasoconstriction on the mechanical interaction between blood vessels and airways. In: Will JA, Dawson CA, Weir EK, Buckner CK, eds. The Pulmonary Circulation in Health and Disease. New York: Academic Press; 1987:321–334.
26. Pride NB, Permutt S, Riley RL, Bromberger-Barnea B. Determinants of maximal expiratory flow from the lungs. J Appl Physiol 1967; 23:646–662.
27. Gold AR, Schwartz AR. The pharyngeal critical pressure—the whys and hows of using nasal continuous positive airway pressure diagnostically. Chest 1996; 110:1077–1088.
28. Gleadhill IC, Schwartz AR, Schubert N, Wise RA, Permutt S, Smith PL. Upper airway collapsibility in snorers and in patients with obstructive hypopnea and apnea. Am Rev Respir Dis 1991; 143:1300–1303.

29. Schwartz AR, Smith PL, Gold AR, Wise RA, Permutt S. Induction of upper airway occlusion in sleeping individuals with subatmospheric nasal pressure. J Appl Physiol 1988; 64:535–542.
30. Schwartz AR, Smith PL, Wise RA, Permutt S. Effect of nasal pressure on upper airway pressure flow relationships. J Appl Physiol 1989; 66:1626–1634.
31. Smith PL, Wise RA, Gold AR, Schwartz AR, Permutt S. Upper airway pressure-flow relationships in obstructive sleep apnea. J Appl Physiol 1988; 64:789–795.
32. Suratt PM, Wilhoit SC, Cooper K. Induction of airway collapse with subatmospheric pressure in awake patients with sleep apnea. J Appl Physiol 1984; 57:140–146.
33. Guilleminault C, Stoohs R, Clerk A, Cetel M, Maistros P. A cause of excessive daytime sleepiness: the upper airway resistance syndrome. Chest 1993; 104:781–787.
34. Hassan, Z., Werber, KM, Pantino, D, Gold, AR. Pharyngeal collapsibility in the upper airway resistance syndrome (UARS). Am J Respir Crit Care Med 1998; 157:A55.
35. Sforza E, Petiau C, Weiss T, Thibault A, Krieger J. Pharyngeal critical pressure in patients with obstructive sleep apnea syndrome. Clinical implications. Am J Respir Crit Care Med 1999; 159:149–157.
36. Marcus CL, McColley SA, Carroll JL, Loughlin GM, Smith PL, Schwartz AR. Upper airway collapsibility in children with obstructive sleep apnea syndrome. J Appl Physiol 1994; 77:918–924.
37. Aronson RM, Onal E, Carley DW, Lopata M. Upper airway and respiratory muscle responses to continuous negative airway pressure. J Appl Physiol 1989; 66:1373–1382.
38. Strohl KP, Redline S. Nasal CPAP therapy, upper airway muscle activation, and obstructive sleep apnea. Am Rev Respir Dis 1986; 134:555–558.
39. Schwartz AR, Thut D, Brower RG, Gauda EB, Roach D, Permutt S, et al. Modulation of maximal inspiratory airflow by neuromuscular activity: Effect of CO_2. J Appl Physiol 1993; 74:1597–1605.
40. Thut DC, Schwartz AR, Roach D, Wise RA, Permutt S, Smith PL. Tracheal and neck position influence upper airway airflow dynamics by altering airway length. J Appl Physiol 1993; 75:2084–2090.
41. Sauerland EK, Harper RM. The human tongue during sleep: electromyographic activity of the genioglossus muscle. Exp Neurol 1976; 51:160–170.
42. Olsen CR, Stevens AE, Price NB, Staub NC. Structural basis for decreased compressibility of constricted trachea and bronchi. J Appl Physiol 1967; 23:35–39.
43. Olsen CR, Stevens AE, McIlroy MB. Rigidity of tracheae and bronchi during muscular constriction. J Appl Physiol 1967; 23:27–34.
44. Schwartz AR, Schubert N, Rothman W, Godley F, Marsh B, Eisele D, et al. Effect of uvulopalatopharyngoplasty on upper airway collapsibility in obstructive sleep apnea. Am Rev Respir Dis 1992; 145:527–532.
45. Lowe AA. Dental appliances for the treatment of snoring and obstructive sleep apnea. In: Kryger M, Roth T, Dement W, eds. Principles and Practice of Sleep Medicine. 2d ed. 1994:722–735.
46. Riley RW, Powell NB, Guilleminault C. Obstructive sleep apnea syndrome: a review of 306 consecutively treated surgical patients. Otolaryngol Head Neck Surg 1993; 108: 117–125.
47. Schmidt-Nowara W, Lowe A, Wiegand L, Cartwright R, Perez-Guerra F, Menn S. Oral appliances for the treatment of snoring and obstructive sleep apnea: a review. Sleep 1995; 18:501–510.
48. Wiegand L, Zwillich CW, Wiegand D, White DP. Changes in upper airway muscle

activation and ventilation during phasic REM sleep in normal men. J Appl Physiol 1991; 71:488–497.
49. Isono S, Morrison DL, Launois SH, Feroah TR, Whitelaw WA, Remmers JE. Static mechanics of the velopharynx of patients with obstructive sleep apnea. J Appl Physiol 1993; 75:148–154.
50. Morrison DL, Launois SH, Isono S, Feroah TR, Whitelaw WA, Remmers JE. Pharyngeal narrowing and closing pressures in patients with obstructive sleep apnea. Am Rev Respir Dis 1993; 148:606–611.
51. Isono S, Tanaka A, Remmers JE, Nishino T. Comparison of static mechanics of passive pharynx between patients with obstructive sleep apnea and normal subjects. Am J Respir Crit Care Med 1995; 151:A667.
52. Isono S, Feroah TR, Morrison DL, Launois SH, Whitelaw WA, Remmers JE. Nasopharyngeal narrowing during inspiratory flow limitation in patients with OSA during sleep. Am Rev Respir Dis 1992; 145:A210–A210.
53. Isono S, Tanaka A, Sho Y, Konno A, Nishino T. Advancement of the mandible improves velopharyngeal airway patency. J Appl Physiol 1995; 79:2132–2138.
54. Isono S, Tanaka A, Tagaito Y, Sho Y, Nishino T. Pharyngeal patency in response to advancement of the mandible in obese anesthetized persons. Anesthesiology 1997; 87: 1055–1062.
55. Leiter JC. Upper airway shape. Is it important in the pathogenesis of obstructive sleep apnea? Am J Respir Crit Care Med 1996; 153:894–898.
56. Rowley JA, Permutt S, Willey SJ, Smith PL, Schwartz AR. Effect of tracheal and tongue displacement on upper airway airflow dynamics. J Appl Physiol 1996; 80: 2171–2178.
57. Hendricks JC, Petrof BJ, Panckeri K, Pack AI. Upper airway dilating muscle hyperactivity during non-rapid eye movement sleep in English bulldogs. Am Rev Respir Dis 1993; 148:185–194.
58. Petrof BJ, Pack AI, Kelly AM, Eby J, Hendricks JC. Pharyngeal myopathy of loaded upper airway in dogs with sleep apnea. J Appl Physiol 1994; 76:1746–1752.
59. Series F, Cote C, Simoneau JA, Gelinas Y, St Pierre S, Leclere J, et al. Physiologic, metabolic, and muscle fiber type characteristics of musculus uvulae in sleep apnea hypopnea syndrome and in snorers. J Clin Invest 1995; 95:20–25.
60. Mezzanotte WS, Tangel DJ, White DP. Waking genioglossal electromyogram in sleep apnea patients versus normal controls (a neuromuscular compensatory mechanism). J Clin Invest 1992; 89:1571–1579.
61. Marcus CL, Omlin KJ, Basinski DJ, Bailey SL, Rachal AB, Von Pechmann WS, et al. Normal polysomnographic values for children and adolescents. Am Rev Respir Dis 1992; 146:1235–1239.
62. Badr MS, Grossman JE, Weber SA. Treatment of refractory sleep apnea with supplemental carbon dioxide. Am J Respir Crit Care Med 1994; 150:561–564.
63. Bruce EN, Mitra J, Cherniack NS. Central and peripheral chemoreceptor inputs to phrenic and hypoglossal motoneurons. J Appl Physiol 1982; 53:1504–1511.
64. Gauda EB, Carroll TP, Schwartz AR, Smith PL, Fitzgerald RS. Mechano- and chemoreceptor modulation of respiratory muscles in response to upper airway negative pressure. J Appl Physiol 1994; 76:2656–2662.
65. Haxhiu MA, Van Lunteren E, Mitra J, Cherniack NS. Responses to chemical stimulation of upper airway muscles and diaphragm in awake cats. J Appl Physiol 1984; 56: 397–403.

66. Henke KG, Arias A, Skatrud JB, Dempsey JA. Inhibition of inspiratory muscle activity during sleep. Chemical and nonchemical influences. Am Rev Respir Dis 1988; 138: 8–15.
67. Mathew OP, Abu-Osba YK, Thach BT. Genioglossus muscle responses to upper airway pressure changes: afferent pathways. J Appl Physiol 1982; 52:445–450.
68. Mathew OP, Abu-Osba YK, Thach BT. Influence of upper airway pressure changes on genioglossus muscle respiratory activity. J Appl Physiol 1982; 51:438–444.
69. Mathew OP. Upper airway negative-pressure effects on respiratory activity of upper airway muscles. J Appl Physiol 1984; 56:500–505.
70. Sant'Ambrogio G, Mathew OP, Fisher JT, Sant'Ambrogio FB. Laryngeal receptors responding to transmural pressure, airflow and local muscle activity. Respir Physiol 1983; 54:317–330.
71. Weiner D, Mitra J, Salamone J, Cherniack NS. Effect of chemical stimuli on nerves supplying upper airway muscles. J Appl Physiol 1982; 52:530–536.
72. Seelagy MM, Schwartz AR, Russ DB, King ED, Wise RA, Smith PL. Reflex modulation of airflow dynamics through the upper airway. J Appl Physiol 1994; 76:2692–2700.
73. Badr MS, Skatrud JB, Simon PM, Dempsey JA. Effect of hypercapnia on total pulmonary resistance during wakefulness and during NREM sleep. Am Rev Respir Dis 1991; 144:406–414.
74. Fouke JM, Teeter JP, Strohl KP. Pressure-volume behavior of the upper airway. J Appl Physiol 1986; 61:912–918.
75. Olson LG, Ulmer LG, Saunders NA. Influence of muscle activity on the elastance of the upper airway of rabbits. J Appl Physiol 1989; 66:755–758.
76. Schwartz AR, Thut D, Russ DB, Seelagy M, Roach D, Brower RG, et al. Effect of electrical stimulation of the hypoglossal nerve on airflow mechanics in the isolated upper airway. Am Rev Respir Dis 1993; 147:1144–1150.
77. Schwartz AR, Eisele DW, Hari A, Testerman R, Erickson D, Smith PL. Electrical stimulation of the lingual musculature in obstructive sleep apnea. J Appl Physiol 1996; 81:643–652.
78. Miki H, Hida W, Chonan T, Kikuchi Y, Takishima T. Effects of submental electrical stimulation during sleep on upper airway patency in patients with obstructive sleep apnea. Am Rev Respir Dis 1989; 140:1285–1289.
79. Miki H, Hida W, Shindoa D, Kikuchi Y, Chonan T, Taguchi O, et al. Effects of the electrical stimulation of the genioglossus on upper airway resistance in anesthetized dogs. Am Rev Respir Dis 1989; 140:1279–1284.
80. Decker MJ, Haaga J, Arnold JL, Atzberger D, Strohl KP. Functional electrical stimulation and respiration during sleep. J Appl Physiol 1993; 75:1053–1061.
81. Bishara H, Odeh M, Schnall RP, Gavriely N, Oliven A. Electrically-activated dilator muscles reduce pharyngeal resistance in anaesthetized dogs with upper airway obstruction. Eur Respir J 1995; 8:1537–1542.
82. Odeh M, Schnall R, Gavriely N, Oliven A. Effect of upper airway muscle contraction on supraglottic resistance and stability. Respir Physiol 1993; 92:139–150.
83. Oliven A, Odeh M, Schnall RP. Improved upper airway patency elicited by electrical stimulation of the hypoglossus nerves. Respiration 1995; 63:213–216.
84. Schnall RP, Pillar G, Kelsen SG, Oliven A. Dilatory effects of upper airway muscle contraction induced by electrical stimulation in awake humans. J Appl Physiol 1995; 78:1950–1956.

85. Eisele DW, Schwartz AR, Hari A, Thut DC, Smith PL. The effects of selective nerve stimulation on upper airway airflow mechanics. Arch Otolaryngol Head Neck Surg 1995; 121:1361–1364.
86. Eisele DW, Smith PL, Alam DS, Schwartz AR. Direct hypoglossal nerve stimulation in obstructive sleep apnea. Arch Otolaryngol Head Neck Surg 1997; 123:57–61.
87. Fregosi RF, Fuller D. Respiratory-related control of extrinsic tongue muscle activity. Respir Physiol 1997; 110:295–306.
88. Fuller D, Mateika JH, Fregosi RF. Co-activation of tongue protrudor and retractor muscles during chemoreceptor stimulation in the rat. J Physiol (Lond) 1998; 507:265–276.
89. Farre R, Peslin R, Montserrat JM, Rotger M, Navajas D. Flow-dependent positive airway pressure to maintain airway patency in sleep apnea-hypopnea syndrome. Am J Respir Crit Care Med 1998; 157(6 Pt 1):1855–1863.
90. Ayappa I, Norman RG, Hosselet J-J, Gruenke RA, Walsleben JA, Rapoport D. Relative occurrence of flow limitation and snoring during continuous positive airway pressure titration. Chest 1998; 114:685–690.
91. Condos R, Norman RG, Krishnasamy I, Peduzzi N, Goldring RM, Rapoport DM. Flow limitation as a noninvasive assessment of residual upper airway resistance during continuous positive airway pressure of obstructive sleep apnea. Am J Respir Crit Care Med 1994; 150:475–480.
92. Chervin RD, Theut S, Bassetti C, Aldrich MS. Compliance with nasal CPAP can be improved by simple interventions. Sleep 1997; 20:284–289.
93. Kribbs NB, Pack AI, Kline LR, Smith PL, Schwartz AR, Schubert NM, et al. Objective measurement of patterns of nasal CPAP use by patients with obstructive sleep apnea. Am Rev Respir Dis 1993; 147:887–895.
94. Meslier N, Lebrun T, Grillier-Lanoir V, Rolland N, Henderick C, Sailly JC, et al. A French survey of 3,225 patients treated with CPAP for obstructive sleep apnoea: benefits, tolerance, compliance and quality of life. Eur Respir J 1998; 12:185–192.
95. Weaver TE, Kribbs NB, Pack AI, Kline LR, Chugh DK, Maislin G, et al. Night-to-night variability in CPAP use over the first three months of treatment. Sleep 1997; 20:278–283.
96. Schwartz AR, Gold AR, Schubert N, Stryzak A, Wise RA, Permutt S, et al. Effect of weight loss on upper airway collapsibility in obstructive sleep apnea. Am Rev Respir Dis 1991; 144:494–498.
97. Schwartz AR, Thut D, Roach D, Smith PL. Effect of hypoglossal nerve stimulation on airflow mechanics in the isolated upper airway. Am Rev Respir Dis 1991; 143: A405.
98. Bonora M, St.John WM, Bledsoe TA. Differential elevation by protriptyline and depression by diazepam of upper airway respiratory motor activity. Am Rev Respir Dis 1985; 31:41–45.
99. Brownell LG, West P, Sweatman P, Acres JC, Kryger MH. Protriptyline in obstructive sleep apnea: a double-blind trial. N Engl J Med 1982; 307:1037–1042.
100. Hanzel DA, Proia NG, Hudgel DW. Response of obstructive sleep apnea to fluoxetine and protriptyline. Chest 1991; 100:416–421.
101. Smith PL, Haponik EF, Allen RP, Bleecker ER. The effects of protriptyline in sleep-disordered breathing. Am J Respir Crit Care Med 1983; 127:8–13.
102. Cartwright RD. Effect of sleep position on sleep apnea severity. Sleep 1984; 7:110–114.

103. Neill AM, Angus SM, Sajkov D, McEvoy RD. Effects of sleep posture on upper airway stability in patients with obstructive sleep apnea. Am J Respir Crit Care Med 1997; 155:199–204.
104. Clark GT, Arand D, Chung E, Tong D. Effect of anterior mandibular positioning on obstructive sleep apnea. Am Rev Respir Dis 1993; 147:624–629.
105. Eveloff SE, Rosenberg CL, Carlisle PC, Millman RP. Efficacy of a Herbst mandibular advancement device in obstructive sleep apnea. Am J Respir Crit Care Med 1994; 149:905–909.
106. Hochban W, Brandenburg U, Peter JH. Surgical treatment of obstructive sleep apnea by maxillomandibular advancement. Sleep 1994; 17:624–629.
107. Lowe A, Fleetham J, Ryan F, Mathews B. Effects of a mandibular repositioning appliance used in the treatment of obstructive sleep apnea on tongue muscle activity. In: Sleep and Respiration. New York: Wiley-Liss, Inc., 1990:395–405.
108. Schwartz AR, O'Donnell CP, Baron J, Schubert N, Alam D, Samadi SD, et al. The hypotonic upper airway in obstructive sleep apnea—Role of structures and neuromuscular activity. Am J Respir Crit Care Med 1998; 157:1051–1057.

3

Sleep-Induced Respiratory Instabilities

JEROME A. DEMPSEY and CURTIS A. SMITH

University of Wisconsin
Madison, Wisconsin

CHRISTINE R. WILSON

Northeastern University
Boston, Massachusetts

PETER R. EASTWOOD

Sir Charles Gairdner Hospital
University of Western Australia
Perth, Western Australia, Australia

MICHAEL C.K. KHOO

University of Southern California
Los Angeles, California

I. Introduction

Key elements in the human ventilatory control system include: (1) the central medullary integrator/pattern generator; (2) sensory inputs from feedback receptors concerned with blood and cell chemistry, the force output or tension developed by the respiratory muscles and airway patency; and (3) the coordination of efferent output to the upper airway and the chest wall pump muscles. In the awake healthy human, the coordination achieved among these elements insures a high degree of precision in the regulation of blood gases and acid/base status and in the mechanical efficiency of each breath in terms of minimizing the amount of work required by the respiratory musculature for a given ventilatory output. Furthermore, any significant disruption in ventilatory output, or in the precision or mechanical efficiency of ventilatory output, is usually short lived. For example, if tidal volume or breathing frequency is changed momentarily—by a sigh, a change in posture or increased mechanical load on the airway or sudden increase in metabolic rate (e.g., with exercise)—the appropriate compensation for these momentary errors are achieved quickly, and homeostasis is restored within a few breaths, and almost always with the subject not even being aware of the brief departure from the normal steady state.

In contrast with this precise, efficient control during wakefulness, the sleeping state predisposes to increased levels of disordered and unstable breathing, and often these instabilities are precipitated over several respiratory cycles and even minutes. That sleep predisposes to significant imprecisions and inefficiencies in the control system, even in the nonclinical, healthy population, is manifest in several ways:

4% of females and 9% of males aged 30–60 years experience more than five apneas or transient under ventilation (hypopneas) per hour of sleep, each with significant oxyhemoglogin desaturation during sleep (1).

Almost all normal humans show a significant alveolar hypoventilation and respiratory acidosis (+2–8 mmHg Pa_{CO2}), which presents throughout sleep.

Resistance to airflow through the upper airway increases significantly in many adult humans during sleep, frequently to levels which are three to five times those while awake. Periodically, as ventilation is *reduced* with the transition from wakefulness to sleep, it is not unusual to see marked *increases* in diaphragm and even accessory respiratory muscle EMG activity, secondary to the hypoventilation and chemoreceptor stimulation associated with increased airway resistance (2,3).

Normal REM sleep causes highly variable, often erratic changes in breathing frequency and tidal volume.

Factors such as the hypoxia of high altitude, aging, or chronic heart failure commonly result in highly unstable and periodic breathing, and these instabilities occur predominately during sleep.

What precipitates this inefficient, imprecise and unstable ventilatory control during sleep—even in healthy individuals? We will briefly review the fundamental effects of sleep on control mechanisms which impact on respiration. At the outset we need to emphasize that our understanding of the mechanisms underlying these instabilities is incomplete in terms of a true comprehensive integrative model, which explains the self-perpetuation of repetitive periodic breathing and even short-term instabilities. What has been established—especially over the past decade—is how individual sensory inputs may contribute to ventilatory inhibition and how changing states of consciousness will impact the magnitude of these inputs and the gain of the controller processing them, thereby promoting breathing pattern instability. Furthermore, theoretical models have been proposed to identify those combinations of conditions that enhance the probability of breathing pattern instability and their perpetuation during sleep.

We will first briefly summarize the fundamental effects of sleep on ventilatory control and then consider how these sleep effects might lead to transient and perpetuated instabilities and periodicities.

II. Fundamental Effects of Sleep on the Ventilatory Control System

A. Removal of Wakefulness Input to the Upper Airway

First, both non-REM and especially REM sleep cause a reduction in tonic efferent input to skeletal muscles which plays an important role in controlling the compliance and therefore the patency of the pharyngeal airway. This reduced input has been observed in the EMG activity of palatal muscles (4) and may originate in a reduced tonic or phasic activity of some medullary neurons, especially those without tight correlation with respiration (5). The mechanical effects of this reduction in tonic upper airway muscle activity varies markedly among healthy sleeping subjects as manifested by increases in inspiratory and sometimes expiratory resistance (R_{UA}), which increases to a measurable extent in most adult subjects and is 10-fold greater than wakefulness in snorers (6). In many (but not all) subjects, this increased R_{UA} accounts for a significant portion of the sleep-induced hypoventilation and the compensatory increase in respiratory pump muscle activity (2,7). In the context of breathing stability, the most important feature of increased R_{UA} is that it is highly unstable throughout sleep (see Fig. 1).

A popular concept is that the upper airway narrowing and increased R_{UA} during sleep occurs because of an imbalance of forces, i.e., the negative pressure developed by the inspiratory muscles sucks in the hypotonic upper airway to a narrower aperture (8). In many cases—especially with the severely obstructive sleep apnea patient—this concept likely explains much of the upper airway obstruction. The fact that the upper airway collapses more readily, i.e., at a much smaller reduction in intrathoracic pressure during sleep vs. wakefulness, also implies the importance of upper airway muscle atonia. On the other hand, there are several instances where muscle atonicity and upper airway resistance do not correlate, such as the absence of significant change in R_{UA} or airway closing pressure between non-REM and REM sleep, even though many upper airway muscles show virtually no tonic (or usually even phasic) upper airway muscle EMG activity in REM. Furthermore, other sleep-induced influences have been shown to have significant effects on upper airway patency. Most importantly, sympathetic efferent vasoconstrictor activity is reduced with the onset of non-REM sleep coincident with the reduction in systemic blood pressure (9), and this reduced efferent sympathetic output may cause vasodilation and vascular engorgement in the upper airway causing airway narrowing and increased R_{UA}. Data supporting this hypothesis are found in the significant reductions in R_{UA} with local topical application of vasoconstrictor substances to the upper airway during sleep (10). Perhaps the increased sympathetic activity associated with REM sleep may also explain the maintained R_{UA} in this state despite the atonicity of upper airway skeletal muscle. Other purely passive mechanical factors, such as caudal traction on the trachea (see below), may also play some role in causing increased R_{UA}, especially when the compliance of the upper airway is high, thereby making its diameter more susceptible to influences from mechanical forces.

B. Loss of Wakefulness Drive to the Pump Muscles

Non REM sleep also results in a reduction in medullary inspiratory neuron activity in cats (5). The consequences of this loss of wakefulness drive to the magnitude of respiratory motor output have been demonstrated by using positive pressure mechanical ventilation during sleep and wakefulness, so as to avoid the confounding effects

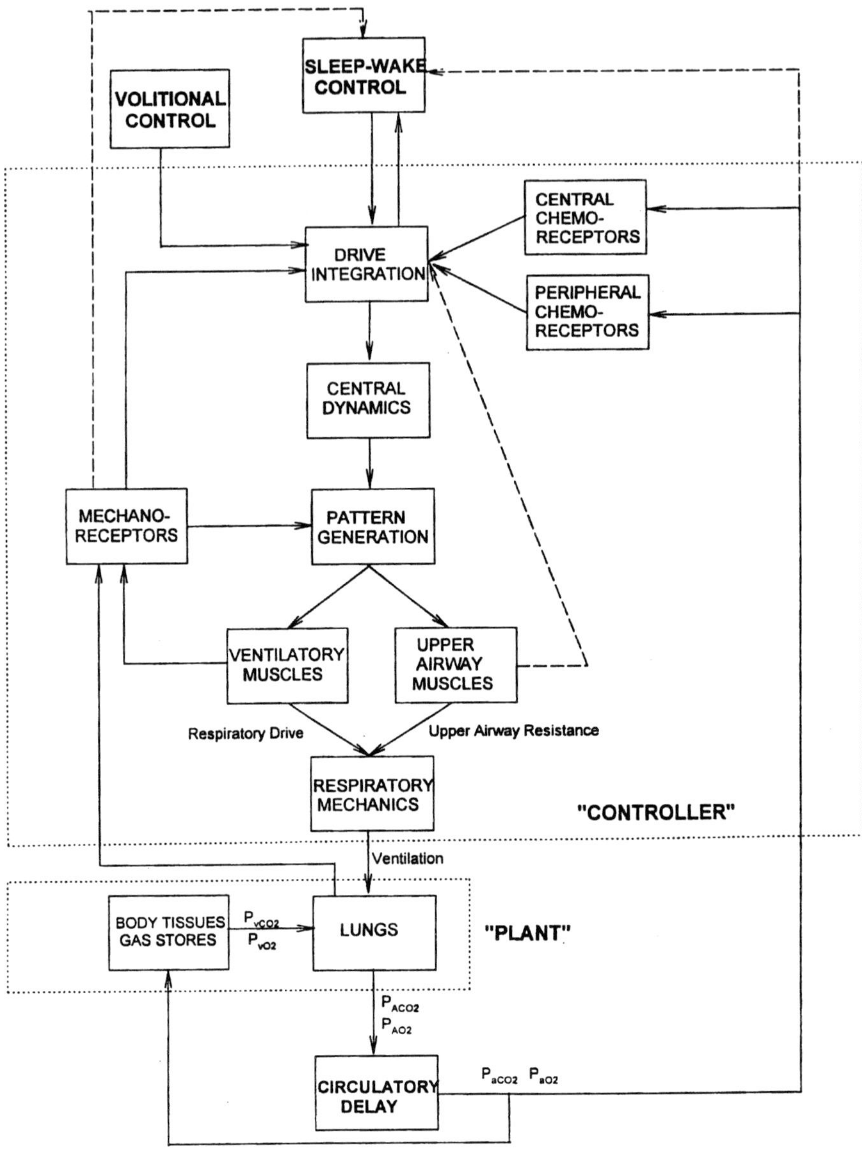

Figure 1 Control theory: schematic diagram of the key factors determining respiratory control stability. Broken arrows represent hypothesized relationships. (From Ref. 52.)

on ventilatory output of sleep-induced changes in airway resistance or chest wall compliance (see above). In this background of constant mechanical ventilation, tidal volume, and frequency: (1) tonic EMG activity of the chest wall expiratory muscles (during central apnea) is reduced in sleeping dogs (11); and (2) in sleeping humans phasic neural respiratory motor output is also reduced at a given Pa_{CO_2} (12). These findings imply that loss of wakefulness causes a significant reduction in input into the respiratory pattern generator from supramedullary areas which reduces respiratory motor output and accounts for some of the sleep-induced hypoventilation and CO_2 retention normally incurred in non-REM sleep. These findings are also consistent with the hypoventilation observed in many intact and tracheotomized sleeping subjects who do not increase their R_{UA} upon transition from awake to sleep (3,12, 13).

REM sleep effects on respiratory motor output are more complex and controversial. In the cat, medullary augmenting inspiratory neurons show substantial increases in activity throughout REM above that observed in non-REM or wakefulness (14,15). Paradoxically, this increased central respiratory drive coexists with marked atonicity of the postural and accessory respiratory muscles in REM; accordingly, it has been suggested that the reduced V_T in REM may be attributed to an uncoupling between neural and mechanical output because of distortion of the atonic chest wall (15). However, in the tracheotomized dog, the reduced V_T in REM corresponded with a reduced diaphragmatic mean EMG activity. That is, respiratory motor output as reflected in the EMG_{di} was tightly coupled to the mechanical ventilatory output, and this neural:mechanical coupling was similar in non-REM and REM (16). The reduced EMG_{di} and corresponding reductions in tracheal pressure or tidal volume during and following obstructive apneas in REM (vs. non-REM) sleep are shown in Figure 2. In addition to these reductions in mean amplitude of the EMG_{di}, many breaths that occur during a high density of eye movements show fractionations (or frequent interruption) of the EMG_{di} (16–18). When these EMG fractionations are of sufficient duration and number, they also caused disruption in pleural pressure development and therefore reduced flow rate and tidal volume (16). So, the phasic events of REM sleep can reduce the amplitude of diaphragm EMG and, in turn, V_T. However, REM events can also be excitatory to breathing frequency, thereby preventing excessive prolongation of T_E in the face of reduced chemical stimuli (see below). The net effect is that eupneic ventilation (and Pa_{CO_2}) is usually quite similar between non-REM and REM, although sometimes PET_{CO_2} (or Pa_{CO_2}) may even be slightly lower in REM (19).

C. Protective Respiratory Reflexes

Protective respiratory reflexes are compromised in sleep. During wakefulness an immediate (200–300 ms) increase in inspiratory motor output occurs in response to added respiratory loads. This immediate response to added resistive or elastic loads does not occur in non-REM sleep (2). Accordingly, V_T will fall transiently when airway resistance increases during sleep and will stay reduced until chemo-

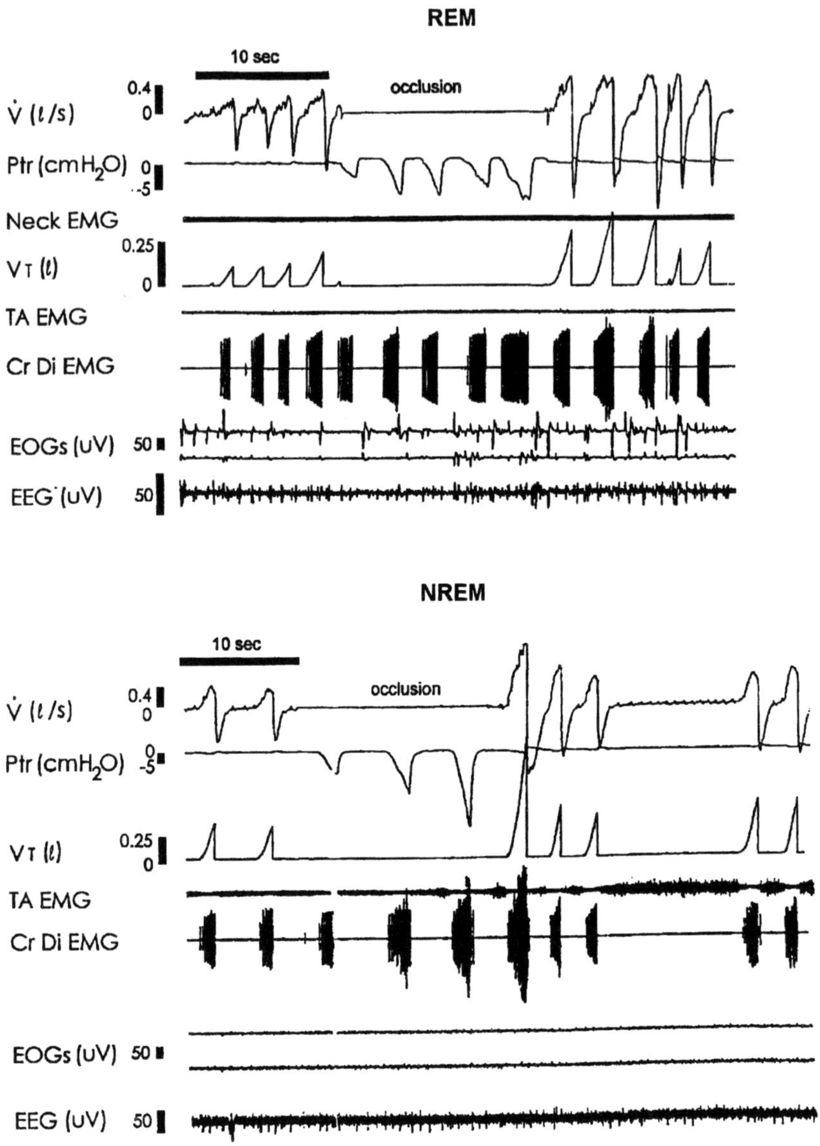

Figure 2 Ventilatory overshoots in non-REM (NREM) and REM sleep in the dog. The trachea is occluded to cause an obstructive event. Note in NREM sleep (bottom) the progressive inspiratory efforts (tracheal pressure and EMG_{di}) in response to the occlusion, followed by a ventilatory overshoot with high V_T, transient hypocapnia, and a subsequent central apnea (also note the tonic abdominal expiratory muscle EMG activity which persisted throughout the central apnea). In REM sleep (top) the respiratory effort increases during the occlusion, but in a nonprogressive erratic manner, the subsequent ventilatory overshoot is depressed and no central apnea follows. (From Ref. 37.)

receptor stimuli slowly rise and inspiratory and expiratory accessory muscles are activated and ventilation is restored. This loss of immediate compensation for respiratory loads accounts for the occurrence of many transient hypopneas in sleep.

Wakefulness input is also important to the response to respiratory muscle unloading. For example, when pressure support is applied to awake humans, tidal volume increases and Pa_{CO2} falls; whereas tidal volume is maintained near constant when pressure support is applied during non-REM sleep, presumably because of a substantial reduction in respiratory motor output (20). Similarly, during prolonged normocapnic or hypocapnic mechanical ventilation at augmented V_T and f, respiratory motor output is reduced substantially or even completely inhibited in the sleeping subject (12,21). This passivity of respiratory motor output during mechanical ventilation is much more difficult to achieve during wakefulness (22–25).

Augmentation of upper airway skeletal muscle EMG (genioglossus and tensor palatini) in response to airway narrowing by negative pressure has been observed in wakefulness, and this serves to stiffen and therefore protect the airway from any further narrowing or collapse. This protective reflex is significantly compromised in non-REM sleep (26) and is lost completely in REM (see also Chap. 5).

D. Additional Sleep-Induced Compromises of Ventilatory Control

In addition to the fundamental neurophysiological changes during sleep outlined above, additional factors would further aggravate disordered breathing. The horizontal position assumed in sleep means FRC will be reduced which will promote a greater O_2 desaturation and rise in Pa_{CO_2} for a given apneic length. This reduced FRC will also mean less caudal traction by the chest wall musculature on the trachea and greater probability of increased and unstable R_{UA} (27,28). The reduced V_A (and raised Pa_{CO_2}) with sleep also means that relatively small further changes in V_A will amplify corresponding disruptions of Pa_{CO_2} (29). Finally, cerebral blood flow tends to increase in sleep, especially REM sleep, which means that for any given arterial P_{CO_2}, the level of brain ECF P_{CO_2} and therefore the stimuli presented to the medullary chemoreceptors will be reduced (30).

III. Factors Inducing Respiratory Stability: Theory

Perpetuation of ventilatory overshoots and undershoots are caused by an as yet incompletely understood and highly complex constellation of factors. Engineering concepts permit us to make some sense conceptually of this oscillatory behavior, by defining the factors that must be present to cause it. The key elements are shown in Figure 1 in a highly simplified model of the ventilatory control system, which includes:

1. The medullary controller, whose gain will determine the magnitude of any corrective action taken in response to a disturbance in gas exchange.

Too small a gain means any corrective actions to a disturbance will be insufficient, whereas an overly high controller gain will tend to overcorrect for any disturbance and lead to its propagation.

2. The plant represents the gas exchanging processes of the lungs. The plant gain quantifies the change in PA_{CO_2} or PA_{O_2} resulting from a given change in ventilation. The smaller the plant gain, the greater the damping of transient fluctuations in ventilation and, thus, the more the stability in breathing pattern. For example, a small lung volume causes a high plant gain and reduced damping because a transient change in ventilation will cause a greater change in PA_{CO_2} and PA_{O_2} than would be the case at higher lung volume.
3. The system delay refers primarily to the time taken for the blood to flow from the lungs to the chemoreceptors. The longer the delay for the chemoreceptors to take corrective action from gas exchange deficiencies, the greater the chances of propagating any disturbance.

In order to produce sustained oscillatory behavior, control theory stipulates that the three factors listed above must be combined in such a way that the overall loop gain magnitude and phase meet certain criteria (29). First, the magnitude of the corrective action must be at least equal to the magnitude of the original disturbance, i.e., loop gain magnitude must be equal to or greater than unity. This may be obtained with a high controller gain or increased plant gain or both. Second, the algebraic sum of all phase shifts (including the effect of pure delays) must be 180 degrees, so that the corrective action is presented 180 degrees out of phase with the disturbance. The frequency with which the unstable or underdamped system oscillates has been likened to a resonant frequency, the value of which depends on the summed contributions of the response times of the individual components and all delays.

It should be emphasized that the basic conditions for instability listed above are strictly valid only when the fluctuations in blood gases and respiration are relatively small. Thus, while this linear model is useful in making predictions as to what conditions might precipitate periodic breathing, nonlinear factors become progressively more important once apnea develops. The latter would determine whether the periodic breathing is self-sustaining or whether stabilizing influences become important enough to dampen out the ventilatory oscillations (see Sec. VI).

Oscillatory behavior is also affected by influences external to the chemoreflex loops. Examples of such external influences include spontaneous sighs or pauses or state changes in ventilatory drive. These influences may produce an effect on ventilation that will be long-lasting or short-lasting, because any changes in ventilation are propagated around the chemoreflex or mechano-reflex loops. Interactions occur between the current effects of the external inputs and the propagated effects of past influences.

IV. Physiological Causes of Ventilatory Overshoots and Undershoots

Instabilities in ventilatory control systems during sleep are highly varied—both in how they are caused and how they are manifested. We divide the ventilatory instabilities into those due primarily to transient changes in upper airway resistance and those that involve overshoots and undershoots in neural feedback mechanisms regulating the timing and/or magnitude of respiratory motor output. Chemoreceptor influences are important elements in either the initiation or the perpetuation of all types of instabilities.

A. Breath-to-Breath Variations in Airway Resistance

During sleep in subjects with mild to moderately high airway resistance wide variations in upper airway resistance often occur because of a changing sleep state and changing coordination of respiratory drive to both upper airway and chest wall *or* to minor changes in posture and neck flexion *or* to changes in caudal taction on the trachea secondary to variations in end-expiratory lung volume (31). We would expect these types of variations in airway resistance to occur most commonly in the lighter, more labile sleep states and in those subjects who already have (in wakefulness) a narrowed airway diameter. In turn, these transient, commonly cyclical breath-to-breath variations in airway resistance become, in the absence of an immediate load-compensating reflex during sleep (see above), a primary cause of hypopneas and apneas—and eventually arousals and sleep discontinuity—even among subjects in nonclinical populations (6,32,33). Sleep-induced modest increases in upper airway resistance (>wakefulness) may be fairly common in healthy subjects; however, it is also likely that a substantial flow-resistive load must be incurred before significant hypopneas will ensue (32). The role of cyclical changes in R_{ua} in periodic breathing is discussed further below.

B. Causes of Ventilatory Overshoot

Neurally mediated apneas and hypopneas commonly occur following transient hyperpneas during sleep. Transient hyperpneas or ventilatory overshoots occur in sleep because of a combination of instabilities in sleep state and airway resistance, which give rise to changes in chemical stimuli and ventilatory responsivity (16,19). For example, an increased P_{CO_2} and decreased P_{O_2} during a sleep-disordered breathing event leads to gradually increasing inspiratory and expiratory efforts against a narrowed or closed upper airway and terminates often in a transient arousal. In turn, the arousal often causes abrupt reduction in upper airway resistance and increased gain of the respiratory pattern generator as sleep effects are suddenly removed resulting in transient ventilatory overshoots (see Fig. 2A). Transient EEG arousals alone, as caused by brief acoustic stimuli during non-REM sleep, have very little systemic effect on ventilation. However, even a very brief transient arousal superimposed on asphyxia causes substantial and more consistent transient increases in tidal volume and greater ventilatory overshoots (33,34). Transient arousals are important in potentiating the ventilatory overshoot, whether these arousals occur prior to the end of the hypopnic or apneic event (in which case the arousal would precipitate event termination) or whether the arousal occurred immediately following event termination (29,33).

Arousal effects might be contributing to the ventilatory (and blood pressure) overshoot following apneas and hypopneas even when these are not measurable in the cortical EEG. Indeed, so-called subcortical (or brain stem) arousals are implicated by the significant blood pressure and heart rate responses, which follow even very mild brief hypopneas with 3% O_2 desaturations and no measurable EEG disturbance. These hypopneas were also commonly followed by ventilatory overshoots, which averaged 50–150% greater than control V_E. Intracellular recordings in the nucleus tractus solitarius show that electrical stimulation of the hypothalamic defense area (perhaps analogous to abrupt subcortical arousals from sleep) has profound facilitory effects on carotid chemoreceptor reflexes (35). Individuals will differ substantially in the magnitude of their ventilatory overshoot, depending upon the sensitivity of their respiratory motor output and their arousability in response to chemo- and mechano-sensory input.

REM sleep will often dampen the ventilatory overshoot following apnea or hypopnea because the phasic inhibitory REM events blunt the tidal volume response to chemoreceptor stimuli. This is noticeable during obstructive apneic events in REM sleep where the intensifying asphyxia will lead to progressive effort by effort increases in diaphragmatic EMG (and in negative pleural pressure) in non-REM sleep, but erratic changes in inspiratory neural drive in REM sleep (16,36) (see Fig. 2). Similarly, ventilatory responses in phasic REM sleep to inhaled CO_2 are erratic with no clear linear slope to the progressively increasing chemical stimulus and while some breaths are clearly augmented, the overall ventilatory response is blunted relative to non-REM wakefulness (19). Again, as in air-breathing eupnea, during airway obstruction, the relationship of pleural pressure development to EMG_{di} amplitude in response to the augmented chemoreceptor stimuli is identical during REM and non-REM sleep (16). Thus, when the pleural pressure response is reduced, so is the EMG_{di}. Of course, a brisk ventilatory overshoot will occur if the apnea or hypopnea that began in REM ends in an arousal or if an arousal occurs early in the postapneic recovery period (37).

Following these actively induced hyperpneas during sleep, several opposing mechanisms determine the amplitude and timing of respiratory motor output. We now present our view on how these mechanisms interact, resulting in continued hyperpnea under some conditions and apnea or hypopnea under others.

C. Stabilizing Effects of Poststimulus, Short-Term Potentiation

It is well established that a continued excitatory, centrally mediated memory effect follows the cessation of almost any type of acute, excitatory sensory input into the medullary pattern generator (38). This has been most often demonstrated in the anesthetized, vagotomized cat by using electrical stimulation of the carotid sinus nerve (CSN) to increase phrenic nerve activity and showing that the augmented activity persists following cessation of CSN stimulation. Use of brief isocapnic hypoxia in the human also demonstrates that the short-term potentiation (STP) mechanism ensures continued excitation of ventilation following stimulus withdrawal during non-REM sleep (at least when PET_{CO_2} is prevented from falling) (39). Given the reduction in R_{ua} during and immediately following chemoreceptor-driven hyperpneas in normal subjects in sleep, it is also likely that efferent phasic and tonic output to the upper airway muscles is an integral part of the STP mechanism (39,40).

With this powerful, centrally mediated, continuing excitatory influence, one would not expect reductions in respiratory motor output, i.e., apnea or hypopnea or increases in R_{ua}, to ever follow transient ventilatory stimulation. Indeed, this important stabilizing mechanism may explain why significant apnea and hypopnea events are not prevalent during sleep in the great majority of healthy subjects despite the potentially destabilizing underlying influences of changing airway mechanics and states of consciousness, along with a reduced FRC and increased Pa_{CO_2}, i.e., increased plant gain. On the other hand, experimentally induced airway obstruction in sleeping humans (41) and dogs (34) can lead to ventilatory overshoot with subsequent central apneas and hypopneas (see Fig. 2). Brief periods of hyperventilation, induced by hypoxia (42) or by mechanical ventilation (43), are also commonly followed by brief prolongation of expiration or reduced V_T. Most relevant to the real world, ventilatory undershoots are commonly observed spontaneously in sleep following transient ventilatory overshoots. This must mean that sensitive inhibitory influences are present which oppose this continued STP (see Sec. VI). There are several candidates for this inhibitory or disfacilatory role based on the physiological changes known to accompany transient hyperpneas.

D. Inhibitory Effects of Hypocapnia

Hypocapnia resulting from ventilatory overshoots has been shown to be a powerful inhibitor of respiratory motor output during sleep. The prevalent concept is that of a highly sensitive apneic threshold during non-REM sleep as demonstrated by the apnea (of 5–10 s duration) which first appears after PET_{CO_2} is lowered 2–4 mmHg (i.e., to waking levels) by 2–4 minutes of passive mechanical ventilation at constant raised V_T and increases in duration progressively with further lowering of P_{CO_2} (23,44). However, it is also important to clarify that these data were obtained with prolonged mechanical ventilation in constant sleep states and they need careful qualification in their application to physiological states where ventilatory overshoots are actively induced and usually very brief. For example, actively induced hyperventilation will cause a continued excitatory STP (see above), which will oppose and therefore blunt any accompanying hypocapnic inhibition.

Mechanical ventilation using the assist control mode has been used to study the effects of hypocapnia in sleeping humans (45) (see Fig. 3). The advantages of

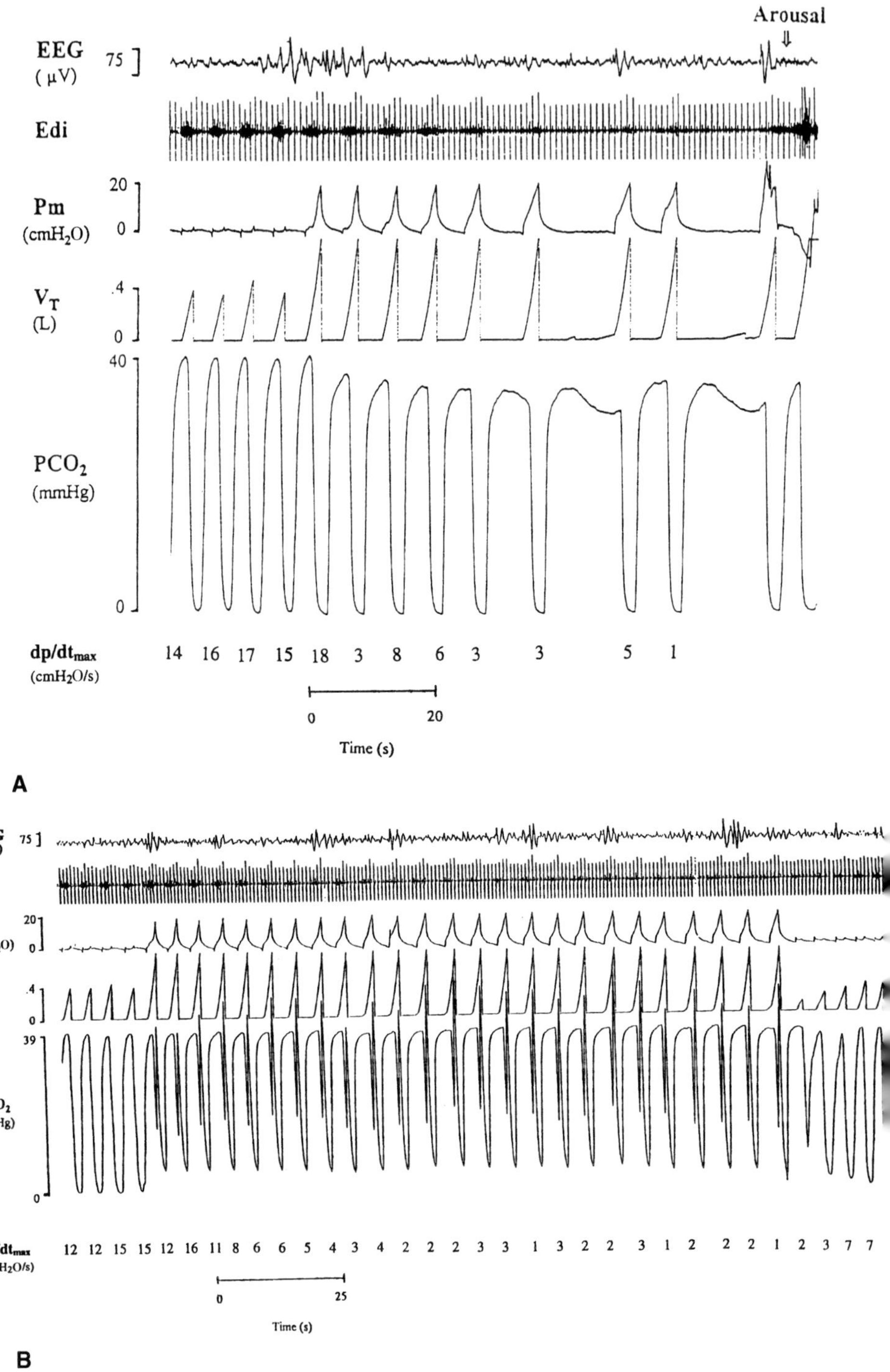

Arousal
EEG (μV) 75
Edi
Pm (cmH$_2$O) 20 0
V_T (L) .4 0
40
PCO_2 (mmHg)
0
dp/dt_{max} (cmH$_2$O/s)
14 16 17 15 18 3 8 6 3 3 5 1
0 20
Time (s)
A
EEG (μV) 75
Edi
Pm (cmH$_2$O) 20 0
V_T (L) .4 0
39
PCO_2 (mmHg)
0
dp/dt_{max} (cmH$_2$O/s)
12 12 15 15 12 16 11 8 6 6 5 4 3 4 2 2 2 3 3 1 3 2 2 3 1 2 2 2 1 2 3 7 7
0 25
Time (s)
B

this approach are that each inspiration is actively initiated by the subject and the time course as well as after effects of hypocapnic inhibition on ventilatory control may be studied. Note in Figure 3A that when tidal volume was raised and $P_{ET_{CO_2}}$ began to gradually fall: (1) the amplitude of respiratory motor output was diminished by the second or third cycle; (2) T_E was prolonged beginning at about the sixth ventilatory cycle (or 30 s of mechanical ventilation); and (3) then apnea and instabilities in breathing pattern ensued after 40 s of assist control mechanical ventilation in hypocapnia. That this T_E prolongation was due solely to hypocapnia was confirmed by companion studies in which the $P_{ET_{CO_2}}$ was held 1–1.5 mmHg > eupnic control (see Fig. 3B). When assist control mechanical ventilation at high V_T is used without permitting hypocapnia, the amplitude of respiratory motor output is reduced over time but remains significantly above zero, therefore breath timing or breath-to-breath stability of breathing pattern is not appreciably changed.

So clearly, small amounts of hypocapnia per se, even when breath initiation is actively induced, will cause apnea and ventilatory instability. These conclusions appear similar to those reached by studying the after effects of several minutes of control mode mechanical ventilation (as mentioned above) under hypocapnic vs. normocapnic conditions. For example, both types of studies tended to show T_E prolongation at about 3–4 mmHg reduction in $P_{ET_{CO_2}}$. However, a major difference between these studies was that for any given reduction in $P_{ET_{CO_2}}$, the longer-duration hypocapnic trials caused a consistent and substantial apnea and the apnea duration increased progressively with further reductions in Pa_{CO_2}, whereas the T_E prolongations during the shorter durations of hypocapnia produced in the assist control trials were shorter and highly variable from trial to trial. The importance of duration of hypocapnia is also suggested by findings in sleeping humans that: (1) brief hypoxic exposure caused transient hypocapnic hyperventilation, which upon cessation of the hypoxia results in reduced V_T or hypopnea but rarely in any significant changes in

Figure 3 (A) Hypocapnic-induced apnea and breathing instability during non-REM sleep in humans. Assist control mode of mechanical ventilation is begun following four breaths of spontaneous breathing. (Note that in this mode the subject actively initiates each inspiration and the ventilator volume was set at ~2× eupneic V_T.) $P_{ET_{CO_2}}$ falls progressively and the amplitude of the EMG_{di} and the instantaneous rate of rise of inspiratory pressure (dP_m/dt_{max}) begins to fall on the second ventilator cycle. After 30–40 s at a reduced $P_{ET_{CO_2}}$, EMG_{di} amplitude is eliminated or near zero and apnea occurs and an unstable breathing pattern ensues until arousal. The apnea appears to result from a progressive dimunition to zero amplitude of the EMG_{di} and of tidal volume, rather than a primary timing effect on expiratory duration, per se. (B) Positive pressure mechanical ventilation at high V_T in normocapnia inhibits respiratory motor output in non-REM sleep. The protocol is identical to that in A except that hypocapnia is prevented as V_T is increased (via added FI_{CO_2}) $P_{ET_{CO_2}}$ (and Pa_{CO_2}) is maintained 1–1.5 mmHg > control. Note that the EMG_{di} amplitude is reduced over time of assist control ventilation to 40–50% of eupneic control levels and remains low (along with a reduced V_T) as eupneic breathing is resumed immediately following cessation of mechanical ventilation. (From Ref. 45.)

breath timing (39); and (2) similarly, brief periods of moderate hypocapnia elicited by control mode mechanical ventilation at increased V_T also resulted in only small reductions in V_T with little or no apnea during the immediate recovery period following cessation of mechanical ventilation (46).

The primary chemoreceptors affected also appear to be important determinants of the inhibitory effects of hypocapnia. With the common type of transient ventilatory overshoot of one to three breaths usually encountered in sleep, Pa_{CO_2} is reduced less than control for about 10–15 seconds (35). Based on time constants of changes in medullary surface pH (47), it is likely that the carotid chemoreceptors (rather than medullary chemoreceptors) are exposed to the most hypocapnia during these transient events. Furthermore, when an isolated, perfused carotid chemoreceptor preparation was used to subject the carotid chemoreceptors alone to reduced P_{CO_2} in the sleeping dog, V_T fell immediately and in a progressive dose-response fashion below eupneic P_{CO_2} levels. At -10 to -15 mmHg carotid body P_{CO_2} below eupnea, the reduction in V_T was 20–40% below eupnea and equal to that obtained with hyperoxia (>500 mmHg) (48). Carotid chemoreceptor hypocapnia alone had little effect on breath timing, even when the carotid sinus nerve sensory input was probably completely inhibited.

Given the relatively small effect of hypocapnia applied solely at the level of the carotid chemoreceptors on breath timing and the importance of the duration of hypocapnia in causing consistent and substantial apneas (see above), we propose that central sleep apneas due primarily to hypocapnia induced by (active) ventilatory overshoots probably require that the medullary chemoreceptors experience significant respiratory alkalosis. Accordingly, given the delay in CO_2 sensing between lung and brain chemoreceptors, we would estimate that the ventilatory overshoot and accompanying hypocapnia must occur for at least one minute to fully inhibit the medullary chemosensors.

So, the evidence for a powerful inhibitory effect of hypocapnia in non-REM sleep is abundant, as shown in sleeping humans and dogs and following both active and passive (or at least partially active) ventilator-induced bouts of hyperventilation. It is also likely that the results from the experimental perturbations mean that hypocapnia is a major cause of real life sleep apneas and hypopneas, whether they occur in isolation or repeatedly as in periodic breathing (see example below). Further evidence in support of this postulate is that supplemental (inspired) CO_2 eliminates central sleep apnea and periodic breathing (49,50)—although it is not conclusive from these latter findings that CO_2, per se, rather than a nonspecific ventilatory stimulus may have been responsible for eliminating the apneas. (We will discuss this second possibility below.) We think there are two major questions remaining before one can equate with certainty the experimental evidence in support of hypocapnia with its purported role as the cause of all normally occurring central apneas and hypopneas and periodicities.

First, as alluded to above, the evidence indicates that apneas would require a reduction in $P_{A_{CO_2}}$ which is sustained and significant in order to provide sufficient inhibition of medullary chemoreceptors, and yet many apneas occur with only very transient reductions in Pa_{CO_2} of <10–15 seconds duration. This discrepancy may mean that some extra-chemoreceptor inhibitory mechanism is involved or that estimates of the apneic threshold do not apply to the dynamic states involving transient hyperpneas and sleep state changes or that medullary chemoreceptors sense changes in Pa_{CO_2} much more quickly than presently believed.

A related question of considerable practical import is what factors affect the magnitude of the hypocapnic-induced apneic threshold relative to the corresponding eupneic P_{CO_2}? Certainly, adding to or subtracting from the background of sensory input into the respiratory controller must influence the P_{CO_2} apneic threshold, but there is very little information on this potentially important influence. For example, many patients with idiopathic central sleep apnea and Cheyne-Stokes respiration are purported to show chronically reduced arterial P_{CO_2} (51). Does this mean, then, that these patients' Pa_{CO_2} is closer to their apneic threshold? . . . or is their absolute apneic threshold value abnormal? . . . or are they more prone to transient ventilatory overshoots and therefore to transient reductions in Pa_{CO_2} because of these extra inputs to breathe which cause their chronic hyperventilation? An apparent contradiction to this alleged effect of chronically reduced Pa_{CO_2} is the reduction in periodic breathing one observes as Pa_{CO_2} is reduced in chronic hypoxia—either over time during acclimatization or in response to pharmacological treatments, which increase drive and reduce P_{CO_2} (see below). Systematic studies of the effects on the apneic threshold of chronically changing the background drive to breathe, perhaps by such means as metabolic acidosis or alkalosis or similar agents, has not been carried out. Subjects may also vary significantly in their responsiveness to any given reduction in Pa_{CO_2}, analogous to the well-established individual variations in the ventilatory response to increased CO_2. Indeed, interindividual variations in the apneic threshold of only ± 1 or 2 mmHg Pa_{CO_2} would make a substantial difference in the prevalence of apneas and instabilities during sleep.

Since the ventilatory overshoot that causes the hypocapnia (under real life circumstances) commonly also involves a simultaneous change in sleep state, then the timing and duration of this transient arousal becomes an important factor in dictating the subsequent effect on ventilatory responses. For example, the abrupt resumption of sleep following the termination of the transient ventilatory overshoot is important in allowing the occurrence of apnea or hypopnea (23,52). Furthermore, if the withdrawal of wakefulness (and therefore, the wakefulness stimulus) is rapid, this may promote longer apneas because of the delay required to elicit compensatory responses from chemoreceptors (52).

In phasic REM sleep—as opposed to non-REM sleep—it is difficult to elicit posthyperventilation apnea. For example, central apneas are rare in REM sleep at high altitude or with idiopathic central sleep apnea syndrome, and the Cheyne-Stokes oscillating pattern common in heart failure is rare in REM (53). This is, in part, due to the blunted ventilatory overshoots in REM (see Fig. 2B), but is also because T_E is not prolonged to the same extent for a given reduction in PET_{CO_2} (38) (see Fig. 4). Thus, in REM sleep the excitatory effects on ponto-medullary respiratory neurons via state-specific REM-related inputs apparently supersede the incoming chemore-

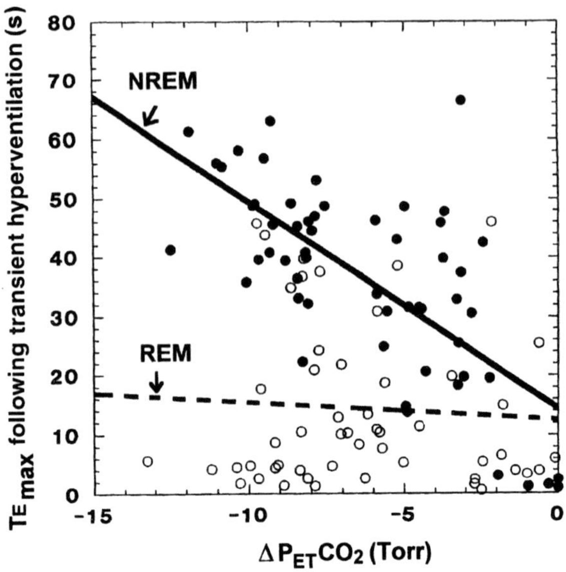

Figure 4 REM sleep effects on the hypocapnic-induced apneic threshold in the dog. The apneas compiled here are those obtained following release of airway occlusion and the subsequent ventilatory overshoots (see Fig. 2). Note that the reduced $P_{ET_{CO_2}}$ caused by the ventilatory overshoot correlates fairly well with the prolonged expiratory time (i.e., apnea length) in NREM, whereas in phasic REM sleep, while some airway occlusion trials do show significant apnea as $P_{ET_{CO_2}}$ is reduced, the great majority do not.

ceptor inputs; these excitatory influences prevent T_E prolongation and (like wakefulness) mask the occurrence of a hypocapnic-induced apneic threshold.

Considering the ventilatory output and neuromechanical coupling in REM sleep, it seems as though this dynamic state may superimpose both inhibitory and excitatory influences on ventilatory control. For example, the V_T response to increased chemical stimuli (or even stimuli present in eupnea) is blunted, whereas the apnea-producing effects of hypocapnia are overridden. While breathing pattern in REM is clearly more erratic than in non-REM under normal physiological circumstances, it must be considered more stable in REM under such altered and normally disruptive conditions as hypoxia or heart failure or airway obstruction. In short, phasic REM sleep apparently dissociates the controller from its usual inputs, whether they may cause excitation or inhibition or disfacilitation of respiratory motor output.

E. Lung Mechanoreceptor Inhibitory Influences

Inhibitory influences from lung stretch incurred during transient hyperpneas might also have continuing or memory-like effects causing apnea or hypopnea when the hyperpnea or stimulation is withdrawn (54). In the dog during non-REM sleep the magnitude of the transient increase in V_T following release of airway obstruction correlated much more closely with the subsequent central apnea than did the associated fall in $P_{ET_{CO_2}}$ (34). Furthermore, in the vagally blocked dog, central apneas following the hyperpneic response to release of airway occlusion were still significant but less than one-third the duration of those in the intact animal (for a given reduction in Pa_{CO_2}) (34). On the other hand, vagotomy had little effect on hypoxic-induced periodic breathing in the anesthetized dog (55).

How important this vagally mediated memory effect is in humans is unknown. Certainly, the Breuer-Hering inhibitory reflex achieved upon passive lung inflation is present in sleeping, intact humans, but does not occur in the lung denervated human (56). However, this inhibition is only obtained at lung volumes above the 1–1.5 range (i.e., >40% of inspiratory capacity) in the human. On the other hand, there is also evidence in sleeping or anesthetized humans that occlusion of the airway at end-expiration during eupneic breathing results in significant prolongation of T_I (57,58). Furthermore, in anesthetized humans very small inflations of <0.5 V_T were shown to cause T_E prolongation (59). These types of data suggest that phasic volume changes may provide significant inhibitory feedback effects on breath timing in humans that are much more sensitive than indicated by the Breuer-Hering static inflation maneuver.

There are several recent mechanical ventilation studies in sleeping humans, which clearly show a significant inhibitory effect primarily on amplitude and to a lesser extent on the timing of respiratory motor output even when Pa_{CO_2} was maintained at normocapneic levels (60,61). In the studies of Henke et al. (47), $P_{ET_{CO_2}}$ was raised 2–4 mmHg greater than eupnea in the sleeping human and EMG_{di} amplitude was still markedly reduced during mechanical ventilation over a wide range of ventilator V_T. A recent study used the assist control mode of mechanical ventilation (i.e., where the subject initiates each inspiration) at increased V_T with Pa_{CO_2} hold slightly greater than eupnea (see Fig. 3B). This approach showed EMG_{di} amplitude to decrease within the first few cycles of mechanical ventilation, and this inhibition of amplitude was enhanced with time over the initial 10–15 ventilator cycles and was maintained over the initial 4–6 breaths following cessation of the mechanical ventilation (62). Breathing frequency changed very little in these studies. Post-mechanical ventilation apnea of substantial length has been elicited by normocapnic mechanical ventilation in sleep, but this effect required increasing ventilator frequencies to slightly greater than eupnea (21). Thus, when the ventilator breath is introduced during early (electrical) expiration, T_E is prolonged and respiratory timing is reset (63,64), and if this high ventilator rate is continued (using the control mode of mechanical ventilation), diaphragm EMG activity is eliminated and tonic EMG is persistent in expiratory muscles throughout the apnea. The apnea persists following cessation of the normocapnic mechanical ventilation even when Pa_{CO_2} has risen several mmHg above the apneic threshold (21,63).

In summary, these mechanical ventilation studies do show nonchemical effects on inhibition of respiratory motor output, especially during sleep. Nonetheless, we think the data to date suggest that hypocapnia is clearly the major cause of central sleep apnea and hypopnea. Neuromechanical inhibition from increased V_T (or respiratory muscle unloading) may play a significant role in reducing the amplitude of respiratory motor output—either by itself or by interacting with transient reductions in Pa_{CO_2}.

The requirement that ventilator frequency must be increased in order to reset respiratory rhythm and cause apnea during normocapnia is pertinent to control of breathing during mechanical ventilation. Furthermore, the persistence of apnea following mechanical ventilation provides insight into the important question of apnea prolongation in the face of high chemical stimuli (see Sec. IV.H). On the other hand, these findings during mechanical ventilation probably have limited relevance to an understanding of the mechanisms initiating real life sleep apnea.

F. Upper Airway Mechanoreceptor Reflexes and Central Apnea

The laryngeal and pharyngeal airways contain receptors which are important to the regulation of both the amplitude and timing of respiratory motor output and to airway tonicity, compliance, and caliber (65). In normal humans, applying a pulse of negative pressure to the intact upper airway (via the mouth) causes activation of genioglossus muscle EMG, and the amplitude of this activation is reduced significantly in non-REM sleep (66). In waking and sleeping dogs the ventilatory response to CO_2 was markedly attenuated by use of the nasal (versus tracheal) breathing routes even when differences in resistance between the two breathing routes were controlled (67). Furthermore, when the upper airway was isolated and the dog was free to breathe through a tracheal stoma, creating a square wave of pressure in the upper airway during expiration, a dual reflex effect resulted, namely, activation of genioglossus muscle activity in wakefulness and non-REM (but not in REM) sleep and a progressive central apnea in all states of consciousness (68). The gain of the apneic length vs. negative pressure relationship was significantly reduced in REM sleep, and although these response gains were similar in wakefulness and non-REM, the animal tolerated much more negative pressures (and therefore longer apneas) in non-REM before arousing and reinitiating inspiration. When the upper airway was exposed (through a endotracheal tube) to the normal ramp of intrathoracic negative pressure generated during inspiration, then the rate of rise of EMG_{di} was slowed, became alinear, and was truncated (69).

It was determined that the threshold of negative pressure required to elicit the central apnea (-5 to -8 cmH_2O) coincided with the closing of the pharyngeal airway and that apnea length increased as pressure was decreased further to cause more and more airway deformation. This effect of airway closure and deformation on central apnea was not affected by complete blockade of the laryngeal reflexes via topical anesthesia, or even by chronic denervation of the superior laryngeal nerve (68,70). These data suggest that the inhibitory reflex effect on breath timing was initiated by deformation of submucosal pharyngeal airway stretch receptors (65), perhaps in a fashion analogous to the intercostal muscle to phrenic inhibitory reflex. Furthermore, the inhibition of inspiration via negative pressure demonstrated a substantial memory effect, depending on the phase of the respiratory cycle during which the airway was closed. This was shown by the use of negative pressure pulses of 300 ms duration (68). When applied during late expiration, the ensuing apnea lasted well beyond the duration of the airway closure (see Fig. 5A), whereas, when applied at any time during inspiration, the inspiration was immediately terminated but restarted immediately after the brief period of upper airway closure. Finally, low-pressure, high-frequency pressure oscillations (akin to those in the snoring human) applied to the upper airway during non-REM sleep also elicited the dual reflex of genioglossus EMG activation (71,72) plus T_E prolongation (71) when applied during expiration and depressed rate of increase in EMG_{di} when applied during inspiration (71) (see Fig. 5B). Unlike the effects of square wave or pulses of negative pressure (see above), these high-frequency oscillations required only very small (noncollapsing) pressures to elicit the dual protective reflex, and the effects were blocked with local topical anesthesia of the airway mucosa. This dual reflex could be important in protecting against complete collapse of the upper airway in snorers in the face of extremely negative intrathoracic pressures.

G. Baroreceptor Stimulation

Transient increases in blood pressure—via sympathetically mediated vasoconstriction and increased cardiac output—routinely accompany the hyperpnea, which coincides with the relief of apnea and/or hypopneas in non-REM and REM sleep, and this increase is usually exaggerated by transient arousal. Baroreceptor stimulation accompanying this increased systemic pressure has been shown to have multiple effects, including ventilatory depression and markedly reduced activation of upper airway abductor muscle EMG activity (73) and even arousal. All of these factors could serve—like hypocapnia and lung stretch (discussed above)—to perpetuate sleep-disordered breathing events.

This hypothesis was tested using extracorporeal perfusion and graded narrowing of the vessel lumen in the isolated carotid sinus region in the sleeping dog (74) (see Fig. 6A). Upon abrupt increases in carotid sinus pressure (P_{CS}), an immediate reduction of V_T was observed that was proportional to the increase in pressure; however, consistent reductions in V_T were not demonstrated until mean P_{CS} was increased 25 mmHg. Even at P_{CS} as high as +50–100 mmHg, V_T and V_E were reduced only 20–25% below control. Increased P_{CS} caused no or little increase in R_{ua} or in cortical EEG. Presumably, then, the reduced tonic and phasic drive to the upper airway with increased baroreceptor stimulation (73) paralleled the reduction in activation of the chest wall pump muscles and upper airway patency was preserved. Another explanation would be that marked reductions in upper airway muscle tone, per se, are not critical to airway patency (75). Phenylephrine bolus infusion was also used in the sleeping human to cause transient increases in systemic BP with very similar results, i.e., transient hypoventilation and no change in R_{ua}, even in snoring subjects who had very high R_{ua} under control conditions in sleep (76) (see Fig. 6B). Given the timing of transient increases in BP which occur immediately following each sleep apnea or hypopnea and the fact that R_{ua} was not affected, we predict that transient increases in BP are not an important link in perpetuating unsta-

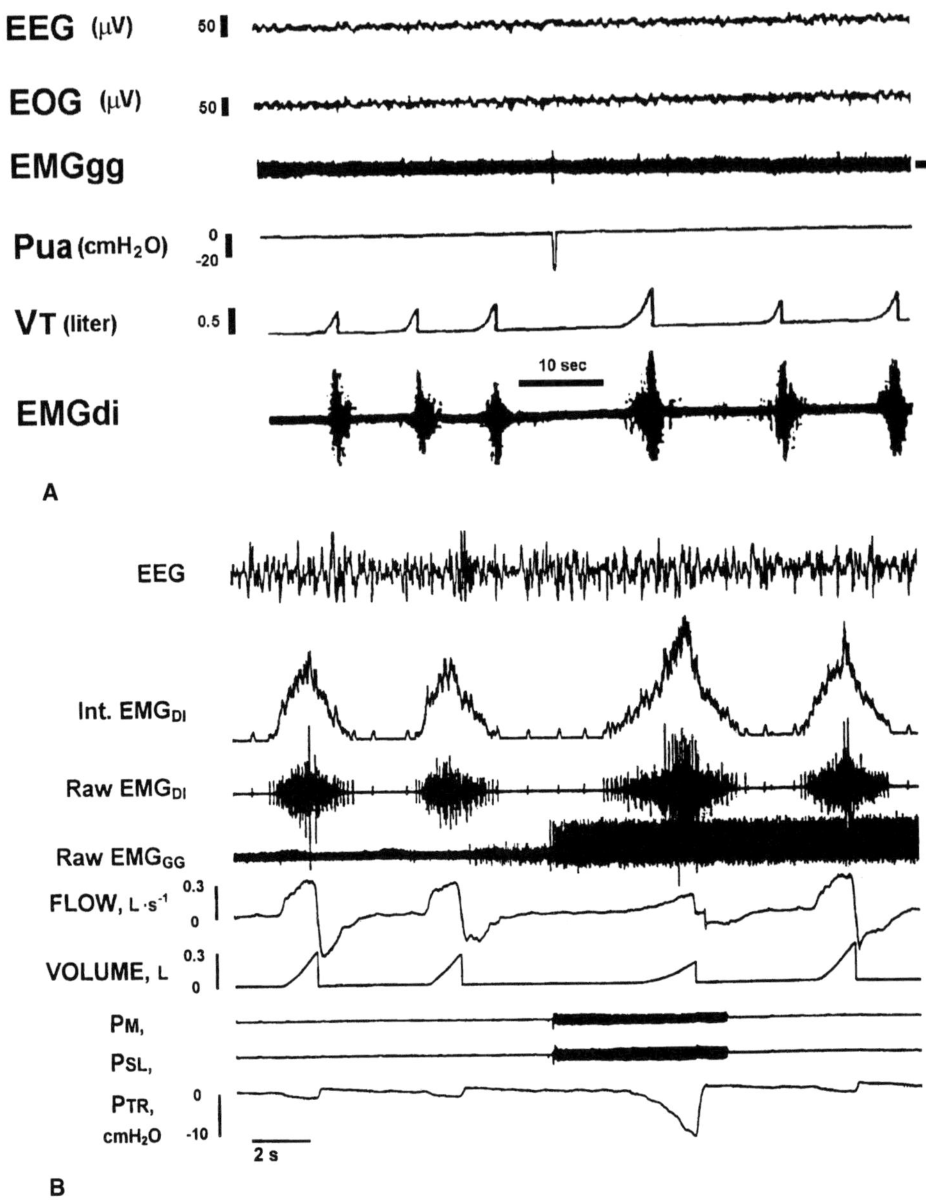

Figure 5 (A) Inhibitory memory or aftereffects of a pulse of negative pressure applied near the end of normal expiration to the isolated upper airway, on prolongation of expiratory time in the sleeping dog breathing via a tracheostomy. Note that the inhibitory effect of this 300 ms pulse of negative pressure on delaying the next inspiratory effort lasts way beyond the application of the negative pressure. (From Ref. 68.) (B) Effects of low pressure (± 1–2 cmH_2O), high-frequency (30 Hz) oscillations applied during expiration to the isolated upper airway of the sleeping dog. The oscillating pressure is seen on the mouth pressure (P_M) and sublaryngeal pressure (P_{SL}) traces. Note that T_E is prolonged and the genioglossus muscle tonic EMG activated during and following the application of the high-frequency pressure oscillations. (From Ref. 71.)

ble breathing. Rather, the inhibitory effect may actually dampen the ventilatory overshoot and help stabilize breathing patterns. On the other hand, there is also recent evidence in rats and humans (77,78) that chronic increases in systemic blood pressure might precipitate sleep-disordered breathing in a positive feedback fashion. The human studies showed that treating the hypertension in severe sleep apneic patients also reduced the severity of the sleep-disordered breathing (78).

H. Apnea Prolongation via Control System Inertia

When central apnea is initiated by (or associated with) a reduction in Pa_{CO_2}, the apnea often persists even after Pa_{CO_2} has returned to well above apneic threshold levels. Why this prolongation? Some of this delay may simply be a reflection of the slower recovery of brain ECF P_{CO_2} following transient hyperpnea and therefore continued hypocapnic inhibition of medullary chemoreceptors at a time when arterial (and carotid chemoreceptor) P_{CO_2} has risen to exceed the apneic threshold. However, there must be an additional nonchemical cause of continued inhibition—because apnea also persists when hypocapnia was not the cause of the apnea, i.e., following prolonged normocapnic passive mechanical ventilation at elevated f_b and V_T during non-REM sleep in humans and dogs (21). When the passive mechanical ventilation was stopped, inspiratory effort was not restored for 20 ± 2 seconds, i.e., until P_{CO_2} had risen 5–10 mmHg greater than eupnea and Pa_{O2} was 15–20 mmHg less than eupnea. Other examples of this inhibitory memory effect in sleeping animals is the prolonged persistent apnea which follows very brief application of a pulse of negative pressure to the upper airway (68) (see Fig. 5A) or the well-known postsigh apnea (79). Electrical stimulation of pulmonary vagal afferents or (especially) the superior laryngeal nerves in newborn animals also causes apnea, which persists beyond the duration of the stimulation (80). The length of these apneas following cessation of sensory input may be influenced by several factors. In the case of the isocapnic mechanical ventilation in sleeping humans, the postventilator apnea was positively related to the magnitude of the tidal volume applied during mechanical ventilation (21); the duration of the passive mechanical ventilation was an additional factor affecting apnea duration (63). With electrical stimulation of the SLN the duration of stimulation was a major determinant of poststimulus apnea duration (80).

This continued inhibition of inspiration represents a centrally mediated hysteresis-like habituation or inertia of the ventilatory control system; in other words, the respiratory rhythm generator seems to be much more difficult to restart once turned off—regardless of the cause of the apnea. The cause of this continued inhibition of inspiratory motor output* is unknown. Because the apnea persists in the face of

---

* Phasic oscillatory neuronal activity has also been observed to be present at various times during apnea (defined by a silent phrenic neurogram) as noted in the glossopharyngeal neurogram and in some bulbar inspiratory neurons (81). These oscillatory patterns reveal the continued presence of central rhythmic respiratory-related output, which is subthreshold for the generation of a breath.

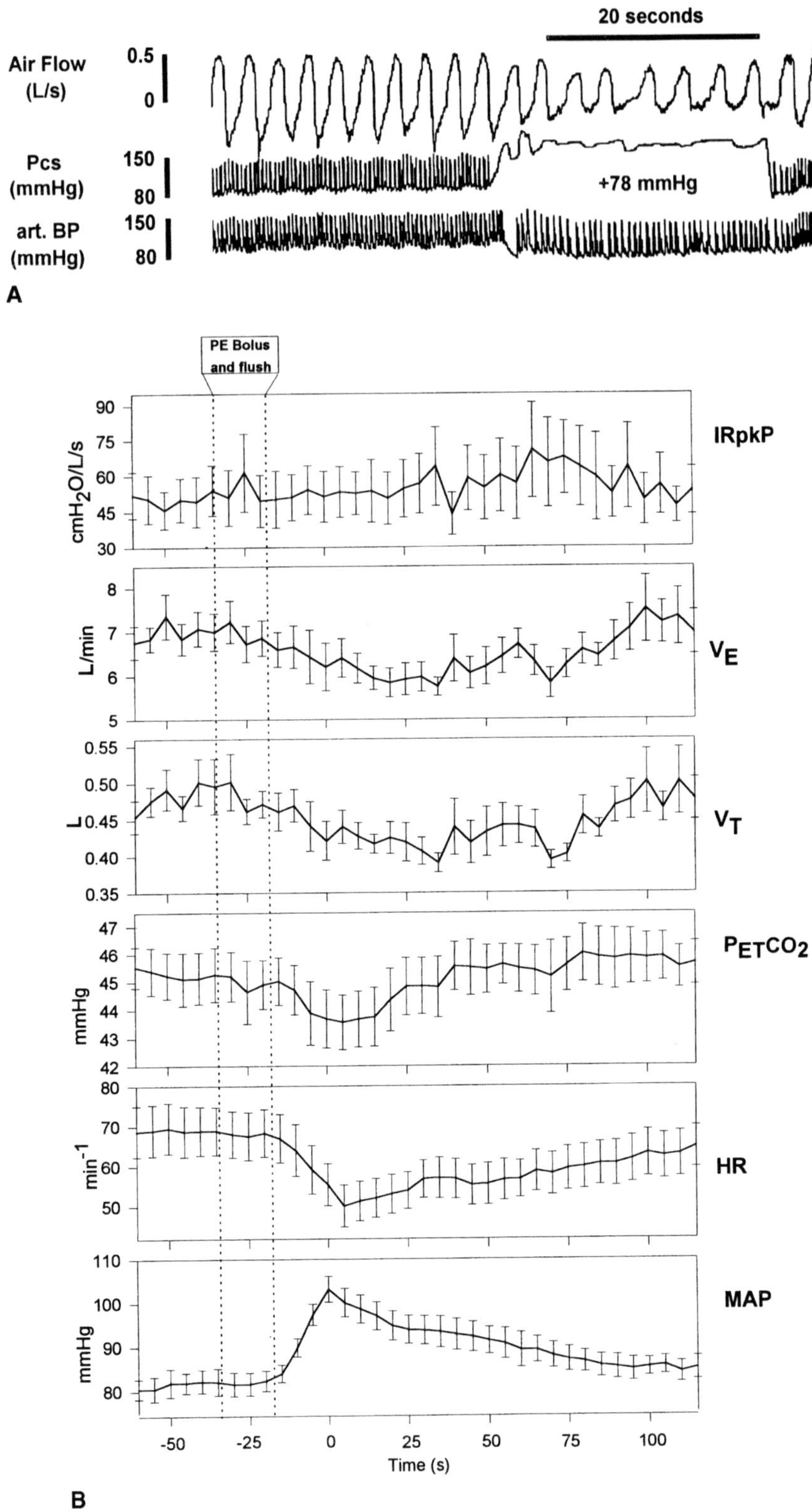
20 seconds
Air Flow (L/s)
0.5
0
Pcs (mmHg)
150
80
+78 mmHg
art. BP (mmHg)
150
80
A
PE Bolus and flush
IRpkP
cmH2O/L/s
90
75
60
45
30
V_E
L/min
8
7
6
5
V_T
L
0.55
0.50
0.45
0.40
0.35
$P_{ET}CO_2$
mmHg
47
46
45
44
43
42
HR
min-1
80
70
60
50
MAP
mmHg
110
100
90
80
-50
-25
0
25
50
75
100
Time (s)
B

rising (and often substantial) chemical stimuli, it appears as though some active inhibitory process would be necessary. In support of this view, many have reported augmented tonic electrical activity to exist in medullary expiratory and postinspiratory neurons (79,82) or in expiratory muscle EMGs of the chest wall or upper airway (11,68,83) during apneas, which are caused reflexly by mechanoreceptor feedback from the lung, chest wall, or upper airway (see Fig. 2A). This tonic expiratory activity may provide persistent reciprocal inhibition of inspiratory neurons; thereby actively prolonging apnea beyond the termination of the influence of the original inhibitory sensory mechanism (84,85). On the other hand, ventilator-induced hypocapnia was recently shown to cause apneas in sleeping cats, and these apneas were usually not accompanied by tonic medullary expiratory activity in non-REM and especially in REM sleep (86). So, the concept of reciprocal inhibition of medullary inspiratory neurons as a means of actively maintaining apneas is certainly not a universal phenomenon, because in these latter-mentioned instances, hypocapnic-induced apnea persisted in the face of quiet, apparently inhibited and/or disfacilitated expiratory neurons (86). On the one hand, it is tempting to speculate that hypocapnic and mechanoreceptor-induced apneas might have entirely different impacts on the respiratory neuronal network. On the other hand, it is also painfully obvious that we do not really understand exactly how *either* of these fundamental types of sensory inputs actually eliminates respiratory rhythm and causes apnea.

V. Types of Sleep-Induced Ventilatory Instabilities

Up to this point we have discussed in isolation several factors operative during sleep, which can lead to ventilatory overshoots and undershoots. Leading candidates promoting these ventilatory instabilities include such disruptive influences as dynamic changes in sleep state, a labile upper airway patency and airway resistance and the absence of immediate compensatory responses of respiratory motor output to increased resistive loads during sleep. In addition, memory-like influences on respiratory motor output persist in the aftermath of each ventilatory overshoot—

Figure 6 Effects of transient changes in systemic blood pressure on the regulation of breathing and upper airway resistance in the sleeping dog (A) and human (B). Note in the dog (A) the increase in pressure in the isolated carotid sinus caused an immediate truncation of inspiratory flow rate and reduced V_T. Systemic blood pressure (BP) fell and heart rate slowed, reflecting that the carotid sinus baroreceptors were effectively stimulated. This evidence of baroreceptor stimulation along with the immediacy of the ventilatory change strongly suggests a causal link between increased carotid sinus pressure and the reduced V_T. In the sleeping human (B) a phenylephrine-induced transient increase in blood pressure caused transient hypoventilation, again with no systematic increase in the resistance of the upper airway (as measured during inspiration at peak pressure, $IR_{PK}P$), even though baseline inspiratory resistance was increased many times awake levels. [From Refs. 74 (A) and 76 (B).]

the excitatory mechanisms promoting ventilatory stability and other sleep-sensitized inhibitory mechanisms, led by hypocapnia, favoring instability of breathing pattern. Just about all persistent breathing instabilities during sleep involve most of these factors to a significant extent as all are tightly linked and often interdependent. Other factors important in determining ventilatory stability include differences in background conditions. For example, the starting anatomy and compliance of the upper airway determines how much it might narrow with changing states of consciousness, and the starting background Pa_{CO_2} might dictate the proximity of the eupneic Pa_{CO_2} (during sleep) to the apneic threshold. Now we will briefly discuss three examples of perpetuated instabilities in breathing pattern during sleep. Another well-known example, that of Cheyne-Stokes respiration associated with chronic heart failure, is discussed in Chapter 14.

A. Example #1: Sleep-Induced Periodic Breathing in the Elderly

Periodic breathing during light stages (I, II) of sleep has been observed in some apparently otherwise healthy aging subjects (32,87,88) at a cycle duration of about 40–60 (see Fig. 7). What might cause these types of instabilities, especially in view of the reduced ventilatory response to chemoreceptor stimuli commonly reported with aging? Pack et al. (88) reasoned that sleep-state stability was less well consolidated in the aged (89) and that aged subjects showed a propensity for oscillations in sleep state, especially across wakefulness and lighter sleep stages. These authors then observed significant (albeit modest in magnitude) cross-correlations between oscillations in EEG frequency and in ventilation in the elderly (87,88). That is, V_E fell as mean EEG frequency fell and vice versa, during sleep stages I and II. These instabilities persisted even in a hyperoxic background. Accordingly, the authors reasoned that this synchronous behavior represented a changing state-dependent contribution of the wakefulness input to the respiratory oscillator.

Hudgel et al. (32,90) examined the role of a changing R_{UA} in this type of periodic breathing. Oscillations in V_T were found to correlate best with a changing R_{UA}—at least in most elderly subjects with periodic breathing (see Fig. 7). In turn, these changes in R_{UA} might also be caused by oscillations in sleep state, only in this scenario the influences of state would primarily be on motor output to the upper airway than to the chest wall musculature. Given the lack of immediate increases in respiratory motor output in response to airway loading (2), one might well expect a transient fall in V_T with increasing loads. Note that all increases in R_{UA} in sleep do not result in transient hypoventilation; it appears to require R_{UA} of about 20 cmH_2O/s in most subjects, but these levels are readily achieved in many sleeping subjects (6,32).

Conceivably, if these state-driven oscillations in R_{UA} were sufficiently brief, they could cause regular periodicities in V_T and V_E and these might be largely independent of any coincident changes in chemoreceptor stimuli. On the other hand, it has also been shown that chemoreceptor stimuli begin to accumulate and increase respiratory motor output beyond the third or fourth loaded respiratory cycle (at re-

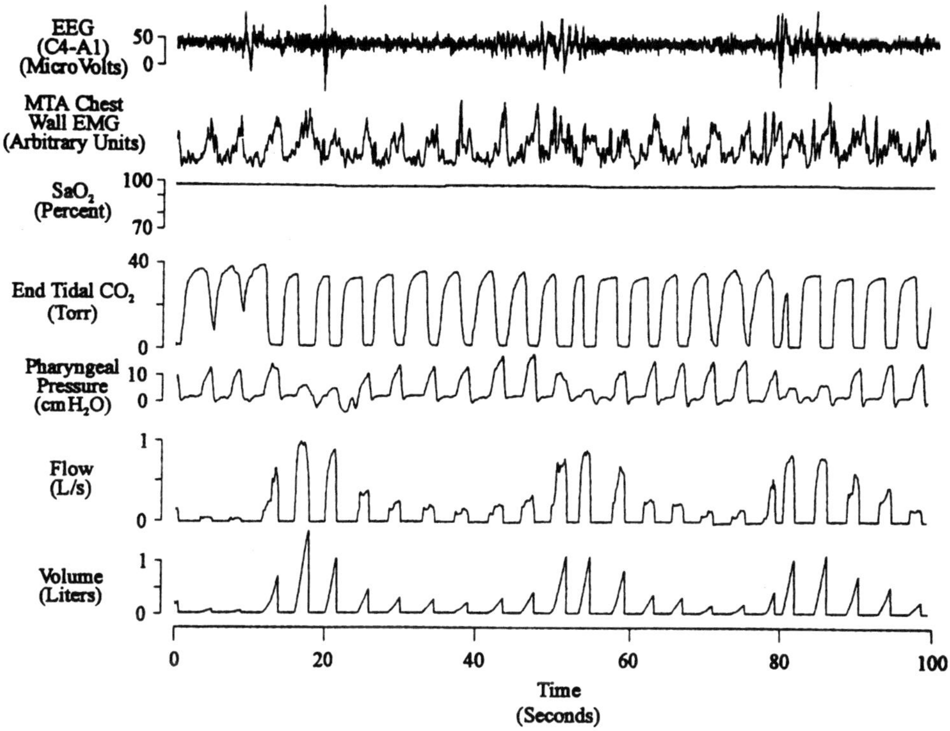

Figure 7 Periodic breathing in the elderly patient in light sleep. Note that the periodicity in breathing coincides with periodicity in changes in upper airway resistance. (From Ref. 32.)

duced V_T) (2). Thus, a changing chemoreceptor drive would likely also make a significant, albeit secondary contribution to ventilatory overshoots and to the magnitude of periodic breathing and even to an oscillating sleep state in these instances. Even barely measurable changes of 1 or 2 mmHg Pa_{CO_2} over time would cause significant oscillations in chemoreceptor output and in the amplitude of respiratory motor output. So, a changing R_{UA} is important in destabilizing periodic breathing in the sleeping elderly, and as such is akin to the pathophysiology of obstructive sleep apnea. Indeed, instabilities both in state and in upper airway caliber may be age dependent.

Other types of periodic breathing might also involve an important contribution from a changing R_{UA}. This has been suggested for some types of Cheyne-Stokes respiration (91) and for hypoxia-induced periodic breathing (92). Certainly changing neural outputs to the pump muscles and the upper airway have been linked in many experiments (93), and, in turn, both are state dependent. We emphasize that the susceptibility to airway narrowing differs markedly among individuals during sleep or with changing afferent outputs. As we explain in the next section, in many human subjects, periodic breathing can also occur without a changing R_{UA} and be driven primarily by changing chemoreceptor stimuli and changing cortical or subcortical sleep states.

B. Example #2: Ventilatory Instability During Sleep in Hypoxia

Sojourners to high altitude commonly experience restlessness and nonrefreshing sleep. Much of this lack of quality sleep can be attributed to the periodic breathing experienced during sleep in hypoxia. The development of periodic breathing during sleep in hypoxia is illustrated in Figure 8. During non-REM or REM sleep in hypoxia, hyperventilation begins immediately upon hypoxic exposure and intensifies with time (49,94). After at least 10 min (but sometimes after only many hours) of hypoxia in the sleeping human, tidal volume begins to oscillate in a waxing and waning pattern. These oscillations keep increasing in magnitude as hypoxia is maintained and Pa_{CO_2} falls further. Usually, then, a large sigh-like augmented inspiration occurs and the subject begins overt periodic breathing cycles of about 15–20 s duration characterized by two or three huge tidal volumes followed by apneas of 5–10 s duration. Arterial oxyhemoglobin saturation swings wildly along the steep part of the oxyhemoglobin dissociation curve.

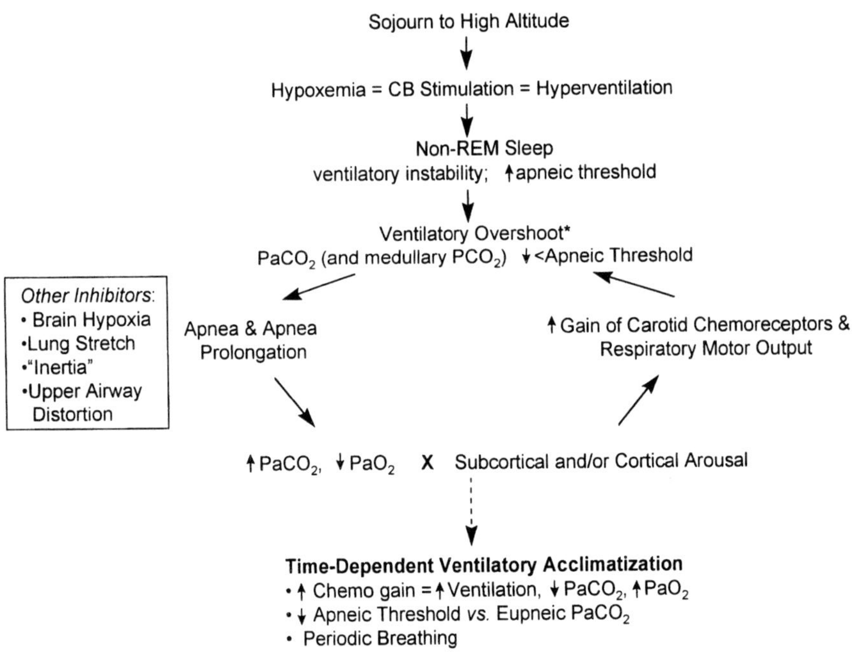

Figure 8 Hypothetical schema to explain perpetuation of periodic breathing during sleep in hypoxia (see text). *Transient ventilatory overshoots due to periodic augmented inspirations, sleep state, or airway resistance changes.

Several factors influence the amount of periodic breathing during sleep in hypoxia. First, not all healthy subjects will experience periodic breathing in hypoxic sleep. For example, some snorers may have a sufficiently high airway resistance in sleep so that hyperventilation during the breath clusters is constrained by the mechanical load, and ventilatory overshoot and hypocapnia sufficient to cause apnea does not occur. Extremes of chemo-responsiveness also will affect periodic breathing; notably, subjects at the very low end of hypoxic ventilatory responsiveness (HVR) tend to have less periodic breathing (as in the high-altitude native) (95). However, sojourners to high altitudes with a wide range of HVR will experience periodic breathing during sleep in hypoxia (49). Second, many days of hypoxic exposure often alleviate much of the periodicity, but it may also persist for very long periods, especially at extreme altitudes. Superimposing additional ventilatory stimuli such as acetazolamide or progesterone or very small amounts of inspired CO_2 also will alleviate much of the periodic breathing in the sleeping sojourner at high altitude (49,94,96,97). Transition from non-REM to REM sleep in hypoxia also results in a dramatic reduction or complete alleviation of periodic breathing.

A Simple Scheme

What causes periodic breathing in hypoxic sleep? Although not entirely settled, we believe the following ingredients are required (see Fig. 8). (Each of these mechanisms were discussed in isolation in prior sections):

- A highly sensitive hypocapnic-induced apneic threshold, which is unmasked during non-REM sleep
- Normal carotid chemoreceptor responsiveness to hypoxemia
- The accumulation of asphyxic stimuli during the apneic period, which displaces the gain of the carotid chemoreceptors to the steeper part of the ventilatory response curve
- Increased gain of the medullary respiratory neurons to sensory input because of the extra input from higher centers added by subcortical (or cortical) "arousal," which occurs just before or after the termination of the apnea
- Mechanisms 2, 3, and 4 combined, leading to a ventilatory overshoot causing hypocapnia, leading to subsequent apnea, etc., thereby perpetuating periodic breathing as long as sleep continues in the hypoxic environment.

That a reduction in Pa_{CO_2} below the apneic threshold is important specifically as a cause of apnea in hypoxic-induced periodic breathing is confirmed by the findings that: (1) the onset of periodic breathing in hypoxic sleep in a given subject occurred at a level of PET_{CO_2} which approximated the subject's separately determined apneic threshold (23); and (2) adding very small amounts of inspired CO_2 via nasal cannula (+1–3 mmHg Pa_{CO_2}, while maintaining PA_{O2} via added N_2 to the inspirate) eliminated the periodic breathing during sleep in hypoxia (49). Apparently, then, the inhibitory effects of the hypocapnia generated by the periodic ventilatory overshoots is sufficient to negate the excitatory effects of the STP generated by carotid chemoreceptor stimulation.

Douglas and Haldane were the first to show near the turn of this century that hypocapnia alone would cause apnea but that hypoxemia needed to accompany the apnea in order to trigger yet another apnea and perpetuate periodic breathing (98). The key here is that sufficient drive to breathe must be incurred during the apnea to cause a subsequent ventilatory overshoot and sufficient hypocapnia to cause the next apnea. With Pa_{CO_2} returning to normal during the apnea, the associated fall in P_{O2} will displace the chemoreceptor stimuli to the steep portion of the carotid chemoreceptor response curve and cause sufficient increase in respiratory motor output for the ventilatory overshoot.

Cortical EEG arousal is observed immediately prior to or following apnea termination in some instances of periodic breathing in hypoxia (99), and this would serve to further increase the magnitude of the ventilatory overshoot. However, cortical EEG arousals do not occur consistently with periodic breathing (49,99). Nevertheless, subcortical or brain stem level of arousal is likely to occur toward the termination of apneic periods as sensory input to the brain stem and mid-brain reach high levels, and this would serve to enhance the chemoreceptor-driven ventilatory drive and ventilatory overshoot in the recovery period (see Sec. IV). It is likely that this combination of effects is operative during periodic breathing in hypoxia. This interactive effect is important to explain the sudden and large increase in ventilatory drive at apnea termination because the suddenness and magnitude of this transient hyperventilation is not typical of rising chemoreceptor stimuli, per se, nor can it be caused solely by transient cortical arousal.

So this combination of ventilatory overshoot driven at high gain by developing asphyxia at the carotid and medullary chemoreceptors plus associated subcortical (and sometimes cortical) arousal, together with a sleep-induced sensitive hypocapnic apneic threshold plus inertial inhibitory mechanisms that prolong apnea, probably explain much of the periodic breathing in the sleeping sojourner at high altitude (see Fig. 8).

Need for More Complexity

There are also some additional considerations which question whether the proposed simple scheme is really the whole answer. First, the proposed key role for a hypocapnic-induced apneic threshold is complicated by the fact that there are several instances where the amount of periodic breathing is actually reduced—rather than worsened—as background eupneic Pa_{CO_2} falls. This stabilization of breathing pattern during sleep occurs over several days sojourn at high altitudes, but this stabilization occurs in the face of an increased level of hyperventilation and hypocapnia (94,96). Several lines of evidence in humans and animal models show that this time-dependent ventilatory acclimatization is attributable to increased gain at the level of the carotid chemoreceptors (100). Thus, this time-dependent stabilization in breathing pattern is especially puzzling because control system theory (see Fig. 1) and comparisons of ventilatory responsiveness among subjects would predict that the propensity for periodic breathing is enhanced (rather than diminished) by increased peripheral chemoreceptor gain. Periodic breathing in sleep is also ameliorated with long-term ventilatory stimulation via hormonal agents or acetazolamide despite causing even more hypocapnia (96,97). Some of this stabilization might be due to less hypoxemia attenuating the hyperventilation. More importantly, removal of breathing periodicity probably occurs because the apneic threshold is reduced more than the decrease in eupneic Pa_{CO_2} induced by the addition of powerful background ventilatory stimuli. This concept of a changing apneic threshold or changes in the gap between eupneic and threshold Pa_{CO_2} have not been explored.

Second, there are other feedback inhibitory influences resulting from lung inflation or transient increases in systemic BP during periodic breathing which could contribute, probably in a minor way in humans, to the apnea that follows the ventilatory overshoot (see Sec. IV. G). Third, the dynamic transient changes in respiratory motor output during periodic breathing may also influence efferent output to and patency of the upper airway. In subjects who already have a high baseline R_{ua}, the transition into hypoxic periodic breathing will cause further marked increases in R_{ua} and even complete airway obstruction. However, in healthy, nonsnoring subjects with relatively low upper airway resistance during sleep, R_{ua} remains unchanged throughout the development and steady state of hypoxic-induced periodic breathing and even when respiratory motor output is very low during ventilator-induced hypocapnia (40,101). Furthermore, even those subjects who experience high R_{ua} during the transition phase into periodic breathing reduced their resistance to normal levels when full-blown periodic breathing had developed. Probably the high chemical stimuli developed during the apnea—along with imperceptible subcortical arousals—provided sufficiently high levels of efferent output to both the upper airway skeletal muscle (motor output) and its vasculature (sympathetic outflow) to ensure airway patency upon apnea termination.

Finally, the background environment of long-term hypoxia (with superimposed asphyxia during the apneas) may provide an additional mechanism of brain hypoxic ventilatory depression as a powerful contributor to the delay of initiation of inspiratory effort and therefore to apnea duration (102). For example, in sleeping humans less than 1 minute of normocapnic hypoxia results in continuing excitatory STP of ventilation following abrupt withdrawal of the hypoxia, but if this normocapnic hypoxia is prolonged for only 4–5 min significant apneas are obtained immediately upon abrupt withdrawal of the hypoxic stimulus (39). These data are strongly suggestive of an important role for (sustained) brain hypoxia in apnea prolongation. Indeed the studies in anesthetized, chemo-denervated animals consistently show marked depression of breathing during hypoxia (103), and in intact animals and humans exposed to hypoxia for >10 minutes a reduction (or roll-off) in ventilatory output commonly occurs and has been attributed to brain hypoxic depression of respiratory motor output (104). However, direct evidence in support of depressive central effects of hypoxia is lacking in the unanesthetized animal. To the contrary, in awake animals, moderate or severe systemic isocapnic hypoxemia: (1) does not cause ventilatory depression in the carotid body denervated animal; and (2) in the goat with carotid chemoreceptors intact and vascularly isolated and perfused with normoxic blood, causes excitation of ventilatory output (105,106).

The role of brain hypoxia in the scheme of ventilatory control in physiological intact preparations and in sleep remains a major unresolved question: How do medullary neurons sense hypoxia? Do hypoxia-sensitive bulbo-spinal medullary neurons facilitate or oppose sensory input from carotid chemoreceptors? Are medullary neurons important in the generation of the respiratory rhythm predominately depressed or excited by hypoxia (107)? How sensitive are these responses and interactions to changing states of consciousness?

C. Example #3: Perpetuation of Sleep-Disordered Breathing—Links Between Central and Obstructive Apneas

Several lines of evidence support a strong causative link between central and obstructive apneas and between central and high-resistance hypopneas. These include: (1) the common occurrence of mixed types of sleep apnea; (2) marked increases in R_{UA} and sometimes even complete occlusion accompanying reduced respiratory motor output in subjects with already compromised airway diameter (92,101); (3) nasal CPAP treatment has been shown to reduce many of the central apneas in patients diagnosed with primary central sleep apnea syndrome and to eliminate the central portion of mixed apneas (108,109); (4) nasal CPAP treatment in some patients with primarily obstructive apneas relieved the obstruction, but a periodic pattern with central apneas persisted. What might explain these links?

Central leading to obstructive apnea may be precipitated by the common effects of a changing sleep state and chemoreceptor stimuli on both upper airway and thoracic pump muscle activation (92). Furthermore, the study of central apneas, either naturally occurring or induced by mechanical hyperventilation, used bronchoscopic imaging during non-REM sleep to show that marked airway narrowing or closure (usually at the level of the velopharynx) commonly occurred early during central apnea prior to the appearance of inspiratory effort (110) (see Fig. 9). Since the airway cannot be sucked closed under these conditions (i.e., in the absence of negative intrathoracic pressure development), perhaps it is pushed closed by the activation of tonic pharyngeal constrictor muscle activity during the apnea, much in the same way as chest wall expiratory muscles and laryngeal adductor muscles are activated tonically upon the initiation of central apnea.

Obstructive or high-resistance breaths leading to central apnea may be precipitated in two ways. First, in non-REM sleep high upper airway resistance (or obstruction) will lead to hypoventilation, asphyxia, and progressive increases in inspiratory efforts (see Fig. 2, top). Thus, respiratory motor output is high at the termination of these high-resistance events, which—especially when combined with transient arousal—will cause ventilatory overshoots. Then, upon return to non-REM sleep (but rarely in REM; see Fig. 2, bottom), if the resultant hypocapnia is below or near the apneic threshold, central apneas or hypopneas will occur. Short-lived ventilatory cycling may also occur.

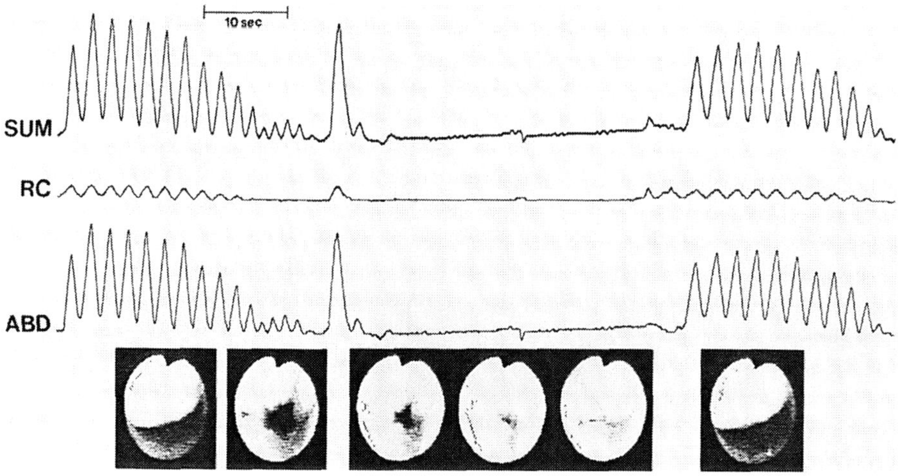

Figure 9 Effects of hypocapnic-induced central apnea on airway closure during non-REM sleep in the human. Note the high tidal volumes produced by mechanical ventilation lead to marked hypoventilation and then central apnea. The airway images are shown throughout the hyperpneic and apneic phase and at the restoration of breathing following an arousal. Note that the airway stays open during the hyperpneic phase, but within 10 seconds or so of the onset of the central apnea the upper airway closed. Other measurements of esophageal pressure showed that the airway closure occurred prior to the reinitiation of an inspiratory effort, i.e., negative esophageal pressure. (From Ref. 110.)

A second, more direct link between airway obstruction (or narrowing) and central apnea (or changes in breath timing) may occur through the inhibitory reflex effects imposed by upper airway obstruction or distortion. The potential for such links is shown by the progressive central apnea caused by negative pressure–induced obstruction of the isolated upper airway in the sleeping dog (68) (see Fig. 5) and by the significant prolongation of T_I and T_E obtained when negative pressure was applied to the isolated upper airway throughout the respiratory cycle (111). Furthermore, correlative data in sleeping humans suggest a link between increases in upper airway resistance during expiration and central apnea (112). Also, exposing the upper airway to the negative pressure normally developed during inspiration caused prolongation of inspiratory time and reduced the rate of rise of EMG_{di} (69). This reflex inhibition of inspiratory motor output increased in strength as inspiration proceeded. Finally, high-frequency pressure oscillations (simulating snoring) also had significant effects on breath timing during sleep. These types of data are consistent with an important role for upper airway reflex receptors in the control of breath timing.

Recognizing the need for more evidence, we propose a positive feedback scheme that enhances and perpetuates sleep-disordered breathing. This process would begin with a reduced respiratory motor output and prolonged expiratory time leading in susceptible individuals to upper airway narrowing and deformation. The resulting stimulation of inhibitory reflex receptors would further delay the onset of the next inspiration and cause central apnea.

Given these proposed types of linkages between the regulation of the muscles of the upper airway and those of the chest wall pump, it is to be expected that reducing airway collapsibility with nasal CPAP would also reduce central apneas either: (1) by preventing the ventilatory overshoots that follow the obstruction; and/or (2) by preventing the inhibition of inspiratory effort presumably caused by airway closure and/or distortion. Conversely, increasing the drive to breathe in carefully selected patients with high upper airway resistance and apparent mixed apneas may well be of significant benefit, especially in preventing the perpetuation of breathing pattern instability (50,113).

VI. Short-Term Memory and Respiratory Stability: Theoretical Considerations

A theme emphasized throughout this review has been the pivotal role in breathing stability played by the opposing memory—like mechanisms of continued excitation vs. inhibition or disfacilitation following withdrawal of ventilatory stimulation. Following a period of hyperpnea, the persisting neural afterdischarge that is the hallmark of short-term potentiation (STP) provides a counterbalancing influence to the hypopnea or apnea that might be expected to occur when the excitatory input is withdrawn. As such, it is generally surmised that STP plays an important role in stabilizing respiratory motor output (101,114). If this is the case, the impairment of STP, either structural or functional, may be necessary for a given individual to develop periodic breathing with apnea. Alternatively, there may exist conditions that attenuate or suppress this mechanism, thereby promoting the likelihood of unstable control. Although STP has been found to be present during non-REM sleep (39), the present evidence suggests that its influence is diminished relative to wakefulness (115). Moreover, the animal and human studies that have demonstrated the existence of STP generally maintained relatively constant levels of end-tidal or arterial P_{CO_2}.

When hypocapnia is allowed to occur during the hyperpneic period, as it does under natural physiological conditions, significant hypoventilatory responses can follow (39). In humans, STP also appears to be masked when moderate levels of hypoxia are sustained for periods longer than a few minutes (39). Animal studies, on the other hand, suggest a much more robust mechanism for STP. The poststimulus increase in respiration is present in anesthetized animals (116), following decerebration (117) or cooling of intermediate areas of the ventral medulla (118), as well as during exposure to various levels of hypercapnia or hypocapnia (119,120). What could account for the apparent discrepancy between the somewhat fragile STP process noted in humans and the seemingly indestructible phenomenon observed in the cat preparation? We believe that a reconciliation of these conflicting observations can be arrived at through a careful review of the certain details obtained in a number of pivotal studies.

We begin first with considerations that relate to the physiological mechanism underlying STP. Eldridge (116) suggested a reverberation hypothesis, postulating that facilatory feedback of nonrespiratory neurons in the reticular formation may help maintain the activity of the respiratory neurons. The available evidence, however, does not support this hypothesis. It now appears that STP is most likely the manifestation of enhanced synaptic transmission resulting from repetitive stimulation of the presynaptic terminals (121,122). Starting with the assumption that the efficacy of presynaptic terminals is increased by a factor that decays exponentially with time, Shen (123) has shown that the dynamic characteristics of STP can be modeled as a static gain placed in parallel with a leaky integrator. The static gain is responsible for the direct effect, converting part of the stimulus virtually instantaneously into a portion of the response. The leaky integrator accounts for the relatively slower afterdischarge, which decays with a time constant on the order of 40 seconds. Models of similar form have been proposed by Eldridge (118) and Poon (124). A key feature of these models is the inclusion of the static gain component. While the attention of most researchers has been focused almost exclusively on the afterdischarge component of STP, one should note that the direct effect can account for half or more of the complete response.

Another set of observations that we believe to be very important is the effect of the conditioning stimulus, or the baseline level of drive, on the magnitude and time course of STP. Eldridge and Gill-Kumar (119) and Vis and Folgering (120) have demonstrated a progressive reduction in the STP response magnitude and time constants as the baseline stimulus level is increased through either hypercapnia or continuous stimulation of the contralateral carotid sinus nerve. On the other hand, with increasing hypocapnia, the apparent magnitude of the STP response to carotid sinus stimulation decreased (119). Below a certain level of P_{CO_2}, the direct effect of the STP response accompanying the start of stimulation disappeared while the time constant of STP development became longer. Upon cessation of the stimulus, the STP response was composed solely of the direct effect; no afterdischarge was visible. These observations can be explained if one accepts the possibility that activation of STP can exist at subthreshold levels of phrenic activity (119). Indeed, data from other studies (125,126) have demonstrated the presence of tonic excitation in respiratory neurons and in expiratory muscle EMG at levels of P_{CO_2} far below the apneic threshold for the phrenic neurogram (see Fig. 2).

Taking the above considerations into account, we have developed a simple model of STP that can allow us to determine its influence on respiratory stability. This model, shown schematically in Figure 10A, contains the essential elements of the static gain and leaky integrator. Equally important, however, is the inclusion of the thresholding and saturation nonlinearity placed at the output end of the model, as well as the nonlinear transformation subsystem situated at the input end. The latter allows the model to account for the progressive reduction in magnitude and time course of the STP response as the baseline stimulus level is increased, as demonstrated in the simulation results presented in Figure 10B. The former subsystem allows for subthreshold dynamics. Thus, under conditions of very low drive (Fig. 10B)

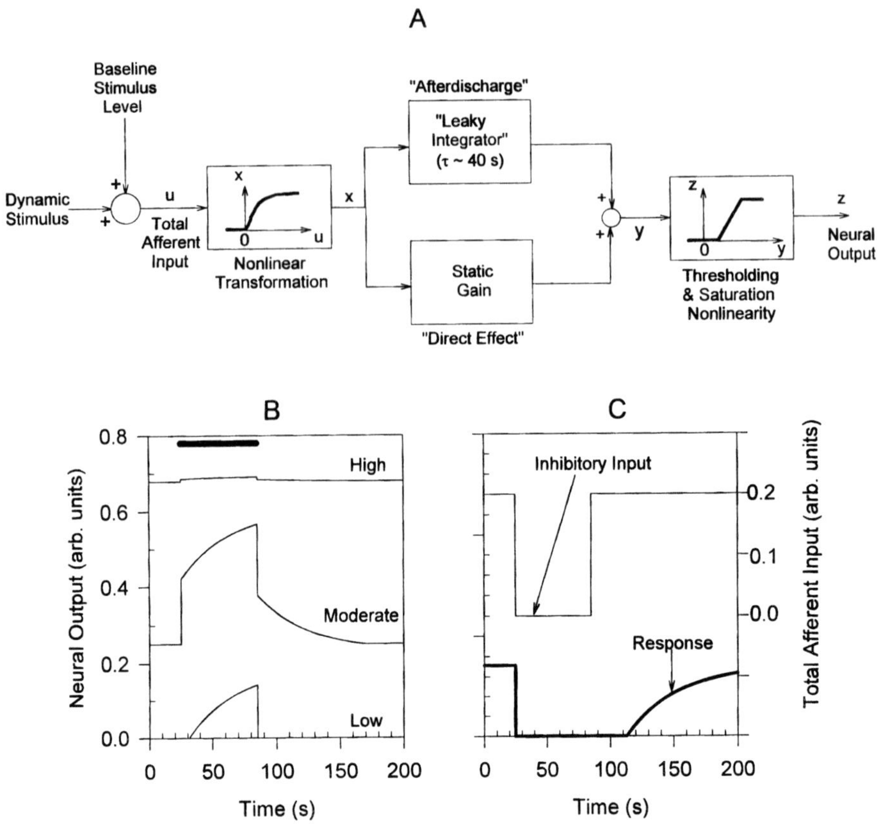

Figure 10 (A) Model of short-term respiratory memory. (B) Predictions of the model to a step stimulus (dark bar) applied at low, moderate, and high levels of conditioning or baseline stimulation. These results quantitatively mimic the STP response at different levels of Pa_{CO_2}. (C) Apnea produced by an inhibitory step input can persist even after withdrawal of the input because the neural activity remains at subthreshold levels.

when phrenic output is silent, application of a step stimulus would still activate STP from a subthreshold level. Phrenic activity is reinitiated only when the model output exceeds threshold, thereby masking the direct effect; similarly, upon cessation of the stimulus, only the direct effect of the STP response is visible, since the afterdischarge phase takes place below threshold.

The relevance of the model to respiratory stability is shown in Figure 10C. Here, a significant inhibitory step input (which could be chemical or neuromechanical in origin) is applied, which leads rapidly to apnea. Decreased stimulation leads to decreased synaptic efficacy, activating the STP process in reverse, but under subthreshold conditions. At time $t = 85$ s, the inhibitory input is withdrawn, invoking the development phase of the STP process. Since much of this continues to occur at subthreshold levels, respiration is not initiated until time t = 115 s. Thus, this mechanism has prolonged the central apnea by 30 s. In summary, the model predicts that STP would exert a stabilizing influence on respiratory motor output when it operates above threshold; however, when part of this process operates at subthreshold levels, its influence on respiratory control can be destabilizing. Furthermore, this subthreshold manifestation of STP presents itself as an inhibitory memory effect and therefore is a potential mechanism that could account for the control system inertia that was discussed earlier.

VII. Summary

Loss of wakefulness as well as variations in the relative state of consciousness throughout sleep have powerful influences on the ventilatory control system which are commonly manifested in unstable breathing patterns. Research over the past two decades has established several state-sensitive influences that predispose to ventilatory instability in sleep, including the increased compliance of the upper airway, the unmasking of a sensitive hypocapnic-induced apneic threshold, the loss of immediate respiratory compensation for mechanical loads, the mechanoreflexes associated with a changing airway patency and/or deformation, and the stabilizing effects of excitatory short-term potentiation vs. counteracting destabilizing effects of chemoreceptor and mechanoreceptor feedback inhibition whose memory-like aftereffects serve to prolong apneas. So, considerable progress has been made in our understanding. However, several fundamental questions remain which prevent a truly integrative, complete understanding of the underlying mechanisms precipitating periodic breathing in sleep:

Concerning the hypocapnic apneic threshold, we do not yet know precisely which chemoreceptors mediate the apnea; in a very practical sense it remains unexplained why transient—as opposed to longer-term—reductions in Pa_{CO_2} cause apnea in sleeping humans.

Does the hypocapnic apneic threshold—in relationship to eupneic Pa_{CO_2}—change in the face of background ventilatory stimuli, and what do these changes mean to enhancing periodic breathing?

How can our knowledge of the profound effects of CO_2 on breathing during sleep be used to develop effective, simple, noninvasive, and nondisruptive treatments of central and mixed apneas?

In sleep, do additional inhibitory factors on the ventilatory control system such as mechanoreceptor feedback, chronic hypertension, and/or brain hypoxia play an important destabilizing role by influencing breathing pattern and upper airway caliber in the sleeping human? To date these mechanisms have received scant attention.

What exactly are the extraneural inputs to the medullary pattern generator which are present in wakefulness and in phasic REM sleep? Specifically, where do they originate in the higher central nervous system? And can their specific influences be modulated pharmacologically to protect against sleep effects on breathing pattern stability and airway tonicity?

What passive or active (neural) mechanisms are responsible for the reduced airway patency and even closure during a central apnea? During breathing, under what conditions do reductions in phrenic motor output also influence airway compliance and patency? Under what circumstances will treating inadequate or unstable neural respiratory motor output alleviate high resistance or obstructive airway events in sleep?

What characteristics differ among individuals to explain why some subjects experience substantial ventilatory overshoots and therefore perpetuate breathing instability in response to combinations of accumulating chemostimulation plus cortical or subcortical arousal? The mechanisms underlying the sensitization of chemoreceptor inputs by changes in state of consciousness remain a mystery.

Acknowledgments

We acknowledge the assistance of Donna Graves and Patricia Kalscheur in the preparation of this manuscript. The original research represented here was supported by grants from NHLBI (R03 HL62686-01 and R01 50531).

References

1. Young T, Palta M, Dempsey J, Skatrud J, Weber S, Badr S. The occurrence of sleep-disordered breathing among middle-aged adults. N Engl J Med 1993; 328(17):1230–1235.
2. Henke KG, Badr MS, Skatrud JB, Dempsey JA. Load compensation and respiratory muscle function during sleep. J Appl Physiol 1992; 72(4):1221–1234.
3. Kay A, Trinder J, Bowes G, Young K. Changes in airway resistance during sleep onset. J Appl Physiol 1994; 76(4):1600–1607.
4. Tangel DJ, Mezzanotte WS, White DP. Influence of sleep on tensor palatini EMG and upper airway resistance in normal men. J Appl Physiol 1991; 70(6):2574–2581.
5. Orem J, Osorio I, Brooks E, Dick T. Activity of respiratory neurons during NREM sleep. J Neurophysiol 1985; 54(5):1144–1156.
6. Skatrud JB, Dempsey JA. Airway resistance and respiratory muscle function in snorers during NREM sleep. J Appl Physiol 1985; 59(2):328–335.
7. Skatrud JB, Dempsey JA, Badr MS, Begle RL. Effects of high airway impedance on CO_2 retention and respiratory muscle activity during NREM sleep. J Appl Physiol 1988; 65:1676–1685.
8. Remmers JE, DeGroot WJ, Sauerland EK, Anch AM. Pathogenesis of upper airway occlusion during sleep. J Appl Physiol 1978; 44:931–938.
9. Somers VK, Dyken ME, Mark, AL, Abboud FM. Sympathetic nerve activity during sleep in normal subjects. N Engl J Med 1993; 328:583–589.

10. Wasicko MJ, Leiter JC, Erlichman JS, Strobel RJ, Bartlett D Jr. Nasal and pharyngeal resistance after topical mucosal vasoconstriction in normal humans. Am Rev Respir Dis 1991; 144:1048–1052.
11. Horner RL, Kozar LF, Kimoff RJ, Phillipson EA. Effects of sleep on the tonic drive to respiratory muscles and the threshold for rhythm generation in the dog. J Physiol 1994; 474(3):525–537.
12. Simon PM, Dempsey JA, Landry DM, Skatrud JB. Effect of sleep on respiratory muscle activity during mechanical ventilation. Am Rev Respir Dis. 1993; 147(1):32–37.
13. Morrell MJ, Harty HR, Adams L, Guz A. Changes in total pulmonary resistance and PCO_2 between wakefulness and sleep in normal human subjects. J Appl Physiol 1995; 78:1339–1349.
14. Orem J. Central respiratory activity in rapid eye movement sleep: augmenting and late inspiratory cells. Sleep 1994; 17(8):1144–1156.
15. Orem J. Excitatory drive to the respiratory system in REM sleep. Sleep 1996; 19: S154–S156.
16. Smith CA, Henderson KS, Xi L, Chow CM, Eastwood PR, Dempsey JA. Neural-mechanical coupling of breathing in REM sleep. J Appl Physiol 1997; 83(6):1923–1932.
17. Hendricks JC, Kline LR. Differential activation within costal diaphragm during rapid eye movement sleep in cats. J Appl Physiol 1991; 70:1194–1200.
18. Netick A, Orem J, Dement W. Neuronal activity specific to REM sleep and its relationship to breathing. Brain Res 1977; 120:197–207.
19. Phillipson EA, Bowes G. Control of breathing during sleep. In: Cherniack NS, Widdicombe JG, eds. Handbook of Physiology: The Respiratory System. Bethesda, MD: American Physiological Society, 1986:649–689.
20. Morrell MJ, Shea SA, Adams L, Guz A. Effect of inspiratory pressure support upon breathing in humans during wakefulness and sleep. Respir Physiol 1993; 93:57–70.
21. Leevers AM, Simon PM, Dempsey JA. Apnea after normocapnic mechanical ventilation during NREM sleep. J Appl Physiol 1994; 77(5):2079–2085.
22. Puddy A, Patrick W, Webster K, Younes M. Respiratory control during volume-cycled ventilation in normal humans. J Appl Physiol 1996; 80:1749–1758.
23. Skatrud JB, Dempsey JA. Interaction of sleep state and chemical stimuli in sustaining rhythmic ventilation. J Appl Physiol 1983; 55:813–822.
24. Fink RB. Influence of cerebral activity in wakefulness on regulation of breathing. J Appl Physiol 1961; 16:15–20.
25. Corfield D, Morrell MJ, Guz A. The nature of breathing during hypocapnia in awake man. Respir Physiol 1995; 101:145–160.
26. Wheatley JR, Mezzanotte WS, Tangel DJ, White DP. Influence of sleep on genioglossus muscle activation by negative pressure in normal men. Am Rev Respir Dis 1993; 148(3):597–605.
27. Van de Graaff WB. Thoracic influence on upper airway patency. J Appl Physiol 1988; 65(5):2124–2131.
28. Begle RL, Skatrud JB, Dempsey JA. Ventilatory compensation for changes in functional residual capacity during sleep. J Appl Physiol 1987; 62(3):1299–1306.
29. Khoo MCK. Periodic breathing and central apnea. In: Altose MD, Kawakami Y, eds. Control of Breathing in Health and Disease. New York: Marcel Dekker, 1999:203–250.
30. Parisi RA, Neubauer JA Santiago TV, Edelman NH. Brain blood flow and control of respiratory muscles during sleep. Acta Biol Med Exp 1986; 11:115–126.

31. Isono S, Remmers JE. Anatomy and physiology of upper airway obstruction. In: Kryger MH, Roth T, Dement WC, eds. Principles and Practice of Sleep Medicine, 2nd ed. London: W. B. Saunders, 1994:632–656.
32. Hudgel DW, Hamilton HB. Respiratory muscle activity during sleep-induced periodic breathing in the elderly. J Appl Physiol 1994; 77(5):2285–2290.
33. Dempsey JA, Smith CA, Harms CA, Chow CM, Saupe KW. Sleep-induced breathing instability. Sleep 1996; 19(3):236–247.
34. Chow CM, Xi L, Smith CA, Saupe KW, Dempsey JA. A volume-dependent apneic threshold during NREM sleep in the dog. J Appl Physiol 1994; 76(6):2315–2325.
35. Silva-Carvalho L, Dawid-Milner MS, Goldsmith GE, Spyer KM. Hypothalamic-evoked effects in cat nucleus tractus solitarius facilitating chemoreceptor reflexes. Exp Physiol 1993; 78(3):425–428.
36. Issa F, Porostocky S. Effects of sleep changes on breathing pattern accompanying sigh breaths. Respir Physiol 1993; 93:175–187.
37. Xi L, Chow CM, Smith CA, Dempsey JA. Effects of REM sleep on the ventilatory response to airway occlusion in the dog. Sleep 1994; 17(8):674–687.
38. Eldridge FL, Millhorn DE. Oscillation, gating, and memory in the respiratory control system. In: Handbook of Physiology. The Respiratory System. Control of Breathing, Vol 2. Bethesda, MD: American Physiological Society, 1986:93–114.
39. Badr MS, Skatrud JB, Dempsey JA. Determinants of poststimulus potentiation in humans during NREM sleep. J Appl Physiol 1992; 73(5):1958–1971.
40. Badr MS, Skatrud JB, Dempsey JA. Effect of chemoreceptor stimulation and inhibition on total pulmonary resistance in humans during NREM sleep. J Appl Physiol 1994; 76(4):1682–1692.
41. Iber C, Davies SF, Chapman RC, Mahowald MM. A possible mechanism for mixed apnea in obstructive sleep apnea. Chest 1986; 89:800–805.
42. Xi L, Smith CA, Saupe KW, Dempsey JA. Effects of memory from vagal feedback on short term potentiation of ventilation in conscious dogs. J Appl Physiol 1993; 462: 547–561.
43. Badr S, Kawak A, Skatrud J, Morrell M, Zahn B, Babcock M. Effect of induced hypocapnic hypopnea on upper airway patency in humans during NREM sleep. Respir Physiol 1997; 110:33–45.
44. Henke KG, Arias A, Skatrud J, Dempsey JA. Inhibition of inspiratory muscle activity during sleep: chemical and non-chemical influences. Am Rev Respir Dis 1988; 138: 8–15.
45. Wilson CR, Satoh M, Skatrud JB, Dempsey JA. Non-chemical inhibition of respiratory motor output during mechanical ventilation in sleeping humans. J Physiol 1999; 518(2):605–618.
46. Badr MS, Kawak A. Post-hyperventilation hypopnea in humans during NREM sleep. Respir Physiol 1996; 103:137–145.
47. Millhorn DE, Eldridge FL, Kiley JP. Oscillations of medullary extracellular fluid pH caused by breathing. Respir Physiol 1984; 55(2):193–203.
48. Smith CA, Saupe KW, Henderson KS, Dempsey JA. Ventilatory effects of specific carotid body hypocapnia in dogs during wakefulness and sleep. J Appl Physiol 1995; 79(3):689–699.
49. Berssenbrugge A, Dempsey J, Iber C, Skatrud J, Wilson P. Mechanisms of hypoxia-induced periodic breathing during sleep in humans. J Physiol (London) 1983; 343: 507–524.

50. Badr MS, Grossman JE, Weber SA. Treatment of refractory sleep apnea with supplemental carbon dioxide. Am J Respir Crit Care Med 1994; 150(2):561–564.
51. Xie A, Wong B, Phillipson EA, Slutsky AS, Bradley TD. Interaction of hyperventilation and arousal in the pathogenesis of idiopathic central sleep apnea. Am J Respir Crit Care Med 1994; 150:489–495.
52. Khoo MCK, Koh SSW, Shin JJW, Westbrook PR, Berry BB. Ventilatory dynamics during transient arousal from NREM sleep: implications for respiratory control stability. J Appl Physiol 1996; 80(5):1475–1484.
53. Hanly PJ, Millar TW, Stejes DC, Baert R, Frais MA, Kryger MH. Respiration and abnormal sleep in patients with congestive heart failure. Chest 1989; 96:480–488.
54. Xi L, Smith CA, Saupe KW, Dempsey JA. Effects of memory from vagal feedback on short-term potentiation of ventilation in conscious dogs. J Physiol (London) 1993; 462:547–561.
55. Cherniack N, Longbardo S, Levine OR, Mellins R, Fishman AP. Periodic breathing in dogs. J Appl Physiol 1966; 21:1847–1854.
56. Iber C, Simon P, Skatrud JB, Mahowald MW, Dempsey JA. The Breuer-Hering reflex in humans. Effects of pulmonary denervation and hypocapnia. Am J Respir Crit Care Med 1995; 152(1):217–224.
57. Polachek J, Strong R, Arens J, Davies C, Metcalf I, Younes M. Phasic vagal influence on inspiratory motor output in anesthetized human subjects. J Appl Physiol 1980; 49: 609–619.
58. Iatridis A, Iber C. The role of neural reflex mechanisms in response to inspiratory motor output in anesthetized human subjects. Am Rev Respir Dis 1992; 145:A405.
59. Gautier H, Bonara M, Gaudy JH. Breuer-Hering reflex and breathing pattern in anesthetized humans and cats. J Appl Physiol 1981; 51:1162–1168.
60. Tobert DG, Simon PM, Stroetz RW, Hubmayr RD. The determinants of respiratory rate during mechanical ventilation. Am J Respir Crit Care Med 1997; 155:485–492.
61. Manchanda S, Leevers AM, Wilson CR, Simon PM, Skatrud JB, Dempsey JA. Frequency and volume thresholds for inhibition of inspiratory motor output during mechanical ventilation. Respir Physiol 1996; 105:1–16.
62. Wilson CR, Satoh M, Skatrud JB, Dempsey JA. Non-chemical inhibition of respiratory motor output during mechanical ventilation in sleeping humans. J Physiol 1999; 518(2):605–618.
63. Satoh M, Eastwood PR, Smith CA, Dempsey JA. Nonchemical elimination of inspiratory motor output via mechanical ventilation in sleep. Am J Respir Crit Care Med 2001; 163:1356–1364.
64. Knox CK. Characteristics of inflation and deflation reflexes during expiration in the cat. J Neurophysiol 1973; 36:284–295.
65. Mathew OP. Control of upper airway muscle activity in regulation of breathing. In: Dempsey JA, Pack AI, eds. Regulation of Breathing. New York: Marcel Dekker, 1994: 1064–1134.
66. Horner, RL. Motor control of the pharyngeal musculature and implications for the pathogenesis of obstructive sleep apnea. Sleep 1996; 19:827–853.
67. Issa FG, Bitner S. Effect of route of breathing on the ventilatory and arousal responses to hypercapnia in awake and sleeping dogs. J Physiol (London) 1993; 465:615–628.
68. Harms CA, Zeng YJ, Smith CA, Vidruk EH, Dempsey JA. Negative pressure-induced deformation of the upper airway causes central apnea in awake and sleeping dogs. J Appl Physiol 1996; 80(5):1528–1539.

69. Eastwood PR, Curran AK, Smith CA, Dempsey JA. Effect of upper airway negative pressure on inspiratory drive during sleep. J Appl Physiol 1998; 84(3):1063–1075.
70. Curran A, Eastwood P, Harms C, Smith C, Dempsey J. Superior laryngeal nerve section alters responses to upper airway distortion in sleeping dogs. J Appl Physiol 1997; 83:768–775.
71. Eastwood PR, Satoh M, Curran AK, Zayas MT, Smith CA, Dempsey JA. Inhibition of inspiratory motor output by high-frequency low-pressure oscillations in the upper airway of sleeping dogs. J Physiol 1999; 517(1):259–271.
72. Plowman L, Lauff DC, Berthon-Jones M, Sullivan CE. Waking and sleeping genioglossus muscle responses to upper airway pressure oscillations in sleeping dogs. J Appl Physiol 1990; 68:2564–2573.
73. Trelease R, Marks J, Harper R. Respiratory inhibition induced by transient hypertension during anesthesia and sleep states. Exp Neurol 1985; 90:173–186.
74. Saupe KW, Smith CA, Henderson KS, Dempsey JA. Effects of raising carotid sinus pressure on upper airway resistance and EEG frequency in sleeping dogs. J Appl Physiol 1995; 78(5):1699–1709.
75. Olson LG, Strohl KP. Non-muscular factors in upper airway patency in the rabbit. Respir Physiol 1988; 71:147–155.
76. Wilson C, Manchanda S, Crabtree D, Skatrud JB, Dempsey JD. An induced blood pressure rise does not alter upper airway resistance in sleeping humans. J Appl Physiol 1998; 84(1):269–276.
77. Mayer J, Weichler U, Herres-Mayer B, Schneider H, Marx U, Peter J. Influence of metroprolol and cilazapril on blood pressure and on sleep apnea activity. J Cardiovasc Pharmacol 1987; 16:952–961.
78. Carley DW, Trbovic S, Radulovacki M. Hydralazine reduces elevated sleep apnea index in spontaneously hypertensive (SHR) rats to equivalence with normotensive Wistar-Kyoto rats. Sleep 1996; 19:363–366.
79. Orem J, Trotter RH. Medullary respiratory neuronal activity during augmented breaths in intact unanesthetized cats. J Appl Physiol 1993; 74:761–769.
80. Lawson EE. Prolonged central respiratory inhibition following reflex-induced apnea. J Appl Physiol 1981; 50:874–879.
81. Batsel HL. Activity of bulbospinal neurons during passive hyperventilation. Exp Neurol 1967; 19:357–374.
82. Remmers JE, Richter DW, Ballantyne D, Bainton CR, Klein JP. Reflex prolongation of stage I expiration. Pfluegers Arch 1986; 407:190–198.
83. Kianicka I, Leroux JF, Praud JP. Thyroarytenoid muscle activity during hypocapnic central apneas in awake nonsedated lambs. J Appl Physiol 1994; 76:1262–1268.
84. Sears TA, Berger AJ, Phillipson EA. Reciprocal tonic activation of inspiratory and expiratory motoneurones by chemical drives. Nature 1982; 299:728–730.
85. Dempsey JD, Leevers LM, Wilson CR, Harms CA, Smith CA. Apnea prolongation via short-term inhibition. Sleep 1996; 19(10):S160–S163.
86. Orem J, Vidruk E. Activity of medullary respiratory neurons during ventilation induced apnea in sleep and wakefulness. J Appl Physiol 1998; 84:922–932.
87. Pack AI, Cola MF, Goldzmidt A, Ogilvie MD, Gottschalk A. Correlation between oscillations in ventilation and frequency content of the electroencephalogram. J Appl Physiol 1992; 72:985–992.
88. Pack AI, Silage DA, Millner RP, Knight H, Shorw ET, Chung DCC. Spectral analysis

of ventilation in elderly subjects awake and asleep. J Appl Physiol 1988; 64:1257–1267.

89. Carskadon MA, Brown ED, Dement WC. Sleep fragmentation in the elderly: relationship to daytime sleep tendency. Neurobiol Aging 1982; 3:321–327.
90. Hudgel DW, Devadatta P, Hamilton H. Pattern of breathing and upper airway mechanics during wakefulness and sleep in healthy elderly humans. J Appl Physiol 1993; 74(5):2198–2204.
91. Dowdell WT, Javaheri S, McGinnis W. Cheyne-Stokes respiration presenting as sleep apnea syndrome. Am Rev Respir Dis 1990; 141:871–879.
92. Hudgel DW, Chapman KR, Faulks C, Hendricks C. Changes in inspiratory muscle electrical activity and upper airway resistance during periodic breathing induced by hypoxia during sleep. Am Rev Respir Dis 1987; 135:899–906.
93. Onal E, Burrows DL, Hart RH, Lopata M. Induction of periodic breathing during sleep causes upper airway obstruction in humans. J Appl Physiol 1986; 61:1438–1443.
94. Berssenbrugge A, Dempsey JA, Skatrud JB. Effects of sleep state on ventilatory acclimatization to chronic hypoxia. J Appl Physiol 1984; 57:1089–1096.
95. Lahiri S. Maret KH, Sherpa MG, Peters RM Jr. Sleep and periodic breathing at high altitude: sherpa native vs sojourners. In: West J, Lahiri S, eds. High Altitude and Man. Bethesda, MD: American Physiological Society, 1984:73–90.
96. Reite M, Jackson D, Cahoon RL, Weil JV. Sleep physiology at high altitude. Electroenceph Clin Neurophysiol 1975; 38:463–471.
97. Sutton JR, Houston CS, Marsell AC. Effect of acetazolamide on hypoxemia during sleep at high altitude. N Engl J Med 1979; 301:1329–1331.
98. Douglas C, Haldane J, Henderson Y, Schneider E. Physiological observations made of Pike's Peak, Colorado with special reference to adaptation to low barometric pressures. Philosophical Trans R Soc Lond 1913; 203:185–381.
99. Khoo MCK, Dynamics of periodic breathing and arousal during sleep at extreme altitude. Respir Physiol 1996; 103:33–43.
100. Bisgard GE, Forster HV. Ventilatory responses to acute and chronic hypoxia. In: Fregly MJ, Blatteis CM, ed. Handbook of Physiology: Environmental Physiology. New York: Oxford University Press, 1996:1207–1239.
101. Warner G, Skatrud JB, Dempsey JA. Effect of hypoxia-induced periodic breathing on upper airway obstruction during sleep. J Appl Physiol 1987; 62:2201–2211.
102. Younes M. The physiological basis of central apnea and periodic breathing. In: Simmons DH, ed. Current Pulmonology. Vol. 10. Chicago: Year Book Medical Publishers, 1989:265–326.
103. Neubauer JA, Melton JE, Edelman HH. Modulation of respiration during brain hypoxia. J Appl Physiol 1990; 68:441–451.
104. Long W, Giesbrecht G, Anthonisen NR. Ventilatory response to moderate hypoxia in awake and chemodenervated cats. J Appl Physiol 1993; 74:805–810.
105. Smith CA, Engwal MJA, Dempsey JA, Bisgard GE. Effects of specific carotid body and brain hypoxia on respiratory muscle control in the awake goat. J Physiol London 1993; 460:623–640.
106. Engwall MJA, Smith CA, Dempsey JA, Bisgard GE. Ventilatory afterdischarge and central respiratory drive interactions in the awake goat. J Appl Physiol 1994; 76(1): 416–423.
107. Haddad GG, Donnelly DF. O_2 deprivation induces a major depolarization in brain stem neurons in the adult but not in the neonatal rat. J Physiol 1990; 429:411–428.

108. Issa FG, Sullivan CE. Reversal of central sleep apnea using nasal CPAP. Chest 1986; 90(2):165–171.
109. Hoffstein V, Slutsky AS. Central sleep apnea reversed by continuous positive airway pressure. Am Rev Respir Dis 1987; 135(5):1210–1212.
110. Badr MS, Toiber F, Skatrud JB, Dempsey JA. Pharyngeal narrowing/occlusion during central sleep apnea. J Appl Physiol 1995; 78:1806–1815.
111. McNamara SG, Issa FG, Szeto E, Sullivan CE. Influence of negative pressure applied to the upper airway on the breathing pattern in unanesthetized awake dogs. Respir Physiol 1986; 65:315–329.
112. Sanders MH, Rogers RM, Pennock BE. Prolonged expiratory phase in sleep apnea. A unifying hypothesis. Am Rev Respir Dis 1985; 131(3):401–408.
113. DeBacker WA, Verbraecken J, Willemen M, Wittesaele W, DeCock W, Van deHeyning P. Central apnea index decreases after prolonged treatment with acetazolamide. Am J Respir Crit Care Med 1995; 151(1):87–91.
114. Eldridge FL. The North Carolina respiratory model: a multipurpose model for studying the control of breathing. In: Khoo MCK, ed. Bioengineering Approaches to Pulmonary Physiology and Medicine. New York: Plenum, 1996:25–49.
115. Gleeson K, Sweet LW. Ventilatory pattern after hypoxic stimulation during wakefulness and NREM sleep. J Appl Physiol 1993; 75:397–404.
116. Eldridge FL. Central neural respiratory stimulatory effect of active respiration. J Appl Physiol 1974; 37:723–735.
117. Eldridge FL. Central neural stimulation of respiration in unanesthetized decerebrate cats. J Appl Physiol 1976; 40:23–28.
118. Eldridge FL. Neural control of breathing during exercise. In: Whipp BJ, Wasserman K, eds. Exercise—Pulmonary Physiology and Pathophysiology. New York: Marcel Dekker, 1991:309–370.
119. Eldridge FL, Gill-Kumar P. Central neural respiratory drive and after discharge. Respir Physiol 1980; 40:49–63.
120. Vis A, Folgering H. Phrenic nerve afterdischarge after electrical stimulation of the carotid sinus nerve in cats. Respir Physiol 1981; 45:217–227.
121. Magleby KL. Synaptic transmission, facilitation, augmentation, potentiation, depression. In: Adelman G, ed. Encyclopedia of Neuroscience, Vol. 2. Boston: Biekhauser, 1987:1170–1174.
122. Zucker RS. Short-term synaptic plasticity. Ann Rev Neurosci 1989; 12:13–31.
123. Shen L. Neural integration by short-term potentiation. Biol Cybern 1989; 61:319–325.
124. Poon CS. Synaptic plasticity and respiratory control. In: Khoo MCK, ed. Bioengineering Approaches to Pulmonary Physiology and Medicine. New York: Plenum, 1996: 93–113.
125. Bainton CR, Kirkwood PA, Sears TA. On the transmission of the stimulating effects of carbon dioxide to the muscles of respiration. J Physiol (Lond) 1978; 280:249–272.
126. Lahiri S, Mokashi A, Delaney RG, Fishman AP. Arterial P_{O2} and P_{CO2} stimulus threshold for carotid chemoreceptors and breathing. Respir Physiol 1978; 34:359–375.

4

Mechanisms of Airway Hypotonia

LESZEK KUBIN and RICHARD O. DAVIES

University of Pennsylvania
Philadelphia, Pennsylvania

I. Introduction

The onset of sleep is associated with a reduction in upper airway patency and an increase in resistance, an effect observed in normal humans and animals, snorers, and patients with obstructive sleep apnea/hypopnea syndrome (OSA) (e.g., Refs. 1–6; see Refs. 7 and 8 for reviews). Patients with OSA commonly have structural abnormalities that result in a narrowed upper airway and collapsible pharynx; but when they are awake, their airway remains continuously patent (except during swallowing, speech, vomiting, etc.). During sleep, however, the cross-sectional area decreases considerably and they experience repeated, clinically significant, obstructive apneas or hypopneas. This sleep-wake state dependence of the disorder points to the involvement of neural mechanisms. The marked increase in resistance is attributed to a sleep-related alteration in the neural control of upper airway striated muscles. In particular, decrements in the activity of upper airway dilator muscles, i.e., those that counteract the collapsing force of the negative pressure generated in the airway during inspiration, are believed to play a permissive role in sleep-related airway obstructions.

The cross-sectional area and resistance of the upper airway are dynamic variables, being determined at any point in time by: (1) the mechanical properties of the upper airway (see Chap. 2); (2) the structures in the upper airways (see Chap. 1);

(3) adhesive forces generated between the walls of the various airway components whenever they come in contact (9–11); and (4) the pattern and magnitude of activity in upper airway muscles. The stiffness and size of the upper airway, in turn, depend on both the level and pattern of upper airway muscle tone and transmural pressures, with the latter depending on the force generated by respiratory pump muscles (diaphragm, intercostals, and abdominals) and the extraluminal pressure in the tissue. The variables controlling upper airway patency are strongly interrelated (12,13). Consequently, studies of the behavior of individual upper airway muscles during sleep are unlikely to be able to explain fully those neuromuscular events that are critical for airway obstructions and their subsequent resolution. Electromyographic studies are informative, however, in that they help to link the mechanical and neural events and provide common ground for interpreting human and animal research, for only in the latter is a precise investigation of central neural events possible. They also provide a window on the central neural mechanisms regulating upper airway motor activity both at the level of, and upstream from, the motor neurons (motoneurons) innervating different muscles. Thus, in this chapter we will first discuss the pattern of sleep-wake cycle–related alterations in the activity of upper airway muscles in normal humans, OSA patients, and experimental animals.

In addition to their respiratory function, upper airway muscles are involved in a number of other behaviors that are predominantly automatic (e.g., swallowing, coughing) or entirely voluntary (e.g., phonation). This multifunctionality requires that the neural pathways controlling upper airway muscles originate from many brain centers and that appropriate neural connections exist to provide for various types of synchronization and sequencing of upper airway muscle activation. Accordingly, four distinct classes of central neuronal systems control upper airway motoneurons: (1) those responsible for centrally generated automatic behaviors (''pattern generators''), including breathing; (2) those transmitting reflexes from peripheral receptors; (3) those related to the level of sleep and arousal; and (4) those for volitional control. Distinct alterations occur in each of these systems in relation to sleep, with additional differences observed between slow-wave [non–rapid eye movement (non-REM)] and REM sleep. These changes will be analyzed in subsequent sections by separately looking at the phasic respiratory, reflex, and sleep state–dependent tonic drives that determine the behavior of upper airway muscles.

The subject of sleep-related changes in the upper airway has been extensively reviewed. Therefore, in this chapter we will emphasize recent developments in the field. Several reviews are particularly relevant to the present material and recommended as sources of complementary information (14–21).

II. Sleep-Related Alterations in the Tone of Individual Upper Airway Muscles

A. Mechanistic Background

Upper airway obstructions in OSA patients occur most commonly in the pharynx (11,22–24), presumably due to the lack of rigid structures supporting this segment

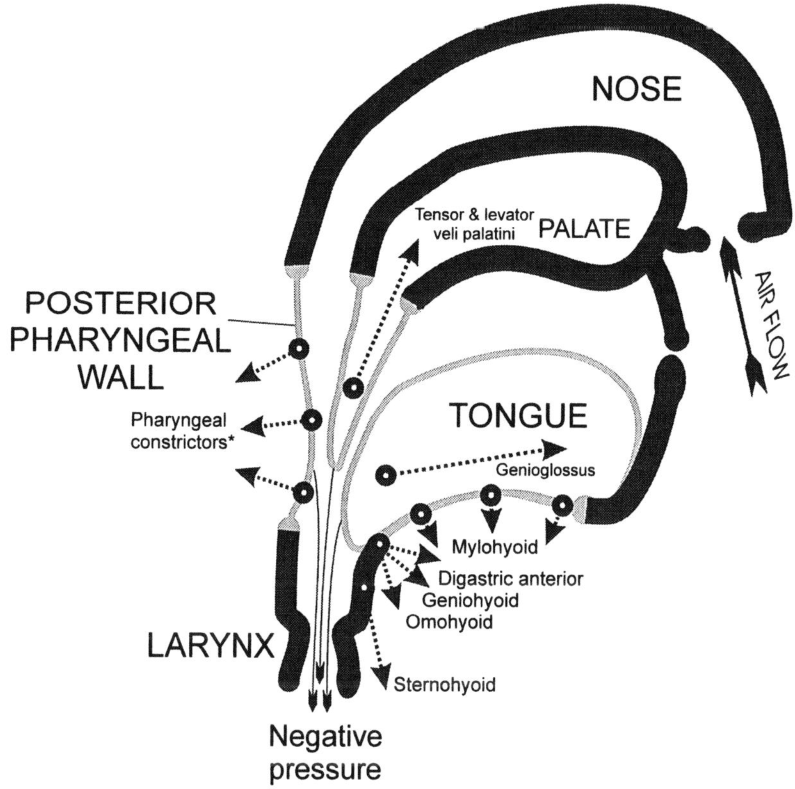

Figure 1 Schematic sagittal cross-section of the upper airway emphasizing that three soft tissue elements—the tongue, the posterior pharyngeal wall, and the soft palate—are pulled toward each other by intraluminal negative pressure. Dashed arrows show approximate directions and sites of attachment of the forces exerted by major muscles that counteract this negative pressure and, therefore, act as pharyngeal dilators. *Pharyngeal constrictors stiffen the posterior pharyngeal wall, and their dilator or constrictor action is position-dependent. Sleep-related changes in the activity of these and other upper airway muscles are summarized in Table 1.

of the airway. Indeed, the schematic view of the pharynx shown in Figure 1 demonstrates that it is the site where three soft tissue elements are pulled inward and toward each other by the centripetal force resulting from the presence of negative pressure in the pharyngeal lumen. Those elements are the posterior pharyngeal wall, the tongue, which acts like a plunger that is sucked into the airway, and the soft palate, which acts like a wedge that is squeezed between the other two. Consequently, those muscles that oppose the airway-narrowing action of negative pressure are the most important controllers of upper airway patency. The nose and larynx, although they are not typical sites of airway obstruction, are important determinants of the magnitude of the negative pressure generated at any given time in the pharyngeal space because they act as pressure dividers between the nasal, pharyngeal, and laryngeal compartments. In addition, those muscles that can pull the airway downward (e.g., sternohyoid and sternothyroid) can counteract the obstruction by increasing the distance between the soft palate and the base of the tongue (25–27), and opening the mouth can terminate an obstruction by relieving the negative pressure in the pharynx (28).

Nasal resistance is about half the total airway resistance (29) and is variable during both wakefulness and sleep (30). However, the walls of the nasal passages are relatively noncompliant, and neurally generated changes in nasal resistance are small (31); thus, various nonneural factors (e.g., mucosal congestion) may have a larger impact on the resistance of this part of the airway than neuromuscular changes (see, however, Ref. 32). Secondarily, increases in nasal resistance will increase the magnitude of the negative pressure generated in the pharynx. Similarly, changes in laryngeal resistance, which in contrast to the nose may be greatly affected by changes in neuromuscular activity (33), can increase or decrease the magnitude of the negative pressure in the pharyngeal portion of the airway. Importantly, the afferent information from receptors in the nose and larynx has more prominent reflex effects on upper airway muscle activity than that from pharyngeal receptors (see Ref. 34 for a review). Thus, the airway compartment where the obstruction is most likely to occur is flanked by less compliant compartments that provide important sensory information about the environment in the upper airway. Consistent with these considerations, sleep-related changes in the activity of pharyngeal and laryngeal dilator muscles have been studied most extensively, as is evident from the data presented in the next section.

B. Changes in Upper Airway Muscle Activity in Normal Subjects in Non-REM and REM Sleep

Table 1 lists 24 upper airway muscles, from the nares through the pharynx and larynx, relevant for the control of airway patency and gives the origin of their motor innervation, their presumed action on airway caliber, and their behavior during quiet wakefulness (W), non-REM sleep, and REM sleep. According to a commonly used convention, the sleep-related changes in the tone of individual upper airway muscles are described relative to the average tone observed during a period of quiet wakefulness preceding sleep. In normal subjects, this approach is limited by the often highly variable activity of some muscles during wakefulness and/or very low level of baseline activity that is difficult to quantify (e.g., Refs. 35–39). To overcome such limitations, recent studies have related the level of activity during different states of sleep to that generated during a maximal voluntary activation (e.g., Refs. 39,40). However, it should be noted that, although the average change in activity determined over several respiratory cycles in a given state may provide a rough measure of hypotonia and the probability of occurrence of an obstruction, a complete airway obstruction is a relatively abrupt event determined by the instantaneous changes in airway muscle activity and pressure gradients, rather than by the time average of muscle activity.

Table 1 shows that the muscles believed to act as dilators have been studied more extensively than constrictors and that the descriptive studies of upper airway muscle behavior across the sleep-wake cycle are far from complete. For certain muscles, this lack of information is due to their poor accessibility for recording. Many studies cited in the table report a decrement in upper airway muscle activity during non-REM sleep and a further decrement during REM sleep. However, for many muscles that have been studied repeatedly in humans and various animal species, there are quantitative and qualitative deviations from this trend, in that no change or an increase in activity is observed, rather than a decrease. In particular, for the genioglossus and posterior crycoarytenoid, a range of behaviors has been reported. No clear pattern of behavior can be identified among pools of muscles when they are grouped either according to the source of their motor innervation or the predominant pattern of respiratory modulation (inspiratory or expiratory).

These inconsistencies may be caused by differences in the ''control'' levels of tonic and respiratory-modulated activities in different studies, which depend, in part, on the route of breathing and subject position and are often manipulated in different experimental protocols (e.g., the level of sleepiness by sleep deprivation, and the respiratory drive by mechanical loading or chemical stimulation). Moreover, in all these studies, mechano- and chemoreceptor reflexes are fully operational, which may substantially modify the pattern of changes initiated centrally at the onset of different stages of sleep. The low baseline activity during wakefulness in normal individuals (e.g., Refs. 35,38,39) may also be an important source of inconsistencies, one that inflates the relative errors of the measurements. However, for the genioglossus, which consistently shows a measurable level of respiratory activity in wakefulness in the majority of studies, the results from normal subjects are still variable (Table 1). In contrast, there appears to be far less variability in the studies of OSA patients in whom the baseline activity is elevated (see Refs. 38,40 and Sec. II.B). Thus, either the disease itself makes upper airway activity drop more consistently during sleep or the elevated baseline activity in OSA patients during wakefulness is in itself an important factor.

C. Upper Airway Muscle Activity in OSA Subjects

Individuals with an anatomically compromised airway have a higher level of activity in their upper airway dilator muscles during wakefulness than normals (38,40,54, 63,64; see, however, Ref. 65). This compensatory increase is not maintained during sleep in humans and is only partly preserved in English bulldogs; consequently, the absolute magnitude of the sleep-related decrease in muscle activity, and increase in airway resistance, is higher in sleep apneics than in normals (38,40). This elevation of upper airway tone in OSA patients during wakefulness helps reveal a strongly suppressant effect of sleep on upper airway muscle activity. Simultaneous recordings

Table 1 Sleep-Related Changes in the Average Level of Activity in Upper Airway Muscles in Normal Subjects

Muscle name	Presumed action on upper airway (**bold = dilating action**)	Nucleus providing motor innervation	Pattern of waking activity	Change during NREM sleep	Change during REM sleep	Ref.
Alae nasi	**Widens nares**	VII	I + t	↓↓	↑↑ or ↓*	h: 31,41
			E + t	↓↓	I:↓, T:↓	r: 42
Tensor veli palatini	Moves **soft palate up** and posterior	V	t + I	↓ or ↓↓	↓↓	h: 36,38,43,44
Levator veli palatini	Moves **soft palate up**	V	I + t or silent	↓		h: 43,45
Palatopharyngeus	Moves soft palate down; pharynx up	XI				
Palatoglossus	Moves tongue up and posterior	XII	I + t	↓		h: 45
Styloglossus	Moves tongue up and posterior	XII				
Genioglossus	Moves **tongue down and anterior**	XII	I + t	↓ or = or ↑	↓ or = or ↓↓*	h: 28,36,38,40, 41,43,44,46–48
			I	↓	↓↓ or ↑	c: 49,50
			I	↓↓ or = ↓	↓↓	d: 153,187
			I		↓↓	g: 86,87
			I or I + t		↓↓	r: 55
Hyoglossus	Moves **tongue down** and posterior	XII				
Stylopharyngeus	Moves up and **widens pharynx**	IX				
Pharyngeal constrictors (eight muscles)	**Stiffen posterior pharyngeal wall**; reduce pharyngeal circumference; move hyoid bone posterior	Nucleus ambiguus (X)	E or silent I (uncharacteristic)	↓ or ↓↓	Silent or irregular	h: 43,39 r: 51
Digastric anterior	Moves **hyoid bone anterior**	VII	t		↓↓	c: 52

Digastric posterior	Moves hyoid bone posterior and lateral	V				
Geniohyoid	Moves **tongue down**; hyoid bone up	XII	I + t	↓↓	↑ or =	h: 5,53
Stylohyoid	Moves hyoid bone up and posterior	VII				
Mylohyoid	**Stiffens floor of the mouth**	V	E			
Omohyoid superior	Moves **hyoid bone down**	C_{1-3} via XII				
Thyrohyoid	Brings closer hyoid bone and thyroid cartilage	C_{1-3} via XII				
Sternohyoid	Moves **hyoid bone down**	C_{1-3} via XII	I I	↓	↑↑ = or ↓	d: 54 r: 51,55
Sternothyroid	Moves **thyroid cartilage down**	C_{1-3} via XII	I	↓	↓↓	r: 55
Posterior cricoarytenoid	**Abducts vocal folds**	Nucleus ambiguus (X)	I + post-I + t I + t I + t I + t	↓ ↓ = =	↓ ↑ ↓↓ ↓↓	h: 56 c: 49,57 l: 58 r: 59,60
Lateral cricoarytenoid	Adducts vocal folds	Nucleus ambiguus (X)	E		↓↓	r: 59,60
Arytenoid	Adducts vocal folds	Nucleus ambiguus (X)	E or I/E + t	↓↓	Silent or irregular	h: 35
Thyroarytenoid	Relaxes vocal folds	Nucleus ambiguus (X)	E + t I or silent E	↓↓ = = or ↓	Silent or irregular ↑ ↓↓	h: 61 l: 58 r: 60
Cricothyroid	Tenses vocal folds	Nucleus ambiguus (X)	I + t I + t I or I/E	= ↓ ↓	↑↑ ↑ I: ↓↓; E: ↓	h: 62 l: 58 r: 42, 59, 60

For each muscle, if available, data from sleep studies in humans are listed first, followed by data from normal, adult, chronically instrumented animals (h, human; c, cat; d, dog; g, goat; l, lamb; r, rat). Changes are described qualitatively relative to the average activity during quiet wakefulness. Symbols and abbreviations: =, no change; ↑ or ↓, small increase or decrease; ↑↑ or ↓↓, large increase or decrease; I, inspiratory; E, expiratory; I/E, phase-spanning; t, tonic; *, phasic REM sleep with intense eye movements.

of upper airway muscle activity and airflow consistently show that flow limitations and occlusions occur at the time when upper airway muscle activity reaches its nadir and that the lowest levels of activity occur during REM sleep (e.g., Refs. 1,66–68). One example is shown in Figure 2.

The neural basis of the increased upper airway motor tone during wakefulness in sleep apneics is not known. One hypothesis is that it is principally a reflex mechanism whereby airway mechanoreceptors sensitive to negative pressure are more strongly stimulated in an anatomically narrow than in a normal airway and provide a stronger reflex excitation to airway dilator motoneurons (38,40). Indeed, the required excitatory reflex pathways are present, and their physiology has been extensively studied (see Sec. III.B and Chap. 5). The observation that positive pressure applied to the upper airway results in a larger drop in the upper airway muscle activity of OSA patients than normal subjects has been interpreted as evidence that OSA patients have either a higher level of activity in upper airway receptors sensitive to negative pressure or a potentiated transmission along the reflex pathway from these receptors to airway dilator motoneurons (38,40). Alternative, or complementary, explanations of the increased level of activity in upper airway muscles in wakefulness in OSA patients are that: (1) the apparently stronger reflex action is secondary to adaptive changes resulting in an increased excitability of the motoneurons

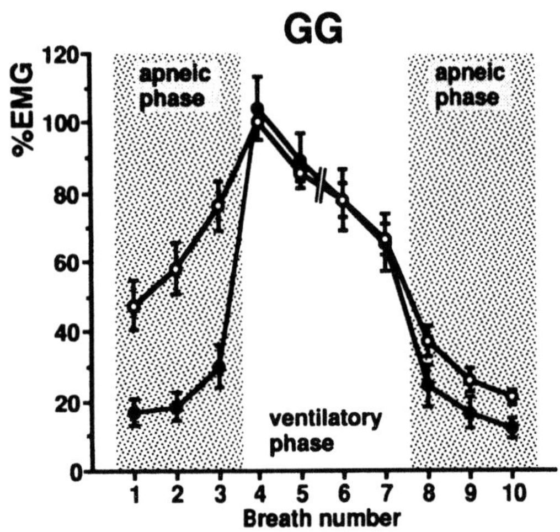

Figure 2 Average breath-to-breath changes in the peak magnitude of genioglossus muscle activity (%EMG) in a group of 12 OSA patients during transitions between obstructive episodes (shaded) and periods with patent airway. Open and filled circles represent data from non-REM sleep and REM sleep, respectively. The EMG magnitude is normalized relative to that during the first unobstructed breath following an obstructive episode during non-REM sleep. Note that apneic episodes coincide with periods of greatly reduced genioglossal muscle activity and that the nadir occurs during obstructive episodes in REM sleep. (From Ref. 67.)

innervating upper airway dilators; (2) an increased central drive is generated by what is referred to as a "wakefulness stimulus" (69,70) (see Sec. III.C for a discussion of its potential neural substrates); or (3) the perception of respiratory resistance leads to a compensatory increase in the tone of upper airway dilator muscles. The last two mechanisms would, by definition, not function during sleep, thus contributing to the larger sleep-related decreases in upper airway motor tone in OSA patients than in normals.

D. State-Dependent Changes in Upper Airway Motor Tone in Reduced Animal Models

Interpretation of the mechanisms leading to electromyographic and mechanical changes occurring with the sleep-wake cycle in instrumented intact humans and animals is complicated by a host of feedback loops provided by mechano- and chemoreceptor reflexes that generally are designed to maintain ventilation at a constant level with respect to metabolic rate, and the neuromechanical coupling between the actions of respiratory pump and upper airway muscles acting through the airway. A radical way to dissociate those peripheral interactions from central effects on upper airway activity is made possible by the use of animals with neuromuscular blockade and artificial ventilation with constant parameters. Such an approach has been extensively used in combination with a reversible pharmacological induction of the neural events characteristic of REM sleep (71,80–82). In those studies, a REM sleep-like postural atonia and depression of activity in upper airway and respiratory pump muscle motoneurons were produced in decerebrate, paralyzed, and artificially ventilated cats following pontine injections of carbachol, a cholinergic agonist, into a specific region of the dorsomedial pontine reticular formation. Since the baseline activity of many upper airway motoneuronal groups is often low and erratic at normocapnic levels in healthy animals and humans, an elevated end-expiratory CO_2 level and/or vagotomy (which releases upper airway motoneurons from tonic vagal inhibition) was utilized. Importantly, in these animals, both chemical and mechanical influences on respiratory output were kept constant, allowing an isolated assessment of the central effects of cholinergic stimulation in the pons on the activity of upper airway motoneurons.

That the changes in respiratory motoneuronal activity observed in this animal model have functional relevance for the changes occurring during natural REM sleep is supported by several lines of evidence:

1. In chronically instrumented, intact cats, carbachol injections into the same region of the pontine tegmentum produce a state having behavioral hallmarks typical of REM sleep, such as cortical desynchronization, hippocampal theta rhythm, eye movements (e.g., Refs. 72,73), and depression of upper airway muscle activity (74).
2. The extracellular level of endogenous acetylcholine increases in this pontine region in chronically instrumented, intact cats during both natural REM sleep (75) and the REM sleep-like state produced by carbachol (76).

3. In decerebrate cats and rats, where only selected signs of REM sleep can be recorded, pontine carbachol has the same effective sites as in chronic animals, and its injection results in postural atonia (77–79), eye movements (80), and a pattern of suppression of the activity of motoneurons innervating different respiratory pump and upper airway muscles similar to that in natural REM sleep in these species (71,81,82).
4. The activity of serotonin-containing neurons of the medullary raphe is suppressed following pontine carbachol injections in decerebrate cats (83), which is similar to the behavior of these cells in intact animals during REM sleep (84,85). Thus, pontine carbachol injections activate an important subset of those pontine mechanisms that are also activated during natural REM sleep.

Studies with the decerebrate cat, carbachol model demonstrate that the magnitude of the suppressant effects activated by cholinergic stimulation in the pons varies greatly among different pools of upper airway motoneurons (82). As shown in Figure 3, the activity of hypoglossal (XII) inspiratory-modulated motoneurons innervating the genioglossus and expiratory-modulated vagal motoneurons innervating the pharyngeal constrictors is almost abolished (depressed to 10–15% of the control activity level), whereas that of inspiratory and postinspiratory laryngeal motoneurons with axons in the recurrent laryngeal nerve are suppressed much less (to 75–80% of the control level). For laryngeal motoneurons, this result is qualitatively compatible with electromyographic studies of the cricothyroid muscle in chronically instrumented intact cats (57). The strong suppression of XII motoneurons is similar to the results of electromyographic studies in intact goats in which the baseline genioglossal activity was increased by hypercapnia or hypoxia (86,87) and in humans during phasic REM sleep (41,43). The suppression of vagal pharyngeal motoneurons is similar to that observed in pharyngeal constrictors in OSA patients (64). An important conclusion from these carbachol studies in decerebrate cats, in which compensatory reflexes from the periphery are eliminated, is that there is a centrally determined pattern of the suppressant effects exerted by pontine cholinergic mechanisms on the activity of different pools of upper airway motoneurons. Other studies in which the carbachol-injected, decerebrate cat model has been used to study the neurochemical mechanisms of the REM sleep-like depression of the activity of XII motoneurons are reviewed in Sec. III.C.

In addition to chronically instrumented, intact, and decerebrate animals, the ability of carbachol to produce REM sleep-like phenomena and respiratory changes has been recently studied in urethane-anesthetized rats (88,89). In contrast to the decerebrate models (71,81,82), in anesthetized rats one can simultaneously record respiratory muscle (or nerve) activity together with changes in cortical and hippocampal EEG. These observations show that the magnitude of the carbachol-induced decrease of genioglossal muscle activity is stronger when accompanied by suprapontine signs of REM sleep, such as cortical desynchronization and hippocampal theta rhythm (88,89). These results suggest that there is a distinct suppressant component

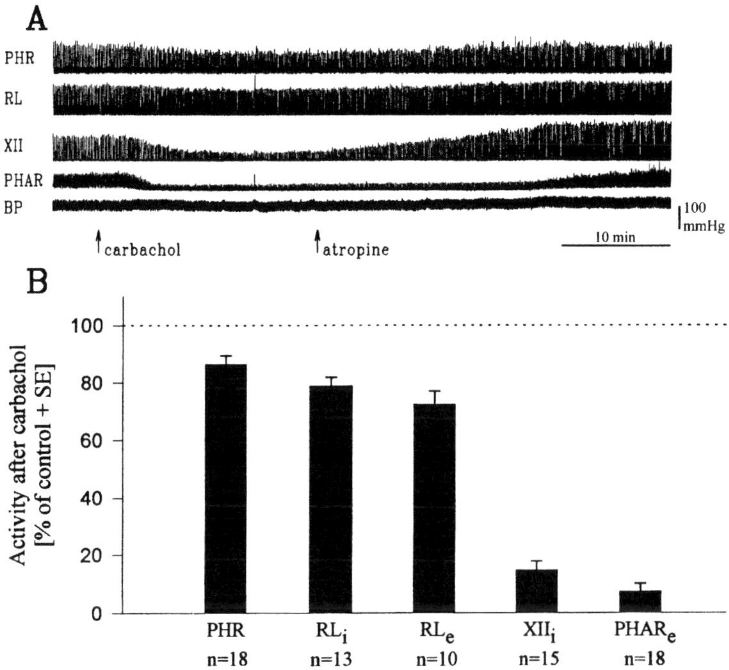

Figure 3 Stereotyped pattern of suppression of activity in respiratory motoneurons during the REM sleep–like atonia produced by a pontine injection of carbachol. (A) Continuous recording of moving averages of phrenic (PHR), recurrent laryngeal (RL), hypoglossal (XII), vagal pharyngeal (PHAR) nerves, and blood pressure (BP) during pontine injection of carbachol and subsequent reversal of the effect by pontine injection of atropine (injections at arrows). Note the small change in the magnitude of PHR and RL nerve activities and the strong decrements of the activities in the nerves innervating pharyngeal muscles (XII and PHAR). (B) Mean data from 10–18 carbachol injections expressed relative to the level of activity before carbachol (dashed line) in individual nerves. The inspiratory and expiratory components of RL nerve activity (RL_i and RL_e) were analyzed separately, and both were only moderately depressed in contrast to the large depression of the inspiratory component of XII and the expiratory component of PHAR activity. The measurements were obtained in paralyzed, vagotomized, and artificially ventilated decerebrate cats. Consequently, the observed pattern of depression of activity in upper airway motoneurons is not corrected by reflexes and reflects the central effects of cholinergic stimulation within the pontine REM sleep–triggering region. In particular, elimination of chemical feedbacks reveals a small depression of phrenic nerve activity, which is absent in spontaneously breathing animals (see Ref. 80). (Modified from Ref. 82.)

acting on genioglossal motoneurons associated with cortical desynchronization and/or theta rhythm. This is in addition to the suppression operating at the brainstem level in both decerebrate animals and those anesthetized rats in which carbachol does not produce electrocortical changes.

III. State-Dependent Changes in Distinct Drives to Upper Airway Motoneurons

The activity of upper airway motoneurons is not generated endogenously; rather, it is the net result of excitatory and inhibitory inputs (drives) that are synaptically transmitted to motoneurons from various premotor sources. The baseline activity of individual upper airway motoneurons and muscles often consists of two features: (1) a tonic component that is present continuously, regardless of the phase of the respiratory cycle; and (2) a phasic component that is bound to a particular portion of the respiratory cycle, such as inspiration, the postinspiratory period, or the late expiratory period. In different muscles, the tonic and phasic components are expressed to various degrees and with a pattern characteristic for the particular muscle. For example, the tensor veli palatini and digastricus muscles show only tonic activity, if any, under normocapnic conditions in wakefulness, but respiratory modulation appears when the respiratory drive is increased by hypercapnia or airway occlusion (36,38). In most upper airway muscles, however, the phasic respiratory and tonic components coexist; e.g., in the genioglossus, inspiratory modulation is superimposed on tonic activity under most conditions. In normal individuals, the peak level of this combined activity is only about 10–15% of the activity generated by maximal voluntary motor efforts involving the tongue (40). The presence of tonic and phasic components of activity in individual upper airway motoneurons demonstrates that the activity of these motoneurons is driven by both respiratory-modulated and tonic central neurons.

One important feature of inspiratory-modulated upper airway motoneurons that distinguishes them from motoneurons that innervate respiratory pump muscles is related to the mode in which their respiratory modulation is produced. In phrenic and intercostal motoneurons, most central respiratory neurons, and expiratory-modulated orofacial motoneurons, respiratory modulation results from a combination of excitatory inputs arriving to motoneurons during their active phase within the respiratory cycle and inhibitory inputs during their inactive phase (see Refs. 90,91). In contrast, intracellular recordings from inspiratory-modulated facial (92), laryngeal (93), and XII (91) motoneurons reveal little or no active phasic inhibition during expiration, i.e., their period of relative inactivity. This lack of reciprocal inhibition in inspiratory-modulated upper airway motoneurons is compatible with their involvement in multiple functions, some of which could be impaired by inhibition occurring during expiration. This feature may positively impact on the ability of upper airway motoneurons to respond with prolonged, tonic activation to various nonrespiratory inputs. Indeed, animal studies demonstrate that periods of activity spanning multiple respiratory cycles can be evoked in individual inspiratory-modulated upper airway motoneurons by brief laryngeal stimulation or chemical stimulation of the respiratory drive (e.g., Refs. 94,95).

In addition to central respiratory and tonic drives, upper airway motoneurons receive reflex drives, with those from central and peripheral chemoreceptors and mechanoreceptors of the respiratory tract being particularly important (see Refs. 15, 96–98 for reviews). These reflex drives are principally tonic, but the phasic nature of the mechanical events in the airway during respiration, and the transmission of these afferent inputs through central respiratory neurons, often make them phasic. Thus, central phasic respiratory, central tonic, and reflex drives represent three functionally distinct inputs to upper airway motoneurons, inputs that may be affected differently by changes in sleep-wake states and that can be separately analyzed (Fig. 4). The relative contribution of each of these three drives to the subthreshold excitability and activity (once the firing threshold is reached) probably varies in a systematic manner among motoneurons innervating different upper airway muscles. This may importantly determine the behavior of different muscles during sleep. Figure 4B–D shows, schematically, three distinct cases.

A. Changes in Central Respiratory Activity

The respiratory drive to the spinal respiratory motoneurons (diaphragm, intercostals, and abdominals) originates in two groups of medullary respiratory cells called the dorsal and ventral respiratory groups and, to some degree, from respiratory neurons of the parabrachial region of the pons (see Refs. 99–102 for reviews of the location of, and connections among, brainstem respiratory neurons). In contrast, little is known about the location and characteristics of those respiratory-modulated neurons that provide the respiratory drive to upper airway motoneurons. For XII motoneurons, inspiratory neurons with axonal projections to the XII motor nucleus are located within, and dorsomedial to, the ventral respiratory group, with some scattered in the reticular formation ventrolateral to the XII nucleus (103,104). This result agrees with anatomical studies in which cells projecting to orofacial motor nuclei were found to originate in this region (105–109). Thus, the ventral respiratory group and adjacent dorsomedial reticular formation are likely to be important sources of respiratory-modulated input to upper airway motoneurons. This is further supported by the presence of rhythmic respiratory activity in XII motoneurons in an in vitro medullary slice from neonatal rats (110). So far, however, no respiratory neurons with demonstrated connections with any of the upper airway motoneurons were studied across the natural sleep-wake cycle. Consequently, our predictions regarding the behavior of such neurons can be only interpreted from studies of respiratory premotor neurons for respiratory pump muscles, other respiratory neurons whose axonal targets remain unknown, and studies of respiratory neurons with identified axonal projections performed in reduced carbachol models of REM sleep–like changes in respiratory output.

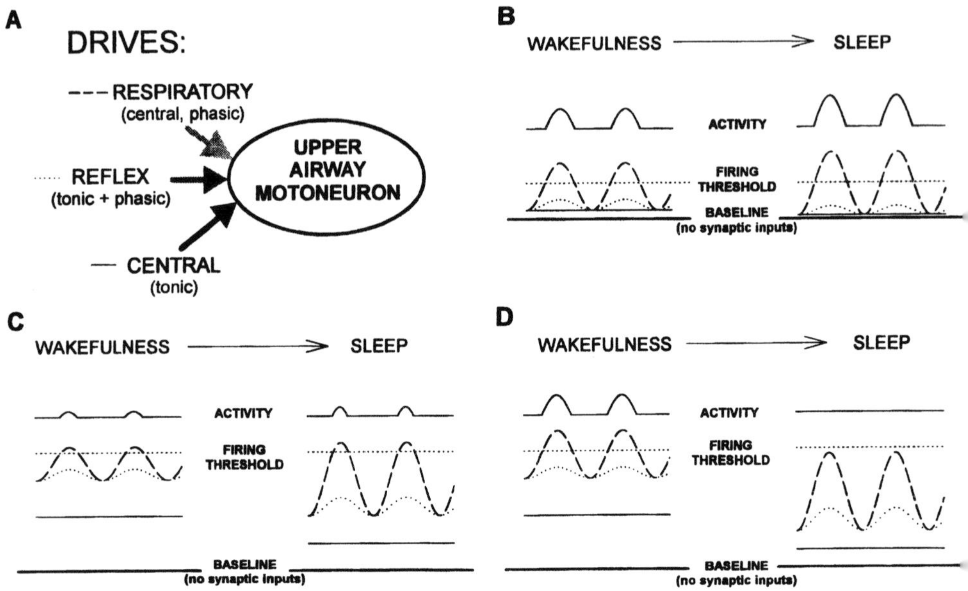

Figure 4 Schematic representation of sleep-related changes in three distinct inputs to upper airway motoneurons and their potential effects on motoneuronal activity. (A) The three distinct excitatory inputs discussed—respiratory, reflex, and central—are shown impinging on an upper airway motoneuron. The central input is tonic only, the reflex input consists of a phasic respiratory and (in C and D) tonic component, and the respiratory input is only phasic. The respiratory input is assumed to increase during sleep, either as a result of increased chemical drive during non-REM sleep or specific excitatory effects exerted on central respiratory neurons during REM sleep. (B–D) The three inputs are additive and depolarize the membrane potential of a motoneuron above the baseline; when membrane potential crosses the threshold, the activity shown in the top trace is evoked. (B) A motoneuron with a strong phasic respiratory, but weak central and reflex inputs during wakefulness. The increase in respiratory input during sleep more than makes up for the loss of the reflex and tonic drives, and the motoneuron becomes more active than during wakefulness. (C) A motoneuron with a moderate phasic respiratory, moderate reflex, and strong central tonic input during wakefulness. A large drop in the tonic input is compensated for during sleep by an increase in the respiratory and the phasic component of the reflex input, and the cell shows almost no change in activity. (D) A motoneuron with a strong phasic respiratory (similar to that in B) and also strong reflex and central inputs during wakefulness. In spite of a large increase in the respiratory input during sleep, the cell becomes silent because of the precipitous drop in the tonic drive. These examples illustrate how distinct inputs and their sleep-related changes may cause quantitatively and qualitatively different changes in the activity of different pools of upper airway motoneurons.

NREM Sleep

Studies in chronically instrumented cats by Orem and collaborators (111–113) and other groups (114–116) demonstrated that non-REM sleep is associated with a small or moderate reduction in the peak firing rate of inspiratory and expiratory neurons located in the region of the ventral respiratory group. In cells having a strong and stable respiratory activity, the average peak firing rate is reduced by 10–20%, and in about 5–15% of the cells there is an increase. The average magnitude of this reduction corresponds to the reduction in the tidal volume and may be also related to the prolonged respiratory cycle time characteristic of non-REM sleep (same number of action potentials over a longer period). In contrast to the strongly respiratory-modulated neurons, cells with a weak and variable respiratory modulation during quiet wakefulness have a relatively large sleep-related reduction in peak firing rate (112). The efferent connections of those neurons were not directly identified, but there can be little doubt that among those with strong respiratory modulation many were premotor to spinal respiratory motoneurons. The weakly respiratory-modulated cells, whose activity was strongly depressed during non-REM sleep, could be premotor to upper airway, respiratory pump motoneurons, or both. Alternatively, they could be upper airway motoneurons themselves or not functionally associated with any respiratory motor output and instead mediate the respiratory modulation of cardiovascular or other functions. Thus, there are relatively consistent decreases in the activity of medullary respiratory cells during non-REM sleep that are large only in neurons having a weak respiratory modulation. A subset of those cells may contribute to the decrements in the respiratory modulation of the activity of upper airway motoneurons and muscles described in Secs. II.B and II.C, provided that appropriate synaptic connections are present.

Many pontine parabrachial respiratory-modulated neurons change their firing rate when the animal enters non-REM sleep; increases or decreases in activity are observed with similar prevalence, with the average being a small decrease (117, 118). The parabrachial region gives origin to projections to the orofacial motor nuclei containing upper airway motoneurons (107,119–121), but interpretation of the sleep-wakefulness data is difficult without knowledge of the efferent connections of those neurons.

Thus, the small or moderate decrease in the activity of central respiratory neurons during non-REM sleep supports the conclusion that at least a part of the decrement in the activity of upper airway motoneurons during this state is caused by the withdrawal of respiratory drive to these motoneurons. The magnitude of this effect in different motoneuronal groups should depend on the relative contribution of the central respiratory and other drives to the excitability of the motoneurons of that particular group.

REM Sleep

In contrast to non-REM sleep, during REM sleep, the average level of activity of medullary respiratory neurons of the cat increases (122–124). This occurs on the background of the highly variable respiratory rhythm and tidal volume characteristic of this state. Thus, in individual respiratory cycles, respiratory cell activity may be much higher or much lower than the average. This variability at the respiratory neuronal level grossly correlates with the breath-to-breath changes in the magnitude of diaphragmatic activity and changes in tracheal pressure (123), which is expected because many of the medullary respiratory cells studied are probably the main source of respiratory drive to the respiratory pump muscles. Correlation of the cell firing rate with the intensity of ponto-geniculo-occipital (PGO) waves suggests that one excitatory component of the effects of REM sleep on medullary respiratory cell activity is related to the pontine networks generating those waves (122). An extrapolation based on this analysis also shows that, during a hypothetical period of REM sleep with no PGO waves (tonic REM sleep), respiratory neurons of the medulla are still under both excitatory and suppressant influences. Respiratory cycles with excited and suppressed respiratory neuronal activity tend to be clustered together, resulting in a quasi-rhythmic alteration between periods of enhanced and suppressed activity (123). Thus, during REM sleep, medullary respiratory neurons are subjected to a combination of excitatory and inhibitory influences whose individual magnitudes show rapid fluctuations. A cluster of several breaths with suppressed central respiratory activity may represent a period of high vulnerability to an obstructive or central apneic event. In addition, a mismatch in either the timing or strength of the central respiratory inputs to respiratory pump motoneurons with respect to upper airway motoneurons may contribute to the collapse of the upper airway due to inadequate muscular compensation for the effect of negative pressure in the airway (125).

The data from intact, chronically instrumented cats are supported by recordings obtained from reduced carbachol models of REM sleep-like changes in respiratory activity (Sec. II.D). In decerebrate cats, the peak firing rate of bulbospinal inspiratory and expiratory neurons of the ventral respiratory group shows, on the average, a moderate decrease following pontine injections of carbachol that produce REM sleep–like postural atonia. However, this decrease is disproportionately small compared to the simultaneously recorded decrements in phrenic, intercostal, and XII nerve activities (126). Moreover, about 20% of the cells increase their activity following pontine carbachol injections, even though the respiratory motor outputs are consistently depressed (71,82).

Similarly, disproportionately small decrements were observed in inspiratory neurons of the ventral respiratory group and adjacent reticular formation with axonal projections to the XII motor nucleus during pontine carbachol–induced decrements in XII nerve activity (104). In this study on urethane-anesthetized rats, XII nerve activity was reduced by 50% following pontine carbachol injections, whereas the peak cell activity decreased on the average by only 5%, and in some cells it increased. These results from a population of cells that are likely to be the source of inspiratory drive to XII motoneurons suggest that, similar to spinal respiratory motoneurons, the inspiratory drive to upper airway motoneurons is not appreciably reduced during REM sleep.

Thus, studies in naturally sleeping cats and in two carbachol models show that there are both excitatory and suppressant effects on central respiratory neurons during REM sleep. The relative magnitudes of these two effects may vary in individual neurons, and probably also with experimental conditions. Since reflex compensations do not occur in the reduced models, these studies unequivocally demonstrate that both excitatory and suppressant inputs impinging on brainstem respiratory neurons during the carbachol-induced, REM sleep–like atonia are generated centrally. The mismatch between the small suppression of central respiratory activity and the significantly larger decrements in the activity of both respiratory pump and upper airway motoneurons indicate that pathways other than respiratory must importantly contribute to the suppression of activity at the motoneuronal level.

Similar to medullary respiratory neurons, many pontine parabrachial respiratory and nonrespiratory neurons show prominent increases in activity during REM sleep (117,127). Cells showing either increases or decreases in activity during natural REM sleep behave similarly during the REM sleep–like state produced by pontine injections of carbachol in chronically instrumented, intact cats (118,127).

In summary, central respiratory drive rarely decreases during natural REM sleep, and, if it does, such decreases occur only intermittently and last a few respiratory cycles. Thus, although we can explain, at least in part, increments in upper airway motor tone during REM sleep on the basis of increases in the activity of central respiratory neurons, an explanation of the decrements seen in many muscles during this stage of sleep based on changes in respiratory activity (Secs. II.B and II.C) requires the assumptions that the synaptic transmission of the respiratory drive to upper airway motoneurons is itself modulated in a state-dependent manner and that such modulation is unevenly distributed among different pools of upper airway motoneurons (potential sources of such modulation are discussed in Sec. III.C). Without such an assumption, we must conclude that upper airway hypotonia during REM sleep is caused by changes in nonrespiratory inputs to upper airway motoneurons.

B. State-Dependent Changes in Reflexes

Important excitatory effects on upper airway dilator muscles originate from central and peripheral arterial chemoreceptors sensitive to changes in pH, P_{CO_2}, and P_{O2} and from receptors located in the upper airway that respond to changes in airway pressure, muscle tension, temperature, and various chemical stimuli. The reflex effects of chemoreceptors occur concurrently in upper airway and respiratory pump muscles, whereas at least certain aspects of reflex actions originating in upper airway receptors are more specifically concerned with the behavior of upper airway muscles. Recent studies of upper airway mechanoreceptor reflexes in humans have highlighted their importance in the maintenance of upper airway motor tone in OSA. These results need to be related to the extensive information about the physiology of airway receptor reflexes derived from studies in experimental animals (see Refs. 15,96,97 for reviews). Therefore, in this section, we will focus on reflexes from airway mechanoreceptors, rather than chemoreflexes. Additional information on this subject is presented in Chapter 5.

Airway Mechanoreceptors and Their Reflex Effects

Of the diverse types of receptors in the upper airway (see Refs. 96,97,128 for reviews), only a few show a slow adaptation to changes in intraluminar pressure suitable for mediating the tonic excitation that negative airway pressure imparts to airway motoneurons. These slowly adapting receptors are stimulated by both negative pressure and low-amplitude, high-frequency ($\pm$2.5 cmH_2O, 10–30 Hz) pressure vibrations like those generated in the airway during snoring (129). Interestingly, a subset of laryngeal and nasal (trigeminal) pressure receptors excited by negative pressure in the airway is also excited when upper airway muscles contract (130,131). Such receptors are called ''drive'' receptors because they are stimulated by a change in configuration of the soft tissue in the airway wall that results from muscular contraction. Thus, they behave as if they were functionally in series with the muscle fibers. The actual location of pressure and ''drive'' receptors within the airway tissue must be superficial, because both their activity and reflex effects on upper airway motoneurons are abolished by anesthetics applied to the airway mucosa (132,133). The apparent prevalence of receptors sensitive to both pressure and muscular contraction probably depends on the level of upper airway muscle tone; enhanced muscle tone, by increasing tissue tension, reduces the threshold for stimulation of receptors by small changes in either variable (129). Therefore, these receptors have a mechanism for the efferent control of their sensitivity to airway pressure changes. This may be particularly relevant for the reflex control of the upper airway in OSA patients. These patients have increased upper airway muscle activity and larger than normal changes in upper airway pressure occurring with the respiratory cycle and during intermittent obstructions.

The activity from those upper airway mechanoreceptors relevant for the reflex control of upper airway muscles is transmitted to the brainstem through the vagus (superior laryngeal branch carrying laryngeal primary sensory afferents), glossopharyngeal (pharynx), and trigeminal (nose) nerves. Although it is necessary to sever all three afferent pathways to abolish the excitatory effects of negative airway pressure on upper airway motoneurons (132,134,135), the most powerful effects originate from the laryngeal region (136). The principal site of central termination of upper airway afferents is the nucleus of the solitary tract, with additional projections to the trigeminal sensory nuclei. Details of the central pathways of reflexes from airway mechanoreceptors innervated by the vagus nerve have been reviewed recently (98). In addition to slowly adapting airway mechanoreceptors, the superior laryngeal nerve carries afferents from receptors of many other modalities that mediate reflexes that protect the airway from irritation and invasion by foreign particles. Electrical stimulation of such afferents inhibits the central respiratory rhythm and may activate coughing and/or swallowing (e.g., Refs. 34,33,137).

Application to the airway lumen of steady negative pressure or pressure oscillations similar to those seen during snoring produces a reflex enhancement of upper airway motoneuronal activity (e.g., Refs. 2,46,136,138–140). Accordingly, receptor unloading by application of positive pressure to the airway, neuromuscular paralysis or upper airway anesthesia reduces genioglossal EMG and XII nerve activity and increases upper airway resistance (132,139,141,142). Such studies demonstrate the presence of an endogenous reflex excitatory drive, presumably originating in the slowly adapting airway pressure receptors. In addition, it suggests that the laryngeal "drive" receptors may be a part of a positive feedback loop that operates between the receptors and upper airway dilator motoneurons, such that enhanced upper airway muscle activity leads to its further enhancement through activation of the appropriate reflex pathway. The higher the upper airway muscle tone, the greater the magnitude of this feedback. Such feedback should primarily involve laryngeal receptors and laryngeal muscles, but, based on what we know about reflexes from laryngeal mechanoreceptors, it will also affect the activity of pharyngeal muscles, as shown in Figure 5. In individuals with a compromised airway (Sec. II.B), this posi-

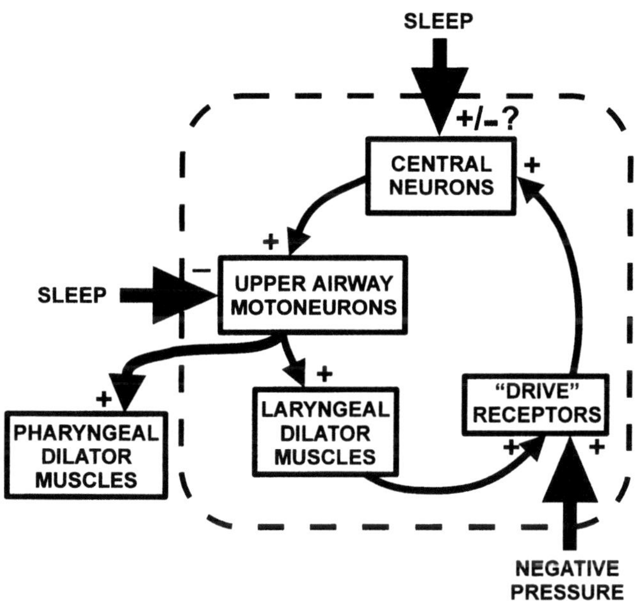

Figure 5 The block diagram of the excitatory reflex pathway between laryngeal "drive" receptors [excited by both negative airway pressure and laryngeal muscle contraction (124)] and upper airway dilators. The diagram emphasizes the positive feedback loop that may operate between the "drive" receptors and laryngeal muscles (enclosed in the dashed box). The functioning of this loop is subjected to the "external" modulatory influences of sleep (predominantly suppressant in motoneurons, and unknown at the level of central neurons transmitting afferent input from the receptors) and negative pressure in the airway. Pharyngeal dilators are also reflexly stimulated by the activity generated within this principally laryngeal reflex pathway. The positive feedback depicted in the diagram may result in an unstable or self-sustaining activity in upper airway dilators. This may be particularly relevant for upper airway control in OSA patients who have elevated upper airway motor tone during wakefulness.

tive feedback may both play an important role in preventing upper airway collapse and make the airway unstable and vulnerable to profound decrements in upper airway muscle tone in response to even small centrally or reflexly initiated decreases in motoneuronal activity. The latter may occur at sleep onset (6,143) or during decreases in the chemical drive to breathe, and may contribute to the observation that increases in upper airway resistance in response to hyperventilatory decrements in respiratory drive are larger in OSA patients than in normal subjects (32,144).

Increases in upper airway mechanoreceptor sensitivity resulting in an increased magnitude of the reflex excitatory effects of negative pressure on upper airway motoneurons can be also induced by aerosols of hypoosmolar solutions delivered to the airway (145,146). These responses may be secondary to the increases in upper airway muscle activity reflexly evoked by stimulation of laryngeal chemoreceptors (cf. Ref. 147). Although the latter receptors are primarily responsible for airway protective reflexes and/or gustatory sensation (34,97), their moderate stimulation may facilitate upper airway motor tone, thereby helping prevent airway obstructions.

In addition to the classical input-output relationships between receptors and effectors, laryngeal afferents are able to produce an increase in the activity of upper airway dilator motoneurons that substantially outlasts the duration of the stimulus. In experimental animals, application of negative pressure pulses to the airway enhances genioglossal EMG or XII nerve activity for a prolonged period (132,139,142). Henke and Sullivan (148) provide a record from an OSA patient in whom a brief period of oscillating pressure applied to the airway during REM sleep produced a prolonged increase of genioglossal EMG and resolution of the apnea with no evidence of arousal. A prolonged activation can be also produced in experimental animals by brief electrical stimulation of the superior laryngeal nerve (149,150). In the cat, the poststimulatory enhancement of XII nerve activity lasts several minutes (Fig. 6A) and occurs without changes in phrenic nerve activity, which distinguishes it from other forms of respiratory potentiation (reviewed in Ref. 151). One function of such a long-lasting poststimulatory enhancement may be to dampen rapid decrements in upper airway tone and thereby stabilize airway patency. Interestingly, however, the increase in XII nerve activity initiated by a brief stimulation of laryngeal afferents can be terminated (''reset'') by stimulation of lingual nerve afferents (Fig. 6B). This confirms the central nature of the enhancement phenomenon and reveals a potentially important ''negative'' contribution of trigeminal afferents to the control of upper airway motor excitability (152). Thus, stimulation of various upper airway receptors has both immediate and prolonged effects on upper airway motor tone. Application of oscillatory pressure stimuli to the airway during sleep represents an interesting and promising step toward taking advantage of these reflexes in the prevention and treatment of OSA (140,148,153).

Upper airway mechanoreceptor reflexes comparable to those in animals have been observed in awake humans. Application of negative pressure to the airway (154–162), high-frequency pressure oscillations (148), or airway occlusions (e.g., Refs. 28,158,163) produce reflex increases in the activity of upper airway muscles.

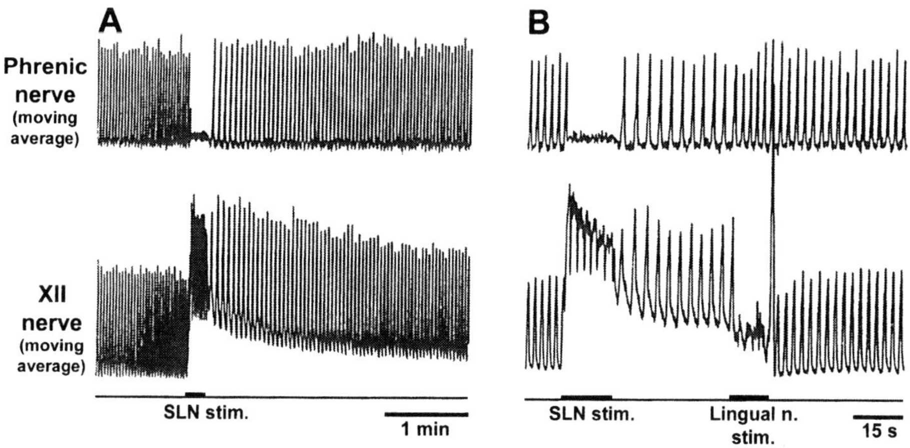

Figure 6 Stimulation of laryngeal afferents has excitatory effects on hypoglossal (XII) motoneurons that outlast the period of stimulation. (A) Compressed records of integrated activity of the phrenic and hypoglossal (XII) nerves before, during, and following electrical stimulation of the superior laryngeal nerve (SLN) with a ~15 s train of pulses. The tonic level and the magnitude of inspiratory modulation of XII nerve activity remain elevated beyond the period of stimulation and exponentially return toward the control over a period of several minutes, while the magnitude of phrenic nerve activity remains almost unchanged (except during the period of stimulation when it is abolished). Such a long-term potentiation of upper airway motor tone initiated by laryngeal afferents may have an important stabilizing effect on airway patency. (B) Another test with SLN stimulation in the same experiment, shown at a more expanded time scale. A brief train of stimuli was applied to the lingual nerve 11 respiratory cycles after the termination of SLN stimulation. The enhancement of XII nerve activity produced by SLN stimulation is ''reset'' by lingual nerve stimulation. Thus, the level of activity in XII motoneurons can vary greatly due to opposing influences exerted by SLN and lingual nerve afferents. (From Ref. 152.)

These responses are predictably reduced following anesthesia of superficial receptors of the glottic, pharyngeal, and nasal airway (160,164). In OSA patients, upper airway anesthesia also attenuates the increase in genioglossal muscle activity occurring during obstructive events in non-REM sleep (165). The magnitude of the reflex excitatory effects of negative pressure in individual airway muscles depends on the route of respiration (e.g., Refs. 135,158,163) and the phase of the respiratory cycle (162).

When short pulses of negative pressure are applied to the airway in wakefulness, the shortest latency of the excitatory response evoked in the genioglossus is compatible with a reflex pathway contained within the lower brainstem and involving few central relay neurons (156,162,166). Thus, there can be little doubt that reflex pathways similar to those described in anesthetized animals are responsible for the observed effects. One caveat with studies in awake subjects, however, is that the central pathways mediating the effects of airway receptors may be more complex than those activated in anesthetized animals and may include components activated by the conscious sensation of the stimulus and/or transmitted centrally by neurons in the reticular formation that are active during wakefulness but silent and unresponsive to sensory stimuli during anesthesia and some stages of sleep. The application of negative pressure stimuli to the mouth in awake humans produces a complex cortical evoked potential whose earliest component has a latency similar to that of the excitation evoked in the genioglossus (167). Thus, the initial portion of the genioglossus response produced during wakefulness is unlikely to be behaviorally controlled, but its later components may have a behavioral contribution or be modified by the conscious sensation of the stimulus. Presumably, any such behavioral contributions would be markedly attenuated during sleep.

Sleep-Dependent Modulation of Upper Airway Reflexes

Even though selected reflexes from upper airway mechanoreceptors have properties that make them suitable for playing a prominent role in the control of upper airway tone, their role in preventing upper airway hypotonia during sleep in OSA patients is controversial. Some studies in awake OSA patients suggest that the reflexes are blunted (159), whereas others identify them as a major mechanism that maintains airway patency (see Ref. 18 and Chap. 5 for reviews). Such differences in results and interpretations can be reconciled only by more studies using comparable protocols.

The questions of whether, and by what mechanisms, upper airway mechanoreceptor reflexes are reduced during sleep in either normal subjects or OSA patients are unanswered. An attenuation may occur at each of the three components of a reflex arc—the receptors, central pathways, and effectors. Regarding the latter, the transmission in the entire reflex pathway will be attenuated, or entirely blocked, when motoneurons become inactive (see Fig. 4D). Thus, motoneurons may act as a filter having a high threshold for the incoming excitatory inputs, while transmission in the afferent limb and the central portion of the reflex pathway may be unaltered. Another level where sleep-related attenuations of reflex transmission may occur in the case of "drive" receptors is the receptor itself, because the activity of these receptors may be reduced secondarily to decrements in the tone of upper airway muscles (see Fig. 5). Like the filtering at the motoneuronal level, the functioning of this mechanism would result from the centrally produced decrements in the excitability of upper airway motoneurons and the resulting decrements in muscle tension. Reflex transmission may be also attenuated due to saturation of activity at either the receptor or the motoneuronal level, but this is unlikely to occur in sleep. An exception to this may be the period just preceding the arousal caused by a severe obstructive event, which may be associated with extreme activation of airway receptors and upper airway motoneurons.

Of the three levels where attenuation in reflex transmission during sleep may occur, the role of central pathways is the most interesting and complex. Reflex transmission may be altered by changes in state through mechanisms such as presynaptic modulation of transmitter release or postsynaptic changes in the excitability of central relay neurons. Since several brainstem neuronal groups (discussed in the next section) show sleep state–dependent changes in activity, have widespread projections within the brainstem, and target neurotransmitter receptors that may be located either pre- or postsynaptically, there is ample potential for central modulation of reflex transmission in a state-dependent manner.

Electrophysiological and neuropharmacological studies indicate that afferent pathways to XII motoneurons may be modulated presynaptically (168–170), albeit the evidence comes from in vitro studies in which the functional identity of the afferent pathway studied cannot be identified and sleep does not occur. In cats, during REM sleep but not non-REM sleep, reflex transmission from trigeminal tooth pulp afferents to second-order trigeminal sensory neurons is suppressed by pre- and/or postsynaptic mechanisms according to some studies (171,172), but another study reported an average increase in both non-REM and REM sleep (173). There is also evidence that the transmission remains unchanged or becomes facilitated during REM sleep in spino-thalamic and spino-cerebellar neurons (174,175). Similarly, the tactile receptive fields and response magnitudes of a majority of spinal dorsal horn neurons are increased (176), and intracellularly recorded monosynaptic excitatory postsynaptic potentials in lumbar motoneurons are larger during REM sleep than in either non-REM sleep or wakefulness (177).

Although some attenuation during either non-REM sleep, REM sleep, or both of various reflexes relevant for respiratory control has often been reported (reviewed in Refs. 178,179), it is usually not possible to distinguish between a genuine state-dependent suppression of reflex transmission occurring centrally and the attenuation that is secondary to a reduced excitability of motoneurons. For example, the average diaphragmatic response to airway occlusion is reduced during REM sleep when compared to non-REM sleep, but an analysis of the breath-to-breath variability of the magnitude of this effect shows that this is an intermittent, and not a tonic, phenomenon (180). Its occurrence may follow the clustering of respiratory cycles with depressed diaphragmatic effort and reduced activity of central respiratory neurons discussed in the preceding section. This type of reflex suppression is related to certain phasic aspects of REM sleep phenomena, rather than to the neural mechanisms maintaining this state. It appears that studies using respiratory timing and/or diaphragmatic activity (whose average magnitude is relatively insensitive to sleep influences) as an output variable show relatively small effects of sleep on reflex transmission. For example, negative pressure pulses applied to the airway during expiration produced similar reflex prolongation of expiration in wakefulness and non-REM sleep, with a small attenuation of this response occurring during REM sleep (137). Similarly, the CO_2 threshold for the resumption of rhythmic respiratory activity does not change across the states of non-REM sleep, REM sleep, and wakefulness (181,182), and the ventilatory sensitivity to CO_2 is the same during NREM sleep and wakefulness in goats (87,183). In one study, apneas and bradycardias in response to instillation of water or inflation of a balloon in the larynx were more pronounced during REM than non-REM sleep when arousal did not occur, whereas arousals themselves were more likely to occur in non-REM than in REM sleep (184). In another study, the latency to the first swallow in response to esophageal acidification was shorter in wakefulness than in non-REM or REM sleep, but within sleep the arousal following esophageal acidification occurred with shorter latency during REM than during non-REM sleep (185). Thus, the stages of sleep may have a differential effect on the arousal threshold and cardiorespiratory reflexes from the larynx. It is also possible that the sleep-related suppression of reflex transmission targets only selected afferent pathways.

With regard to reflex responses to airway negative pressure in upper airway muscles, the data are conflicting. Most studies show that these reflexes remain present, albeit attenuated, in the genioglossal muscle activity during non-REM sleep, or both non-REM and REM sleep, in chronically instrumented animals (153,186,187), normal humans (148,188), and OSA patients (148,189). Upper airway receptors also importantly contribute to arousal from both non-REM and REM sleep (190–195), thus showing that sensory modalities from the upper airway are being transmitted and sensed centrally. One group concluded, however, that the sensory input from the upper airway makes a negligible contribution to arousal in severe snorers and OSA patients (196,197), and in a few studies the genioglossal muscle response to negative pressure was nearly abolished during non-REM sleep (154,157,166). Paradoxically, in one study in normal humans, the genioglossus excitatory response to an inspiratory resistive load was absent during wakefulness, but present during NREM sleep (36).

In summary, despite some discrepancies in the experimental results, reflexes from airway mechanoreceptors probably play an important role in maintaining the activity of upper airway motoneurons during both sleep and wakefulness. Their magnitude varies with changes in the sleep-wake cycle as a result of both state-dependent changes in other central drives to upper airway motoneurons and sleep-specific central processes that may modulate transmission in selected reflex pathways. On the top of this, OSA itself may lead to distinct alterations in reflex transmission occurring at the receptor, central pathway, and/or effector level. To study and interpret the latter, we need a better understanding of the mechanisms underlying the state-dependent modulation of the transmission of the relevant reflexes in normal experimental animals and human subjects.

C. Changes in Central Tonic Drives

Several distinct neuronal groups in the pontomedullary reticular formation have predictable and well-characterized changes in activity with the sleep-wake cycle and anatomically proven connections with upper airway motoneurons. For some of these neuronal groups, the neurotransmitters that they utilize in communicating with their postsynaptic targets are also known. Of these, the level of activity in serotonin (5-HT)- and norepinephrine (NE)-containing neurons of the brainstem decreases during non-REM and even more so during REM sleep (198–200). In contrast, pontine acetylcholine (ACh)-containing and other neurochemically unidentified neurons of the ponto-medullary reticular formation selectively increase their activity during REM sleep (or during both REM sleep and wakefulness), while their activity is lowest during non-REM sleep (201–204; see Refs. 205–208 for reviews). Consequently, one would expect that, if selected brainstem neurons excite upper airway motoneurons and have sleep-related decreases in activity, this excitation would be withdrawn during sleep. Such a mechanism is called disfacilitation. On the other hand, those neurons having increased activity during sleep may contribute to decrements in upper airway motor activity through the mechanism of sleep state-specific inhibition. The evidence for these two modes of state-dependent effects is reviewed in the following sections.

Sleep-Related Withdrawal of Excitatory Drives (Disfacilitation)

Both 5-HT- and NE-containing afferent fibers abound in the upper airway motor nuclei (209–214), and the net effect of applying either transmitter onto orofacial, including upper airway, motoneurons is excitation (215–223), even though both amines may act through numerous receptor subtypes, of which only some produce excitatory effects (see Refs. 224–228 for reviews of NE and 5-HT receptor classification and pharmacology).

Raphe Neurons: Role of Serotonin, Thyrotropin-Releasing Hormone, and Substance P

The serotonergic input to upper airway motoneurons originates in the pallidus, obscurus, and parapyramidal nuclei of the medullary raphe (120,121,229–232). These neurons, distributed along the midline of the medulla and physiologically identified as 5-HT-containing neurons using well-established criteria (83,233), are most active during wakefulness, slightly decrease their activity during non-REM sleep, and then show a dramatic decrease at the onset of, and throughout, REM sleep (84,85). Indeed, the REM sleep–related decreases in the activity of caudal medullary raphe neurons appear to be more profound than those in pontine and more rostral medullary raphe cells (see Fig. 16 in Ref. 198). Thus, a significant portion of their excitatory input to upper airway motoneurons may be withdrawn, particularly during REM sleep.

The excitatory effects of 5-HT onto upper airway motoneurons are mediated by more than one type of receptor and through several cellular mechanisms. The excitatory effects mediated by 5-HT_2 receptors are the best documented (both 2A and 2C subtypes are probably involved). These receptors are present in high concentrations in orofacial motor nuclei, as demonstrated by receptor autoradiography (234), receptor immunohistochemistry (235,236), and the presence of the corresponding receptor mRNA (237–239). Functional pharmacological studies also show that the excitation of orofacial motoneurons is mediated by more than one 5-HT_2 receptor subtype (219,220,240). 5-HT_2 receptors are coupled to phosphoinositol second messenger systems and increase motoneuronal activity by directly (postsynaptically) depolarizing the membrane through closure of K^+ channels and opening other cation channels. The two mechanisms have different dynamic properties and can be pharmacologically dissociated (219).

Pharmacological antagonism of 5-HT$_2$ receptors leads to a significant decrement in upper airway motor tone in animal models having increased upper airway activity. This was observed in decerebrate cats in which XII nerve activity was initially enhanced by vagotomy and hypercapnia (220), and in English bulldogs (241), where the geniohyoid EMG is elevated, compared to normal dogs, in association with the anatomically narrowed upper airway that is characteristic of this breed (242). In both studies, the reductions in activity following methysergide, a broad-spectrum 5-HT antagonist, were about 50%. Importantly, in the cat studies, the serotonergic antagonists were injected directly into the XII nucleus, demonstrating that a major portion of the endogenous serotonergic excitatory action is exerted within the nucleus, rather than at other premotor sites (220). The neural nature of this endogenous drive was further supported in the cat by microdialysis studies in which the extracellular level of 5-HT in the XII nucleus region decreased during both the carbachol-induced REM sleep–like atonia and pharmacological inhibition of the activity of 5-HT-containing cells (243). In addition, serotonergic neurons in the medullary raphe having axonal projections to the XII nucleus were silenced during the carbachol-induced XII nerve atonia (83). In the same animal model, the injection of 5-HT into the XII nucleus significantly attenuated the carbachol-induced depression of XII nerve activity (244) (Fig. 7). The magnitude of this effect was compatible with the reduction of the spontaneous XII nerve activity produced by serotonergic antagonists and corresponded to about half of the magnitude of suppression of XII nerve activity produced by pontine carbachol (244). Thus, the withdrawal of serotonergic excitatory effects mediated by 5-HT$_2$ receptors makes an important, although only a partial, contribution to the carbachol-induced decrement in XII nerve activity; other mechanisms must also play a role. Based on these studies, enhancing the serotonergic excitation of upper airway motoneurons during sleep could be of therapeutic value in OSA patients, especially if one were able to control the time and site of delivery of appropriate drugs in a manner that avoids their side effects on the sleep-wake cycle and behavior. Attempts to enhance the level of central 5-HT by reuptake blockers or L-tryptophan administration have so far yielded mixed results (245,246). Pharmacological approaches to the treatment of OSA are further discussed in Chapter 24.

In addition to 5-HT$_2$ receptors, ligand binding and/or mRNA studies demonstrate the presence of other 5-HT receptors, such as 5-HT$_{1A}$, 5-HT$_{1B}$, and 5-HT$_3$, in the XII (239,247–249) and other orofacial motor nuclei (e.g., Refs. 249–251). Of those, stimulation of 5-HT$_{1A}$ receptors by systemic administration of a selective agonist has complex effects on motor activity (e.g., Ref. 240). However, in adult animals there are no obvious functional effects on the activity of orofacial motoneurons when 5-HT$_{1A}$ agonists are applied directly onto motoneurons (219,220, 240,252,253), and there is no evidence for the presence of 5-HT$_{1A}$ receptor protein (254) or mRNA (239) in upper airway motor nuclei. [5-HT$_{1A}$ receptors and their mRNA are present in XII motoneurons of neonatal rats, but the expression of these

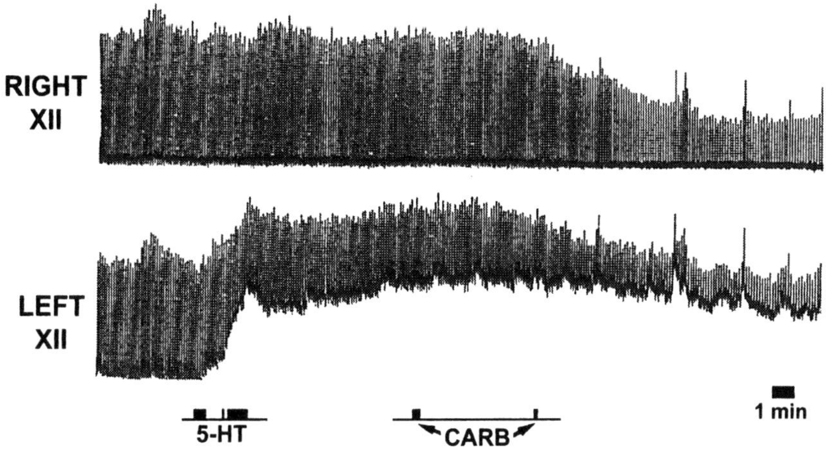

Figure 7 Stimulation of hypoglossal (XII) motoneurons with serotonin (5-HT) counteracts the depression of their activity during the REM sleep–like atonia produced by a pontine injection of carbachol. The activity of the right and left XII nerves was simultaneously recorded in a decerebrate, paralyzed, and artificially ventilated cat. The activity of the left nerve was initially enhanced by a microinjection of 5-HT into the left XII nucleus (at the marker). 5-HT enhanced the activity on one side only, indicating that the action of the drug was contained within one XII nucleus. Subsequently, two successive injections of carbachol into the pons produced the characteristic, REM sleep–like, depression of XII nerve activity, especially on the right side. However, the decay of the tonic level of the left XII nerve activity (bottom of the trace) is very small. (From Ref. 244.)

receptors decreases considerably by postnatal day 28, and 5-HT$_{1A}$ receptor agonists no longer modulate XII motoneuronal firing behavior in vitro (255) in agreement with in vivo studies in adult animals (252).]

In contrast to 5-HT$_{1A}$ receptors that disappear from the XII nucleus in mature animals, 5-HT$_{1D}$ receptors located within the XII nucleus are active in both neonatal and adult rats. Their stimulation is associated with either net enhancement (168) or reduction (170,252) of the excitability of XII motoneurons. Since in other systems these receptors are often localized presynaptically, where they modulate the release of various transmitters from axon terminals, the direction and magnitude of their effect may depend on the set of afferent pathways to motoneurons that are active under the given experimental conditions. The receptors may be also located postsynaptically on XII motoneurons, as suggested by high abundance of their mRNA in the XII nucleus (239). In anesthetized rats and decerebrate cats, microinjection of a 5-HT$_{1B}$ agonist onto XII motoneurons results in a moderate suppression (about 20%) of XII nerve activity (252; our unpublished observations). Extrapolation of these results to sleep states, when 5-HT-containing neurons have reduced firing rates, suggests that a reduced stimulation of 5-HT$_{1B}$ receptors located within the XII nucleus could lead to a moderate enhancement of XII motoneuronal activity. The magnitude of this effect is less than the reduction in spontaneous XII nerve activity produced by antagonism of the endogenous excitatory effects mediated primarily by 5-HT_2 receptors (220). No information is available on the function of the 5-HT_3 receptors present in the XII and other upper airway motor nuclei (239,249,250).

Serotonergic neurons have very extensive axonal projections within the brainstem (256). Thus, the sleep-wake cycle variations in the release of 5-HT may affect upper airway motor tone by acting not only on motoneurons but also at numerous premotor sites. In particular, serotonergic terminals, receptors and/or functional effects of 5-HT have been demonstrated in medullary respiratory neurons (257) and central viscerosensory nuclei mediating upper airway reflexes (251,258,259).

In contrast to orofacial motoneurons, the net effect of 5-HT on medullary respiratory neurons is inhibitory (260,261); the inhibition is due, at least in part, to a direct action mediated by 5-HT_{1A} receptors on inspiratory (262) and expiratory neurons (263). Some expiratory, postinspiratory, and inspiratory neurons may be also excited by 5-HT (260,264,265), presumably through 5-HT_2 receptors. The predominance of inhibitory effects suggests that the sleep-related decrement in the activity of brainstem serotonergic cells will lead, on the one hand, to the withdrawal of a direct serotonergic excitatory input to upper airway motoneurons and, on the other hand, to the withdrawal of serotonergic inhibition that is exerted on their respiratory premotor neurons (Fig. 8). Through such a dual action of 5-HT during sleep, the central respiratory drive to motoneurons would be enhanced at the same time that the direct serotonergic excitation of motoneurons is withdrawn. Thus, an increase in respiratory drive may compensate, to some extent, for the decrease in tonic drive. This is schematically illustrated in Figure 4C. Although most individual components of this scheme have been reported, the presence of endogenous inhibitory effects of 5-HT on respiratory neurons remains to be demonstrated and its magnitude measured.

Microinjection of 5-HT into the XII nucleus did not change the response of XII motoneurons to negative pressure pulses applied to the upper airway of decerebrate cats (266), suggesting that the transmission of this particular reflex is not modulated by 5-HT at the motoneuronal level. However, there are serotonergic projections to brainstem viscerosensory nuclei that transmit afferent information from upper airway receptors (e.g., Refs. 251,258,259). In particular, serotonergic medullary raphe neurons with projections to the nucleus of the solitary tract decrease their activity during carbachol-induced atonia (83). Thus, the potential for sleep-related serotonergic modulation of transmission of upper airway reflexes is present, although the specific neuroanatomical and neuropharmacological substrates of such modulation await investigation.

In addition to 5-HT, serotonergic neurons contain, and may co-release from their axon terminals, various combinations of amino acid (glutamate, GABA) and peptide transmitters, including thyrotropin-releasing hormone (TRH) and substance P (SP) (267–270). Both SP- and TRH-containing terminals (271–276) and SP and TRH receptors (248,277,278) are present within orofacial motor nuclei, and both

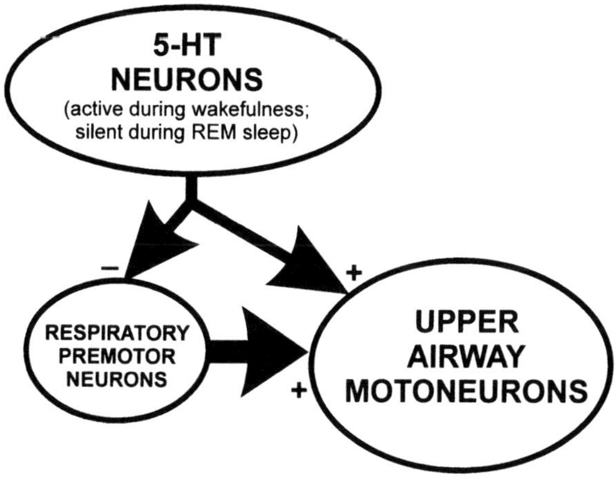

Figure 8 Serotonin (5-HT) has predominantly excitatory (+) effects on upper airway motoneurons, whereas it is predominantly inhibitory (−) to medullary respiratory neurons, some of which are the source of respiratory drive to upper airway motoneurons (premotor neurons). This diagram shows how sleep-related decrements in the activity of 5-HT-containing neurons may simultaneously lead to the withdrawal of tonic serotonergic excitation at the motoneuronal level (disfacilitation) and enhancement of the respiratory drive relayed to the motoneurons through their premotor respiratory neurons. The relative contribution of these two opposite actions of 5-HT may vary among different pools of upper airway motoneurons. Consequently, during sleep, motoneurons with weak respiratory and strong tonic (serotonergic) drive will be suppressed, whereas those with a strong respiratory and weak tonic drive may have no change or even an increase in activity.

peptides are excitatory to upper airway motoneurons (279–284). Since it has been proposed that the release of peptides from the axon terminals of raphe neurons may require higher levels of activity than does the release of 5-HT (285) and that complex pre- and postsynaptic interactions may take place among the co-released transmitters and peptides at the site of their release (286,287), it is not known under what conditions TRH and SP can have endogenous excitatory effects on upper airway motoneurons. Appropriate studies with antagonists have not been performed due to the lack of suitable pharmacological tools. The firing rate of caudal raphe cells increases by 50–100% above the 1–4 Hz typically seen during quiet wakefulness in association with strong motor and respiratory efforts; in some cells, the firing behavior becomes less regular and shows a phasic pattern temporally related to rhythmic movements (288). This raises the possibility that TRH and/or SP are released around the time of enhanced respiratory effort; e.g., during the arousals caused by airway occlusion. The powerful effects of these peptides when applied exogenously onto upper airway motoneurons warrant more research and suggest therapeutic potential.

Most considerations regarding the effects of 5-HT and other transmitters released by neurons having sleep-wake–dependent activity focus on the qualitative nature of their effects. However, at least for the raphe system, both neuroanatomical and neurophysiological data show that substantial differences exist in the density of the innervation of, and magnitude of the serotonergic effects on, different motoneuronal pools. These differences are of interest because they may be related to the differences in the effect of sleep on different upper airway muscles (Secs. II.B and II.D). In the XII nucleus, serotonergic terminals are more frequently closely apposed to the distal dendrites than to the proximal dendrites or cell bodies of XII motoneurons (149,210); the same was observed for TRH-containing terminals (273). In addition, the overall density of 5-HT or TRH terminals, including those likely to make synaptic contacts with motoneurons, was higher in the vicinity of laryngeal than XII or facial motoneurons (214,273). One interpretation of these data is that 5-HT and TRH are likely to exert stronger effects on laryngeal than other orofacial motoneurons. In support of this, the duration of the excitatory postsynaptic potentials produced in trigeminal masseter and mylohyoid motoneurons by electrical stimulation within the medullary raphe positively correlated with the density of serotonergic innervation (289), and the magnitude of the effect of iontophoretically applied 5-HT on masseter and digastric motoneurons was proportional to the density of serotonergic terminals in the corresponding portions of the trigeminal motor nucleus (217). However, another study designed to compare the sensitivity to iontophoretically applied 5-HT between XII and laryngeal motoneurons reported that, relative to their control firing rates, XII motoneurons were excited more strongly than laryngeal motoneurons (223). In addition, a comparison of the absolute increases in firing rate showed that the excitatory effect developed faster in XII than laryngeal motoneurons (223). Such results could not be predicted on the basis of the anatomical measures of the densities of the serotonergic innervation of the compared motoneuronal pools; they did, however, correlate with the stronger suppression of XII than laryngeal motoneurons observed in the same animal model following pontine injections of carbachol (Sec. II.D), and with most observations of the behavior of the corresponding upper airway muscles during natural REM sleep (Secs. II.B and II.C). One reason for the discrepancy between the density of synaptic contacts and the magnitude of the pharmacological effect of 5-HT is the presence of high densities of 5-HT terminals in the XII and other orofacial motor nuclei that do not make identifiable synaptic contacts and, therefore, may participate in what is called ''volume transmission'' (290). In this type of transmission, transmitters are released into the extracellular space and must diffuse much larger distances to reach their receptors than is the case in a classical synapse. Such ''free'' 5-HT terminals may account for about 75% of the serotonergic innervation of the XII nucleus (210), compared with less than 25% of such terminals on trigeminal motoneurons (291). Since axon terminals with no synaptic specializations were so numerous, volume transmission appears to be the prevalent form of serotonergic transmission in the XII motor nucleus. This would be consistent with 5-HT playing a role of a global, state-dependent modulator of the excitability of XII motoneurons, with only a small fraction of 5-HT terminals engaged in spatially selective actions through classical synapses.

Norepinephrine

Similar to serotonergic neurons, brainstem norepinephrine (NE)-containing cells have gradually decreasing firing rates with the progression from active wakefulness to REM sleep (199,200) and project to orofacial motoneurons (120,121,212, 213,292). NE has a net excitatory effect on upper airway motoneurons (219,221,284, 293,294). One caveat here is that our predictions regarding the sleep-state dependence and other behaviors of NE-containing neurons are largely based on the comprehensive studies of locus coeruleus neurons, especially in rats where they form a compact and highly homogeneous neuronal group (see Refs. 295,296 for reviews). However, noradrenergic projections to orofacial motoneurons originate primarily from the pontine reticular formation ventral to the locus coeruleus (locus subcoeruleus, the pontine parabrachial region, and the A5 group), rather than the locus coeruleus itself (107,120,121,211,292). Thus, although there is evidence that the activity of subcoeruleus NE-containing neurons also decreases during sleep (200), such studies are far less extensive than those of 5-HT containing neurons, and assumptions that the effects of NE on upper airway motoneurons vary with the sleep-wake cycle must be made cautiously.

Like 5-HT, the effects of NE on upper airway motoneurons may be exerted through multiple receptors located either postsynaptically on the motoneurons or presynaptically, on interneurons or afferent pathways to the motor nuclei. Postsynaptic excitatory effects are probably mediated by α_1- and/or β-adrenoceptors (294,297). mRNA for all α_1-adrenoceptor subtypes (α_{1A}, α_{1B}, α_{1D}) and binding sites for β-adrenoceptors are present in the orofacial motor nuclei, although the latter receptors may be largely located on astrocytes (298–301). Presynaptic effects may be mediated by α_2-adrenoceptor subtypes, which suppress the release of various endogenous transmitters (302,303); therefore, the direction of their effect will depend on the nature of the affected afferent pathway. α_2-Adrenoceptors may also be located postsynaptically on motoneurons (297). The effect of α_2-adrenoceptor agonists applied to the XII nucleus region in vitro is an inhibition of XII nerve activity (304), but the effect decreases with development (303). In situ hybridization and immunohistochemical studies show that of the three α_2-adrenoceptor subtypes (α_{2A}, α_{2B}, α_{2C}), only the α_{2C} adrenoceptor subtype is present in upper airway motor nuclei in sizable amounts (305–307). Thus, the excitatory effects of NE on upper airway motoneurons are likely to be mediated by α_1- and β-adrenoceptors, whereas α_2-adrenoceptors may exert more prominent role at various premotor sites, including those relevant for the control of respiratory rate (260,308–310).

One prominent feature of locus coeruleus neurons is their high sensitivity to stimuli that are novel or otherwise require a protective reaction, e.g., hypercapnia, hypotension, or pain (295,296). On presentation of novel somatosensory stimuli, locus coeruleus neurons often respond in a highly phasic, rapidly adapting manner. Extrapolation of the properties of locus coeruleus neurons to noradrenergic neurons controlling upper airway motoneurons suggests that the noradrenergic input to motoneurons may be particularly important for transmission of transient excitatory inputs at times of high sensory stimulation, including arousals that terminate obstructive episodes. By functioning in this manner, the noradrenergic neurons would complement the action of 5-HT neurons, which provide a tonic, wakefulness-related drive to upper airway motoneurons (see the preceding section). This functional distinction between the roles of 5-HT and NE remains, however, hypothetical.

Acetylcholine

Brainstem acetylcholine (ACh)-containing neurons, especially those in the pons, have state-dependent activity patterns. Some are maximally active during both wakefulness and REM sleep, whereas others have activity increases only during REM sleep (see Ref. 311). The recent demonstrations of pre- and postsynaptic cholinergic effects in orofacial motoneurons (169,312) raise the possibility that ACh may play an important role in regulating the excitability of upper airway motoneurons in a state-dependent manner. In particular, postsynaptic excitatory effects are mediated in XII and VII motoneurons by nicotinic cholinergic receptors (312). However, the source(s) of the cholinergic innervation of upper airway motoneurons and the firing behavior of such ACh premotor neurons need to be determined in order to properly interpret the role of ACh in motoneuronal control, especially within the framework of its potential sleep dependence.

State-Dependent Active Inhibition

The active, postsynaptic inhibition of motoneurons, mediated by inhibitory amino acids, has been extensively investigated in relation to the atonia of postural muscles during REM sleep. Glycine is the mediator of the REM sleep–specific, inhibitory postsynaptic potentials present in lumbar postural motoneurons throughout (313–315), or at least at the transition into (316), the atonia of REM sleep. Consistent with the inhibition being mediated by glycine, which opens Cl^- channels, the membrane resistance of lumbar motoneurons decreases during natural REM sleep (317,318) and during the postural atonia produced by pontine carbachol (77). Based on these studies and earlier experiments with electrical stimulation of the pontomedullary reticular formation, it is believed that REM sleep activates a descending inhibitory system whose origin is in the dorsomedial pontine reticular formation (corresponding to the pontine sites where carbachol is effective) and that contains two successive synaptic relays, one in the medial medullary reticular formation and one in the spinal cord (see Refs. 319,320 for reviews). Substantiating this, neurons showing REM sleep–specific increases in activity were observed in the ventromedial medullary reticular formation (201,203,321–323), and stimulation of cells in this region with glutamate evokes a generalized postural atonia (78).

In support of a major role of REM sleep–specific glycinergic inhibition of lumbar motoneurons, the iontophoretic application strychnine, a glycine receptor antagonist, nearly abolishes both changes in membrane resistance and the REM sleep–specific inhibitory postsynaptic potentials in lumbar motoneurons of chronically instrumented, intact cats (315). This result still remains to be reconciled with the extensive evidence that other pathways mediating excitatory or inhibitory effects and showing prominent sleep state dependence also impinge directly on spinal motoneurons. In particular, spinal motoneurons are innervated by descending fibers from the serotonergic neurons of the medullary raphe and noradrenergic neurons of the locus coeruleus (see Refs. 280,324,325). The serotonergic terminals also contain peptide transmitters such as TRH and SP (see Refs. 280,326). As with upper airway motoneurons (see above), these four transmitters have net excitatory effects on spinal motoneurons (see Refs. 280,327). Interestingly, serotonergic fibers make a substantial number of contacts with lumbar motoneurons, averaging more than 1500 contacts per motoneuron (328). This represents a significant portion (about 5%) of the total contacts, more than group Ia afferent synapses from muscle spindles. Thus, one would expect that, when monaminergic neuronal firing decreases greatly during REM sleep, disfacilitation of spinal motoneurons occurs, adding to the effect of glycinergic active inhibition.

A glycine-mediated hyperpolarization is also present in XII and trigeminal motoneurons during the carbachol-induced atonia of REM sleep, indicating that upper airway motoneurons are subjected to a postsynaptic inhibition similar to that seen in lumbar motoneurons (52,329). However, in contrast to lumbar motoneurons, other neurotransmitters have been shown to play a major role in mediating the REM sleep–related suppression of activity in upper airway motoneurons, whereas the magnitude of glycinergic inhibition may be more limited. Support for this comes from the following. First, microinjections of antagonists of amino acid–mediated inhibition (strychnine for glycine receptors, and bicuculline or picrotoxin for $GABA_A$ receptors) into the trigeminal motor nucleus reduces the suppressant effect of REM sleep on reflexly evoked motoneuronal responses by less than 20% (330). Second, the pontine carbachol–induced depression of the spontaneous activity of XII motoneurons in decerebrate cats is little affected by microinjections of either strychnine (Fig. 9) or bicuculline into the XII nucleus, whereas a reflexly evoked inhibition due to lingual nerve stimulation is abolished (331). Finally, the glycine-containing neurons that project to the trigeminal motor nucleus are not located in those sites of the medullary reticular formation from which REM sleep–like atonia is produced in spinal motoneurons (332,333). Thus, in spite of the presence of very dense glycinergic afferents in all upper airway motor nuclei (334), a major role of this neurotransmitter is probably to mediate various reflex inhibitory influences onto upper airway motoneurons (see Refs. 335,336). Similar evidence exists that activation of $GABA_A$ receptors (blocked by bicuculline) does not make major contribution to the REM sleep atonia of XII motoneurons (331).

The activation of pontine cholinergic neurons during REM sleep may also engage presynaptic mechanisms leading to a suppression of activity in upper airway motoneurons. One example of this has been demonstrated in recordings from XII motoneurons in a medullary slice preparation from juvenile rats; the addition of M_2 muscarinic cholinergic receptor agonists to the bath suppresses spontaneous and

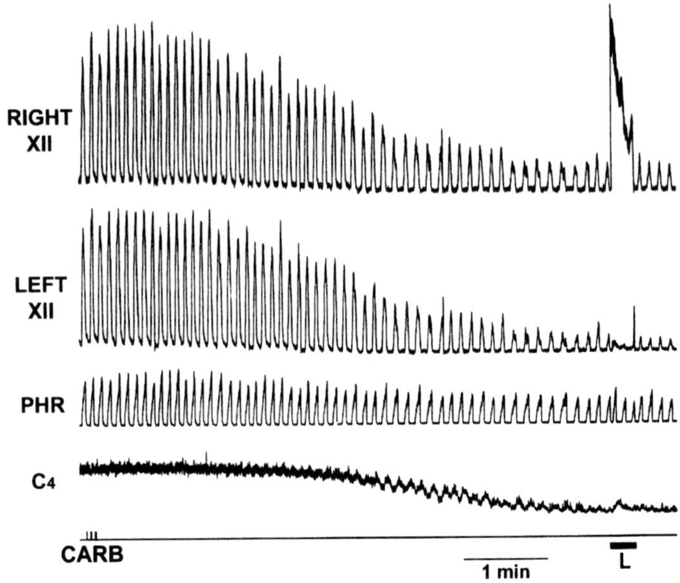

Figure 9 Antagonism of glycine-mediated inhibition does not prevent the carbachol-induced depression of hypoglossal (XII) nerve activity. In this experiment, strychnine (a blocker of glycine receptors) was microinjected twice into the right XII nucleus in a decerebrate, paralyzed, vagotomized, and artificially ventilated cat (3 and 16 min before the beginning of the record). The traces show the integrated activities of both XII nerves, phrenic nerve (PHR), and the C_4 nerve branch innervating dorsal neck muscles (representing postural activity). Carbachol, injected into the pons at the beginning of the trace, initiates the REM sleep–like suppression of the activity of all nerves. The activity of both XII nerves is similarly suppressed in spite of the earlier injection of strychnine into the right XII motor nucleus. The large, transient increase in the activity of the right XII nerve at the end of the trace is produced by electrical stimulation of the lingual nerve (bar marked ''L'') and was used in this study as one of the controls for the persistence of glycinergic blockade (see the original publication for details). (Modified from Ref. 331.)

evoked excitatory postsynaptic potentials mediated by glutamate (see Ref. 169) (Fig. 10). Since this occurs without changes in the postsynaptic properties of the motoneurons and is associated with a reduction in the frequency, but not amplitude, of spontaneous postsynaptic currents, the effect is probably due to decreased glutamate release from presynaptic terminals. Through this presynaptic inhibitory mechanism, acetylcholine has the potential to exert REM sleep–related depressant effects on orofacial motoneurons. Unlike the permissive (disfacilitatory) mechanisms discussed in the two preceding sections, this one would be actively engaged during REM sleep (and/or wakefulness, when brainstem cholinergic systems are also active), yet it would not require the participation of inhibitory amino acids such as glycine or GABA.

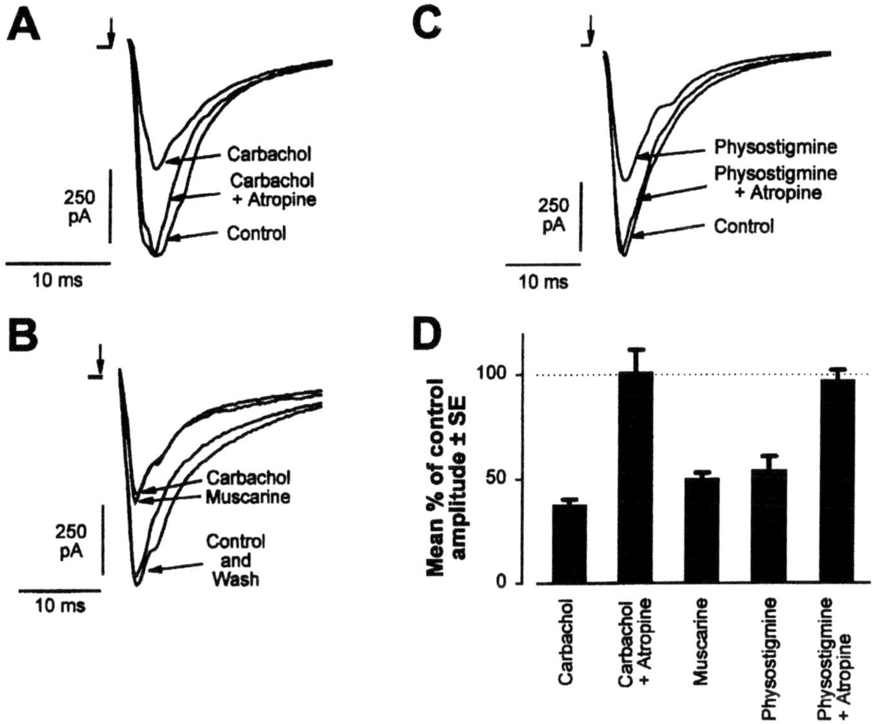

Figure 10 Synaptic excitatory currents, evoked in hypoglossal (XII) motoneurons by electrical stimulation of the medullary reticular formation and mediated by glutamate receptors, are reduced by cholinergic agonists. This cholinergic modulation is exerted presynaptically, by means of a reduction in transmitter release from glutamatergic synapses on XII motoneurons. Since cholinergic brainstem neurons are activated during REM sleep and wakefulness, this demonstrates the potential of the cholinergic system to suppress, in a state-dependent manner, excitatory inputs to upper airway motoneurons. Data from an in vitro medullary slice from a juvenile rat. (A–C) Changes in the amplitude of the evoked current produced by superfusion of the slice with different cholinergic drugs. The magnitude of the evoked current is reduced by carbachol, a broad-spectrum cholinergic agonist (A), muscarine (B), and physostigmine, an inhibitor of endogenous acetylcholinesterase (C). The effects are blocked by atropine, a muscarinic antagonist. (D) Average data from 3–22 XII motoneurons studied with different drugs. (From Ref. 169.)

D. Effect of Sleep Deprivation on the Control of the Upper Airway

Sleep deprivation may have a distinct effect on the control of orofacial motoneurons, as evidenced by the observation that it impairs speech, including its motor aspects (337). Related to this, and of particular relevance to OSA, are the observations that sleep-related decrements in the activity of upper airway motoneurons or the frequency and severity of obstructive apneic episodes are more profound in sleep-deprived than in control subjects (338–342). Although the neurochemical basis of this remains to be elucidated, these effects may be mediated by hypothalamic neurons whose activity is strongly dependent on both the accumulation of sleep debt and circadian time (e.g., Refs. 343–345). A determination of the interactions between the mechanisms of sleepiness and those controlling upper airway motoneurons is critical for our understanding of the pathophysiology of OSA.

IV. Summary and Conclusions

In this chapter, we covered selected physiological mechanisms that, under normal conditions, are important for the maintenance of upper airway motor tone during wakefulness and/or contribute to the loss of this tone during sleep. Those mechanisms were considered as distinct ''drives'' that may undergo state-specific changes upon transitions from wakefulness to non-REM sleep and REM sleep and discussed largely on the basis of data from animals and humans without symptoms of OSA. The reason for such an approach was our conviction that clinically significant upper airway atonias and hypotonias are physiological phenomena superimposed on an anatomically altered upper airway. Indeed, many observations pertinent to the clinical picture of OSA can be explained by assuming that a reduced airway size must lead to a reflex and/or behavioral ''upregulation'' of upper airway motor tone that will then show larger than normal decreases during sleep because the starting level is higher. In addition, however, there is evidence that an altered pattern of the use of, and an increased demand on, upper airway motoneurons in OSA patients leads to alterations in the physiology of various aspects of the central and reflex control of upper airway motoneurons. For example, an intermittently occurring extremely strong activation of upper airway muscles may lead to muscle hypertrophy and injury (346–349), and enhanced stimulation of upper airway mechanoreceptors may result in not only the physiological phenomenon of reflex habituation (350) but also changes in the protein content of afferent nerve endings in the airway mucosa (351). A chronic need to cope with sleep fragmentation, sleep deprivation, and recurring hypoxemia may cause additional changes in upper airway motor control, some of which can be demonstrated even in individuals whose upper airway is normal (e.g., the preceding section). Thus, the load imposed on breathing by the narrow upper airway of OSA patients will activate many of the same mechanisms that are present in normal individuals as well as others that are absent or potentially present, but rarely activated.

Attempts to distinguish between the physiological mechanisms that are normally present and the pathological mechanisms peculiar to OSA are hampered by the limited availability of adequate animal models. English bulldogs (242) and instrumented dogs with externally applied tracheal occlusions (352) are, so far, the only models with which one can dissect selected mechanisms that may be specific to OSA (see Chap. 16). New models are needed to facilitate investigations into various aspects of the neuroanatomical, neurochemical, and molecular alterations in the neural control of the upper airway resulting from altered upper airway anatomy.

Current treatments for OSA aim to enlarge the airway. The most common treatment, continuous positive airway pressure (CPAP), eliminates, rather than takes advantage of, physiological mechanisms controlling the upper airway, for the positive airway pressure reflexly reduces upper airway dilator muscle activity (40,139, 160,353). Thus, there is a need to devise treatments that will apply the new information about the physiology and pharmacology of upper airway control. Based on the data reviewed in this chapter, two new strategies could be utilized: increasing the aminergic stimulation of upper airway motoneurons during sleep and enhancing the reflex excitatory drives to upper airway motoneurons.

Acknowledgments

The authors' research was supported by grants HL-47600, HL-42236, and HL-60287 from the National Heart, Lung, and Blood Institute of the National Institutes of Health.

References

1. Remmers JE, DeGroot WJ, Sauerland EK, Anch AM. Pathogenesis of upper airway occlusion during sleep. J Appl Physiol 1978; 44:931–938.
2. Brouillette RT, Thach BT. A neuromuscular mechanism maintaining extrathoracic airway patency. J Appl Physiol 1979; 46:772–779.
3. Anch AM, Remmers JE, Sauerland EK, DeGroot WJ. Oropharyngeal patency during waking and sleep in the Pickwickian syndrome: electromyographic activity of the tensor veli palatini. Electromyogr Clin Neurophysiol 1981; 21:317–330.
4. Lopes JM, Tabachnik E, Muller NL, Levison H, Bryan AC. Total airway resistance and respiratory muscle activity during sleep. J Appl Physiol 1983; 54:773–777.
5. Wiegand DA, Latz B, Zwillich CW, Wiegand L. Upper airway resistance and geniohyoid muscle activity in normal men during wakefulness and sleep. J Appl Physiol 1990; 69:1252–1261.
6. Kay A, Trinder J, Bowes G, Kim Y. Changes in airway resistance during sleep onset. J Appl Physiol 1994; 76:1600–1607.
7. Douglas NJ. Control of ventilation during sleep. In: Kryger MH, Roth T, Dement WC, eds. Principles and Practice of Sleep Medicine. Philadelphia: Saunders, 1994:204–211.
8. Badr MS. Effect of ventilatory drive on upper airway patency in humans during NREM sleep. Respir Physiol 1996; 103:1–10.
9. Reed WR, Roberts JL, Thach BT. Factors influencing regional patency and configuration of the human infant upper airway. J Appl Physiol 1985; 58:635–644.
10. Olson LG, Strohl KP. Airway secretions influence upper airway patency in the rabbit. Am Rev Respir Dis 1988; 137:1379–1381.
11. Van der Touw T, Crawford ABH, Wheatley JR. Effects of a synthetic lung surfactant on pharyngeal patency in awake human subjects. J Appl Physiol 1997; 82:78–85.
12. Leiter JC, Knuth SL, Bartlett D, Jr. Dependence of pharyngeal resistance on genioglossal EMG activity, nasal resistance, and airflow. J Appl Physiol 1992; 73:584–590.

13. Isono S, Feroah TR, Hajduk EA, Brant R, Whitelaw WA, Remmers JE. Interaction of cross-sectional area, driving pressure, and airflow of passive velopharynx. J Appl Physiol 1997; 83:851–859.
14. Phillipson EA, Bowes G. Control of breathing during sleep. In: Cherniack NS, Widdicombe JG, eds. Handbook of Physiology. Section 3: The Respiratory System. Volume II: Control of Breathing, Part I. Bethesda, MD: American Physiological Society, 1986: 649–689.
15. Iscoe SD. Central control of the upper airway. In: Mathew OP, Sant'Ambrogio G, eds. Respiratory Function of the Upper Airway. New York: Marcel Dekker, 1988:125–192.
16. Kuna ST, Sant'Ambrogio G. Pathophysiology of upper airway closure during sleep. J Am Med Assoc 1991; 266:1384–1389.
17. Isono S, Remmers JE. Anatomy and physiology of upper airway obstruction. In: Kryger MH, Roth T, Dement WC, eds. Principles and Practice of Sleep Medicine. Philadelphia: Saunders, 1994:642–656.
18. White DP. Pathophysiology of obstructive sleep apnoea. Thorax 1995; 50:797–804.
19. Lydic R. Respiratory modulation by nonrespiratory neurons. In: Schwartz WJ, ed. Sleep Science: Integrating Basic Research and Clinical Practice. Basel: Karger, 1997: 117–142.
20. Deegan PC, McNicholas WT. Pathophysiology of obstructive sleep apnoea. Eur Respir J 1995; 8:1161–1178.
21. Horner RL. Motor control of the pharyngeal musculature and implications for the pathogenesis of obstructive sleep apnea. Sleep 1996; 19:827–853.
22. Hudgel DW. Variable site of airway narrowing among obstructive sleep apnea patients. J Appl Physiol 1986; 61:1403–1409.
23. Chaban R, Cole P, Hoffstein V. Site of upper airway obstruction in patients with idiopathic obstructive sleep apnea. Laryngoscope 1988; 98:641–647.
24. Shepard JW, Jr., Thawley SE. Localization of upper airway collapse during sleep in patients with obstructive sleep apnea. Am Rev Respir Dis 1990; 141:1350–1355.
25. Roberts JL, Reed WR, Thach BT. Pharyngeal airway-stabilizing function of sternohyoid and sternothyroid muscles in the rabbit. J Appl Physiol 1984; 57:1790–1795.
26. Strohl KP, Olson LG. Concerning the importance of pharyngeal muscles in the maintenance of upper airway patency during sleep. Chest 1987; 92:918–920.
27. Rowley JA, Permutt S, Willey S, Smith PL, Schwartz AR. Effect of tracheal and tongue displacement on upper airway airflow dynamics. J Appl Physiol 1996; 80:2171–2178.
28. Kuna ST, Smickley J. Response of genioglosus muscle activity to nasal airway occlusion in normal sleeping adults. J Appl Physiol 1988; 64:347–353.
29. Proctor DF. The upper airways. I. Nasal physiology and defense of the lungs. Am Rev Respir Dis 1977; 115:97–129.
30. Hudgel DW, Robertson DW. Nasal resistance during wakefulness and sleep in normal man. Acta Otolaryngol 1984; 98:130–135.
31. Wheatley JR, Tangel DJ, Mezzanotte WS, White DP. Influence of sleep on alae nasi EMG and nasal resistance in normal men. J Appl Physiol 1993; 75:626–632.
32. Sériès F, Cormier Y, Desmeules M, La Forge J. Effects of respiratory drive on upper airways in sleep apnea patients and normal subjects. J Appl Physiol 1989; 67:973–979.
33. Bartlett D, Jr. Respiratory functions of the larynx. Physiol Rev 1989; 69:33–57.

34. Widdicombe JG. Reflexes from the upper respiratory tract. In: Cherniack NS, Widdicombe JG, eds. Handbook of Physiology. Section 3: The Respiratory System. Vol. II: Control of Breathing, Part 1. Bethesda, MD: American Physiological Society, 1986: 363–394.
35. Kuna ST, Insalaco G, Villeponteaux RD. Arytenoideus muscle activity in normal adult humans during wakefulness and sleep. J Appl Physiol 1991; 70:1655–1664.
36. Tangel DJ, Mezzanotte WS, Sandberg EJ, White DP. Influences of NREM sleep on the activity of tonic vs. inspiratory phasic muscles in normal men. J Appl Physiol 1992; 73:1058–1066.
37. Carlson DM, Carley DW, Önal E, Lopata M, Basner RC. Acoustically induced cortical arousal increases phasic pharyngeal muscle and diaphragmatic EMG in NREM sleep. J Appl Physiol 1994; 76:1553–1559.
38. Mezzanotte WS, Tangel DJ, White DP. Influence of sleep onset on upper-airway muscle activity in apnea patients versus normal controls. Am J Respir Crit Care Med 1996; 153:1880–1887.
39. Kuna ST, Smickley JS, Vanoye CR. Respiratory-related pharyngeal constrictor muscle activity in normal human adults. Am J Respir Crit Care Med 1997; 155:1991–1999.
40. Mezzanotte WS, Tangel DJ, White DP. Waking genioglossal electromyogram in sleep apnea patients versus normal controls (a neuromuscular compensatory mechanism). J Clin Invest 1992; 89:1571–1579.
41. Wiegand L, Zwillich CW, Wiegand D, White DP. Changes in upper airway muscle activation and ventilation during phasic REM sleep in normal men. J Appl Physiol 1991; 71:488–497.
42. Sherrey JH, Megirian D. State dependence of upper airway respiratory motoneurons: functions of the cricothyroid and nasolabial muscles of the unanesthetized rat. Electroencephalogr Clin Neurophysiol 1977; 43:218–228.
43. Sauerland EK, Orr WC, Hairston LE. EMG patterns of oropharyngeal muscles during respiration in wakefulness and sleep. Electromyogr Clin Neurophysiol 1981; 21:307–316.
44. Worsnop C, Kay A, Pierce R, Kim Y, Trinder J. Activity of respiratory pump and upper airway muscles during sleep onset. J Appl Physiol 1998; 85:908–920.
45. Tangel DJ, Mezzanotte WS, White DP. Influences of NREM sleep on activity of palatoglossus and levator palatini muscles in normal men. J Appl Physiol 1995; 78:689–695.
46. Sauerland EK, Harper RM. The human tongue during sleep: electromyographic activity of the genioglossus muscle. Exp Neurol 1976; 51:160–170.
47. Chokroverty S. Phasic tongue movements in human rapid-eye-movement sleep. Neurology 1980; 30:665–668.
48. Basner RC, Ringler J, Schwartzstein RM, Weinberger SE, Weiss JW. Phasic electromyographic activity of the genioglossus increases in normals during slow-wave sleep. Respir Physiol 1991; 83:189–200.
49. Haxhiu MA, van Lunteren E, Mitra J, Cherniack NS. Comparison of the response of diaphragm and upper airway dilating muscle activity in sleeping cats. Respir Physiol 1987; 70:183–193.
50. Richard CA, Harper RM. Respiratory-related activity in hypoglossal neurons across sleep-waking states in cats. Brain Res 1991; 542:167–170.
51. Sherrey JH, Pollard MJ, Megirian D. Respiratory functions of the inferior pharyngeal constrictor and sternohyoid muscles during sleep. Exp Neurol 1986; 92:267–277.

52. Pedroarena C, Castillo P, Chase MH, Morales FR. The control of jaw-opener motoneurons during active sleep. Brain Res 1994; 653:31–38.
53. Wiegand DA, Latz B, Zwillich CW, Wiegand L. Geniohyoid muscle activity in normal men during wakefulness and sleep. J Appl Physiol 1990; 69:1262–1269.
54. Hendricks JC, Petrof BJ, Panckeri K, Pack AI. Upper airway dilating muscle hyperactivity during non-rapid eye movement sleep in English bulldogs. Am Rev Respir Dis 1993; 148:185–194.
55. Megirian D, Hinrichsen CFL, Sherrey JH. Respiratory roles of genioglossus, sternothyroid, and sternohyoid muscles during sleep. Exp Neurol 1985; 90:118–128.
56. Kuna ST, Smickley JS, Insalaco G. Posterior cricoarytenoid muscle activity during wakefulness and sleep in normal adults. J Appl Physiol 1990; 68:1746–1754.
57. Orem J, Lydic R. Upper airway function during sleep and wakefulness: experimental studies on normal and anesthetized cats. Sleep 1978; 1:49–68.
58. Kianicka I, Praud J-P. Influence of sleep states on laryngeal and abdominal muscle response to upper airway occlusion in lambs. Ped Res 1997; 41:862–871.
59. Sherrey JH, Megirian D. Respiratory EMG activity of the posterior cricoarytenoid, cricothyroid and diaphragm muscles during sleep. Respir Physiol 1980; 39:355–365.
60. Megirian D, Sherrey JH. Respiratory functions of the laryngeal muscles during sleep. Sleep 1980; 3:289–298.
61. Kuna ST, Insalaco G, Woodson GE. Thyroarytenoid muscle activity during wakefulness and sleep in normal adults. J Appl Physiol 1988; 65:1332–1339.
62. Kuna ST, Smickley JS, Vanoye CR, McMillan TH. Cricothyroid muscle activity during sleep in normal adult humans. J Appl Physiol 1994; 76:2326–2332.
63. Suratt PM, McTier RF, Wilhoit SC. Upper airway muscle activation is augmented in patients with obstructive sleep apnea compared with that in normal subjects. Am Rev Respir Dis 1988; 137:889–894.
64. Kuna T, Smickley JS. Superior pharyngeal constrictor activation in obstructive sleep apnea. Am J Respir Crit Care Med 1997; 156:874–880.
65. Douglas NJ, Jan MA, Yildirim N, Warren PM, Drummond GB. Effect of posture and breathing route on genioglossal electromyogram activity in normal subjects and in patients with the sleep apnea/hypopnea syndrome. Am Rev Respir Dis 1993; 148: 1341–1345.
66. Önal E, Lopata M, O'Connor T. Pathogenesis of apneas in hypersomnia-sleep apnea syndrome. Am Rev Respir Dis 1982; 125:167–174.
67. Okabe S, Hida W, Kikuchi Y, Taguchi O, Takishima T, Shirato K. Upper airway muscle activity during REM and non-REM sleep of patients with obstructive apnea. Chest 1994; 106:767–773.
68. Carlson DM, Önal E, Carley DW, Lopata M, Basner RC. Palatal muscle electromyogram activity in obstructive sleep apnea. Am J Respir Crit Care Med 1995; 152:1022–1027.
69. Fink BR. Influence of cerebral activity in wakefulness on regulation of breathing. J Appl Physiol 1961; 16:15–20.
70. Orem J. The nature of the wakefulness stimulus for breathing. In: Suratt P, Remmers JE, eds. Sleep and Respiration. New York: Wiley-Liss, 1990:23–31.
71. Kimura H, Kubin L, Davies RO, Pack AI. Cholinergic stimulation of the pons depresses respiration in decerebrate cats. J Appl Physiol 1990; 69:2280–2289.
72. Vanni-Mercier G, Sakai K, Lin JS, Jouvet M. Mapping of cholinoceptive brainstem

structures responsible for the generation of paradoxical sleep in the cat. Arch Ital Biol 1989; 127:133–164.

73. Yamamoto K, Mamelak AN, Quattrochi JJ, Hobson JA. A cholinoceptive desynchronized sleep induction zone in the anterodorsal pontine tegmentum: locus of the sensitive region. Neuroscience 1990; 39:279–293.
74. Lydic R, Baghdoyan HA, Zwillich CW. State-dependent hypotonia in posterior cricoarytenoid muscles of the larynx caused by cholinoceptive reticular mechanisms. FASEB J 1989; 3:1625–1631.
75. Kodama T, Takahashi Y, Honda Y. Enhancement of acetylcholine release during paradoxical sleep in the dorsal tegmental field of the cat brain stem. Neurosci Lett 1990; 114:277–282.
76. Lydic R, Baghdoyan HA, Lorinc Z. Microdialysis of cat pons reveals enhanced acetylcholine release during state-dependent respiratory depression. Am J Physiol 1991; 261: R766–R770.
77. Morales FR, Engelhardt JK, Soja PJ, Pereda AE, Chase MH. Motoneuron properties during motor inhibition produced by microinjection of carbachol into the pontine reticular formation of the decerebrate cat. J Neurophysiol 1987; 57:1118–1129.
78. Lai YY, Siegel JM. Cardiovascular and muscle tone changes produced by microinjection of cholinergic and glutamatergic agonists in dorsolateral pons and medial medulla. Brain Res 1990; 514:27–36.
79. Takakusaki K, Matsuyama K, Kobayashi Y, Kohyama J, Mori S. Pontine microinjection of carbachol and critical zone for inducing postural atonia in reflexively standing decerebrate cats. Neurosci Lett 1993; 153:185–188.
80. Tojima H, Kubin L, Kimura H, Davies RO. Spontaneous ventilation and respiratory motor output during carbachol-induced atonia of REM sleep in the decerebrate cat. Sleep 1992; 15:404–414.
81. Taguchi O, Kubin L, Pack AI. Evocation of postural atonia and respiratory depression by pontine carbachol in the decerebrate rat. Brain Res 1992; 595:107–115.
82. Fenik V, Davies RO, Pack AI, Kubin L. Differential suppression of upper airway motor activity during carbachol-induced, REM sleep-like atonia. Am J Physiol 1998; 275: R1013–R1024.
83. Woch G, Davies RO, Pack AI, Kubin L. Behaviour of raphe cells projecting to the dorsomedial medulla during carbachol-induced atonia in the cat. J Physiol (Lond) 1996; 490:745–758.
84. Trulson ME, Trulson VM. Activity of nucleus raphe pallidus neurons across the sleep-waking cycle in freely moving cats. Brain Res 1982; 237:232–237.
85. Heym J, Steinfels GF, Jacobs BL. Activity of serotonin-containing neurons in the nucleus raphe pallidus of freely moving cats. Brain Res 1982; 251:259–276.
86. Parisi RA, Neubauer JA, Frank MM, Edelman NH, Santiago TV. Correlation between genioglossal and diaphragmatic responses to hypercapnia during sleep. Am Rev Respir Dis 1987; 135:378–382.
87. Parisi RA, Santiago TV, Edelman NH. Genioglossal and diaphragmatic EMG responses to hypoxia during sleep. Am Rev Respir Dis 1988; 138:610–616.
88. Horner RL, Kubin L. Pontine carbachol elicits multiple rapid eye movement sleep-like neural events in urethane-anesthetized rats. Neuroscience 1999; 93:215–226.
89. Fenik V, Ogawa H, Davies RO, Kubin L. The activity of locus coeruleus (LC) neurons is reduced in urethane-anesthetized rats during carbachol-induced episodes of REM sleep-like suppression of upper airway motor tone. Soc Neurosci Abstr 1999; 25:2144.

90. Lynn RB, Kreider MS, Miselis RR. Thyrotropin-releasing hormone-immunoreactive projections to the dorsal motor nucleus and the nucleus of the solitary tract of the rat. J Comp Neurol 1991; 311:271–288.
91. Woch G, Kubin L. Non-reciprocal control of rhythmic activity in respiratory-modulated XII motoneurons. NeuroReport 1995; 6:2085–2088.
92. Huangfu D, Koshiya N, Guyenet PG. Central respiratory modulation of facial motoneurons in rats. Neurosci Lett 1993; 151:224–228.
93. Barillot JC, Grélot L, Reddad S, Bianchi AL. Discharge patterns of laryngeal motoneurones in the cat: an intracellular study. Brain Res 1990; 509:99–106.
94. Hwang J-C, Bartlett D, Jr., St. John WM. Characterization of respiratory-modulated activities of hypoglossal motoneurons. J Appl Physiol 1983; 55:793–798.
95. Withington-Wray DJ, Mifflin SW, Spyer KM. Intracellular analysis of respiratory-modulated hypoglossal motoneurons in the cat. Neuroscience 1988; 25:1041–1051.
96. Mathew OP, Sant'Ambrogio FB. Laryngeal reflexes. In: Mathew OP, Sant'Ambrogio G, eds. Respiratory Function of the Upper Airway. New York: Marcel Dekker, Inc., 1988:259–302.
97. Sant'Ambrogio G, Tsubone H, Sant'Ambrogio FB. Sensory information from the upper airway: role in the control of breathing. Respir Physiol 1995; 102:1–16.
98. Kubin L, Davies RO. Central pathways of pulmonary and airway vagal afferents. In: Dempsey JA, Pack AI, eds. Regulation of Breathing. New York: Marcel Dekker, 1995: 219–284.
99. Feldman JL. Neurophysiology of breathing in mammals. In: Bloom FE, ed. Handbook of Physiology. The Nervous System IV. Intrinsic Regulatory Systems of the Brain. Bethesda, MD: American Physiological Society, 1986:463–524.
100. Ezure K. Synaptic connections between medullary respiratory neurons and considerations on the genesis of respiratory rhythm. Prog Neurobiol 1990; 35:429–450.
101. Monteau R, Hilaire G. Spinal respiratory motoneurons. Prog Neurobiol 1991; 37:83–144.
102. Duffin J, Ezure K, Lipski J. Breathing rhythm generation: focus on the rostral ventrolateral medulla. News Physiol Sci 1995; 10:133–140.
103. Ono T, Ishiwata Y, Inaba N, Kuroda T, Nakamura Y. Hypoglossal premotor neurons with rhythmical inspiratory-related activity in the cat: localization and projection to the phrenic nucleus. Exp Brain Res 1994; 98:1–12.
104. Woch G, Ogawa H, Davies RO, Kubin L. Behavior of hypoglossal inspiratory premotor neurons during the carbachol-induced, REM sleep-like suppression of upper airway motoneurons. Exp Brain Res 2000; 130:508–520.
105. Yamada H, Ezure K, Manabe M. Efferent projections of inspiratory neurons of the ventral respiratory group. A dual labeling study in the rat. Brain Res 1988; 455:283–294.
106. Takada M, Itoh K, Yasui Y, Mitani A, Nomura S, Mizuno N. Distribution of premotor neurons for the hypoglossal nucleus in the cat. Neurosci Lett 1984; 52:141–146.
107. Dobbins EG, Feldman JL. Differential innervation of protruder and retractor muscles of the tongue in rat. J Comp Neurol 1995; 357:376–394.
108. Ugolini G. Specificity of rabies virus as a transneuronal tracer of motor networks: transfer from hypoglossal motoneurons to connected second-order and higher order central nervous system cell groups. J Comp Neurol 1995; 356:457–480.
109. Fay RA, Norgren R. Identification of rat brainstem multisynaptic connections to the

oral motor nuclei using pseudorabies virus III. Lingual muscle motor systems. Brain Res Rev 1997; 25:291–311.

110. Smith JC, Ellenberger HH, Ballanyi K, Richter DW, Feldman JL. Pre-Bötzinger complex: a brainstem region that may generate respiratory rhythm in mammals. Science 1991; 254:726–729.

111. Orem J, Montplaisir J, Dement WC. Changes in the activity of respiratory neurons during sleep. Brain Res 1974; 82:309–315.

112. Orem J, Osorio I, Brooks E, Dick TE. Activity of respiratory neurons during NREM sleep. J Neurophysiol 1985; 54:1144–1156.

113. Orem JM. Respiratory neuronal activity in sleep. In: Edelman NH, Santiago TV, eds. Breathing Disorders of Sleep. New York: Churchill Livingstone, 1986:19–44.

114. Puizillout J-J, Ternaux J-P. Variations d'activités toniques, phasiques et respiratoires, au niveau bulbaire pendant l'endormement de la préparation 'encéphale isolé.' Brain Res 1974; 66:67–83.

115. Foutz AS, Boudinot E, Morin-Surun M-P, Champagnat J, Gonsalves SF, Denavit-Saubié M. Excitability of ''silent'' respiratory neurons during sleep-waking states: an iontophoretic study in undrugged chronic cats. Brain Res 1987; 404:10–20.

116. Chang F.-C.T. Modification of medullary respiratory-related discharge patterns by behaviors and states of arousal. Brain Res 1992; 571:281–292.

117. Sieck GC, Harper RM. Pneumotaxic area neuronal discharge during sleep-waking states in the cat. Exp Neurol 1980; 67:79–102.

118. Gilbert KA, Lydic R. Parabrachial neuron discharge in the cat is altered during the carbachol-induced REM sleep-like state (DCarb). Neurosci Lett 1990; 120:241–244.

119. Travers JB, Norgren R. Afferent projections to the oral motor nuclei in the rat. J Comp Neurol 1983; 220:280–298.

120. Fort P, Sakai K, Luppi P-H, Salvert D, Jouvet M. Monoaminergic, peptidergic, and cholinergic afferents to the cat facial nucleus as evidenced by a double immunostaining method with unconjugated cholera toxin as a retrograde tracer. J Comp Neurol 1989; 283:285–302.

121. Fort P, Luppi P-H, Sakai K, Salvert D, Jouvet M. Nuclei of origin of monoaminergic, peptidergic, and cholinergic afferents to the cat trigeminal motor nucleus: a double-labeling study with cholera-toxin as a retrograde tracer. J Comp Neurol 1990; 301: 262–275.

122. Orem J. Medullary respiratory neuron activity: relationship to tonic and phasic REM sleep. J Appl Physiol 1980; 48:54–65.

123. Orem J. Central respiratory activity in rapid eye movement sleep: augmenting and late inspiratory cells. Sleep 1994; 17:665–673.

124. Orem J. Excitatory drive to the respiratory system in REM sleep. Sleep 1996; 19: S154–S156.

125. Hudgel DW, Harasick T. Fluctuation in timing of upper airway and chest wall inspiratory muscle activity in obstructive sleep apnea. J Appl Physiol 1990; 69:443–450.

126. Kubin L, Kimura H, Tojima H, Pack AI, Davies RO. Behavior of VRG neurons during the atonia of REM sleep induced by pontine carbachol in decerebrate cats. Brain Res 1992; 592:91–100.

127. Gilbert KA, Lydic R. Pontine cholinergic reticular mechanisms cause state-dependent changes in the discharge of parabrachial neurons. Am J Physiol 1994; 266:R136–R150.

128. Widdicombe J, Sant'Ambrogio G, Mathew OP. Nerve receptors of the upper airway. In: Mathew OP, Sant'Ambrogio G, eds. Respiratory Function of the Upper Airway. New York: Marcel Dekker, Inc., 1988:193–231.
129. Zhang S, Mathew OP. Response of laryngeal mechanoreceptors to high-frequency pressure oscillation. J Appl Physiol 1992; 73:219–223.
130. Mathew OP, Sant'Ambrogio G, Fisher JT, Sant'Ambrogio FB. Respiratory afferent activity in the superior laryngeal nerves. Respir Physiol 1984; 58:41–50.
131. Wallois F, Macron JM, Jounieaux V, Duron B. Trigeminal nasal receptors related to respiration and to various stimuli in cats. Respir Physiol 1991; 85:111–125.
132. Mathew OP, Abu-Osba YK, Thach BT. Genioglossus muscle responses to upper airway pressure changes: afferent pathways. J Appl Physiol 1982; 52:445–450.
133. Sant'Ambrogio G, Mathew OP, Sant'Ambrogio FB. Role of intrinsic muscles and tracheal motion in modulating laryngeal receptors. Respir Physiol 1985; 61:289–300.
134. Hwang J-C, St. John WM, Bartlett D, Jr. Afferent pathways for hypoglossal and phrenic responses to changes in upper airway pressure. Respir Physiol 1984; 55:341–354.
135. van Lunteren E, Van de Graaff WB, Parker DM, Mitra J, Haxhiu MA, Strohl KP, et al. Nasal and laryngeal reflex responses to negative upper airway pressure. J Appl Physiol 1984; 56:746–752.
136. Amis TC, O'Neill N, Wheatley JR, Van der Touw T, Di Somma E, Brancatisano A. Soft palate muscle response to negative upper airway pressure. J Appl Physiol 1999; 86:523–530.
137. Harms CA, Zeng Y-J, Smith CA, Vidruk EH, Dempsey JA. Negative pressure-induced deformation of the upper airway causes central apnea in awake and sleeping dogs. J Appl Physiol 1996; 80:1528–1539.
138. Brouillette RT, Thach BT. Control of genioglossus muscle inspiratory activity. J Appl Physiol 1980; 49:801–808.
139. Mathew OP, Abu-Osba YK, Thach BT. Influence of upper airway pressure changes on genioglossus muscle respiratory activity. J Appl Physiol 1982; 52:438–444.
140. Brancatisano A, Van der Touw T, O'Neill N, Amis TC. Influence of upper airway pressure oscillations on soft palate muscle electromyographic activity. J Appl Physiol 1996; 81:1190–1196.
141. DeWeese EL, Sullivan TY. Effects of upper airway anesthesia on pharyngeal patency during sleep. J Appl Physiol 1988; 64:1346–1353.
142. Janczewski WA. Muscle relaxation attenuates the reflex response to laryngeal negative pressure. Respir Physiol 1997; 107:219–230.
143. Colrain IM, Trinder J, Fraser G, Wilson GV. Ventilation during sleep onset. J Appl Physiol 1987; 63:2067–2074.
144. Badr MS, Kawak A, Skatrud JB, Morrell MJ, Zahn BR, Babcock MA. Effect of induced hypocapnic hypopnea on upper airway patency in humans during NREM sleep. Respir Physiol 1997; 110:33–45.
145. Sant'Ambrogio FB, Anderson JW, Kuna ST, Sant'Ambrogio G. Effect of changes in airway surface liquid on laryngeal receptors and muscles. Respir Physiol 1995; 101: 31–39.
146. Kuna ST, Sant'Ambrogio FB, Sant'Ambrogio G. Effect of airway surface liquid composition on laryngeal muscle activation. Sleep 1996; 19:180–183.
147. Dickman JD, Smith DV. Response properties of fibers in the hamster superior laryngeal nerve. Brain Res 1988; 450:25–38.

148. Henke KG, Sullivan CE. Effects of high-frequency oscillating pressures on upper airway muscles in humans. J Appl Physiol 1993; 75:856–862.
149. Jiang C, Mitchell GS, Lipski J. Prolonged augmentation of respiratory discharge in hypoglossal motoneurons following superior laryngeal nerve stimulation. Brain Res 1991; 538:215–225.
150. Hayashi F, McCrimmon DR. Respiratory motor responses to cranial nerve afferent stimulation in rats. Am J Physiol 1996; 271:R1054–R1062.
151. Eldridge FL, Millhorn DE. Oscillation, gating, and memory in the respiratory control system. In: Cherniack NS, Widdicombe JG, eds. Handbook of Physiology. Section 3: The Respiratory System. Vol. II: Control of Breathing, Part 1. Bethesda, MD: American Physiological Society, 1986:93–114.
152. Tojima H, Kubin L, Davies RO, Pack AI. Reflex control of upper airway patency: role of serotonin (5HT). Am Rev Respir Dis 1992; 145:A212.
153. Plowman L, Lauff DC, Berthon-Jones M, Sullivan CE. Waking and genioglossal muscle responses to upper airway pressure oscillation in sleeping dogs. J Appl Physiol 1990; 68:2564–2573.
154. Aronson RM, Önal E, Carley DW, Lopata M. Upper airway and respiratory muscle responses to continuous negative airway pressure. J Appl Physiol 1989; 66:1373–1382.
155. Leiter JC, Daubenspeck JA. Selective reflex activation of the genioglossus in humans. J Appl Physiol 1990; 68:2581–2587.
156. Horner RL, Innes JA, Murphy K, Guz A. Evidence for reflex upper airway dilator muscle activation by sudden negative airway pressure in man. J Physiol (Lond) 1991; 436:15–29.
157. Wheatley JR, Tangel DJ, Mezzanotte WS, White DP. Influence of sleep on response to negative airway pressure of tensor palatini muscle and retropalatal airway. J Appl Physiol 1993; 75:2117–2124.
158. Mortimore IL, Douglas NJ. Palatopharyngeus has respiratory activity and responds to negative pressure in sleep apnoeics. Eur Respir J 1996; 9:773–778.
159. Mortimore IL, Douglas NJ. Palatal muscle EMG response to negative pressure in awake sleep apneic and control subjects. Am J Respir Crit Care Med 1997; 156:867–873.
160. Morrison DL, Launois SH, Isono S, Feroah TR, Whitelaw WA, Remmers JE. Pharyngeal narrowing and closing pressures in patients with obstructive sleep apnea. Am Rev Respir Dis 1993; 148:606–611.
161. Philip-Joët F, Marc I, Sériès F. Effects of genioglossal response to negative airway pressure on upper airway collapsibility during sleep. J Appl Physiol 1996; 80:1466–1474.
162. Tantucci C, Mehiri S, Duguet A, Similowski T, Arnulf I, Zelter M, et al. Application of negative expiratory pressure during expiration and activity of genioglossus in humans. J Appl Physiol 1998; 84:1076–1082.
163. Tangel DJ, Mezzanotte WS, White DP. Respiratory-related control of palatoglossus and levator palatini muscle activity. J Appl Physiol 1995; 78:680–688.
164. Horner RL, Innes JA, Holden HB, Guz A. Afferent pathway(s) for pharyngeal dilator reflex to negative pressure in man: a study using upper airway anaesthesia. J Physiol (Lond) 1991; 436:31–44.
165. Berry RB, McNellis MI, Kouchi K, Light RW. Upper airway anesthesia reduces phasic genioglosus activity during sleep apnea. Am J Respir Crit Care Med 1997; 156:127–132.

166. Wheatley JR, Mezzanotte WS, Tangel DJ, White DP. Influence of sleep on genioglossus muscle activation by negative pressure in normal men. Am Rev Respir Dis 1993; 148:597–605.
167. Strobel RJ, Daubenspeck JA. Early and late respiratory-related cortical potentials evoked by pressure pulse stimuli in humans. J Appl Physiol 1993; 74:1484–1491.
168. Umemiya M, Berger AJ. Presynaptic inhibition by serotonin of glycinergic inhibitory currents in the rat brain stem. J Neurophysiol 1995; 73:1192–1200.
169. Bellingham MC, Berger AJ. Presynaptic depression of excitatory synaptic inputs to rat hypoglossal motoneurons by muscarinic M2 receptors. J Neurophysiol 1996; 76: 3758–3770.
170. Singer JH, Bellingham MC, Berger AJ. Presynaptic inhibition of glutamatergic synaptic transmission to rat motoneurons by serotonin. J Neurophysiol 1996; 76:799–807.
171. Cairns BE, Fragoso MC, Soja PJ. Active-sleep-related suppression of feline trigeminal sensory neurons: evidence implicating presynaptic inhibition via a process of primary afferent depolarization. J Neurophysiol 1996; 75, 3:1152–1162.
172. Cairns BE, Fragoso MC, Soja PJ. Activity of rostral trigeminal sensory neurons in the cat during wakefulness and sleep. J Neurophysiol 1995; 73, 6:2486–2498.
173. Satoh T, Yamada S, Yokota T, Ohshima T, Kitayama S. Modulation during sleep of the cat trigeminal neurons responding to tooth pulp stimulation. Physiol Behav 1987; 39:395–398.
174. Carli G, Diete-Spiff K, Pompeiano O. Transmission of sensory information through the lemniscal pathway during sleep. Arch Ital Biol 1967; 105:31–51.
175. Xi MC, Yamuy J, Liu R-H, Morales FR, Chase MH. Dorsal spinocerebellar tract neuron are not subjected to postsynaptic inhibition during carbachol-induced motor inhibition. J Neurophysiol 1997; 78:137–144.
176. Kishikawa K, Uchida H, Yamamori Y, Collins JG. Low-threshold neuronal activity of spinal dorsal horn neurons increases during REM sleep in cats: comparison with effects of anesthesia. J Neurophysiol 1995; 74:763–769.
177. Glenn LL, Dement WC. Group I excitatory and inhibitory potentials in hindlimb motoneurons during wakefulness and sleep. J Neurophysiol 1981; 46:1089–1101.
178. Henke KG, Badr MS, Skatrud JB, Dempsey JA. Load compensation and respiratory muscle function during sleep. J Appl Physiol 1992; 72:1221–1234.
179. Berry RB, Gleeson K. Respiratory arousal from sleep: mechanisms and significance. Sleep 1997; 20:654–675.
180. Smith CA, Henderson KS, Xi L, Chow C-M, Eastwood PR, Dempsey JA. Neural-mechanical coupling of breathing in REM sleep. J Appl Physiol 1997; 83:1923–1932.
181. Issa FG, Bitner S. Effect of route of breathing on the ventilatory and arousal responses to hypercapnia in awake and sleeping dogs. J Physiol (Lond) 1993; 465:615–628.
182. Horner RL, Kozar LF, Kimoff RJ, Phillipson EA. Effects of sleep on the tonic drive to respiratory muscle and the threshold for rhythm generation in the dog. J Physiol (Lond) 1994; 474:525–537.
183. Parisi RA, Edelman NH, Santiago TV. Central respiratory carbon dioxide chemosensitivity does not decrease during sleep. Am Rev Respir Dis 1992; 145:832–836.
184. Sullivan CE, Murphy E, Kozar LF, Phillipson EA. Waking and ventilatory responses to laryngeal stimulation in sleeping dogs. J Appl Physiol 1978; 45:681–689.
185. Orr WC, Johnson LF. Responses to different levels of esophageal acidification during waking and sleep. Digest Dis Sci 1998; 43:241–245.

186. Orem J, Dick T, Norris P. Laryngeal and diaphragmatic responses to airway occlusion in sleep and wakefulness. Electroencephalogr Clin Neurophysiol 1980; 50:151–164.
187. Issa FG, Edwards P, Szeto E, Lauff D, Sullivan CE. Genioglossus and breathing responses to airway occlusion: effect of sleep and route of occlusion. J Appl Physiol 1988; 64:543–549.
188. Horner RL, Innes JA, Morrell MJ, Shea SA, Guz A. The effect of sleep on reflex genioglossus muscle activation by stimuli of negative airway pressure in humans. J Physiol (Lond) 1994; 476:141–151.
189. Okabe S, Chonan T, Hida W, Satoh M, Kikuchi Y, Takishima T. Role of chemical drive in recruiting upper airway and inspiratory intercostal muscles in patients with obstructive sleep apnea. Am Rev Respir Dis 1993; 147:190–195.
190. Yasuma F, Kozar LF, Kimoff RJ, Bradley TD, Phillipson EA. Interaction of chemical and mechanical respiratory stimuli in the arousal response to hypoxia in sleeping dogs. Am Rev Respir Dis 1991; 143:1274–1277.
191. Issa FG, Sullivan CE. Arousal and breathing responses to airway occlusion in healthy sleeping adults. J Appl Physiol 1983; 55:1113–1119.
192. Issa FG, McNamara SG, Sullivan CE. Arousal responses to airway occlusion in sleeping dogs: comparison of nasal and tracheal occlusions. J Appl Physiol 1987; 62:1832–1836.
193. Basner RC, Ringler J, Garpestad E, Schwartzstein RM, Sparrow D, Weinberger SE, et al. Upper airway anesthesia delays arousal from airway occlusion induced during human NREM sleep. J Appl Physiol 1992; 73:642–648.
194. McNicholas WT, Coffey M, McDonnell T, O'Regan R, Fitzgerald MX. Upper airway obstruction during sleep in normal subjects after selective topical oropharyngeal anesthesia. Am Rev Respir Dis 1987; 135:1316–1319.
195. Berry RB, Kouchi KG, Bower JL, Light RW. Effect of upper airway anesthesia on obstructive sleep apnea. Am J Respir Crit Care Med 1995; 151:1857–1861.
196. Chadwick GA, Crowley P, Fitzgerald MX, O'Regan RG, McNicholas WT. Obstructive sleep apnea following topical oropharyngeal anesthesia in loud snorers. Am Rev Respir Dis 1991; 143:810–813.
197. Deegan PC, Mulloy E, McNicholas WT. Topical oropharyngeal anesthesia in patients with obstructive sleep apnea. Am J Respir Crit Care Med 1995; 151:1108–1112.
198. Jacobs BL, Azmitia EC. Structure and function of the brain serotonin system. Physiol Rev 1992; 72:165–229.
199. Aston-Jones G, Bloom FE. Activity of norepinephrine-containing locus coeruleus neurons in behaving rats anticipates fluctuations in the sleep-waking cycle. J Neurosci 1981; 1:876–886.
200. Reiner PB. Correlational analysis of central noradrenergic neuronal activity and sympathetic tone in behaving cats. Brain Res 1986; 378:86–96.
201. Kanamori N, Sakai K, Jouvet M. Neuronal activity specific to paradoxical sleep in the ventromedial medullary reticular formation of unrestrained cats. Brain Res 1980; 189: 251–255.
202. Sakai K, Sastre J-P, Kanamori N, Jouvet M. State-specific neurons in the ponto-medullary reticular formation with special reference to the postural atonia during paradoxical sleep in the cat. In: Pompeiano O, Ajmone Marsan C, eds. Brain Mechanisms of Perceptual Awareness and Purposeful Behavior. New York: Raven, 1981:405–429.
203. Steriade M, Sakai K, Jouvet M. Bulbo-thalamic neurons related to thalamocortical activation processes during paradoxical sleep. Exp Brain Res 1984; 54:463–475.

204. Steriade M, Datta S, Paré D, Oakson G, Curro Dossi R. Neuronal activities in brainstem cholinergic nuclei related to tonic activation processes in thalamocortical systems. J Neurosci 1990; 10:2541–2559.
205. Sakai K. Executive mechanisms of paradoxical sleep. Arch Ital Biol 1988; 126:239–257.
206. Jones BE. Paradoxical sleep and its chemical/structural substrates in the brain. Neuroscience 1991; 40:637–656.
207. Reiner PB. Are mesopontine cholinergic neurons either necessary or sufficient components of the ascending reticular activating system? Semin Neurosci 1995; 7:355–359.
208. Baghdoyan HA. Cholinergic mechanisms regulating REM sleep. In: Schwartz WJ, ed. Sleep Science: Integrating Basic Research and Clinical Practice. Basel: Karger, 1997: 88–116.
209. Aldes LD, Chronister RC, Marco LA, Haycock JW, Thibault J. Differential distribution of biogenic amines in the hypoglossal nucleus of the rat. Exp Brain Res 1988; 73: 305–314.
210. Aldes LD, Marco LA, Chronister RB. Serotonin-containing axon terminals in the hypoglossal nucleus of the rat. An immuno-electronmicroscopic study. Brain Res Bull 1989; 23:249–256.
211. Aldes LD. Topographically organized projections from the nucleus subceruleus to the hypoglossal nucleus in the rat: a light and electron microscopic study with complementary axonal transport techniques. J Comp Neurol 1990; 302:643–656.
212. Aldes LD, Chronister RB, Shelton C, III, Haycock JW, Marco LA, Wong DL. Catecholamine innervation of the rat hypoglossal nucleus. Brain Res Bull 1988; 21:305–312.
213. Aldes LD, Shaw B, Chronister RB, Haycock JW. Catecholamine-containing axon terminals in the hypoglossal nucleus of the rat: an immuno-electronmicroscopic study. Exp Brain Res 1990; 81:167–178.
214. Arita H, Sakamoto M, Hirokawa Y, Okado N. Serotonin innervation patterns differ among the various medullary motoneuronal groups involved in upper airway control. Exp Brain Res 1993; 95:100–110.
215. McCall RB, Aghajanian GK. Serotonergic facilitation of facial motoneuron excitation. Brain Res 1979; 169:11–27.
216. Katakura N, Chandler SH. An iontophoretic analysis of the pharmacologic mechanisms responsible for trigeminal motoneuronal discharge during masticatory-like activity in the guinea pig. J Neurophysiol 1990; 63:356–369.
217. Kurasawa I, Toda K, Nakamura Y. Non-reciprocal facilitation of trigeminal motoneurons innervating jaw-closing and jaw-opening muscles induced by iontophoretic application of serotonin in the guinea pig. Brain Res 1990; 515:126–134.
218. Ribeiro-do-Valle LE, Metzler CW, Jacobs BL. Facilitation of masseter EMG and masseteric (jaw-closure) reflex by serotonin in behaving cats. Brain Res 1991; 550:197–204.
219. Larkman PM, Kelly JS. Ionic mechanisms mediating 5-hydroxytryptamine- and noradrenaline-evoked depolarization of adult rat facial motoneurones. J Physiol (Lond) 1992; 456:473–490.
220. Kubin L, Tojima H, Davies RO, Pack AI. Serotonergic excitatory drive to hypoglossal motoneurons in the decerebrate cat. Neurosci Lett 1992; 139:243–248.
221. Al-Zubaidy ZA, Erickson RL, Greer JJ. Serotonergic and noradrenergic effects on

respiratory neural discharge in the medullary slice preparation of neonatal rats. Pflügers Arch 1996; 431:942–949.
222. Rose D, Khater-Boidin J, Toussaint P, Duron B. Central effects of 5-HT on respiratory and hypoglossal activities in the adult cat. Respir Physiol 1995; 101:59–69.
223. Fenik V, Kubin L, Okabe S, Pack AI, Davies RO. Differential sensitivity of laryngeal and pharyngeal motoneurons to iontophoretic application of serotonin. Neuroscience 1997; 81:873–885.
224. Bylund DB, Eikenberg DC, Hieble JP, Langer SZ, Lefkowitz RJ, Minneman KP, et al. International Union of Pharmacology nomenclature of adrenoceptors. Pharmacol Rev 1994; 46:121–136.
225. Hieble JP, Bylund DB, Clarke DE, Eikenburg DC, Langer SZ, Lefkowitz RJ, et al. International Union of Pharmacology. X. Recommendation for nomenclature of α_1-adrenoceptors: consensus update. Pharmacol Rev 1995; 47:267–270.
226. Zifa E, Fillion G. 5-Hydroxytryptamine receptors. Pharmacol Rev 1992; 44:401–458.
227. Saxena PR. Serotonin receptors: subtypes, functional responses and therapeutical relevance. Pharmacol Ther 1995; 66:339–368.
228. Hoyer D, Martin G. 5-HT receptor classification and nomenclature: towards a harmonization with the human genome. Neuropharmacology 1997; 36:419–428.
229. Holtman JR, Jr., Marion LJ, Speck DF. Origin of serotonin-containing projections to the ventral respiratory group in the rat. Neuroscience 1990; 37:541–552.
230. Manaker S, Tischler LJ. Origin of serotonergic afferents to the hypoglossal nucleus in the rat. J Comp Neurol 1993; 334:466–476.
231. Li Y-Q, Takada M, Mizuno N. The sites of origin of serotoninergic afferent fibers in the trigeminal motor, facial, and hypoglossal nuclei in the rat. Neurosci Res 1993; 17: 307–313.
232. Connelly CA, Ellenberger HH, Feldman JL. Are there serotonergic projections from raphe and retrotrapezoid nuclei to the ventral respiratory group in the rat? Neurosci Lett 1989; 105:34–40.
233. McCall RB, Clement ME. Identification of serotonergic and sympathetic neurons in medullary raphe nuclei. Brain Res 1989; 477:172–182.
234. Pazos A, Probst A, Palacios JM. Serotonin receptors in the human brain—IV. Autoradiographic mapping of serotonin-2 receptors. Neuroscience 1987; 21:123–139.
235. Sharma A, Punhani T, Fone KCF. Distribution of the 5-hydroxytryptamine (2c) receptor protein in adult rat brain and spinal cord determined using a receptor-directed antibody: effect of 5,7-dihydroxytryptamine. Synapse 1997; 27:45–56.
236. Fay R, Kubin L. Pontomedullary distribution of 5-HT_{2A} receptor-like protein in the rat. J Comp Neurol 2000; 418:323–345.
237. Mengod G, Pompeiano M, Martínez-Mir MI, Palacios JM. Localization of the mRNA for the 5-HT_2 receptor by in situ hybridization histochemistry. Correlation with the distribution of receptor sites. Brain Res 1990; 524:139–143.
238. Wright DE, Seroogy KB, Lundgren KH, Davis BM, Jennes L. Comparative localization of serotonin$_{1A}$, $_{1C}$, and $_2$ receptor subtype mRNAs in rat brain. J Comp Neurol 1995; 351:357–373.
239. Okabe S, Mackiewicz M, Kubin L. Serotonin receptor mRNA expression in the hypoglossal motor nucleus. Respir Physiol 1997; 110:151–160.
240. Aghajanian GK, Sprouse JS, Sheldon P, Rasmussen K. Electrophysiology of the central serotonin system: receptor subtypes and transducer mechanisms. Ann NY Acad Sci 1990; 600:93–103.

241. Veasey SC, Panckeri KA, Hoffman EA, Pack AI, Hendricks JC. The effects of serotonin antagonists in an animal model of sleep-disordered breathing. Am J Respir Crit Care Med 1996; 153:776–786.
242. Hendricks JC, Kline LR, Kovalski RJ, O'Brien JA, Morrison AR, Pack AI. The English bulldog: a natural model of sleep-disordered breathing. J Appl Physiol 1987; 63:1344–1350.
243. Kubin L, Reignier C, Tojima H, Taguchi O, Pack AI, Davies RO. Changes in serotonin level in the hypoglossal nucleus region during carbachol-induced atonia. Brain Res 1994; 645:291–302.
244. Kubin L, Tojima H, Reignier C, Pack AI, Davies RO. Interaction of serotonergic excitatory drive to hypoglossal motoneurons with carbachol-induced, REM sleep-like atonia. Sleep 1996; 19:187–195.
245. Hanzel DA, Proia NG, Hudgel DW. Response of obstructive sleep apnea to fluoxetine and protriptyline. Chest 1991; 100:416–421.
246. Schmidt HS. L-tryptophan in the treatment of impaired respiration during sleep. Bull Eur Physiol Respir 1982; 19:625–629.
247. Thor KB, Blitz-Siebert A, Helke CJ. Autoradiographic localization of $5HT_1$ binding sites in the medulla oblongata of the rat. Synapse 1992; 10:185–205.
248. Manaker S, Zucchi PC. Autoradiographic localization of neurotransmitter binding sites in the hypoglossal and motor trigeminal nuclei of the rat. Synapse 1998; 28:44–59.
249. Morales M, Battenberg E, de Lecea L, Sanna PP, Bloom FE. Cellular and subcellular immunolocalization of the type 3 serotonin receptor in the rat central nervous system. Mol Brain Res 1996; 36:251–260.
250. Kolta A, Dubuc R, Lund JP. An immunocytochemical and autoradiographic investigation of the serotoninergic innervation of trigeminal mesencephalic and motor nuclei in the rabbit. Neuroscience 1993; 53:1113–1126.
251. Thor KB, Blitz-Siebert A, Helke CJ. Autoradiographic localization of $5HT_1$ binding sites in autonomic areas of the rat dorsomedial medulla oblongata. Synapse 1992; 10: 217–227.
252. Okabe S, Kubin L. Role of $5HT_1$ receptors in the control of hypoglossal motoneurons in vivo. Sleep 1996; 19:S150–S153.
253. Bayliss DA, Viana F, Talley EM, Berger AJ. Neuromodulation of hypoglossal motoneurons: cellular and developmental mechanisms. Respir Physiol 1997; 110:139–150.
254. Kia HK, Miquel M-C, Brisorgueil M-J, Davel G, Riad M, Mestikawy SE, et al. Immunocytochemical localization of serotonin(1A) receptors in the rat central nervous system. J Comp Neurol 1996; 365:289–305.
255. Talley EM, Sadr NN, Bayliss DA. Postnatal development of serotonergic innervation, $5\text{-}HT_{1A}$ receptor expression, and 5-HT responses in rat motoneurons. J Neurosci 1997; 17:4473–4485.
256. Steinbusch HWM. Distribution of serotonin—immunoreactivity in the central nervous system of the rat-cell bodies and terminals. Neuroscience 1981; 6:557–618.
257. Voss MD, de Castro D, Lipski J, Pilowsky PM, Jiang C. Serotonin immunoreactive boutons form close appositions with respiratory neurons of the dorsal respiratory group in the cat. J Comp Neurol 1990; 295:208–218.
258. Thor KB, Helke CJ. Serotonin- and substance P-containing projections to the nucleus tractus solitarii of the rat. J Comp Neurol 1987; 265:275–293.
259. Manaker S, Verderame HM. Organization of serotonin 1A and 1B receptors in the nucleus of the solitary tract. J Comp Neurol 1990; 301:535–553.

260. Champagnat J, Denavit-Saubié M, Henry JL, Leviel V. Catecholaminergic depressant effects on bulbar respiratory mechanisms. Brain Res 1979; 160:57–68.
261. Arita H, Ochiishi M. Opposing effects of 5-hydroxytryptamine on two types of medullary inspiratory neurons with distinct firing patterns. J Neurophysiol 1991; 66:285–292.
262. Lalley PM. The excitability and rhythm of medullary respiratory neurons in the cat are altered by the serotonin receptor agonist 5-methoxy-*N,N*,dimethyltryptamine. Brain Res 1994; 648:87–98.
263. Lalley PM, Bischoff A-M, Richter DW. 5-HT-1A receptor-mediated modulation of medullary expiratory neurons in the cat. J Physiol (Lond) 1994; 476:117–130.
264. Lalley PM, Bischoff AM, Schwarzacher W, Richter DW. 5-HT_2 receptor-controlled modulation of medullary respiratory neurones in the cat. J Physiol (Lond) 1995; 487: 653–661.
265. Rampin O, Pierrefiche O, Denavit-Saubié M. Effects of serotonin and substance P on bulbar respiratory neurons in vivo. Brain Res 1993; 622:185–193.
266. Douse MA, White DP. Serotonergic effects on hypoglossal neural activity and reflex responses. Brain Res 1996; 726:213–222.
267. Arvidsson J, Cullheim S, Ulfhake B, Bennett GW, Fone KCF, Cuello AC, et al. 5-Hydroxytryptamine, substance P, and thyrotropin-releasing hormone in the adult cat spinal cord segment L_7: immunohistochemical and chemical studies. Synapse 1990; 6:237–270.
268. Nicholas AP, Pieribone VA, Arvidsson U, Hökfelt T. Serotonin-, substance P- and glutamate/aspartate-like immunoreactivities in medullo-spinal pathways of rat and primate. Neuroscience 1992; 48:545–559.
269. Kachidian P, Poulat P, Marlier L, Privat A. Immunohistochemical evidence for the coexistence of substance P, thyrotropin-releasing hormone, GABA, methionin-enkephalin, and leucin-enkephalin in the serotonergic neurons of the caudal raphe nuclei: A dual labeling in the rat. J Neurosci Res 1991; 30:521–530.
270. Henry JN, Manaker S. Colocalization of substance P or enkephalin in serotonergic neuronal afferents to the hypoglossal nucleus in the rat. J Comp Neurol 1998; 391: 491–505.
271. Holtman JR, Jr. Immunohistochemical localization of serotonin- and substance P-containing fibers around respiratory muscle motoneurons in the nucleus ambiguus of the cat. Neuroscience 1988; 26:169–178.
272. Tallaksen-Greene SJ, Elde R, Wessendorf MW. Regional distribution of serotonin and substance P co-existing in nerve fibers and terminals in the brainstem of the rat. Neuroscience 1993; 53:1127–1142.
273. Sun Q-J, Pilowsky P, Llewellyn-Smith IJ. Thyrotropin-releasing hormone inputs are preferentially directed towards respiratory motoneurons in rat nucleus ambiguus. J Comp Neurol 1995; 362:320–330.
274. Gatti PJ, Coleman WC, Shirahata M, Johnson T, Massari VJ. Synaptic interactions of retrogradely labeled hypoglossal motoneurons with substance P-like immunoreactive nerve terminals in the cat: a dual-labeling electron microscopic study. Exp Brain Res 1996; 110:175–182.
275. Gatti PJ, Llewellyn-Smith IJ, Sun Q-J, Chalmers D, Pilowsky P. Substance P-immunoreactive boutons closely appose inspiratory protruder hypoglossal motoneurons in the cat. Brain Res 1999; 834:155–159.

276. Hinrichsen CFL, Weston S. Substance P in the hypoglossal nucleus of the rat. Arch Oral Biol 1999; 44:683–691.
277. Manaker S, Rizio G. Autoradiographic localization of thyrotropin-releasing hormone and substance P receptors in the rat dorsal vagal complex. J Comp Neurol 1989; 290: 516–526.
278. Nakaya Y, Kaneko T, Shigemoto R, Nakanishi S, Mizuno N. Immunohistochemical localization of substance P receptor in the central nervous system of the adult rat. J Comp Neurol 1994; 347:249–274.
279. White SR, Crane GK, Jackson DA. Thyrotropin-releasing hormone (TRH) effects on spinal cord neuronal excitability. Ann NY Acad Sci 1989; 553:337–350.
280. White SR, Fung SJ, Jackson DA, Imel KM. Serotonin, norepinephrine and associated neuropeptides: effects on somatic motoneuron excitability. Prog Brain Res 1996; 107: 183–199.
281. Rekling JC. Excitatory effects of thyrotropin-releasing hormone (TRH) in hypoglossal motoneurons. Brain Res 1990; 510:175–179.
282. Bayliss DA, Viana F, Berger AJ. Mechanisms underlying excitatory effects of thyrotropin-releasing hormone on rat hypoglossal motoneurons in vitro. J Neurophysiol 1992; 68:1733–1745.
283. Magalang UJ, Okabe S, Kubin L. Microinjection of the TRH analogue MK-771 into the rat hypoglossal nucleus induces a biphasic excitation. Sleep Res 1996; 25:16.
284. Funk GD, Smith JC, Feldman JL. Development of thyrotropin-releasing hormone and norepinephrine potentiation of inspiratory-related hypoglossal motoneuron discharge in neonatal and juvenile mice in vitro. J Neurophysiol 1994; 72:2538–2541.
285. Iverfeldt K, Serfözö P, Diaz Arnesto L, Bartfai T. Differential release of coexisting neurotransmitters: frequency dependence of the efflux of substance P, thyrotropin releasing hormone and [^{3}H] serotonin from tissue slices of rat ventral spinal cord. Acta Physiol Scand 1989; 137:63–71.
286. Hökfelt T, Johansson O, Goldstein M. Chemical anatomy of the brain. Science 1984; 225:1326–1334.
287. Millhorn DE, Hökfelt T, Szymeczek CL, Bayliss DA, Seroogy KB. Cellular, molecular and developmental aspects of chemical synaptic transmission. In: Haddad GG, Farber JP, eds. Developmental Neurobiology of Breathing. New York: Marcel Dekker, 1991: 11–70.
288. Veasey SC, Fornal CA, Metzler CW, Jacobs BL. Response of serotonergic caudal raphe neurons in relation to specific motor activities in freely moving cats. J Neurosci 1995; 15:5346–5359.
289. Nagase Y, Moritani M, Nakagawa S, Yoshida A, Takemura M, Zhang L-F, et al. Serotonergic axonal contacts on identified cat trigeminal motoneurons and their correlation with medullary raphe nucleus stimulation. J Comp Neurol 1997; 384:443–455.
290. Agnati LF, Zoli M, Stromberg I, Fuxe K. Intercellular communication in the brain: wiring versus volume transmission. Neuroscience 1995; 69:711–726.
291. Saha S, Appenteng K, Batten TFC. Light and electron microscopical localisation of 5-HT-immunoreactive boutons in the rat trigeminal motor nucleus. Brain Res 1991; 559:145–148.
292. Aldes LD, Chapman ME, Chronister RB, Haycock JW. Sources of noradrenergic afferents to the hypoglossal nucleus in the rat. Brain Res Bull 1992; 29:931–942.
293. Stafford IL, Jacobs BL. Noradrenergic modulation of the masseteric reflex in behaving cats. I. Pharmacological studies. J Neurosci 1990; 10:91–98.

294. Nishimura Y, Muramatsu M, Asahara T, Tanaka T, Yamamoto T. Electrophysiological properties and their modulation by norepinephrine in the ambiguus neurons of the guinea pig. Brain Res 1995; 702:213–222.
295. Aston-Jones G, Shipley MT, Chouvet G, Ennis M, van Bockstaele E, Pieribone V, et al. Afferent regulation of locus coeruleus neurons: anatomy, physiology and pharmacology. Prog Brain Res 1991; 88:47–75.
296. Aston-Jones G, Rajkowski J, Kubiak P, Valentino RJ, Shipley MT. Role of the locus coeruleus in emotional activation. Prog Brain Res 1996; 107:379–402.
297. Parkis MA, Bayliss DA, Berger AJ. Actions of norepinephrine on rat hypoglossal motoneurons. J Neurophysiol 1995; 74:1911–1919.
298. Day HEW, Campeau S, Watson SJ, Jr., Akil H. Distribution of α_{1A}-, α_{1B}- and α_{1D}-adrenergic receptor mRNA in the rat brain and spinal cord. J Chem Neuroanat 1997; 13:115–139.
299. Shao Y, Sutin J. Expression of adrenergic receptors in individual astrocytes and motor neurons isolated from the adult rat brain. Glia 1992; 6:108–117.
300. Shao Y, Sutin J. Noradrenergic facilitation of motor neurons: localization of adrenergic receptors in neurons and nonneuronal cells in the trigeminal motor nucleus. Exp Neurol 1991; 114:216–227.
301. Rainbow TC, Parsons B, Wolfe BB. Quantitative autoradiography of α_1- and α_2-adrenergic receptors in rat brain. Proc Natl Acad Sci USA 1984; 81:1585–1589.
302. Trombley PQ, Shepherd GM. Noradrenergic inhibition of synaptic transmission between mitral and granule cells in mammalian olfactory bulb cultures. J Neurosci 1992; 12:3985–3991.
303. Selvaratnam SR, Parkis MA, Funk GD. Developmental modulation of mouse hypoglossal nerve inspiratory output in vitro by noradrenergic receptor agonists. Brain Res 1998; 805:104–115.
304. Parkis MA, Berger AJ. Clonidine reduces hyperpolarization-activated inward current (I_h) in rat hypoglossal motoneurons. Brain Res 1997; 769:108–118.
305. Scheinin M, Lomasney JW, Hayden-Hixson DM, Schambra UB, Caron MG, Lefkowitz RJ, et al. Distribution of α_2-adrenergic receptor subtype gene expression in rat brain. Mol Brain Res 1994; 21:133–149.
306. Talley EM, Rosin DL, Lee A, Guyenet PG, Lynch KR. Distribution of α_{2A}-adrenergic receptor-like immunoreactivity in the rat central nervous system. J Comp Neurol 1996; 372:111–134.
307. Rosin DL, Talley EM, Lee A, Stornetta RL, Gaylinn BD, Guyenet PG, et al. Distribution of α_{2C}-adrenergic receptor-like immunoreactivity in the rat central nervous system. J Comp Neurol 1996; 372:135–165.
308. Hilaire G, Monteau R, Errchidi S. Possible modulation of the medullary respiratory rhythm generator by the noradrenergic A_5 area: an in vitro study in the newborn rat. Brain Res 1989; 485:325–332.
309. Errchidi S, Hilaire G, Monteau R. Permanent release of noradrenaline modulates respiratory frequency in the newborn rat: an in vitro study. J Physiol (Lond) 1990; 429: 497–510.
310. Johnson SM, Smith JC, Feldman JL. Modulation of respiratory rhythm in vitro: role of $G_{i/o}$ protein-mediated mechanisms. J Appl Physiol 1996; 80:2120–2133.
311. Thakkar MM, Strecker RE, McCarley RW. Behavioral state control through differential serotonergic inhibition in the mesopontine cholinergic nuclei: a simultaneous unit recording and microdialysis study. J Neurosci 1998; 18:5490–5497.

312. Zaninetti M, Tribollet E, Bertrand D, Raggenbass M. Presence of functional neuronal nicotinic acetylcholine receptors in brainstem motoneurons of the rat. Eur J Neurosci 1999; 11:2737–2748.
313. Morales FR, Boxer P, Chase MH. Behavioral state-specific inhibitory postsynaptic potentials impinge on cat lumbar motoneurons during active sleep. Exp Neurol 1987; 98:418–435.
314. Chase MH, Soja PJ, Morales FR. Evidence that glycine mediates the postsynaptic potentials that inhibit lumbar motoneurons during the atonia of active sleep. J Neurosci 1989; 9:743–751.
315. Soja PJ, López-Rodríguez F, Morales FR, Chase MH. The postsynaptic inhibitory control of lumbar motoneurons during the atonia of active sleep: effect of strychnine on motoneuron properties. J Neurosci 1991; 11:2804–2811.
316. Glenn LL, Dement WC. Membrane potential, synaptic activity, and excitability of hindlimb motoneurons during wakefulness and sleep. J Neurophysiol 1981; 46:839–854.
317. Glenn LL, Dement WC. Membrane resistance and rheobase of hindlimb motoneurons during wakefulness and sleep. J Neurophysiol 1981; 46:1076–1088.
318. Morales F, Chase MH. Postsynaptic control of lumbar motoneuron excitability during active sleep in the chronic cat. Brain Res 1981; 225:279–295.
319. Chase MH, Morales F. The atonia and myoclonia of active (REM) sleep. Annu Rev Psychol 1990; 41:557–584.
320. Mori S. Contribution of postural muscle tone to full expression of posture and locomotor movements: multi-faceted analyses of its setting brainstem-spinal cord mechanisms in the cat. Jpn J Physiol 1989; 39:785–809.
321. Netick A, Orem J, Dement W. Neuronal activity specific to REM sleep and its relationship to breathing. Brain Res 1977; 120:197–207.
322. Takakusaki K, Ohta Y, Mori S. Single medullary reticulospinal neurons exert postsynaptic inhibitory effects via inhibitory interneurons upon alpha-motoneurons innervating cat hindlimb muscles. Exp Brain Res 1989; 74:11–23.
323. Takakusaki K, Shimoda N, Matsuyama K, Mori S. Discharge properties of medullary reticulospinal neurons during postural changes induced by intrapontine injections of carbachol, atropine and serotonin, and their functional linkages to hindlimb motoneurons in cats. Exp Brain Res 1994; 99:361–374.
324. Wu W, Wessendorf W. Organization of the serotonergic innervation of spinal neurons in rats—I. Neuropeptide coexistence in varicosities innervating some spinothalamic tract neurons but not in those innervating postsynaptic dorsal column neurons. Neuroscience 1992; 50:885–898.
325. Holstege JC. The ventro-medial medullary projections to spinal motoneurons: ultrastructure, transmitters and functional aspects. Prog Brain Res 1996; 107:159–181.
326. Wu W, Elde R, Wessendorf MW. Organization of the serotonergic innervation of spinal neurons in rats—III. Differential serotonergic innervation of somatic and parasympathetic preganglionic motoneurons as determined by patterns of co-existing peptides. Neuroscience 1993; 55:223–233.
327. Kiehn O. Plateau potentials and active integration in the 'final common pathway' for motor behavior. Trends Neurosci 1991; 14:68–73.
328. Alvarez JF, Pearson JC, Harrington D, Dewey D, Torbeck L, Fyffe REW. Distribution of 5-hydroxytryptamine-immunoreactive boutons on α-motoneurons in the lumbar spinal cord of adult cats. J Comp Neurol 1998; 393:69–83.

329. Yamuy J, Fung SJ, Xi M, Morales FR, Chase MH. Hypoglossal motoneurons are postsynaptically inhibited during carbachol-induced rapid eye movement sleep. Neuroscience 1999; 94:11–15.
330. Soja PJ, Finch DM, Chase MH. Effect of inhibitory amino acid antagonists on masseteric reflex suppression during active sleep. Exp Neurol 1987; 96:178–193.
331. Kubin L, Kimura H, Tojima H, Davies RO, Pack AI. Suppression of hypoglossal motoneurons during the carbachol-induced atonia of REM sleep is not caused by fast synaptic inhibition. Brain Res 1993; 611:300–312.
332. Rampon C, Peyron C, Petit J-M, Fort P, Gervasoni D, Luppi P-H. Origin of the glycinergic innervation of the rat trigeminal motor nucleus. NeuroReport 1996; 7:3081–3085.
333. Turman J, Chandler SH. Immunohistochemical evidence for GABA and glycine-containing trigeminal premotoneurons in the guinea pig. Synapse 1994; 18:7–20.
334. Rampon C, Luppi P-H, Fort P, Peyron C, Jouvet M. Distribution of glycine-immunoreactive cell bodies and fibers in the rat brain. Neuroscience 1996; 75:737–755.
335. Lowe AA. The neural regulation of tongue movements. Prog Neurobiol 1981; 15:295–344.
336. Takata M. Two types of inhibitory postsynaptic potentials in the hypoglossal motoneurons. Prog Neurobiol 1993; 40:385–411.
337. Harrison Y, Horne JA. Sleep deprivation affects speech. Sleep 1997; 20:871–877.
338. Guilleminault C, Rosekind M. The arousal threshold: sleep deprivation, sleep fragmentation, and obstructive sleep apnea. Bull Eur Physiopath Respir 1981; 17:341–349.
339. Leiter JC, Knuth SL, Bartlett D, Jr. The effect of sleep deprivation on activity of the genioglossus muscle. Am Rev Respir Dis 1985; 132:1242–1245.
340. O'Donnell CP, King ED, Schwartz AR, Smith PL, Robotham JL. Effect of sleep deprivation on responses to airway obstruction in the sleeping dog. J Appl Physiol 1994; 77:1811–1818.
341. Persson HE, Svanborg E. Sleep deprivation worsens obstructive sleep apnea. Chest 1996; 109:645–650.
342. Kimoff RJ. Sleep fragmentation in obstructive sleep apnea. Sleep 1996; 19:S61–S66.
343. Sherin JE, Shiromani PJ, McCarley RW, Saper CB. Activation of ventrolateral preoptic neurons during sleep. Science 1996; 271:216–219.
344. Yeh ER, Erokwu B, LaManna JC, Haxhiu MA. The paraventricular nucleus of the hypothalamus influences respiratory timing and activity in the rat. Neurosci Lett 1997; 232:63–66.
345. Szymusiak R. Magnocellular nuclei of the basal forebrain: substrates of sleep and arousal regulation. Sleep 1995; 18:478–500.
346. Petrof BJ, Pack AI, Kelly AM, Eby J, Hendricks JC. Pharyngeal myopathy of loaded upper airway in dogs with sleep apnea. J Appl Physiol 1994; 76:1746–1752.
347. Edström L, Larsson H, Larsson L. Neurogenic effects on the palatopharyngeal muscle in patients with obstructive sleep apnoea: a muscle biopsy study. J Neurol Neurosurg Psych 1992; 55:916–920.
348. Sériès F, Simoneau J-A, St.Pierre S, Marc I. Characteristics of the genioglossus and musculus uvulae in sleep apnea hypopnea syndrome and in snorers. Am J Respir Crit Care Med 1996; 153:1870–1874.
349. Friberg D, Ansved T, Borg K, Carlsson-Norlander B, Larsson H, Svanborg E. Histological indications of a progressive snorers disease in the upper airway muscles. Am J Respir Crit Care Med 1998; 157:586–593.

350. Mifflin SW. Intensity and frequency dependence of laryngeal afferent inputs to respiratory hypoglossal motoneurons. J Appl Physiol 1997; 83:1890–1899.
351. Friberg D, Gazelius B, Hökfelt T, Nordlander B. Abnormal afferent nerve endings in the soft palatal mucosa of sleep apnoics and habitual snorers. Reg Peptides 1997; 71: 29–36.
352. Kimoff JR, Makino H, Horner RL, Kozar LF, Lue F, Slutsky AS, et al. Canine model of obstructive sleep apnea: model description and preliminary application. J Appl Physiol 1994; 76:1810–1817.
353. Deegan PC, Nolan P, Carey M, McNicholas WT. Effects of positive airway pressure on upper airway dilator muscle activity and ventilatory timing. J Appl Physiol 1996; 81:470–479.

5

Airway Reflexes
Changes with Sleep

DAVID P. WHITE

Brigham and Women's Hospital
and Harvard Medical School
Boston, Massachusetts

I. Introduction

The principal event in the development of obstructive sleep apnea is a collapse or near-collapse of the pharyngeal airway during sleep. As a result, understanding the mechanisms that control upper airway patency while awake and how such mechanisms are impacted by sleep is essential if one is to grasp the pathophysiology of this disorder. Therefore, all such mechanisms will be discussed briefly in the beginning of this chapter with a particular focus on the control of the pharyngeal musculature. Thereafter, reflex mechanisms involved in the control of these muscles and how such reflexes are affected by sleep will be addressed at length.

The pharyngeal airway between the choanae (end of the nasal septum) and the epiglottis has little rigid or bony support and is, therefore, substantially dependent on nonstructural mechanisms (primarily muscle activation) to maintain patency. Because this is the site of airway collapse during sleep in the apneic individual, understanding these mechanisms is important in understanding the disorder. This should not imply that airway anatomy is unimportant. Bones and soft tissue clearly define the basic size and structure of the pharyngeal airway and the extent to which muscular mechanisms must be activated to avoid collapse. Therefore, an anatomically large airway will likely require little muscle activation, while a small one may constantly need such support to maintain patency. As a result, individual anatomy in many ways defines the propensity of the airway to collapse (1,2). However, anatomy does not change over the sleep-wake cycle, indicating that nonstructural influences (muscular and other) dictate the state-related nature of this disorder.

The principal nonstructural determinants of upper airway luminal size in humans are the pharyngeal dilator muscles. Substantial evidence suggests that the activity of these muscles is quite important in the maintenance of airway patency (3–5). Most, but not all, such pharyngeal dilator muscles have an inspiratory phasic pattern of activation (6–10). Increased contraction during inspiration (Fig. 1) offsets the negative intrapharyngeal pressure at this point in the respiratory cycle, thereby avoiding collapse (5). There are numerous pharyngeal muscles with complex anatomy and intricate relationships, with some, but not all, of these muscles being demonstrated in Figure 2. However, only a few such muscles have been studied in any detail, leaving us with an incomplete understanding of their control and interactions.

Several other factors may also influence the patency and collapsibility of the

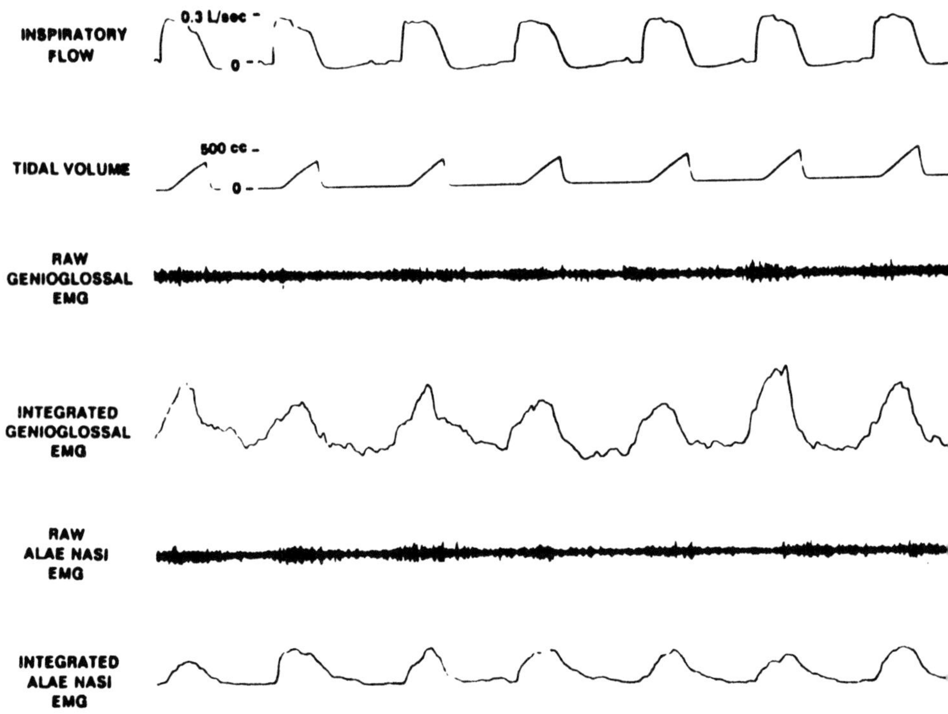

Figure 1 Sample recording from a normal subject during stage 2 non–rapid-eye-movement (non-REM) sleep. Raw and integrated (moving-time–averaged) genioglossal and alae nasi EMG signals show phasic activation during inspiration (corresponding to a positive deflection in respiratory flow signal). (From Ref. 46.)

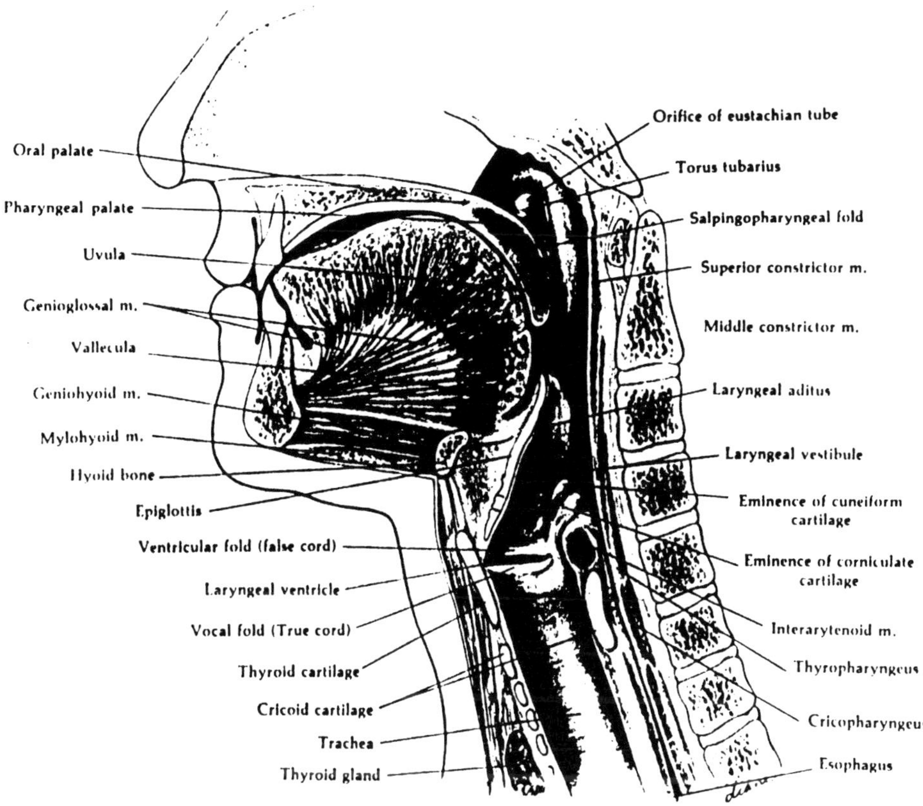

Figure 2 Parasagittal section of the pharynx, larynx, and mouth of a male adult. This figure demonstrates some, but not all, of the muscles involved in the maintenance of pharyngeal patency. The complexity of the airway and muscular interactions is evident. (From Ref. 97.)

upper airway. First, considerable animal data suggest that increasing airway length or increased tracheal traction on the upper airway may substantially improve airflow characteristics and reduce collapsibility (11,12). In at least one such study, upper airway muscle activation (tongue displacement) actually had little influence on airway patency until tracheal traction was applied (13). This would suggest that lung volume (the principal determinant of airway length and tracheal traction) may importantly influence the dynamics of the upper airway. However, these mechanisms have not been carefully studied to date in humans. Second, pharyngeal mucosal perfusion can also affect airway patency. Imaging and physiological studies suggest that the application of vasoconstrictors to the mucosa increases pharyngeal luminal size (14). Edema is likely to have the opposite effect. Finally, the surface characteristics of the airway (surface tension) may affect pharyngeal collapsibility. A recent study suggests that a synthetic lung surfactant preparation (low surface tension) applied to the upper airway of normal subjects substantially reduced collapsibility and improved the ability of the airway to reopen once closed (15). However, the actual importance of this latter mechanism (and airway perfusion as well) remains unclear at this time.

II. Control of the Pharyngeal Musculature During Wakefulness

As stated above, the pharyngeal musculature importantly influences the patency of the human upper airway. Therefore, the mechanisms controlling the activity of these muscles can have a substantial impact on airway size. Although there are numerous pharyngeal muscles, we will focus on the genioglossus because it is the dilator muscle that has been studied most extensively. In the basal state, as described above (6,16), this muscle demonstrates an inspiratory phasic pattern of activation (Fig. 1), which is present to some extent even in the absence of airway negative pressure or other local stimuli (17). This was demonstrated in laryngectomized patients breathing exclusively through their tracheostomy (17). Therefore, central neural mechanisms not dependent on afferent stimuli from the upper airway maintain some activity in this muscle during both inspiration and expiration.

Against this background of centrally generated neural input, local airway mechanisms can also substantially influence genioglossal activation and the activity of other upper airway muscles as well. It has been known for some time that the application of negative pressure to the isolated upper airway of an animal leads to an increase in the activity of the genioglossus muscle (18,19). In anesthetized rabbits severing the superior laryngeal nerve substantially attenuated this reflex, and the addition of upper airway topical anesthesia largely abolished it (20). This would suggest that laryngeal mucosal receptors are driving this reflex. However, a recent study in dogs indicated that topical anesthesia of the entire upper airway could not abolish this reflex, and the authors argue that spindles or ''submucosal mechanoreceptors'' may play an important role (21). Muscle spindles have actually been demonstrated in the tongue musculature of primates (22,23) with increased afferent activity in response to stretching of the tongue anteriorally in cats (24). The importance of this mechanism in controlling genioglossal activation remains unclear. Therefore, a variety of mechanisms are available to respond to changes in airway pressure. A similar short-latency negative pressure reflex has been demonstrated in humans (25,26) following the rapid application of pulses of negative pressure (Fig. 3). This reflex can also be substantially attenuated in normal humans by combined nasopharyngeal anesthesia and injection of the superior laryngeal nerve, suggesting that laryngeal and mucosal receptors are important in mediating this reflex (25). A similar reflex has been demonstrated in other upper airway dilator muscles as well (27,28). It is this reflex that will be the focus of this chapter.

The information provided above suggests that several mechanisms may be driving this upper airway negative pressure reflex. There are likely mucosal mechanoreceptors responsible for at least a portion of the reflex, with most evidence sug-

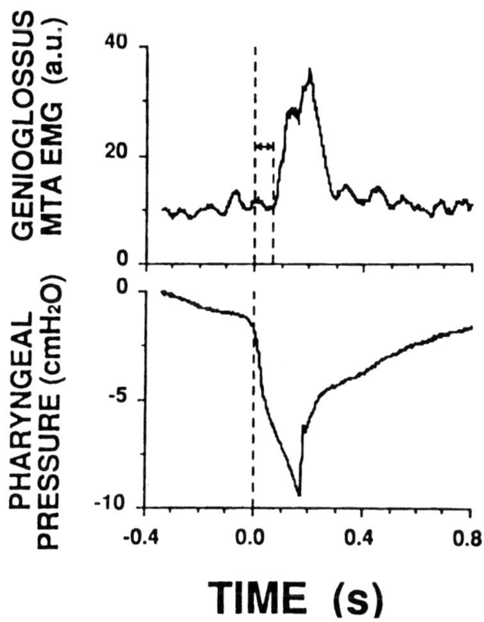

Figure 3 Representative computer recording of genioglossal moving-time-average (MTA) electromyogram (EMG) and pharyngeal pressure in one normal subject during a negative pressure generation. Vertical dashed lines indicate negative pressure onset in both panels. Second vertical dashed line in top panel denotes onset of increasing genioglossal EMG activity. (From Ref. 26.)

gesting that the afferent pathway from these receptors is through the superior laryngeal nerve (20,25). However, severing this nerve in rabbits did not completely abolish the reflex [particularly when negative pressure was applied through the nose (20)], nor did blocking the superior laryngeal nerve in humans (25). Nasopharyngeal anesthesia further attenuated the reflex in humans (25) and largely abolished it in some animals (20). In addition, negative airway pressure in the rat has been demonstrated to increase the discharge of single fiber afferents in the anterior ethmoidal nerve [a branch of the trigeminal (29)]. Therefore, nasopharyngeal and laryngeal mucosal mechanoreceptors with afferents through the trigeminal and superior laryngeal nerves, respectively, are likely important mediators of this reflex. However, there is little evidence for afferents originating in the oropharyngeal airway (glossopharyngeal nerve) playing a substantial role in negative pressure muscle activation (30). Finally, as stated above, muscle spindles located in pharyngeal dilator muscles may provide an additional mechanism by which negative pressure could lead to augmented muscle activity.

A number of additional mechanisms influencing upper airway muscle activation will be addressed briefly. First, standard chemical respiratory stimuli (hypoxia and hypercapnia) can increase genioglossal electromyogram (EMG) (31,32) and EMG of other upper airway muscles as well (7). Second, there are pulmonary vagal influences on genioglossal/hypoglossal activity. Lung inflation leads to a graded inhibition of genioglossal EMG or hypoglossal neural activity (33,34). When such inflation is prevented by airway occlusion or by vagal blockade, genioglossal activity increases. Third, there is a relationship between blood pressure and genioglossal activation. Maneuvers that increase baroreceptor output (increased blood pressure, change of posture, etc.) inhibit genioglossal/hypoglossal activity (35,36). Finally, one recent study suggests that the female hormones estrogen and progesterone may increase upper airway muscle EMG (37). In that study, women had considerably greater genioglossal activity than men during wakefulness (37), with recent data suggesting that this was mediated by the female hormones (38). Therefore, the genioglossus is subject to a variety of inputs that precisely control its activity, thereby maintaining airway patency.

A. Waking Pharyngeal Muscle Activity in the Apnea Patient

There is an increasing body of evidence indicating that the pharyngeal dilator muscles of the apnea patient have increased activity during wakefulness when compared to normal, nonapneic individuals. These data take two forms. First, studies in which the genioglossal EMG has been normalized to a percent of maximal activity indicate that this muscle in the apnea patient is functioning at a much higher percent of maximum than that of controls (Fig. 4). This has been demonstrated for the tensor

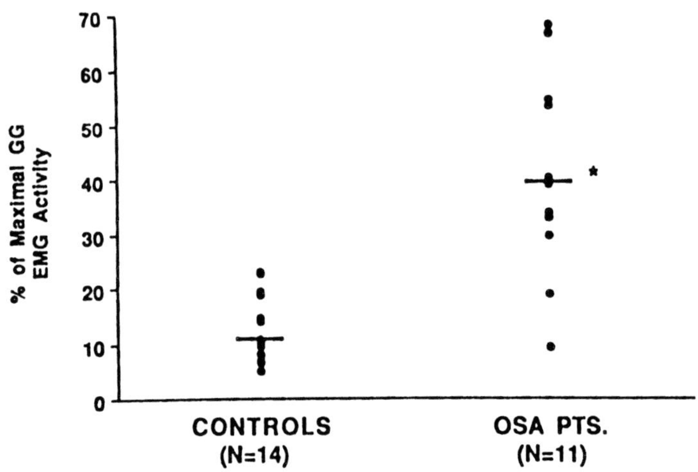

Figure 4 Peak phasic GG EMG, expressed as a percentage of maximal activity, is demonstrated for 14 controls and 11 obstructive apnea patients during basal breathing. The genioglossus functions at a higher percentage of maximum in obstructive sleep apnea patients compared to controls. $^{*}p < 0.05$ vs. controls. (From Ref. 39.)

palatini as well (40). A similar observation was made in the English bulldog, an animal model of obstructive sleep apnea (41). Second, studies of the musculus uvula comparing apnea patients to nonapneic snorers demonstrated increased muscle area (hypertrophy), muscle tension development, and anaerobic enzymatic capability in the apnea patients (42). Thus, this muscle in the apnea patient is highly "trained." All such data suggest that some mechanism is leading to increased activity in these upper airway muscles in the apneic individual.

What is driving the augmented muscle activity in these patients is unclear. However, it seems highly probably that this represents some form of neuromuscular compensation for the deficient pharyngeal anatomy in this patient group. There are overwhelming data indicating that the majority of apnea patients have a small pharyngeal airway (1,2). This was originally demonstrated in 1983 using computed tomography (CT) imaging (2) and has been confirmed repetitively using increasingly sophisticated imaging technologies during wakefulness (1). In addition, studies conducted during sleep (43) examining the passive human upper airway (no or little muscle activation) have confirmed the anatomically small airway of the apnea patient. The source or cause of the deficient anatomy is highly variable in some cases relating to obesity and fat deposition around the airway, while in others it may be a product of tonsillar hypertrophy or bony abnormalities (micrognathia). Regardless of the cause, most evidence suggests that apnea patients have a structurally small airway while awake, which collapses when they go to sleep.

Although it seems logical that the previously described augmented dilator muscle activity is a response to the deficient anatomy, how reduced airway size leads to neuromuscular compensation remains unclear. Possibilities include neural mechanoreceptive reflexes, chemoreflexes (responsive to hypoxia or hypercapnia), or possibly a "learned" behavior. These possibilities will all be discussed at length below.

III. Sleep Effects on Upper Airway Muscle Activity

A. Normal Subjects

Despite the importance of pharyngeal dilator muscles in the maintenance of airway patency and their probable role in the development of obstructive apnea during sleep, the impact of sleep on the activity of these muscles in normal individuals has not been adequately defined. There is abundant evidence that the resistance to airflow across the pharyngeal airway increases during sleep in virtually all normal individuals (6,44). However, the muscle correlates of this increasing resistance have been somewhat more difficult to demonstrate.

Studies of the genioglossus muscle demonstrate reduced activity in the immediate wake-sleep transition, although the decrements are small (40). However, over time, genioglossal activity recovers and is often higher during stable non-REM sleep (particularly during stages 3 and 4 sleep) than is encountered during wakefulness (45), although this observation has not been carefully controlled for changes in tidal volume. This is the case despite increased airflow resistance. These observations suggest that decreased genioglossal activation is not responsible for the rising airflow resistance, at least during stable NREM sleep. During REM sleep, genioglossal activity is quite variable depending on the proximity to rapid eye movements (46). In the immediate temporal proximity to such eye movements, genioglossal EMG is substantially inhibited (Fig. 5). However, during tonic REM sleep, the EMG level is quite similar to that encountered during non-REM sleep. The explanation for this varied effect of sleep on genioglossal activity remains unclear. However, one can speculate as to its cause. In the immediate wake-sleep transition, decreased genioglossal EMG (GGEMG) likely results from withdrawal of central neural input that

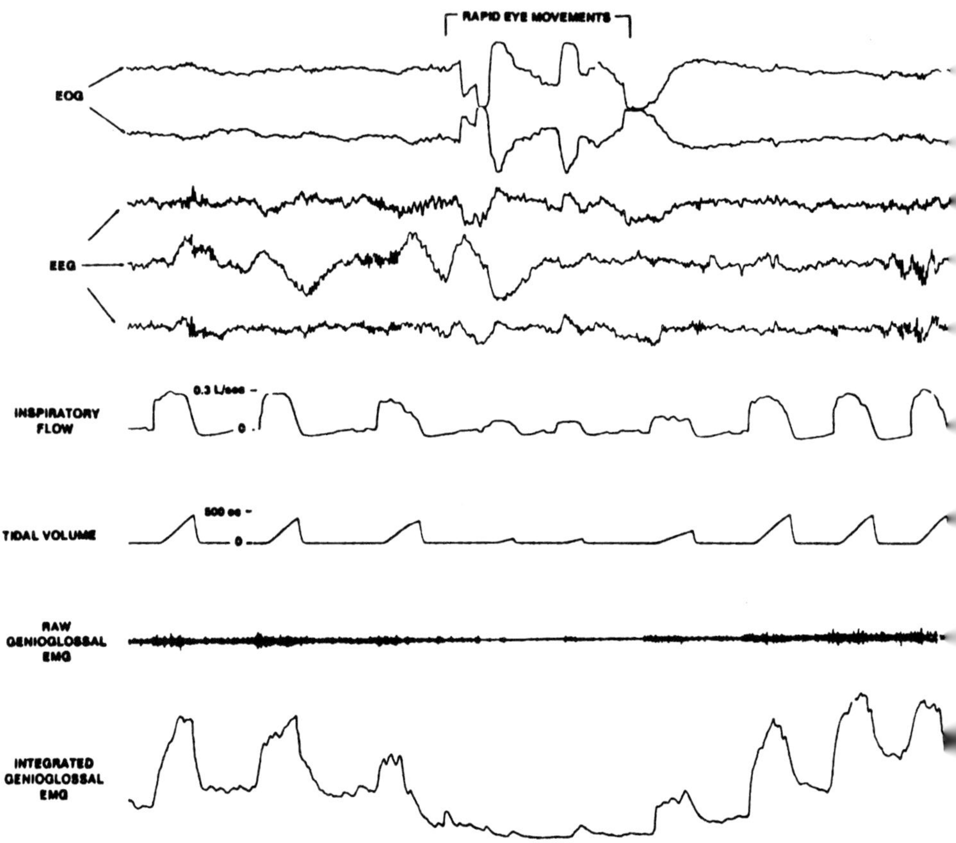

Figure 5 Depicted are EOG (electro-oculogram), EEG (electroencephalogram), inspiratory flow plus integrated tidal volume, and raw plus integrated (moving time average) genioglossal EMG. The effect of rapid eye movements on genioglossal EMG are seen. Note abrupt decline in the raw and integrated genioglossal EMG during a burst of eye movements. (From Ref. 46.)

requires wakefulness for its maintenance, i.e., the wakefulness stimulus (47). Other upper airway muscles lose activity as well (see below). However, over time, due to hypoventilation and rising airflow resistance, P_{CO_2} rises. This likely stimulates genioglossal activity back to waking levels or above. The activity of other upper airway muscles (see below) remains suppressed, contributing to the elevated pharyngeal resistance. Therefore, genioglossal activity is stimulated (response to CO_2), yet airflow resistance remains elevated (depressed dilator muscle activity, not genioglossus). During tonic REM sleep, mechanisms similar to those in non-REM sleep are likely active. Therefore, sleep is likely to have a complex effect on genioglossal activation.

The activity of other upper airway muscles is variably influenced by sleep. The geniohyoid muscle (which extends from the mandible to the hyoid and influences hyoid bone position) demonstrates inspiratory phasic activation during wakefulness and sleep with diminished activity being observed during both non-REM and REM sleep when compared to wakefulness (8). Of note, it was primarily a decrement in tonic muscle activity that was observed during sleep with a general maintenance of inspiratory activation. Similarly, the palatoglossus and levator palatini muscles (which importantly influence palatal position and route of breathing) both generally lose activity during sleep, although palatoglossal activity recovered to near waking levels during stage 3 and 4 sleep (48). More impressively, the tensor palatini (a palatal muscle that may position the palate off the posterior pharyngeal wall) demonstrated substantial decrements during all stages of non-REM sleep, being only about 20–25% as active during stages 3 and 4 sleep as during wakefulness (9,10). In this study a direct correlation was observed between falling tensor palatini EMG and rising airflow resistance. Of note, the tensor palatini did not demonstrate inspiratory phasic activation during wakefulness or sleep. This has led to speculation that sleep may have a greater impact on the control of tonic muscle activity than inspiratory phasic activation (10). This concept is compatible with the observation in chronically instrumented cats that inspiratory phasic respiratory neurons largely maintain activity levels during sleep while tonic or nonphasic respiratory neurons are substantially attenuated (47).

Thus, studies in normal subjects indicate that sleep has a highly variable influence on pharyngeal muscle activation. Most muscles demonstrate a relatively modest impact of sleep, although this was certainly not the case for the tensor palatini, whose activity fell dramatically (9). On the other hand, the genioglossus muscle was minimally affected by sleep (45). Therefore, the influence of sleep on these muscles is complex but leads to a substantial impact on airflow resistance.

B. Obstructive Apnea Patients

Most evidence to date suggests that sleep has a more profound impact on pharyngeal dilator muscle activity in the apnea patient than in the normal control. Because virtually all such studies have focused on the genioglossal muscle, it will be primarily discussed. The original studies addressing the pathophysiology of obstructive sleep apnea reported a substantial decrement in genioglossal activity in the apnea patient associated with sleep onset and airway collapse (49). It was assumed that this falling muscle activity was responsible for the diminished airway patency. However, these patients were generally studied during periods of apnea and hyperpnea with episodic hypoxia, hypercapnia, and probably hypocapnia. All could influence muscle activity. As a result, the isolated effect of sleep on this muscle in the apnea patient was not clarified by these studies.

More recently, genioglossal and tensor palatini EMGs have been examined in the discreet transition from stable wakefulness to early non-REM sleep in apneic individuals (40). This study indicates that, in general, apnea patients have a substantially greater decrement in both genioglossal and tensor palatini EMG (Fig. 6) following sleep onset than occurs in normal controls. In most patients, both EMGs fell

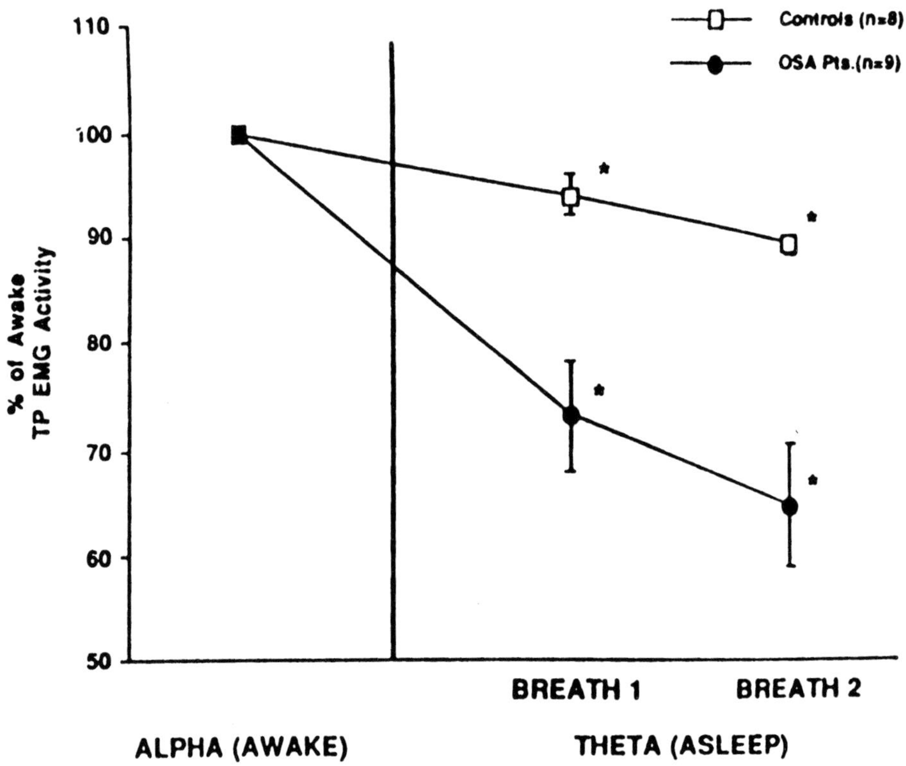

Figure 6 Depicted is the effect of sleep onset [transition from alpha (wakefulness) to non-REM sleep (theta)] on tensor palatini (TP) muscle activity. The first two breaths after this transition are demonstrated. Note the small but significant decrement in EMG in normal controls and the much greater reduction in activity in the apnea patients. $*p < 0.05$ less than awake (alpha) value. (From Ref. 40.)

to about 60% of the waking value by breath 2 (after the alpha-theta transition), while they were closer to 90% of the waking value in the control group at this time point. As a result, sleep onset has a different impact on the pharyngeal musculature in apnea patients when compared to controls.

Why apnea patients have these large changes in muscle activity at sleep onset in unclear. One could certainly argue that this represents a diminution or loss of the neuromuscular compensation present during wakefulness in these patients. In support of this concept is the observation that actual muscle activity levels (% of maximum) in these patients are not dropping below normal during sleep but are actually moving closer toward normal (40). This, therefore, makes it somewhat hard to argue that the primary abnormality in sleep apnea is a pathological sleep-induced loss of pharyngeal muscle activity. The apnea patient still has supra-normal muscle activation present during sleep. However, this activity (although elevated) is simply inadequate to maintain airway patency due to deficient airway anatomy. The mechanisms responsible for this loss of muscle activity during sleep will be discussed below.

IV. Sleep Effects on Pharyngeal Muscle Reflexes

There has been considerable interest of late in sleep effects on pharyngeal muscle reflexes as many investigators believe it is these reflexes that drive the neuromuscular compensation present in the apnea patient during wakefulness. If this is the case, a reduction or complete loss of these reflexes during sleep could explain the decrements in upper airway muscle activity that occur at sleep onset in apnea patients. Thus, a reflex-driven neuromuscular mechanism could be highly state dependent.

It has been known for many years that postural reflexes are substantially reduced or lost during sleep (50). Available evidence indicates this to be a product of reduced gamma efferent output to muscle spindles during sleep, thereby reducing spindle-mediated muscle activation in response to stretch or lengthening (51). Therefore, if the upper airway muscle response to negative pressure is driven by muscle spindles, one might expect a substantial attenuation in this response during sleep. However, as discussed above, most evidence suggests that this upper airway reflex is activated by laryngeal and nasal mucosal receptors, and the impact of sleep on this specific type of receptor mechanism has not been carefully studied.

In the last few years, several reports have emerged indicating a substantial impact of sleep on the genioglossal response to negative airway pressure in humans. Wheatley et al. (26,27) observed a large decrement in this response during stable stages 2, 3, and 4 sleep, as did Horner et al. (52) (Fig. 7). To the extent that this reflex is driven by mucosal mechanoreceptors, these mechanisms (like the spindle-driven ones) appear to be substantially state dependent as well. In a recent study, Shea et al. (53) reported a small but statistically insignificant decrement in this reflex in the wake-sleep transition but an actual inhibition of genioglossal muscle activation during REM sleep in response to negative pressure. Thus, REM sleep may be a particularly vulnerable time for pharyngeal airway protection leading to frequent apneas during REM sleep, as has been commonly reported.

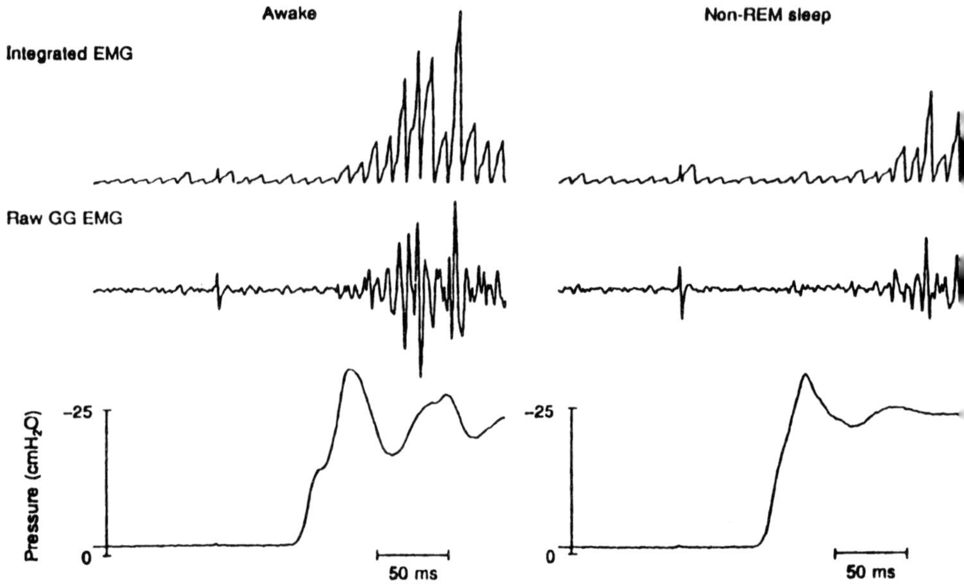

Figure 7 Single response in one normal subject of the genioglossal (GG) muscle in response to negative pressure during wakefulness and non-REM sleep. Note the increased latency and decreased magnitude of the EMG response during sleep. (From Ref. 52.)

Despite this clear impact of sleep on directly measured genioglossal reflex activation, a recent study in apnea patients suggests that these reflex mechanisms are not entirely lost (54). It has been known for years that the genioglossal EMG gradually increases over the course of an obstructive apnea with a final large EMG burst occurring at the time of arousal in association with airway reopening (49). Whether the gradually incrementing genioglossal activity was a product of the increasing hypoxia and hypercapnia associated with apnea or resulted more from the large negative pressure swings in the upper airway has remained unclear. However, a recent study by Berry et al. (54) suggests the latter at least plays a role. They observed a reduced slope of increasing genioglossal EMG over time during apnea following topical upper airway anesthesia in apnea patients. In addition, the steady increment in EMG over time previously observed in the genioglossus was not always observed. The authors concluded from these observations that the negative upper airway pressure occurring with each ventilatory effort during apnea was activating mechanoreceptors leading to rising genioglossal EMG, even though these patients were asleep. Topical anesthesia reduced this influence. Therefore, functionally important neural reflex responsiveness likely remains in the genioglossus during non-REM sleep, although large negative pressure swings may be required to activate it.

The animal literature suggests that slightly different events may be occurring. A recent study in dogs indicates that the genioglossus can be activated by negative upper airway pressure during wakefulness and that this reflex persists into non-REM sleep although greater negative pressure was required to activate it (21). During REM sleep, no reflex could be elicited. Whether these results are truly different from what was observed in humans is debatable. If Wheatley et al. (26,29) had used greater negative pressure in humans during non-REM sleep, a more impressive reflex may have been elicited. This may be relevant because apnea patients commonly develop airway pressures below negative 30 cmH_2O during obstructive events. As stated above, recent studies of humans during REM sleep indicate that genioglossal activation was actually inhibited in response to negative pressure (53) rather than being augmented. Why this was not observed in animals is unclear. However, REM sleep may be a particularly vulnerable time in both animals and humans.

V. The Negative Pressure Reflex and Sleep Apnea Pathogenesis

From the discussion above, it should be clear that a number of concepts regarding upper airway motor control and sleep apnea are fairly well established.

1. Most obstructive sleep apnea patients:
   Have an anatomically small upper airway.
   Have augmented pharyngeal dilator muscle activity present during wakefulness.
   Have substantial decrements in upper airway muscle activity at sleep onset in association with pharyngeal closure.
2. Pharyngeal dilator muscles:
   Respond to pulses of negative pressure with increased activity.
   Demonstrate a substantial attenuation of this reflex during sleep, particularly stable non-REM and REM sleep.

Does this mean that the negative pressure reflex is driving the neuromuscular compensation in the apnea patient during wakefulness, thereby compensating for deficient anatomy? Is it loss of this reflex during sleep that leads to falling muscle activity in the apnea patients and pharyngeal closure? Neither of these questions can be answered with the currently available information. However, the evidence for and against these concepts is provided below.

There are a number of observations suggesting that upper airway reflex mechanisms may be modulating the neuromuscular compensation of the apnea patient. First, the application of positive pressure (CPAP) to the pharyngeal airway of the apnea patient during wakefulness leads to a substantial reduction in genioglossal EMG to near normal (non–sleep apnea) levels (39) (Fig. 8). It would seem logical that a neuromuscular mechanism driven by negative airway pressure could be turned off or inactivated by positive pressure, thereby returning muscle activity to normal levels. This observation, therefore, supports a role for this reflex. In addition, there is a reasonable temporal relationship between sleep effects on the upper airway reflex in normal subjects and sleep effects on airway patency in apnea patients (see

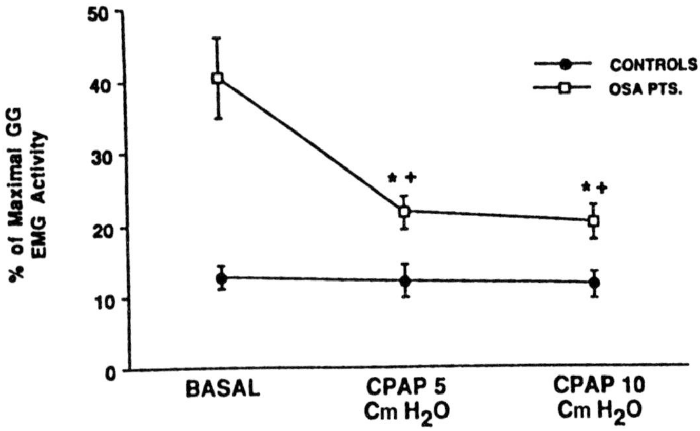

Figure 8 Depicted is the mean genioglossal (GG) muscle response to the application of continuous positive airway pressure (CPAP) during wakefulness in normal controls and obstructive sleep apnea patients. Note the substantial decrement in EMG in the apnea patients, but little change in the controls. $^{*}p < 0.05$ vs. controls; $^{+}p < 0.05$ vs. basal. (From Ref. 39.)

Table 1). This association assumes that sleep has a similar impact on the negative pressure reflex in apnea patients as was observed in normal humans and animals. Although this has not been demonstrated, it is likely to be the case.

During wakefulness, the reflex is active as is neuromuscular compensation in the apnea patient. The impact of the sleep-wake transition on the reflex seems to be small, but apnea frequency is substantial. During REM sleep, the reflex is substantially reduced or abolished [based on both animal data (21) and studies of normal humans (53)] at a time when apnea frequency is quite high. On the other hand, during stable NREM sleep the reflex is markedly diminished (data from normal subjects) (26,27,52,55), at least at the negative pressure levels tested, yet apneas rarely occur. This later dissociation, however, could result from mechanisms unrelated to sleep effects on the negative pressure reflex. Most apnea patients rarely reach stable non-REM sleep due to recurrent apnea-induced arousal. In addition, CO_2 stimulation of upper airway muscle activity could sustain airway patency during

Table 1

	Awake	Sleep-wake transition	Stable NREM sleep	REM sleep
Negative pressure reflex	Active	?	↓	↓↓ or absent[a]
Apnea frequency	0	↑	↓	↑↑

[a] Based on animal and human studies.

non-REM sleep in some patients (6). One would have to conclude, therefore, that apneas generally occur at a time when the reflex is diminished or absent (REM sleep) and are rare when the reflex is active (awake). Non-REM sleep is more confusing and will require further study. It should be noted that normal subjects lose or have a reduced negative pressure reflex during sleep yet do not develop overt apnea. This likely results from their anatomically larger airway, which does not require reflex-driven dilator muscle activity to maintain patency. Therefore, upper airway anesthesia during sleep in normal subjects does not commonly lead to frequent apneas or hypopneas (56,57). Similarly, upper airway anesthesia in apnea patients would not be expected to increase apnea frequency as the reflex is already diminished or absent during sleep and is not likely subject to further decrement. Recent studies support this concept (58,59).

Conversely, there are also reasons to doubt a relationship between this reflex and the pharyngeal neuromuscular compensation of the apnea patient. The most compelling reason relates to the absence of a clear stimulus for the reflex during wakefulness in the apneic individual. As addressed above, negative airway pressure has been the most reliable method of activating this reflex, although airway deformation or muscle stretch may well be what is actually detected. In most studies somewhere between -8 (26,27) and -25 (52) cmH_2O negative pressure has been required to activate this muscle. However, during wakefulness, such levels of negative pressure are rarely encountered during tidal breathing in normal humans (60). Although not formally studied, in our experience apnea patients generate only minimally greater negative airway pressure while awake than do normal individuals. In addition, the application of small external resistive loads to normal subjects, thereby increasing intrapharyngeal negative pressure, does not lead to the immediate augmentation of the genioglossal EMG to the levels encountered in the apnea patient. Therefore, it is difficult to argue that the negative airway pressure occurring during tidal breathing in the apnea patient is driving the neuromuscular compensation present during wakefulness.

On the other hand, preliminary data from our laboratory indicate that dense naso-, oropharyngeal anesthesia leads to a reduction in basal genioglossal activity during wakefulness in both normal controls and apnea patients. Similarly, DeWeese and Sullivan (56) observed increased airflow resistance in normal subjects following topical oro-, laryngopharyngeal anesthesia. This would suggest that intrapharyngeal stimuli (mucosal receptors) are driving some of the activity in these muscles. In addition, studies conducted in animals indicate that pressure receptors located in the larynx (with afferents in the superior laryngeal nerve) are activated during spontaneous inspiration and can be augmented by airway occlusion (61–63). With loss of integrity of the superior laryngeal nerve, inspiratory phasic activity of the genioglossus muscle is often lost in the cat (64). Therefore, there are receptors present in the upper airway that can respond to relatively small changes in intrapharyngeal pressure.

In conclusion, the current data suggest a relationship between reflex mechanisms in the pharyngeal airway and the neuromuscular compensation present in the apnea patient. However, not all data support this concept. In addition, we have yet to precisely define the receptor mechanism responsible for either this reflex (65–67) or the neuromuscular compensation of the apnea patient. The afferent pathways also need further definition. Therefore, considerable work is still needed in this area.

VI. Sleep and Central Neuromodulation of Pharyngeal Airway Reflexes

As the precise receptors and afferents responsible for mediating the upper airway negative pressure reflex have not been completely defined, it is difficult, at a basic level, to definitively address how sleep might modulate this reflex. However, if we assume that afferents in the superior laryngeal and trigeminal nerves are involved in this process, it is possible to speculate about these mechanisms.

Several neuromodulatory systems have been shown to be substantially affected by sleep. These include the serotonergic (raphe nuclei) (68,69), noradrenergic (locus coeruleus) (70,71), and cholinergic (pedunculopontine and lateral dorsal tegmentum) (72,73) systems. Both serotonergic and noradrenergic cells gradually decrease their firing frequency with sleep onset and reach their lowest level during REM sleep (68–71). Cholinergic cells, on the other hand, lose activity precipitously at sleep onset with some cells demonstrating a recovery of activity during REM sleep (72,73). Because the role of these cholinergic cells in upper airway motor control is poorly studied at this time, they will not be addressed further.

The serotonergic system has been studied fairly extensively as a possible modulator of upper airway motor activity. It has been well demonstrated that serotonergic raphe cells project directly to the hypoglossal (74,75) and trigeminal nuclei (76,77) and that 5-HT provides a tonic excitatory or facilitory input to these upper airway motor neurons (78). In vivo studies show a substantial increase in tonic hypoglossal neuron activity when serotonin is applied at the hypoglossal nucleus (78), while in vitro data indicate that serotonin depolarizes these motor neurons and increases the slope of injected current versus firing frequency (79). In addition, a recent study showed diminished basal hypoglossal neural activity and responsiveness to negative pressure when serotonin antagonists were applied at the hypoglossal nucleus (80). Therefore, 5-HT may modulate both the basal tonic activity of these neurons and their ability to respond to excitatory input (potentially the reflex) by its actions at the motor nucleus. In addition, there is reason to believe that serotonergic mechanisms could influence afferent input to these motor neurons as well. As stated previously, at least a portion of the afferent mechanisms illicited by negative pressure occur through the superior laryngeal nerve (61–63). Superior laryngeal afferents have been demonstrated to reach the hypoglossal nucleus by pathways through the nucleus of the solitary tract (23). It has also been demonstrated that raphe neurons project to this solitary tract nucleus as well (81). Therefore, it is possible that 5-HT may influence sensory synaptic transmission in the nucleus of the solitary tract, thereby producing a reflex that is highly sensitive to state.

Some of these same principles apply to the noradrenergic system (locus coeruleus, or LC) as well. As stated, LC neurons have a highly state-dependent firing pattern with substantially reduced activity during non-REM sleep and little firing during REM (70,71). In addition, neurons from the subcoeruleus have been demonstrated to project to both the hypoglossal (82,83) and trigeminal nuclei (84). Finally, noradrenaline both depolarizes hypoglossal motor neurons and augments the slope of injected current versus firing frequency in a fashion similar to 5-HT (85). Therefore, as with 5-HT, the potential for a state-related impact on basal motor activity and reflex responsiveness is substantial.

VII. Other Upper Airway Reflexes

Numerous reflex mechanisms present in the upper airway influence not only the activity of airway dilator muscles (86), but ventilatory timing (87), the sensation of dyspnea (88), and a variety of circulatory functions as well (89,90). These range from the diving reflex in response to water (or cold) around or in the nose, which leads to bradycardia, laryngeal closure, and a centralization (less flow to the skin and extremities) of the circulation to laryngeal reflexes mediated through the superior laryngeal nerve leading to decreased respiratory frequency or even apnea (87). There are also chemoreflex mechanisms that can influence both upper airway muscle activation and respiration in general (31,32). These mechanisms are responsive to falling arterial P_{O_2} (carotid body) and rising P_{CO_2} (carotid body and medullary chemoreceptors) and airway CO_2. Although many of these mechanisms may influence respiration during sleep, little is known about their interaction with state and their impact on disordered breathing. However, two such reflexes are probably worth further discussion, although their mechanism and importance are less well defined than the negative pressure response.

First, there is some literature indicating the presence of a nasal reflex that can influence respiratory pattern during sleep (91,92) although neither the receptor activated nor the afferent mechanism have been defined. In support of such a reflex was the observation that nasal anesthesia led to a substantial increase in the frequency of central apneas during sleep in normal subjects (91). This observation would suggest that such receptors stimulate ventilation and that by inhibiting them (anesthesia) respiration can be reduced or intermittently abolished. A study by McNicholas et al. (92) supports this concept. They observed that added nasal flow (4 L/min of compressed air) led to increased minute ventilation during sleep while mouth breathing (no nasal flow) led to reduced respiration. On the other hand, McNicholas et al. (57) did not report an increase in the number of central apneas during sleep following nasal anesthesia. Other studies, conducted during wakefulness, suggest that nasal airflow actually inhibits respiration (88). As a result, the mechanism and importance of this nasal reflex in ventilatory control awake and asleep remains to be defined.

Second, there is some evidence in both animals and humans supporting an upper airway reflex that inhibits respiration. It has been demonstrated for years that stimulation of the superior laryngeal nerve leads to inhibition of diaphragmatic and intercostal muscle activity and can lead to apnea if the stimulus is strong enough (89). More recently, the application of negative pressure to the upper airway in a variety of animal preparations has been observed to have a similar effect—diaphragmatic inhibition (80,89). Therefore, upper airway negative pressure may stimulate upper airway muscles, but it commonly inhibits the respiratory pump muscles. This reflex was recently examined during natural sleep in dogs. Harms et al. reported that negative upper airway pressure sufficient to close or deform the airway inhibited respiration during wakefulness, non-REM sleep, and REM sleep (21). In addition, brief pulses of negative pressure also inhibited respiration even after the negative pressure was discontinued. These observations would suggest that pharyngeal deformation or closure may not only increase the resistance to airflow, but inhibit respiration as well.

There are some data in humans supporting this inhibitory reflex. Studies by Thach et al. (93,94) revealed that the application of negative pressure to the upper airway of tracheostomized infants led to an inhibition of respiratory pump muscle activity manifested as diminished peak flow, tidal volume, and negative airway pressure. Respiratory timing could also be influenced, although frank apnea was not encountered. Whether these results apply to the adult human is unclear.

Studies in adults have less directly addressed this issue but are suggestive. Issa and Sullivan made a number of observations in a small group of patients with predominantly central sleep apnea (95). First, central apneas became largely obstructive when the patients move from the supine to the lateral decubitus position. Second, the application of fairly high levels of nasal CPAP could abolish virtually all observed central apneas yielding rhythmic respiration. Lower pressures resulted in obstructive events. Finally, oropharyngeal anesthesia in several of these patients converted central apneas to either a normal ventilatory pattern or pure obstructive effects. From these observations the authors concluded that a reflex inhibition of respiration occurred during sleep secondary to activation of a supraglottic receptor responsive to airway collapse. Hoffstein and Slutsky (96) also reported the successful elimination of central apnea with nasal CPAP. Although these studies in humans certainly do not prove the existence of such a reflex, they suggest that such mechanisms may exist, which could, in part, explain the frequent simultaneous occurrence of central and obstructive apneas.

VIII. Conclusions

Current data suggest that upper airway reflex mechanisms (primarily activated by negative pressure) and the influence of sleep on such mechanisms may play an important role in the pathophysiology of obstructive sleep apnea. It seems clear that inadequate pharyngeal anatomy leads to the activation of neuromuscular compensatory mechanisms during wakefulness and that such mechanisms cannot be maintained during sleep. Although some evidence supports the concept that this augmented muscle activity in apnea patients during wakefulness is driven by the upper airway negative pressure reflex, this has not been thoroughly documented. In addition, the influence of sleep on this reflex has been only partially defined. Finally, the basic neural mechanisms controlling this negative pressure reflex and how state (sleep) modulates such mechanisms are only beginning to be investigated. Therefore, considerable additional work is needed in this area if we are to both understand the pathophysiology of obstructive sleep apnea and realistically approach pharmacological therapy.

References

1. Schwab RJ, Gefter WB, Hoffman FA, Gupta KB, Pack AI. Dynamic upper airway imaging during awake respiration in normal subjects and patients with sleep disordered breathing. Am Rev Respir Dis 1993; 148:1375–1400.
2. Haponik E, Smith P, Bohlman M, Allan R, Goldman S, Bleecker E. Computerized tomography in obstructive sleep apnea: correlation of airway size with physiology during sleep and wakefulness. Am Rev Respir Dis 1983; 127:221–226.
3. Schwartz AR, Thut DC, Brower RG, Gauda EB, Roach D, Permutt S, Smith PL. Modulation of maximal inspiratory airflow by neuromuscular activity: effect of CO_2. J Appl Physiol 1993; 74:1597–1605.
4. Brouillette RT, Thach BT. A neuromuscular mechanism maintaining extrathoracic airway patency. J Appl Physiol 1979; 46:772–779.
5. Leiter JC, Knuth SL, Bartlett D. Dependence of pharyngeal resistance on genioglossal EMG activity, nasal resistance and airflow. J Appl Physiol 1992; 73:584–590.
6. Weigand L, Zwillich CW, White DP. Collapsibility of the human upper airway during normal sleep. J Appl Physiol 1989; 66:1800–1808.
7. Tangel DJ, Mezzanotte WS, White DP. Respiratory-related control of palatoglossus and levator palatini muscle activity. J Appl Physiol 1995; 78:680–688.
8. Wiegand DA, Latz B, Zwillich CW, Weigand L. Geniohyoid muscle activity in normal men during wakefulness and sleep. J Appl Physiol 1990; 69:1262–1269.
9. Tangel DJ, Mezzanotte WS, White, DP. The influence of sleep on tensor palatini EMG and upper airway resistance in normal subjects. J Appl Physiol 1991; 70:2574–2581.
10. Tangel DJ, Mezzanotte WS, Sandberg EJ, White DP. The influence of sleep on the activity of tonic postural versus inspiratory phasic muscles in normal men. J Appl Physiol 1992; 73:1058–1066.
11. Van de Graaff WB. Thoracic influence on upper airway patency. J Appl Physiol 1988; 65:2123–2131.
12. Schwartz AR, Rowley JA, Thut DC, Permutt S, Smith PL. Structural basis for alterations in upper airway collapsibility. Sleep 1996; 19:S184–S188.
13. Rowley JA, Permutt S, Willey S, Smith PL, Schwartz AR. Effect of tracheal and tongue displacement on upper airway airflow dynamics. J Appl Physiol 1996; 80:2171–2178.
14. Wasicko MJ, Hutt DA, Parisi RA, Neubauer JA, Mezrich R, Edelman NH. The role

of vascular tone in the control of upper airway collapsibility. Am Rev Respir Dis 1990; 141:1569–1577.
15. Van Der Touw T, Crawford ABH, Wheatley JR. Effects of a synthetic lung surfactant on pharyngeal patency in awake human subjects. J Appl Physiol 1997; 82:78–85.
16. Sauerland EK, Orr WC, Hairston LE. EMG patterns of oropharyngeal muscles during respiration in wakefulness and sleep. Electromyogr Clin Neurophysiol 1981; 21:307–316.
17. Innes JA, Morrell MA, Koboyaski I, Hamilton RD, Guz A. Central and reflex control of genioglossus in subjects who underwent laryngectomy. J Appl Physiol 1995; 78: 2180–2186.
18. Mathew OP. Upper airway negative-pressure effects on respiratory activity of upper airway muscles. J Appl Physiol 1984; 56:500–505.
19. Mathew OP, Abu-Osba YK, Thach BT. Influence of upper airway pressure changes on genioglossus muscle respiratory activity. J Appl Physiol 1982; 52:438–444.
20. Mathew OP, Abu-Osba YK, Thach BT. Genioglossus muscle responses to upper airway pressure changes: Afferent pathways. J Appl Physiol 1982; 52:445–450.
21. Harms CA, Zeng Y, Smith CA, Vidruk EH, Dempsey JA. Negative pressure-induced deformation of the upper airway causes central apnea in awake and sleeping dogs. J Appl Physiol 1996; 80:1528–1539.
22. Bowman JP. The Muscle Spindle and Neural Control of the Tongue. Springfield, IL: Charles C Thomas, 1971.
23. Lowe AA. Tongue movement—brainstem mechanisms and clinical postulates. Brain Behav Evol 1984; 25:128–137.
24. Brancatisano A, Davis P, Van der Touw T, Wheatley J. Role of upper airway negative pressure on proprioceptive afferents from the tongue. J Appl Physiol 1999; 86:1396–1401.
25. Horner RL, Innes JA, Holden HB, Guz A. Afferent pathways for pharyngeal dilator reflex to negative pressure in man: a study using upper airway anesthesia. J Physiol (Lond) 1991; 436:31–44.
26. Wheatley JR, Mezzanotte WS, Tangel DJ, White DP. Influence of sleep on genioglossus muscle activation by negative pressure in normal men. Am Rev Respir Dis 1993; 148: 597–605.
27. Wheatley JR, Tangel DJ, Mezzanotte WS, White DP. Influence of sleep on response to negative airway pressure of tensor palatini muscle and retropalatal airway. J Appl Physiol 1993; 75:2117–2124.
28. Mortimore IL, Douglas NJ. Palatopharyngeus has respiratory activity and responds to negative pressure in sleep apnoeics. Eur Respir J 1996; 9:773–778.
29. Tsubone H. Nasal ''pressure'' receptors. Jpn J Vet Sci 1990; 52:225–232.
30. Hwang JC, St. John WM, Bartlett D, Jr. Receptors responding to changes in upper airway pressure. Respir Physiol 1984; 55:355–366.
31. Onal E, Lopata M, O'Connor TD. Diaphragmatic and genioglossal electromyogram responses to isocapnic hypoxia in humans. Am Rev Respir Dis 1981; 124:215–217.
32. Onal E, Lopata M, O'Connor TD. Diaphragmatic and genioglossal electromyogram response to CO_2 rebreathing in humans. J Appl Physiol 1981; 50:1052–1055.
33. Kuna ST. Inhibition of inspiratory upper airway motoneuron activity by phasic volume feedback. J Appl Physiol 1986; 60:1373–1379.

34. van Lunteren E, Strohl KP, Parker DM, Bruce EN, Van de Graaff WR, Cherniack NS. Phasic volume-related feedback on upper airway muscle activity. J Appl Physiol 1984; 56:730–736.
35. Salamone JA, Strohl KP, Weiner DM, Mitra J, Cherniack NS. Cranial and phrenic nerve responses to changes in systemic blood pressure. J Appl Physiol 1983; 55:61–68.
36. Garpestad E, Basner RC, Ringler J, Lilly J, Schwartzstein R, Weinberger S, Weiss JW. Phenylephrine-induced hypertension acutely decreases genioglossal EMG activity in awake humans. J Appl Physiol 1992; 72:110–115.
37. Popovic RM, White DP. Influence of gender on waking genioglossal EMG and upper airway resistance. Am J Respir Crit Care Med 1995; 152:725–731.
38. Popovic RM, White DP. Upper airway muscle activity in normal women: Influence of hormonal status. J Appl Physiol 1998; 84:1055–1062.
39. Mezzanotte WS, Tangel DJ, White DP. Waking genioglossal EMG in sleep apnea patients versus normal controls (a neuromuscular compensatory mechanism). J Clin Invest 1992; 89:1571–1579.
40. Mezzanotte WS, Tangel DJ, White DP. Waking and sleeping upper airway muscle activity in apnea patients versus normal controls. Am J Respir Crit Care Med 1996; 153: 1880–1887.
41. Hendricks JC, Petrof B, Panckeri K, Pack AI. Upper airway dilating muscle hyperactivity during non-rapid eye movement sleep in English bulldogs. Am Rev Respir Dis 1993; 148:185–194.
42. Series F, Cote C, Simoneau JA, Gelinas Y, St. Pierre S, Leclerc R, Ferland R, Marc I. Physiologic and metabolic profile of musculus uvulae in sleep apnea syndrome and in snorers. J Clin Invest 1995; 95:20–25.
43. Isoni S, Remmers J, Tanaka A, Sho Y, Sato J, Nishno T. Anatomy of pharynx in patients with obstructive sleep apnea and in normal subjects. J Appl Physiol 1997; 82:1319–1326.
44. Hudgel DW, Martin RJ, Johnson B, Hill P. Mechanics of the respiratory system and breathing pattern during sleep in normal humans. J Appl Physiol 1984; 56:133.
45. Basner RC, Ringler J, Schwartzstein RM, Weinberger SE, Weiss JW. Phasic electromyographic activity of the genioglossus increases in normals during slow-wave sleep. Respir Physiol 1991; 83:189–200.
46. Wiegand L, Zwillich CW, Wiegand D, White DP. Changes in upper airway muscle activation and ventilation during phasic REM sleep in normal men. J Appl Physiol 1991; 71:488–497.
47. Orem J. The nature of the wakefulness stimulus for breathing. Prog Clin Biol Res 1990; 345:23–30.
48. Tangel DJ, Mezzanotte WS, White DP. The influence of NREM sleep on the activity of the palatoglossus and levator palatini muscles in normal men. J Appl Physiol 1995; 78:689–695.
49. Remmers JE, de Groot WJ, Sauerland EK, Anch AM. Pathogenesis of upper airway occlusion during sleep. J Appl Physiol 1978; 44:931–938.
50. Tuttle WW. The effect of sleep upon the patellar tendon reflex. Am J Physiol 1924; 68:345–348.
51. Buchwald JS, Eldred E. Relation between gamma efferent discharge and cortical activity. Electroenceph Clin Neurophysiol 1961; 13:243–247.
52. Horner RL, Innes JA, Morrell MJ, Shea SA, Buz A. The effect of sleep on reflex genio-

glossus muscle activation by stimuli of negative airway pressure in humans. J Physiol (Lond) 1994; 476:141–151.
53. Shea SA, Edwards JK, White DP. Effect of wake-sleep transitions and rapid eye movement sleep on pharyngeal muscle response to negative pressure in humans. J Physiol 1999; 520(3):897–908.
54. Berry RB, McNellis MI, Kouchi K, Light RW. Upper airway anesthesia reduces phasic genioglossal activity during sleep apnea. Am J Respir Crit Care Med 1997; 156:127–132.
55. Issa FG, Edwards P, Szeto E, Lauff D, Sullivan CE. Genioglossus and breathing responses to airway occlusion: effect of sleep and route of occlusion. J Appl Physiol 1988; 64:543–549.
56. DeWeese EL, Sullivan TY. Effects of upper airway anesthesia on pharyngeal patency during sleep. J Appl Physiol 1988; 64:1346–1353.
57. McNicholas WT, Coffey M, McDonnell T, O'Regan R, Fitzgerald MX. Upper airway obstruction during sleep in normal subjects after selective topical oropharyngeal anesthesia. Am Rev Respir Dis 1987; 135:1316–1319.
58. Deegan PC, Mulloy E, McNicholas WT. Topical oropharyngeal anesthesia in patients with obstructive sleep apnea. Am J Respir Crit Care Med 1995; 151:1108–1112.
59. Berry RB, Kouchi KG, Bower JL, Light RW. Effect of upper airway anesthesia on obstructive sleep apnea. Am J Respir Crit Care Med 1995; 151:1857–1861.
60. Proctor DF. Modifications of breathing for phonation. In: Macklem PT, Mead J, eds. Handbook of Physiology, Sec. 3, The Respiratory Systems, Vol. 3, Mechanics of Respiration. Bethesda, MD: American Physiological Society, 1986:597–604.
61. Mathew OP, Sant'Ambrogio G. Fisher JT, Sant'Ambrogio FB. Laryngeal pressure receptors. Respir Physiol 1984; 57:113–122.
62. Mathew OP, Sant'Ambrogio G, Fisher JT, Sant'Ambrogio FB. Respiratory afferent activity in the superior laryngeal nerves. Respir Physiol 1984; 58:41–50.
63. Sant'Ambrogio G, Mathew OP, Fisher JT, Sant'Ambrogio FB. Laryngeal receptors responding to transmural pressure, airflow and local muscle activity. Res Physiol 1983; 54:317–330.
64. Nolan P, Bradford A, O'Regan RG, McKeogh D. The effects of changes in laryngeal airway CO_2 concentration on genioglossus muscle activity in the anesthetized cat. Exp Physiol 1990; 75:271–274.
65. Sant'Ambrogio G, Tsubone H, Sant' Ambrogio FB. Sensory information from the upper airway: role in the control of breathing. Resp Physiol 1995; 102:1–16.
66. Kubin L, Davies RO. Central pathways of pulmonary and airway vagal afferents. In: Dempsey JA, Pack AI, eds. Regulation of Breathing. New York: Marcel Dekker, 1994: 219–284.
67. Iscoe SD. Central control of the upper airway. In: Mathew OP, Sant'Ambrogio G, eds. Respiratory Function of the Upper Airway. New York: Marcel Dekker, 1998:125–192.
68. Trulson ME, Trulson VM. Activity of nucleus raphe pallidus neurons across the sleep-waking cycle in freely moving cats. Brain Res 1982; 237:232–237.
69. Fornal C, Auerbach S, Jacobs BL. Activity of serotonin-containing neurons in nucleus raphe magnus in freely moving cats. Exp Neurol 1985; 88:590–608.
70. Aston-Jones G, Bloom FE. Activity of norepinephrine-containing locus coeruleus neurons in behaving rats anticipates fluctuations in the sleep-waking cycle. J Neurosci 1981; 1:876–886.

71. Foote SL, Bloom FE, Aston-Jones G. Nucleus locus coeruleus: new evidence of anatomical and physiological specificity. Physiol Rev 1983; 63:844–914.
72. Steriade M, Datta S, Pare D, Oakson G, Curro Dossi R. Neuronal activities in brainstem cholinergic nuclei related to tonic activation processes in thalamocortical systems. J Neurosci 1990; 10:2541–2559.
73. Steriade M, McCarley RW. Brainstem Control of Wakefulness and Sleep. New York: Plenum Press, 1990.
74. Manaker S, Tischler LJ, Morrison AR. Raphespinal and reticulospinal collaterals to the hypoglossal nucleus in the rat. J Comp Neurol 1992; 322:68–78.
75. Manaker S, Tischler LJ. Origin of serotonergic afferents to the hypoglossal nucleus in the rat. J Comp Neurol 1993; 334:466–476.
76. Fort P, Luppi P-H, Sakai K, Salvert D, Jouvet M. Nuclei of origin of monoaminergic, peptidergic, and cholinergic afferents to the cat trigeminal motor nucleus: A double-labeling study with cholera toxin as a retrograde tracer. J Comp Neurol 1990; 301:262–275.
77. Li YQ, Takada M, Mizuno N. The sites of origin of serotonergic afference fibers in the trigeminal motor, facial, and hypoglossal nuclei in the rat. Neurosci Res 1993; 17:307–313.
78. Kubin L, Tojima H, Davies RO, Pack AI. Serotonergic excitatory drive to hypoglossal motoneurons in the decerebrate cat. Neurosci Lett 1992; 139:243–248.
79. Berger AJ, Bayliss DA, Viana F. Modulation of neonatal rat hypoglossal motoneuron excitability by serotonin. Neurosci Lett 1992; 143:164–168.
80. Douse MA, White DP. Serotonergic effects on hypoglossal neural activity and reflex responses. Brain Res 1996; 726:213–222.
81. Thor KB, Helke CJ. Serotonin- and substance P-containing projections to the nucleus tractus solitarii of the rat. J Comp Neurol 1987; 265:275–293.
82. Aldes LD, Chapman ME, Chronister RB, Haycock JW. Sources of noradrenergic afferents to the hypoglossal nucleus in the rat. Brain Res Bull 1992; 29:931–942.
83. Aldes LD. Topographically organized projections from the nucleus subcoeruleus to the hypoglossal nucleus in the rat: a light and electron microscopic study with complementary axonal transport techniques. J Comp Neurol 1990; 302:643–656.
84. Travers JB, Norgren R. Afferent projections to the oral motor nuclei in the rat. J Comp Neurol 1983; 220:280–298.
85. Parkis MA, Bayliss DA, Berger AJ. Actions of norephinephrine on rat hypoglossal motoneurons. J Neurophysiol 1995; 74:1911–1919.
86. Mathew OP, Gosh TK. Role of airway afferents on upper airway muscle activity. In: Dempsey JA, Pack AI, eds. Regulation of Breathing. New York: Marcel Dekker, 1995: 511–541.
87. Mathew OP, Abu-Osba YK, Thach BT. Influence of upper airway pressure changes on respiratory frequency. Respir Physiol 1982; 49:223–233.
88. McBride B, Whitelaw WA. A physiologic stimulus to upper airway receptors in humans. J Appl Physiol 1981; 51:1189–1197.
89. Widdicombe JC. Upper respiratory tract reflexes. In: Cherniack NS, Widdicombe JG, eds. Handbook of Physiology, Sec. 3, The Respiratory System, Volume 2, Control of Breathing. Bethesda, MD: The American Physiologic Society, 1986:363–394.
90. Folgering H, Olivier O. The diving response depresses ventilation in man. Clin Respir Physiol 1985; 21:143–147.

91. White DP, Cadieux RJ, Lombard RM, Bixler EO, Kales A, Zwillich CW. The effects of nasal anesthesia on breathing during sleep. Am Rev Respir Dis 1985; 132:972–975.
92. McNicholas WT, Coffey M, Boyle T. Effects of nasal airflow on breathing during sleep in normal humans. Am Rev Respir Dis 1993; 147:620–623.
93. Thach BT, Schefft GC, Pickens DL, Menon AP. Influence of upper airway negative pressure reflex on response to airway occlusion in sleeping infants. J Appl Physiol 1989; 67:749–755.
94. Thach BT, Menon AP, Schefft GL. Effects of negative upper airway pressure on pattern of breathing in sleeping infants. J Appl Physiol 1989; 66:1599–1605.
95. Issa FG, Sullivan CE. Reversal of central sleep apnea using nasal CPAP. Chest 1986; 90:165–171.
96. Hoffstein V, Slutsky AS. Central sleep apnea reversed by continuous positive airway pressure. Am Rev Respir Dis 1987; 135:1210–1212.
97. Bosma JF, Donna MW, Tanuka E, Robertson D. Anatomy of the pharynx, pertinent to swallowing. Dysphagia 1986; 1:23–33.

6

Arousal Mechanisms and Autonomic Consequences

RICHARD L. HORNER

University of Toronto
Toronto, Ontario, Canada

I. Overview

In a variety of species, including humans, sleep onset is typically characterized by gradual changes in cortical electroencephalographic (EEG) activity and progressive loss of postural muscle tone (1–6). However, these changes at sleep onset contrast markedly with those normally observed at spontaneous awakening from sleep when abrupt activation of the EEG and postural muscle tone occur (1–3,7,8). Awakenings are also normally accompanied by large brief changes in autonomic output producing transient surges in heart rate (HR), blood pressure (BP), and ventilation ($\dot{V}$), which then decline in subsequent wakefulness (8–12). An example of the effects of awakening on HR and $\dot{V}$ is shown in Figure 1. Since these cardiorespiratory responses occur even during normal spontaneous awakenings and without any overt behavioral activity (e.g., gross body movements or locomotion), it is apparent that the magnitude of cardiorespiratory changes at wake onset exceed obvious physiological need and are not a simple reversal of the changes that occur at sleep onset.

The most dramatic examples of the cardiorespiratory responses to awakening from sleep are those that accompany the repetitive arousals in patients with sleep-related breathing disorders. For example, in patients with obstructive sleep apnea,

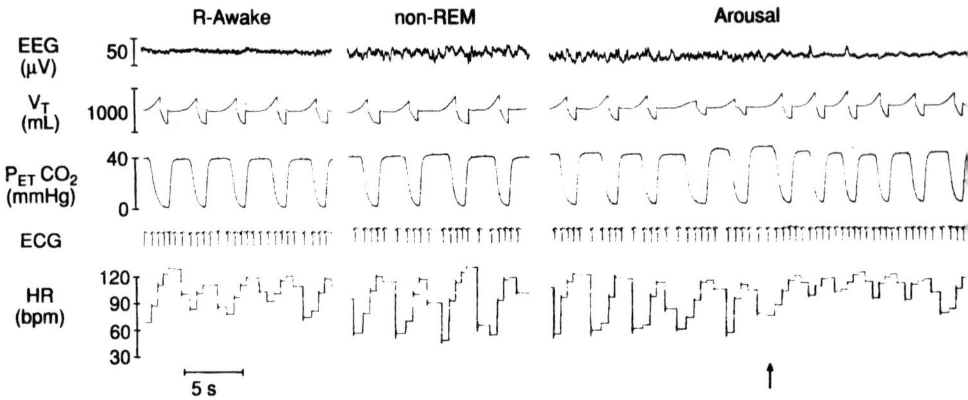

Figure 1 Example of transient increase in heart rate and ventilation upon spontaneous awakening from sleep. The traces show changes in heart rate and ventilation between periods of established wakefulness (R-Awake) and non-REM sleep (left panels), and at the transition from non-REM sleep to wakefulness (right panels, point of awakening indicated by arrow). The traces are from a spontaneously breathing dog. Mean heart rate and ventilation are increased in established wakefulness compared to non-REM, but awakening from sleep produced notable transient heart rate acceleration and increased ventilation, which then decline in subsequent established wakefulness. No body movements or evidence of overt behavioral arousal are noticeable at awakening. EEG, Electroencephalogram; V_T, tidal volume; $P_{ET}CO_2$, end-tidal P_{CO_2}; ECG, electrocardiogram; HR, instantaneous heart rate. (From Ref. 8.)

the repetitive large increases in HR and BP associated with arousal from sleep and resolution of apneas are thought to increase the risk for development of adverse cardiovascular events such as angina, myocardial infarction, stroke, and systemic hypertension (13,14). The mechanisms associated with arousal from sleep are thought to be predominantly responsible for these cardiovascular responses at the end of obstructive apneas rather than the hypoxemia (15). In patients with central and mixed apneas, the large increases in $\dot{V}$ that accompany arousal from sleep can predispose to subsequent apneas (12).

This chapter summarizes the neural processes engaged at awakening from sleep and the autonomic mechanisms that may be responsible for producing the large HR, BP, and $\dot{V}$ responses. Emphasis is placed on the processes involved in normal spontaneous awakenings because determining the influences of state-dependent processes on autonomic outputs is confounded in situations of sleep-disordered breathing. This is because the changes in arterial blood gases, breathing pattern, lung volume, and respiratory load associated with sleep-disordered breathing events can themselves affect autonomic outputs and obscure the primary effect of the change in sleep-wake state. Moreover, it is proposed that focusing on the neural mechanisms and autonomic consequences of normal arousals from sleep yields new insights into the nature of the awake state, specifically how wake onset differs from subsequent periods of wakefulness and why this may contribute to large brief cardiorespiratory activation. As such, this chapter includes a description of the changes in activity at the transition from sleep to wakefulness of brain-stem neuronal systems that are integral to the reticular activating system and sleep-wake regulation. Based on this analysis, and contrasting these effects with subsequent periods of established wakefulness, it is proposed that the moments just after awakening are fundamentally different from periods of established wakefulness that have been the major focus of attention in the past. Indeed, evidence suggests that a neurophysiologically distinct, transiently heightened awake state exists at wake onset compared to later wakefulness. This conclusion leads to important modifications of those physiological models that are currently used to explain the HR, BP, and $\dot{V}$ responses to awakening.

II. State-Dependent Changes in Cardiorespiratory Outputs

Figure 2 illustrates the well-described overall changes in HR, BP, and $\dot{V}$ between wakefulness, non–rapid-eye-movement (non-REM) sleep, and REM sleep. Compared to steady-state wakefulness, non-REM sleep is generally associated with reductions in HR, BP, and $\dot{V}$, whereas further decreases occur during tonic REM sleep and phasic REM events produce phasic increases. Over the last several decades there have been many investigations into the mechanisms responsible for the overall changes in cardiorespiratory activity in the different sleep-wake states. These studies have focused on state-dependent changes in respiratory muscle activity, upper airway resistance, ventilatory responses to altered blood gases and resistive loads, and, importantly, the impact of sleep on central respiratory neurons (for reviews, see Refs. 16–23). The effects of sleep-wake state on HR and BP, and the hemodynamic factors contributing to these changes, have also been studied extensively (16,24).

However, upon examination of these previous studies, it is striking that by far the most attention has been paid to investigating cardiorespiratory control mechanisms in steady-state sleep-wake periods, whereas comparatively little attention has been paid to the mechanisms underlying the HR, BP, and $\dot{V}$ changes at transitional states such as arousal from sleep. Indeed, where the responses at awakening from sleep have been considered, the prevailing assumption is that the difference in control mechanisms identified for the established sleep-wake states is responsible for the surges in those physiological variables at awakening. However, as described in this chapter, focusing on the neural processes engaged at awakening from sleep, and the autonomic mechanisms underlying the cardiorespiratory responses, reveals important differences between the state of wakefulness in the period immediately after wake onset compared to subsequent periods of established wakefulness. Since these considerations lead to some important modifications of the current models that are used to explain the HR, BP, and V responses to awakening from sleep, these current models and their limitations are discussed in the following sections.

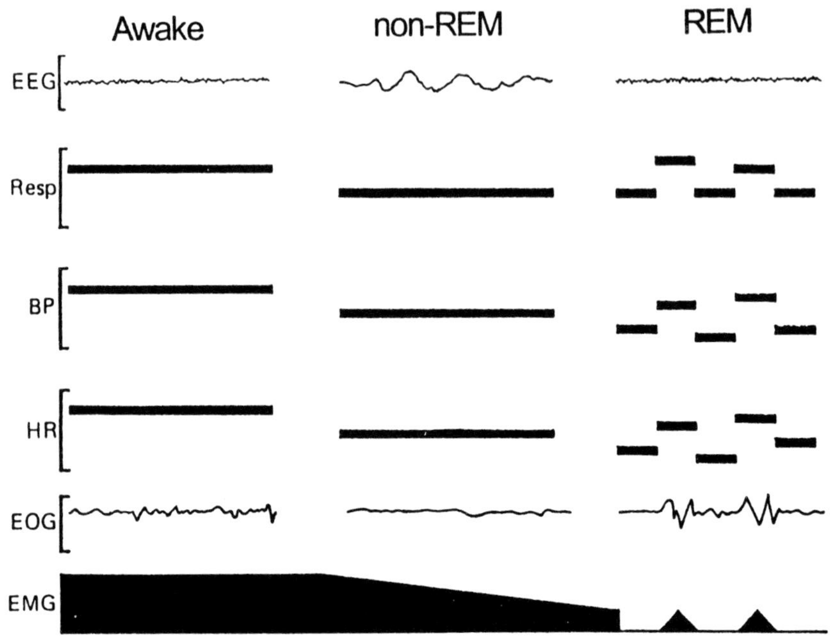

Figure 2 Overall changes in mean ventilation (Resp), blood pressure (BP), and heart rate (HR) between established periods of wakefulness (Awake), non-REM sleep, and REM sleep. The general changes in appearance of the electroencephalogram (EEG), electro-oculogram (EOG), and neck electromyogram (EMG) are also shown schematically for the different sleep-wake states. Note the phasic changes in cardiorespiratory outputs associated with phasic REM events (i.e., eye movements and muscle twitches). (Adapted from Ref. 16.)

III. Current Models Used to Explain Transient Cardiorespiratory Activation at Awakening

A. Ventilatory Response to Awakening

The large stimulatory effect of awakening from sleep on $\dot{V}$ is usually explained in terms of both a change in set-point for Pa_{CO_2} between sleep and wakefulness and a difference in the hypercapnic ventilatory response between these two states (for reviews, see Refs. 18,25). This scheme is summarized in Figure 3. As shown in this figure, the steady-state value for Pa_{CO_2} in wakefulness (i.e., the set-point) is approximately 40 mmHg, which is sufficient to maintain resting $\dot{V}$ at normal waking levels (e.g., 5 L/min). However, in sleep there is reduced $\dot{V}$ and increased Pa_{CO_2} because of (1) an increase in the level of Pa_{CO_2} required to maintain spontaneous breathing (18,26,27), (2) reduced ventilatory responses to the increased CO_2 (5,18,28,29), (3) increased upper airway resistance (19,30–33), (4) reduced compensatory responses to this respiratory load (19,32,34,35), and (5) decreased tonic drive to respiratory

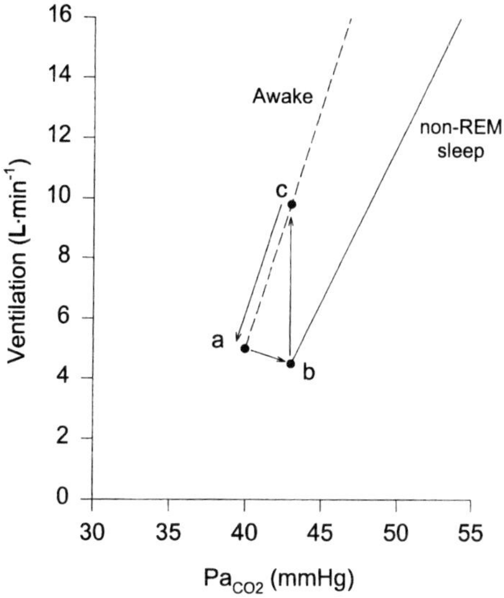

Figure 3 Traditional model used to explain the surge in ventilation at awakening from sleep based upon sleep-wake related differences in the set-point for Pa_{CO_2} and the hypercapnic ventilatory response. Points a and b indicate the change in Pa_{CO_2} and ventilation between wakefulness and non-REM sleep, and the dashed and solid lines represent the ventilatory responses to CO_2 in these states. Upon awakening from sleep (at point b), the prevailing Pa_{CO_2} is initially hypercapnic for the levels normally encountered in wakefulness, and this discrepancy drives ventilation to point c in accordance with the waking hypercapnic ventilatory response. The transient nature of the increased ventilation at awakening is then explained by the time course of the decrease in CO_2 and ventilation produced by the waking hypercapnic ventilatory response. In this model, the key component mediating the surge in ventilation at awakening from sleep is the state-related change in CO_2 drive to breathe. (Adapted from Ref. 25. Points a and b and the slopes of the hypercapnic ventilatory response from Refs. 18,28,169.)

neurons and motoneurons (21,36–38). However, an important consequence of this difference in Pa_{CO_2} between sleep and wakefulness is that if sudden awakening occurs, then the Pa_{CO_2} that was previously present during sleep initially represents a hypercapnic stimulus for the levels normally encountered in wakefulness. This inappropriately high level of CO_2 then drives $\dot{V}$ to a level determined by the waking CO_2 response curve and produces a relative hyperpnea (Fig. 3). Under normoxic conditions the sleep-related changes in Pa_{O_2} would have minimal effect on the ventilatory response to awakening (18). The surge in $\dot{V}$ at wake onset still occurs in animals without an upper airway (18), suggesting that a change in upper airway resistance is also not a major factor mediating the transient increase in $\dot{V}$.

Therefore, the current model used to explain the hyperpnea at awakening from sleep is explained purely in terms of the waking CO_2 response, whereas the transient nature of the increased $\dot{V}$ is explained by the time course of the decrease in CO_2 and $\dot{V}$ produced by the hypercapnic ventilatory response. However, for the reasons outlined in Sec. IV, it is unlikely that this mechanism fully explains the surge in $\dot{V}$ at wake onset.

B. Cardiovascular Responses to Awakening

The changes in HR and BP across sleep-wake states are largely dependent upon intact vagal and sympathetic innervations (8,39,40). However, determination of the precise autonomic mechanisms involved in state-dependent cardiovascular changes has been facilitated by those studies that have documented actual changes in sympathetic and parasympathetic outputs across sleep-wake states. In some studies, direct recording of autonomic nervous system activity has been performed, e.g., microneurography has been used to document sleep-related changes in muscle sympathetic nerve activity in humans (41–44), and chronic recordings of renal sympathetic activity have been performed in animals (9). Other studies have inferred sleep-related changes in autonomic activity by observing changes in HR and BP with blockade of one (or other) branch of the autonomic nervous system (e.g., Refs. 8,45,46). Spectral analysis techniques have also proved useful in gaining insight into sleep-related changes in autonomic output (e.g., Refs. 47,48).

Although each of these approaches has yielded valuable information regarding the neural basis for sleep-related cardiovascular changes, each technique has its own advantages and disadvantages. For example, interpretation of changes in autonomic output from microneurographic recordings of muscle sympathetic nerve activity is somewhat limited because only one branch of the autonomic nervous system is recorded, and because this sympathetic branch shows characteristic differences across sleep-wake states compared to the sympathetic output to other vascular beds. For example, in REM sleep, muscle sympathetic nerve activity is increased (41–43), whereas renal sympathetic activity is decreased (9). A differential distribution of sympathetic output to different vascular beds has also been observed in a pharmacological model of REM sleep where the REM-like state was associated with increased sympathetic output to vasoconstrictor fibers of hindlimb skeletal muscle but decreased output to the cardiac, renal, splanchnic, and lumbar sympathetic nerves (49). The overall effect of this differential distribution of sympathetic output in REM sleep is a net vasodilation in the major resistance vessels, which contributes to the overall decrease in BP in REM sleep (16,24). Transient vasoconstriction in the skeletal muscle vasculature is thought to be an important contributor to the transient increases in BP in phasic REM sleep (16,24,50).

Spectral analysis of HR variability has also been used to determine the prevailing balance of sympathetic and parasympathetic activities (51,52), and this approach has been applied to sleep (e.g., Refs. 47,48). However, the results of such studies, performed during spontaneous breathing, are somewhat complicated because interpretation relies on the validity of several assumptions that may be affected by the influences of sleep and its disturbance (52). In particular, changes in sleep-wake state are associated with significant changes in other physiological variables, e.g., blood gases, lung volume, breathing pattern, and respiratory effort (e.g., Refs. 18,19), each of which can independently influence sympathetic and parasympathetic outflow (52–55) and therefore obscure the primary state-dependent effects on autonomic activity. However, most important for studies during sleep, particularly in patients with sleep-related breathing disorders, are the wide fluctuations in respiratory rate that can accompany sleep onset and arousals from sleep. In these cases, interpretation becomes complicated because the large fluctuations in respiratory rate that occur can fully encompass the frequency ranges used to separate the sympathetic and parasympathetic components of HR variability (52,56).

Despite these caveats, the results of studies using the variety of techniques described above, in a variety of species, suggest that steady-state wakefulness exerts a tonic stimulatory effect on the sympathetic output to the heart and blood vessels (8,41–43,47,48). However, there are far fewer data regarding the acute effects of awakening from sleep on sympathetic output. One study in intact cats has reported that spontaneous arousals from non-REM sleep are associated with large increases in renal sympathetic nerve activity (9), and in humans the occurrence of K complexes during sleep are associated with transient increases in muscle sympathetic nerve activity (41–44). Since K complexes during sleep are thought to be markers of an endogenous arousal/alerting response (57), these observations are consistent with the suggestion that arousal-related mechanisms lead to sympathetic activation. This mechanism has been recently confirmed in naturally sleeping dogs (8) and humans (44), where increased sympathetic drive to the heart and muscle blood vessels, respectively, were demonstrated at awakening from sleep. Constant mechanical $\dot{V}$ was used in the former study (8) to highlight the independent effects of a change in sleep-wake state on sympathetic output, i.e., avoiding state-dependent changes in breathing pattern, lung volume, and blood gases, which can affect autonomic output (52–55) and obscure the primary effect of the state change. An example of the dramatic effect of arousal from sleep on sympathetic output is shown in Figure 4.

In contrast to the several lines of evidence indicating a stimulatory effect of wakefulness on sympathetic output, the effects of wakefulness on parasympathetic output are less clear-cut. Several studies in animals and humans suggest that established wakefulness is associated with a tonic withdrawal of parasympathetic drive to the heart and that this is an important contributor to the increased HR when awake (45–47; see Refs. 16,24,58 for reviews). However, a major factor contributing to this parasympathetic withdrawal is probably a change in respiratory activity. For example, upper airway resistance increases in sleep (19,20,30,31,33), and this leads to increased respiratory efforts in response to the load (20). These increased efforts can themselves lead to an increased vagal contribution to HR variability by the central mechanisms associated with respiratory sinus arrhythmia (59–62). Any respiratory slowing in sleep would also increase the magnitude of the vagal contribution to heart rate variability (63).

That sleep-related changes in blood gases, breathing effort, and breathing pattern can importantly contribute to the parasympathetic control of HR was demon-

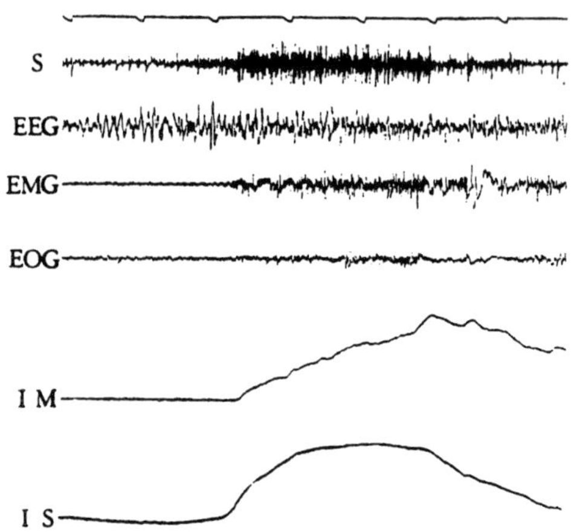

Figure 4 Large increase in renal sympathetic nerve activity upon spontaneous awakening from non-REM sleep in an unrestrained cat. The point of arousal can be taken as the onset of increased neck muscle activity (see EMG channel) and EEG desynchronization. S, Raw sympathetic nerve activity; IS, integrated sympathetic nerve activity; IM, integrated neck muscle activity; other abbreviations as for Figure 2. Time marks show 1-s intervals. (From Ref. 9.)

strated by a recent study in dogs in which breathing rate and depth and blood gases were controlled by constant mechanical $\dot{V}$, while HR changes were monitored during spontaneous fluctuations in sleep-wake state with blockade of the cardiac sympathetic innervation (8). Under these conditions, there was a minimal change in the parasympathetic influence on HR between non-REM sleep and steady-state wakefulness, showing that changes in breathing pattern importantly contribute to the vagal withdrawal and increased HR observed in established wakefulness (8) (Fig. 5). However, vagal influences have major contributions to the HR acceleration observed at awakening from sleep, even in the absence of changes in breathing pattern (8). Indeed, the condition of mechanical $\dot{V}$ to keep constant the respiratory influences on autonomic activity serves to highlight the fact that a simple awakening from sleep acts as a large stimulus for transient vagal withdrawal and HR acceleration (Fig. 5). As can also be observed in Figure 5, the HR at awakening from sleep can even increase to the levels observed during mild exercise, even though there is no evidence of overt behavioral arousal, such as movements, at awakening. The decrease in cardiac vagal activity after presentation of ''natural arousing stimuli'' in cats (40) supports the result that arousal phenomena lead to vagal withdrawal, although the number and types of stimuli applied to how many cats is unclear in that study, as is whether the stimuli were actually applied in wakefulness or sleep. Overall, the large transient parasympathetic withdrawal to the heart (8) and the increased sympathetic drive to the heart and blood vessels (8,9) would explain the large brief BP and HR responses to awakening.

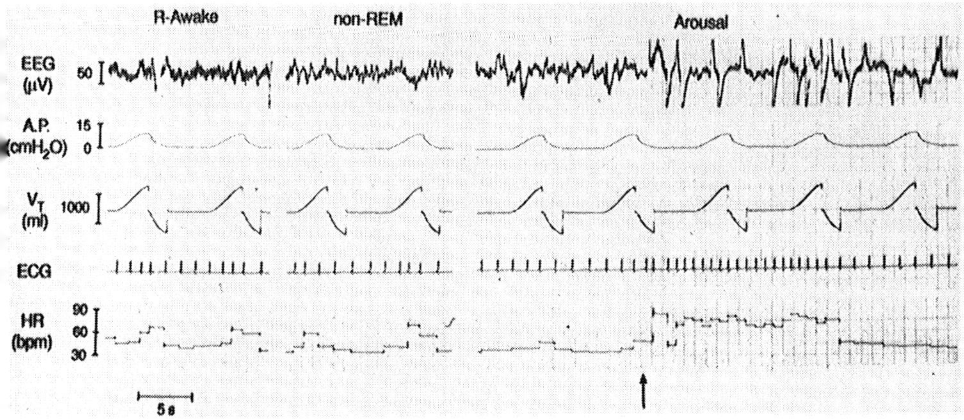

Figure 5 Example showing the differential effects of established wakefulness versus transitions into wakefulness on the parasympathetic control of heart rate. The traces show changes in heart rate between periods of established wakefulness (R-Awake) and non-REM sleep (left panels) and at the transition from non-REM sleep to wakefulness (right panel, point of awakening indicated by arrow). The traces are from a dog undergoing constant mechanical ventilation with blockade of the cardiac sympathetic innervation, i.e., leaving only the parasympathetic innervation active. Mean heart rate changed minimally between steady-state wakefulness and non-REM sleep, but awakening from sleep produced significant vagal withdrawal and large increases in heart rate. No body movements of evidence of overt behavioral arousal were noticeable at awakening; the large voltage deflections on the EEG trace are artifacts due to eye movements. The swings in airway pressure (A.P.) are produced by mechanical ventilation. Other abbreviations as for Figure 1. (From Ref. 8.)

As discussed above, differences in the set-point for Pa_{CO_2} and a change in the hypercapnic ventilatory response can be used to explain (at least in part) the increased $\dot{V}$ at awakening from sleep (Fig. 3). Application of such a model to the control of HR and BP may similarly be used to explain the hemodynamic effects of awakening. The decreased muscle sympathetic nerve activity in non-REM sleep compared to wakefulness, in association with a decreased BP and HR (41–43), suggests that sleep is associated with a change in baroreceptor function. Indeed, there are data to suggest that there is a downward resetting of the baroreflex in non-REM sleep compared to wakefulness, and this appears to be accompanied by increased baroreflex sensitivity (64,65), although this latter effect is not observed consistently (66). Figure 6 illustrates how changes in the set-point and sensitivity of the baroreflex between wakefulness and sleep could explain increased HR and BP at awakening. In this scheme, because the set-point for mean arterial BP is lower during sleep and the sensitivity of the baroreflex may be slightly higher (64,65), the BP upon a sudden awakening from sleep will initially represent a hypotensive stimulus compared to the levels normally encountered in wakefulness. This inappropriately low BP will drive compensatory mechanisms to increase BP, and there will also be some

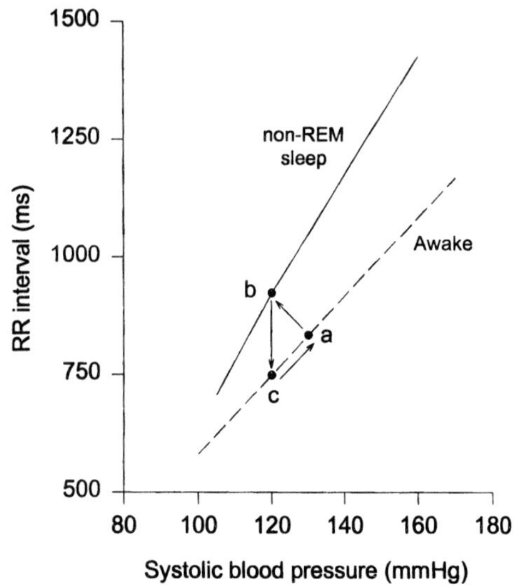

Figure 6 Hemodynamic model that may explain some of the increased heart rate and blood pressure at awakening from sleep. This model is based on the differences between wakefulness and sleep in the set-point and sensitivity of the baroreflex and is an adaptation of the ventilatory model shown in Figure 3. Points a and b indicate typical changes in heart rate (plotted as RR interval) and blood pressure between wakefulness and non-REM sleep, and the dashed and solid lines represent baroreflex sensitivities in these states (64). Systolic pressure is shown on the abscissa because this is typically used to quantify baroreflex responses (e.g., Refs. 64–66,95). Upon awakening from sleep (at point b), the level of systolic pressure will initially represent a hypotensive stimulus compared to the levels normally encountered in wakefulness, and this inappropriate level will drive compensatory mechanisms to increase blood pressure (i.e., from c to a). There will also be some increase in heart rate due to differences in the set-point of the baroreflex curves between sleep and wakefulness. In this model, the transient nature of the blood pressure and heart rate change at awakening is explained in terms of a difference in the set-point of the baroreflex between wakefulness and sleep and possibly an overshoot of the waking set-point.

increase in HR due to differences in the set-point of the curves between sleep and wakefulness (Fig. 6). In this model, the transient nature of the BP and HR surge at awakening would have to be explained in terms of a difference in the baroreflex set-point between wakefulness and sleep and possibly an overshoot of the waking set-point. However, as discussed below, neither this hemodynamic model (Fig. 6) nor the ventilatory model (Fig. 3) is likely to be able to fully explain the surges in HR, BP, and $\dot{V}$ at awakening.

IV. Limitations of Current Ventilatory and Hemodynamic Models in Explaining the Cardiorespiratory Responses to Awakening

A. Limitations of Ventilatory Model

As shown in Figure 3, the surge in $\dot{V}$ at awakening from sleep has been attributed to the differences in set-point for Pa_{CO_2} between sleep and wakefulness and the hypercapnic ventilatory response. In this scheme, the higher Pa_{CO_2} that is present during sleep leads to the CO_2 at awakening being initially hypercapnic, and this produces increased $\dot{V}$. Therefore, the key component of this model is a state-dependent change in the chemical drive to breathe. However, a ventilatory stimulus unrelated to prevailing levels of Pa_{CO_2} probably also contributes to the increased $\dot{V}$ at wake onset. Such an effect is apparent during hypocapnia produced by constant mechanical $\dot{V}$ when the act of awakening itself can provide a stimulus to breathe, even at levels of hypocapnia sufficient to abolish all spontaneous breathing movements both prior to the awakening and in subsequent periods of established wakefulness (8,27). An example of such a response to awakening is shown in Figure 7. Interestingly, similar transient drives to breathe, unrelated to the levels of blood gases, are also observed in phasic REM sleep (36,67).

That stimuli can provide potent excitation of breathing, even when applied at levels of blood gases well below the threshold for central respiratory activity, and in the absence of a chemical drive to breathe, has been observed in many previous studies (e.g., Refs. 36,68–70). Indeed, it is a long-held view that nonchemical inputs can replace some of the central and peripheral chemoreceptor inputs and still yield a total drive that exceeds the threshold for respiratory rhythm generation (68,71). The types of stimuli that can typically produce such increases in respiratory output, independently of a chemical drive to breathe, are those normally associated with alerting responses or those known to produce reticular activation and an aroused state, e.g., pinching, prodding, or sciatic nerve stimulation (68,69). The ventilatory responses to these nonclassical respiratory stimuli are similar to those produced by direct electrical activation of the reticular activating system, an effect that can stimulate respiratory motor output and trigger inspiration (21,72–75). Interestingly, the degree of respiratory activation following reticular stimulation decreases slowly after termination of the stimuli (75,76), an effect similar to the phenomenon of after discharge (21,68,77–79; see Ref. 21 for discussion). That arousal stimuli can stimulate $\dot{V}$ independently of chemical respiratory stimulation is also demonstrated by studies in patients with congenital central hypoventilation syndrome who lack ventilatory chemosensitivity (for review, see Ref. 80). In these patients mental stimulation leads to an increased $\dot{V}$ to a similar degree as that observed in control subjects (81).

Detailed consideration of the effects of awakening from sleep on the activity of reticular activating system neurons is given in Sec. V. However, some initial comments are relevant here given that the studies performed by Orem and colleagues have shown that state-dependent discharge of brain-stem reticular formation neurons

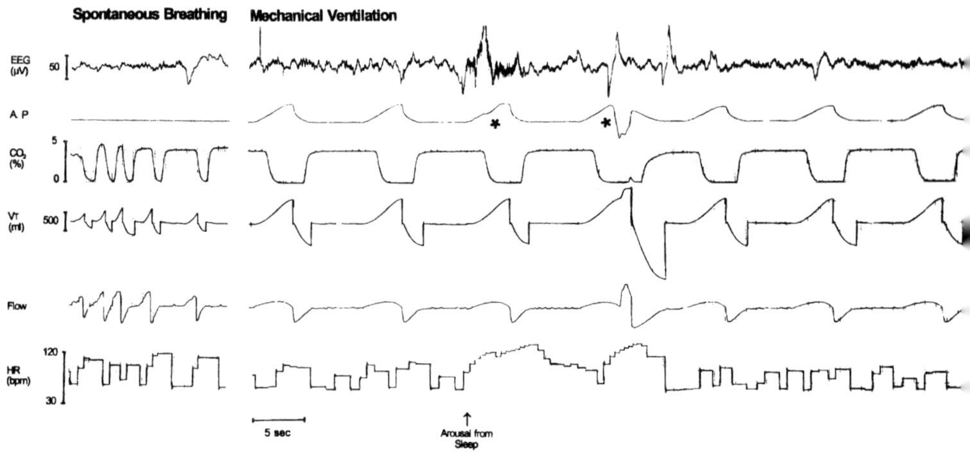

Figure 7 Example of transient stimulation of spontaneous breathing upon awakening from sleep, despite a level of hypocapnia sufficient to abolish all spontaneous breathing movements both prior to the awakening and in subsequent periods of established wakefulness. The traces are from a dog undergoing constant mechanical ventilation to an end-tidal CO_2 just below spontaneous breathing levels. This level of mechanical ventilation is sufficient to abolish all spontaneous breathing movements in sleep and established wakefulness, as judged by the smooth and reproducible flow and pressure traces produced by the ventilator (36,70). However, awakening from sleep provides a transient stimulus to breathe as shown by the downward (inspiratory) deflections in the airway pressure trace (indicated by *) and the increased inspiratory flow and tidal volume. The arrow indicates the point of spontaneous awakening. Abbreviations as for Figures 1 and 5. (From Horner and Phillipson, unpublished data.)

is important for state-related modulation of medullary respiratory neuronal activity and motor output (see Ref. 21 for review). Neurons of the brain-stem reticular formation generally show decreased activity in non-REM sleep compared to wakefulness, with increased activity in REM (see Refs. 17,21,82–84 for reviews). Aroused states in humans are also associated with activation of the midbrain reticular formation as shown by positron emission tomography (85). These state-dependent changes in reticular neuronal activity are relevant because in chronically instrumented intact cats, medullary respiratory neurons also show characteristic changes in activity with sleep-wake states. In particular, respiratory-related neurons that are more tonically active during wakefulness show decreased discharge in non-REM sleep, and some even become inactive, whereas cells with a strong respiratory-related phasic discharge, presumably tightly coupled to the respiratory rhythm generator, are less affected by sleep (21,37). Importantly, iontophoresis of glutamate to reexcite those tonic respiratory neurons most affected by non-REM sleep reveals the persistence of a respiratory-related pattern (i.e., a pattern that was subthreshold before glutamate), a result which suggests that these medullary respiratory cells are critically dependent upon tonic excitatory processes associated with wakefulness for their respiratory activity (86). The tonic, nonrespiratory input to medullary respiratory neurons when awake (i.e., the ''wakefulness stimulus''), is thought to arise from the reticular formation (18,21). That electrical stimulation of the midbrain reticular formation in anesthetized or decerebrate animals converts the activity of several respiratory muscles or motor nerves from a sleep-like pattern to one more like wakefulness supports this concept (21,72–75). As such, a decrease in the magnitude of these tonic excitatory influences on medullary respiratory neurons would produce decreased $\dot{V}$ in non-REM sleep compared to wakefulness (21,37). This concept is supported by the observation that non-REM sleep is associated with reduced tonic drive to respiratory muscle, an effect that can be observed independently of a change in phasic drive associated with respiratory rhythm (36).

In REM sleep, the level of medullary respiratory neuronal discharge is greater than in non-REM sleep (21,87,88), and there is considerable variation around the mean level of discharge in REM associated with tonic and phasic events (87,88). The increased medullary respiratory neuronal discharge in REM sleep suggests that central respiratory drive is increased during this state (21,87). However, since tidal volume is often lowest during REM, this increased central respiratory drive must be opposed by inhibitory influences acting at the level of the motoneuron (21,89). Indeed, these REM sleep–related inhibitory mechanisms may be similar to those acting at postural motoneurons (90,91). Since these inhibitory mechanisms can express themselves to varying degrees in REM sleep and produce transient fluctuations in motoneuron excitability in postural and respiratory motoneurons (21,36,87,89–91), these transient fluctuations in drive probably importantly contribute to the irregular and erratic respiratory output that typifies REM sleep.

In summary, neuronal processes associated with reticular activation can exert major influences on respiratory neurons and motor output. In addition, observations suggest that processes associated with spontaneous awakenings and alerting reactions can themselves provide a transient stimulus to breathe, even at levels of blood gases sufficient to abolish spontaneous breathing before and after the arousal reaction. These observations suggest that differences in the set-point for Pa_{CO_2} and the hypercapnic ventilatory response between sleep and wakefulness probably only partly explain the increased $\dot{V}$ at arousal from sleep. A revised model to explain the increased $\dot{V}$ at awakening is proposed at the end of this section, after a discussion of the limitations of the current hemodynamic model described below.

B. Limitations of Hemodynamic Model

Changes in the set-point and sensitivity of the baroreflex between sleep and wakefulness (64–66) may explain the tonic stimulatory effect of wakefulness on HR and BP (Fig. 6). However, although the relevance of this mechanism in explaining the phasic increases in HR and BP at awakening from sleep needs to be formerly tested, it is unlikely that this model can be used to fully explain these responses for the reasons outlined below. First, increases in HR and BP are observed during wakefulness in baroreceptor denervated animals (92), indicating the presence of a direct centrally mediated effect of sleep-wake state on cardiac autonomic activity and vasomotor tone that can occur independently of the baroreflex. Furthermore, the HR and BP changes that occur with changes in sleep-wake state are larger after baroreceptor denervation than before (92), suggesting that the baroreflex normally buffers the cardiovascular effects of a change in sleep-wake state. Moreover, HR increases dramatically upon awakening from sleep at a time when BP also increases significantly (Fig. 1). The large increase in HR, despite the surge in BP, suggests that the baroreflex may in fact be partially uncoupled at awakening. This suggestion is supported by the result that during sleep, pharmacologically induced BP increases produce typical baroreflex-induced decreases in HR unless sleep is disturbed by a K complex (64). At this time, BP continues to increase, but this is now accompanied by a significant increase in HR (Fig. 8). This result suggests that phasic arousal or alerting reactions can uncouple baroreflex-induced slowing of the heart. Similar observations have been made during arousal associated with the defense reaction (93; see Ref. 94 for review) and mental arousal (65). Spontaneous K complexes during sleep also lead to significant increases in HR, BP, as well as muscle sympathetic nerve activity (41–44).

Taken together, these observations suggest that wakefulness likely exerts an inhibitory effect on the baroreflex control of HR and that this effect leads to the change in set-point and sensitivity in wakefulness compared to sleep and uncoupling of the baroreflex in states of arousal (64,65,93,94). This effect may also explain why only about 15% of spontaneous fluctuations in RR intervals and arterial pressures follow the directions predicted by the baroreflex in wakefulness (95) and why both HR and BP show such large increases at awakening from sleep.

C. A Revised Model to Explain Cardiorespiratory Responses to Awakening from Sleep

As discussed above, the current ventilatory and hemodynamic models probably do not fully explain the large brief cardiorespiratory activation produced by awakening from sleep, or why these changes exceed obvious physiological need and those observed in later periods of established wakefulness. A chief reason for this discrepancy is probably that a major assumption of these models is that the sole factor responsible for the large brief cardiorespiratory activation at awakening is the difference in control mechanisms between the states of sleep and wakefulness. In the ventilatory model this difference relates to the prevailing levels of Pa_{CO_2} and the hypercapnic ventilatory responses between sleep and wakefulness (Fig. 3), whereas in the hemodynamic model this difference relates to changes in the prevailing levels of BP and effects on the baroreflex (Fig. 6).

However, common to both these models is the basic assumption that the period of wakefulness that occurs immediately after sleep is functionally similar to subsequent periods of established wakefulness, i.e., the major factor contributing to the cardio-respiratory activation is the inappropriate level of the physiological variable

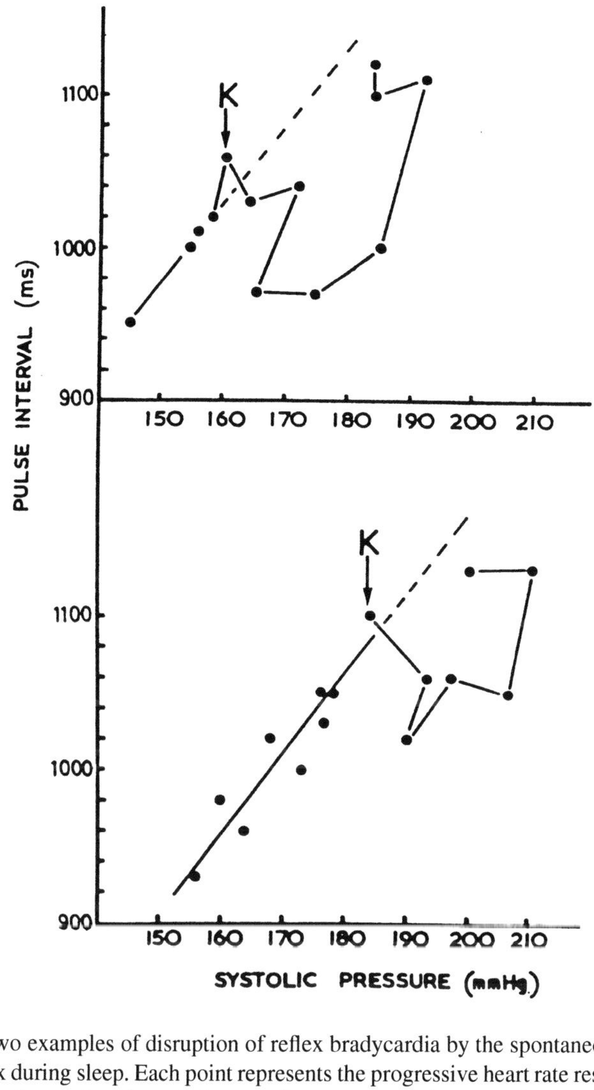

Figure 8 Two examples of disruption of reflex bradycardia by the spontaneous occurrence of a K complex during sleep. Each point represents the progressive heart rate response (plotted as pulse interval) as a function of the systolic pressure of the preceding beat. The increase in blood pressure was produced by intravenous injection of angiotensin. The slope of the response (solid line) indicates baroreflex sensitivity. Note that following the K complex, baroreflex-induced slowing of the heart was disrupted (i.e., deviated from the preceding baroreflex response line) and heart rate increased along with blood pressure. (From Ref. 64.)

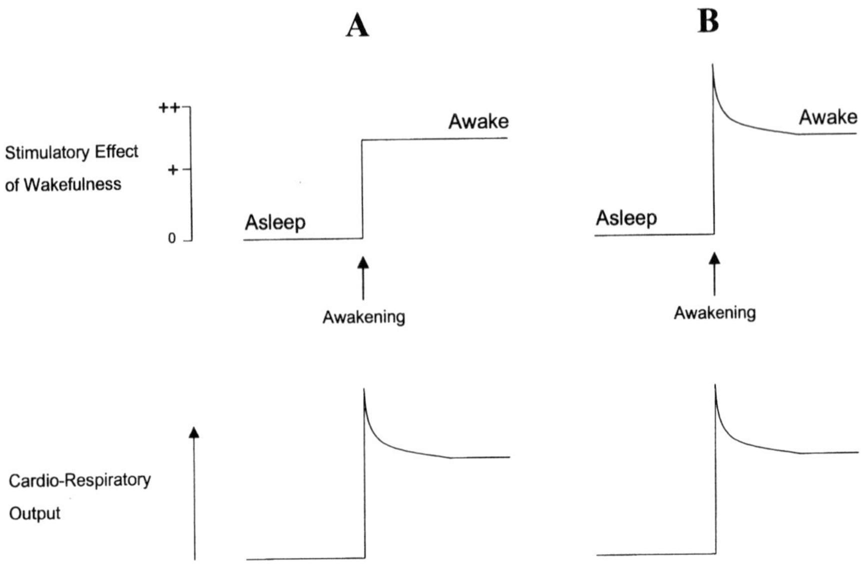

Figure 9 Alternative, but not mutually exclusive, models that may account for the large brief cardiorespiratory activation at awakening from sleep. (A) The difference in physiological control mechanisms between sleep and wakefulness, with an inappropriate level of the physiological variable at wake onset, importantly contributes to the cardiorespiratory activation at awakening. In this scheme, the stimulatory effect of wakefulness (i.e., the wakefulness stimulus) is the same at wake onset compared to subsequent wakefulness. (B) The property of the awake state at wake onset importantly contributes to cardiorespiratory activation by providing a transiently increased wakefulness stimulus. See text for further discussion. The magnitude and time constant of the depicted changes are arbitrary and were chosen simply to highlight the differences between the two models.

(Pa_{CO_2} or BP) at wake onset compared to previous sleep (Fig. 9A). However, if the period of wakefulness at wake onset is functionally distinct from subsequent periods of wakefulness, and even associated with a transiently heightened awake state, this may importantly contribute to the autonomic responses at awakening and the large cardiorespiratory responses (Fig. 9B). This is an important distinction because it places a major emphasis on the role of wakefulness in contributing to the cardiorespiratory responses rather than the change from sleep to waking per se. For example, the phrase ''arousal from sleep'' implies (probably falsely given the considerations described in the next section) that a state change from sleep to wakefulness is the key factor contributing to the resulting autonomic responses, whereas the state change may, in fact, be more importantly involved in producing a transiently aroused awake state compared to subsequent wakefulness. In this case the state change would be more correctly described as a transition from sleep into aroused wakefulness. This transiently aroused awake state may then provide a potent ''wakefulness stimulus'' contributing a transient excitation of respiratory neurons and sympathetic outflow and transient vagal withdrawal and baroreflex uncoupling (see previous sections for effects of wakefulness on these parameters). As such, these effects would importantly contribute to the large brief cardiorespiratory activation observed at wake onset. Evidence supporting the concept that awakening from sleep is associated with the spontaneous generation of a neurophysiologically distinct, transiently aroused awake state, compared to subsequent wakefulness, is described below.

V. Pattern of Reticular Activating System Neuronal Activity at Awakening from Sleep

A. Basic Organization of the Reticular Activating System

There have been major advances regarding the brain-stem sites and neurochemical substrates underlying the generation of brain activity characterizing sleep and wakefulness. Following initial identification of the reticular activating system as sites in the brainstem where electrical stimulation could produce cortical activation (96), advances in immunohistochemical techniques have led to the identification of several anatomically and chemically distinct cell groups as comprising this ascending activation system. These groups include serotonergic [i.e., 5-hydroxytryptamine (5-HT)–containing] dorsal raphe (DR) neurons, noradrenergic locus coeruleus (LC) neurons, and cholinergic neurons of the laterodorsal and pedunculopontine tegmental nuclei (LDT and PPT, respectively). Substantia nigra and ventral tegmental area dopaminergic neurons, tuberomamillary hypothalamic histaminergic neurons, and basal forebrain cholinergic neurons are also thought to comprise this ascending activation system (see Refs. 84,97–101 for reviews). Activation of these systems promote EEG desynchronization via depolarization of thalamic relay neurons, which produces tonic firing (for reviews, see Refs. 98,100,102,103). However, these different cell groups vary in the extent of their thalamic projections. For example, the major projection for cholinergic LDT and PPT neurons is the thalamus, whereas other systems such as the LC have more widespread connections (see Refs. 98,104 for discussion).

The major role of the cholinergic LDT and PPT neurons in depolarizing thalamic relay neurons and promoting EEG activation is suggested by their prominent discharge in the two states associated with cortical desynchronization, i.e., wakefulness and REM sleep (105–107). In contrast, DR and LC discharge is minimal in REM sleep but high in wakefulness (108–112). This and other evidence, e.g., measurement of acetylcholine release in the thalamus during sleep and wakefulness (113), has led to the concept that activation of LDT and PPT cholinergic neurons importantly contributes to cortical activation and EEG desynchronization in states of wakefulness and arousal (84,97–100,102). However, this does not suggest that DR and LC neurons are unimportant because discharge of these neurons is thought to be highly relevant to other important aspects of brain activity in states of wakefulness and arousal. LC neurons are thought to play an important role in modifying vigilance and sensory responsiveness (114,115), whereas DR neurons are thought to be importantly involved in facilitation of gross motor responses (116,117). This separation of function highlights the possibility that discrete neuronal systems comprising the ascending arousal systems may contribute distinct properties associated with the waking brain. This concept, as it relates to the processes engaged at awakening from sleep, is discussed in more detail in the following sections.

A simplified diagram of the connectivity between components of the brainstem reticular activating system is shown in Figure 10. This figure is a modification of that described by Reese et al. (104) and includes the major changes in firing pattern across sleep-wake states described above. There is evidence that the DR inputs to LDT/PPT neurons (118) are inhibitory, with 5-HT_{1A}-like receptors mediating the inhibition (119–122). LC inputs to LDT/PPT neurons are also inhibitory (123). Other relevant interactions are inhibitory 5-HT inputs to LC neurons (124) and excitatory cholinergic inputs to LC neurons (125–128).

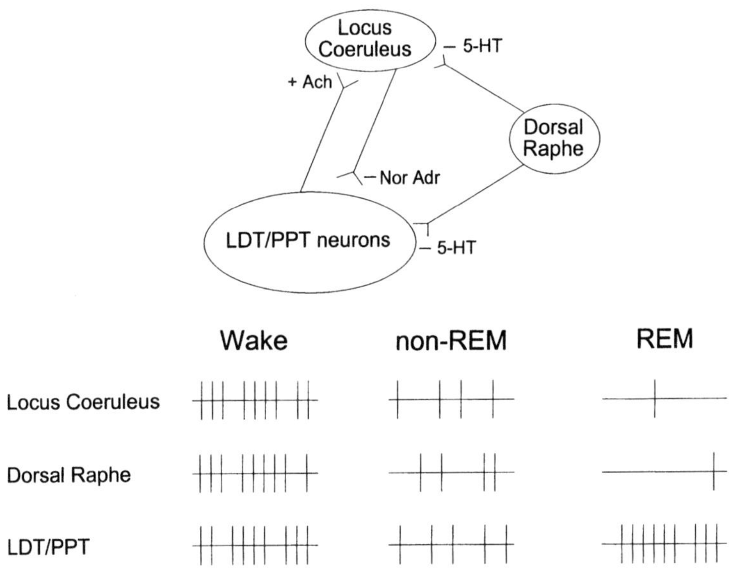

Figure 10 A simplified diagram of the connectivity between components of the brainstem reticular activating system. Ascending and descending projections are not shown. Also shown in this figure is a schema of the general changes in discharge across sleep-wake states of the neuronal groups comprising the reticular activating system. See text for further discussion. Ach, acetylcholine; Nor Adr, noradrenaline; 5-HT, 5-hydroxytryptamine; +, excitatory connections; –, inhibitory connections; LDT/PPT, laterodorsal and pedunculopontine tegmental nuclei. (Adapted from Ref. 104.)

B. Distinct Firing Patterns of Reticular Activating System Neurons at Wake Onset Compared to Subsequent Wakefulness

As shown in Figure 10 and described above, established wakefulness is associated with increased firing of DR (108–110), LC (111), and LDT/PPT (105–107) neurons compared to non-REM sleep. In REM sleep, DR and LC firing is minimal (108–111), whereas some LDT/PPT neurons become active (105–107) and probably contribute to the EEG desynchrony typically associated with REM. However, as described below, there are also some major changes in firing patterns of these neuronal groups at transitions between sleep-wake states particularly at awakening from sleep.

Large transient increases in discharge occur at spontaneous awakening from REM sleep for the majority of DR neurons (109,112) and at awakening from non-REM and REM sleep for LC neurons (111). However, of major importance to this discussion is that the discharge rates at wake onset far exceed the discharge rates in subsequent periods of established wakefulness both for DR neurons (Fig. 11) and LC neurons (Fig. 12) and remarkably even reach levels similar to that observed during experimenter-induced phasic arousal reactions, e.g., after startle or alerting stimuli (109,111,112). Another noticeable feature of the large DR and LC discharge at spontaneous awakening is that the discharge progressively increases in the few seconds before wake onset and reaches a maximum in the few seconds following awakening (109,111,112). For awakenings elicited by external sensory stimuli (e.g., sound), these large increases in firing accompany the awakening but do not precede it (109,111,112). Since it is thought that LC neurons play an important role in modifying vigilance and sensory responsiveness (114,115), while DR neurons facilitate gross motor output (116,117), the large increases in firing of these neuronal groups in the few seconds before and after awakening suggest that the central nervous system may be especially "geared up" to receive and respond to sensory inputs at wake onset compared to other states, even subsequent wakefulness. The enhanced responsiveness of visual cortex neurons to visual inputs upon awakening (102,129) supports this concept. It has even been suggested that these bursts of LC and DR activity at awakening may serve a protective function, e.g., preparing an animal to respond immediately to sensory stimuli, which may even be potentially threatening (111,112,130). In this context, the abrupt changes in EEG activity and activation of postural muscle tone at awakening (1–4,7,8) and the large cardiorespiratory changes (8–12) would be appropriate physiological responses. Further evidence to support the concept that wake onset is associated with the spontaneous activation of a distinct, transiently aroused awake state is discussed below.

C. Spontaneous Activation of a Distinct Arousal State at Wake Onset

In the previous section it was proposed that the firing patterns of DR and LC neurons at awakening from sleep are consistent with the hypothesis that the neuronal mecha-

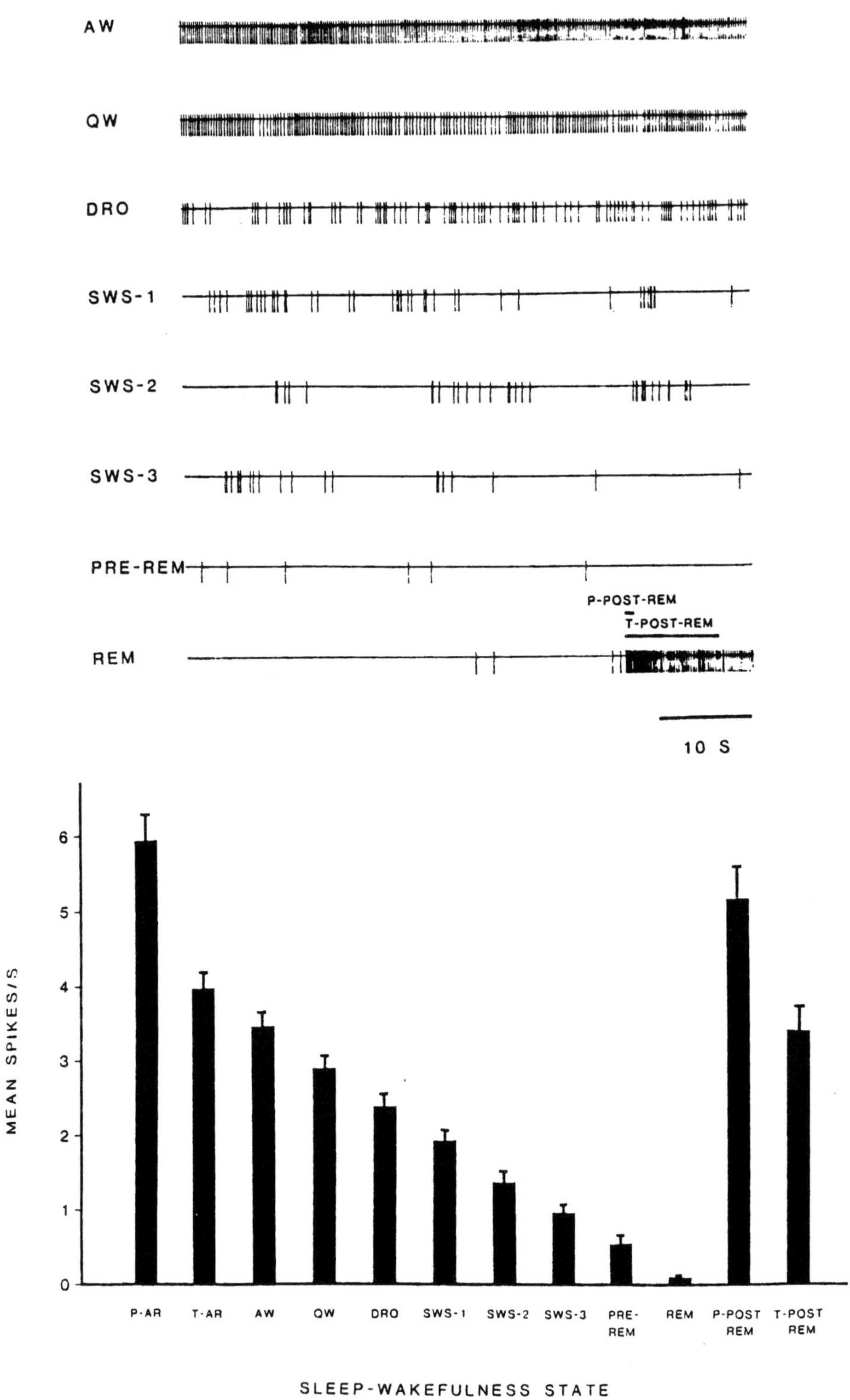
AW
QW
DRO
SWS-1
SWS-2
SWS-3
PRE-REM
P-POST-REM
T-POST-REM
REM
10 S
MEAN SPIKES/S
0
1
2
3
4
5
6
P-AR
T-AR
AW
QW
DRO
SWS-1
SWS-2
SWS-3
PRE-REM
REM
P-POST REM
T-POST REM
SLEEP-WAKEFULNESS STATE

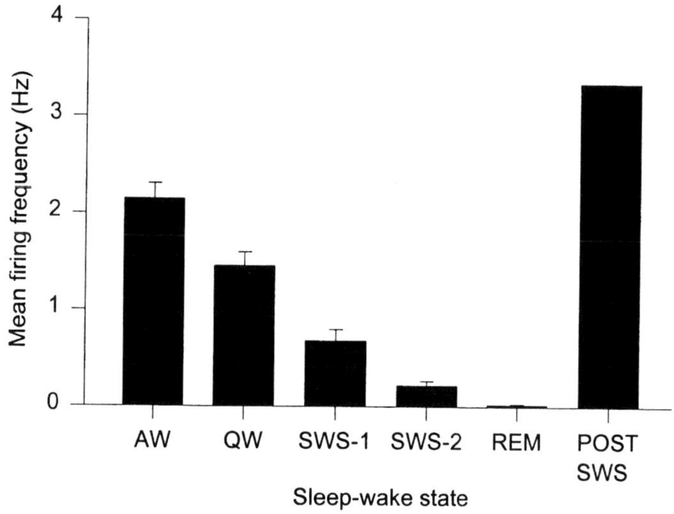

Figure 12 Locus coeruleus neuronal activity across sleep-wake states in rats. Mean discharge rates (±SEM) are shown for different sleep-wake states (abbreviations as for Fig. 11). Note the decreased discharge upon progression from wakefulness to non-REM sleep, with minimal firing in REM. Also note the large transient increases in discharge at spontaneous awakening from non-REM sleep, to levels that exceed even those in active wakefulness. (Adapted from Ref. 111.)

nisms engaged at wake onset indicate the spontaneous generation of a transiently aroused awake state compared to subsequent wakefulness. Given the functions of these neuronal groups in facilitating sensorimotor responsiveness (114–117), it would be expected then that wake onset would be associated with enhanced central nervous system responses to sensory stimuli. This hypothesis was tested in a recent study using the acoustic startle reflex (131). The startle reflex is a standard unconditioned reflex elicited by a sudden loud noise producing whole body movement (Fig. 13A). This reflex is observed in a wide variety of species, including humans, and

Figure 11 Dorsal raphe neuronal activity across sleep-wake states in freely moving cats. Unit activity is shown on the left panel, and mean discharge rates (±SEM) are shown on the right. Note the decreased discharge upon progression from wakefulness to non-REM sleep, with minimal firing in REM. Also note the large transient increases in discharge at spontaneous awakening from REM sleep, to levels which even exceed those in active wakefulness. P-AR, Phasic arousal produced in wakefulness by loud (112 dB) auditory stimulus; T-AR, tonic arousal in the period immediately after the loud stimulus; AW, active wakefulness; QW, quiet wakefulness; DRO, drowsy; SWS-1, SWS-2, SWS-3, progressively deepening slow wave (non-REM) sleep; PRE-REM, transition to REM sleep; REM, REM sleep; P-POST REM, first second at the end of a REM period; T-POST REM, period of wakefulness immediately after REM sleep. (From Ref. 109.)

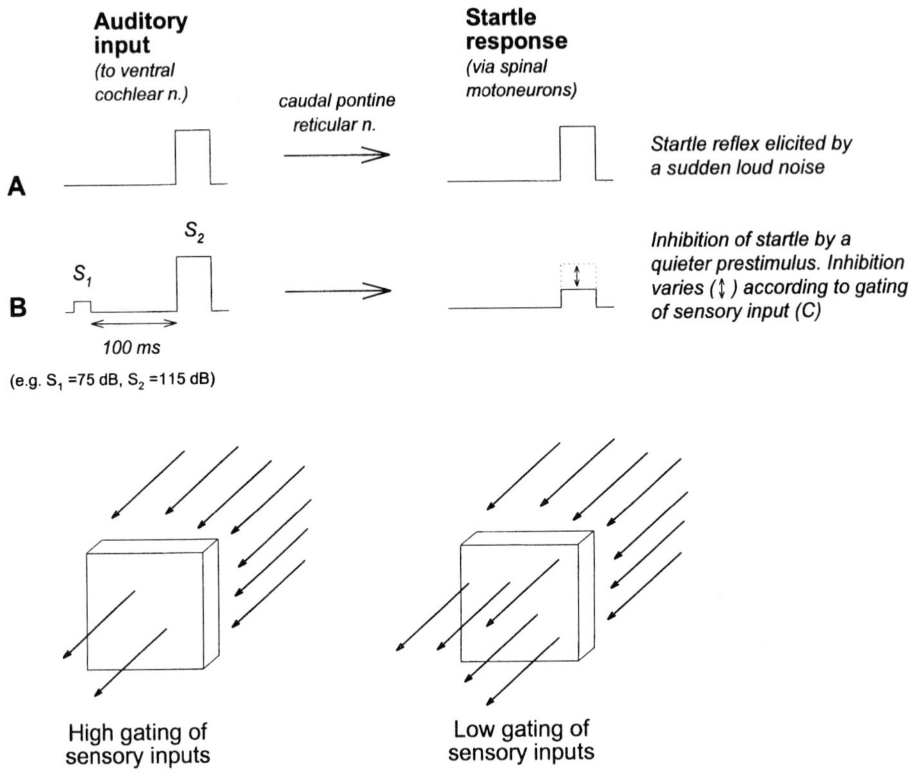

Figure 13 Schema showing elements of the acoustic startle reflex and its modulation by sensory inputs. The acoustic startle reflex is elicited by a sudden loud noise producing whole body movement and is mediated by a serial brainstem circuit comprising the ventral cochlear nucleus, the caudal pontine reticular nucleus and spinal motoneurons (A). A classic feature of this reflex is the diminution of startle responses when a quieter stimulus (S_1) is presented immediately before the loud stimulus (S_2) (B). This phenomenon, known as prepulse inhibition, is used as a measure of sensorimotor gating (C). The magnitude of prepulse inhibition of startle responses varies according to the degree of sensorimotor gating and arousal state. See text for further details.

likely serves a protective function, e.g., by facilitating fight or flight (132). Anatomical and electrophysiological studies have shown that the startle reflex is mediated by a serial brainstem circuit comprising at least three central relays: the ventral cochlear nucleus, the caudal pontine reticular nucleus, and spinal motoneurons (133,134) (Fig. 13A). Given the simple circuitry of this reflex, it serves as a useful model to investigate neuronal influences on mammalian behavior (133,134). In particular, the central relay station of this reflex is influenced by state-dependent neuronal processes (see below). Another important feature of the startle reflex is that it can be modulated under specific conditions, e.g., diminution of the startle response when a quieter stimulus is presented immediately before the loud stimulus (135 137) (Fig. 13B). This robust phenomenon, known as prepulse inhibition, is used as a measure of sensorimotor gating (Fig. 13C), with reduced prepulse inhibition indicating reduced gating of this elementary motor response to a sudden intense sensory input. Reduced prepulse inhibition occurs in clinical disorders where there is an inability to inhibit attention to incoming sensory information (136,137) and also occurs in documented states of aroused wakefulness (138). Reduced prepulse inhibition of startle responses at wake onset compared to later established wakefulness would indicate enhanced sensorimotor responsiveness and support the concept that this period is associated with a transiently aroused awake state.

In rats equipped with electrodes for chronic recording of sleep-wake state and body movement, the startle reflex was elicited by a sudden loud auditory tone (115 dB, 40 ms duration) (Fig. 13A). Prepulse inhibition was elicited by a barely audible tone (74 dB, 20 ms duration) preceding the loud tone by 100 ms (Fig. 13B). Stimuli were applied either 3–10 s after spontaneous awakenings or in established wakefulness (>30 s). Figure 14 shows an example of the effects of awake state on responses to the startle stimuli alone (top traces) and responses to the paired stimuli producing prepulse inhibition (lower traces). Compared to established wakefulness, the magnitude of the startle reflex was similar at wake onset from non-REM and REM sleep. This result suggests that there was no difference in the effects of awake state *directly* on the relays of the primary acoustic startle circuit. However, awakening from non-REM sleep reduced prepulse inhibition (i.e., responses to the paired stimuli were larger) compared to established wakefulness (Fig. 14). For the group of rats this effect was statistically significant for wake onset from non-REM sleep, but the reductions in prepulse inhibition were intermediate, and more variable, at wake onset from REM sleep and not statistically different from those in established wakefulness (131).

Since reduced prepulse inhibition of startle responses occurs in states of aroused wakefulness (138), the similar effects produced at awakening from non-REM sleep supports the notion that the processes associated with wake onset are involved in the spontaneous generation of a transiently aroused awake state compared to subsequent wakefulness (131). Moreover, the reduced prepulse inhibition of startle responses at wake onset from non-REM shows that the central neural mechanisms engaged at awakening from non-REM *indirectly* influence the relays of the startle circuit, i.e., by mechanisms involved in sensorimotor gating. Since these circuits have been established and involve state-dependent neurons of the reticular activating system (see below), this result provides a means to gain further insight into the neuronal processes engaged at awakening and their functional consequences.

D. Neural Processes Engaged at Awakening and the Functional Consequences

Giant cells in the caudal pontine reticular nucleus are critical for the generation of startle responses (139–142) (Fig. 13A), and prepulse inhibition ultimately occurs

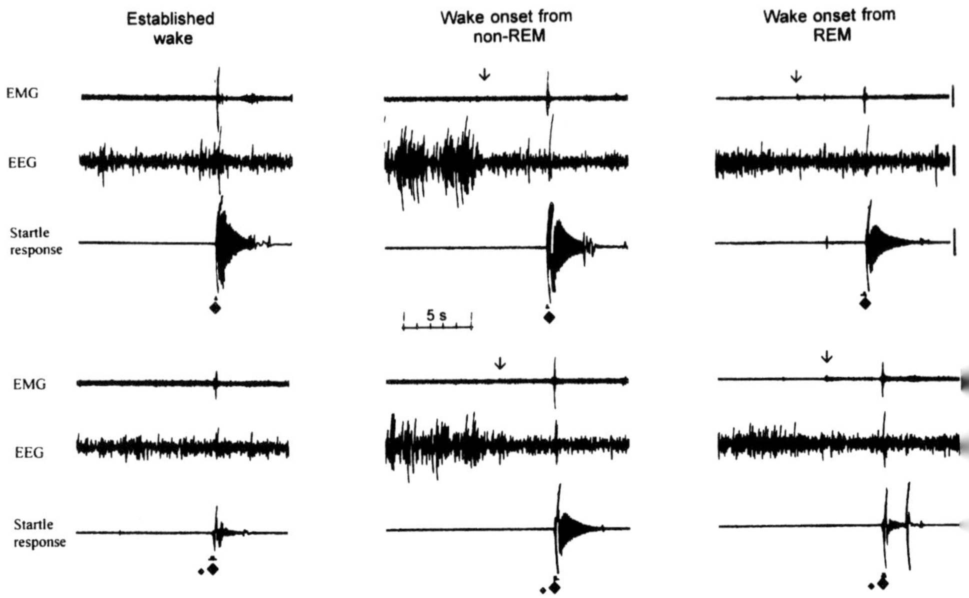

Figure 14 Example of the effects of awake state on the startle reflex and its modulation by sensory inputs. Responses to the startle stimuli alone (i.e., S_2 from Fig. 14) are shown on the top traces (startle stimuli applied at ◆). Responses to the paired stimuli producing prepulse inhibition (i.e., $S_1 + S_2$) are shown on the lower traces (stimuli applied at ♦◆). The initial large pen deflection immediately after the stimulus (latencies < 10 ms) indicates the startle response as measured by body movement. The startle response in established wakefulness was similar to that at wake onset from non-REM and REM sleep. However, awakening from non-REM sleep reduced prepulse inhibition (i.e., responses to the paired stimuli were larger) compared to established wakefulness. The arrows indicate the point of spontaneous awakenings. Responses are shown on a slow time scale to illustrate the changes in sleep-wake states. Calibration bars for the EEG and neck EMG are 200 μV, and for startle 2 mV. The second large pen deflection in the panel on the bottom right is due to a sudden spontaneous change in body position. (From Ref. 131.)

at the synapses onto these cells (134) by decreasing their firing responses to auditory stimuli (139). Prepulse inhibition can be produced by various neuronal circuits, such as those involving the medial prefrontal cortex (143), hippocampus (144), nucleus accumbens and ventral pallidum (137), inferior colliculus (145), as well as cholinergic cells of the PPT (146,147). However, despite this apparent complexity, PPT neurons are thought to be the final common output pathway mediating prepulse inhibition of startle responses (146,147).

Unit recordings of PPT neurons (104,148) show that a large number of cells exhibit acoustic sensitivities in the range of 50–60 dB, with some firing at slightly higher thresholds (70–80 dB). Cholinergic PPT neurons project to the caudal pontine

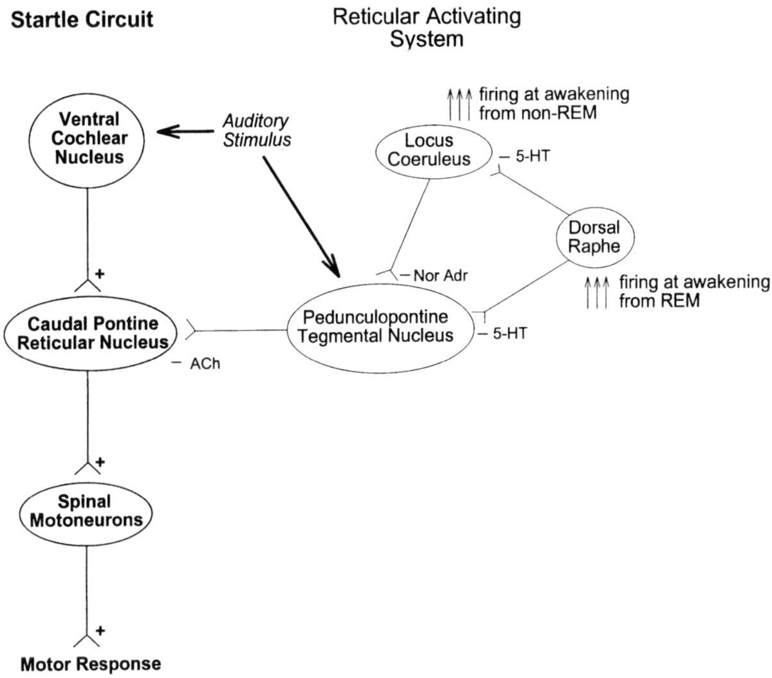

Figure 15 Diagram to show the wiring of the acoustic startle circuit and the interaction of this circuit with sleep-wake related neurons of the reticular activating system (as depicted in Fig. 10). The reticular activating system influences the startle circuit via the pedunculopontine tegmental nucleus, which is also the final common output pathway mediating prepulse inhibition of startle responses. See text for further details. Abbreviations as for Figure 10.

reticular nucleus and inhibit acoustically responsive neurons (146). However, unlike PPT neurons, acoustically responsive caudal pontine reticular neurons typically fire only in response to high threshold (>80 dB) auditory stimuli (134,139). This differential sensitivity of PPT and caudal pontine reticular neurons suggests that the latter group is important in mediating startle responses to high-intensity auditory stimuli, while the former group is important in inhibiting these responses following the initial presentation of a low threshold auditory stimulus (i.e., prepulse inhibition). Further evidence that the PPT is importantly involved in the prepulse inhibition of startle responses is demonstrated by the disruption of this inhibition (but not startle responses per se) following PPT lesions, with the magnitude of effect related to lesion size (146,147). These observations add further weight to the suggestion that the neural processes engaged at awakening from non-REM sleep modulate the activity of the PPT and that this effect mediates the effects of wake onset on prepulse inhibition of startle responses (131).

Figure 15 shows the wiring of the acoustic startle circuit (133,134) and the interaction of this circuit with sleep-wake related neurons of the reticular activating system identified in Figure 10. Although PPT neurons are importantly involved in mediating prepulse inhibition (see above), their activity is also known to change in relation to sleep-wake state, cortical desynchronization, as well as ponto-geniculo-occipital waves, i.e., states associated with arousal and alerting (Sec. V.A) (105,107,149,150). The PPT also has established interactions with DR and LC neurons, whose firing patterns at awakening (109,111,112) are consistent with the hypotheses that the neural mechanisms engaged at wake onset are characteristically different from those in subsequent wakefulness, and that wake onset is associated with a transiently heightened awake state (see above). Indeed, the large transient increases in firing of LC and DR neurons at awakening, along with the identified inhibitory projections of these neurons to the PPT, would explain the reduced prepulse inhibition of startle responses at wake onset compared to subsequent wakefulness. In this scheme the pronounced discharges of these neuronal groups at awakening would inhibit PPT neurons and their responses to the low-intensity auditory stimuli. This would then produce less inhibition of the startle response as the loud auditory stimulus subsequently progressed through the higher threshold acoustic startle circuit (see Ref. 131) (Fig. 15). Although this hypothesis remains to be formally tested, if LC neurons do have an important role in mediating enhanced sensory responsiveness at awakening from sleep, this would explain why the inhibition of startle responses was markedly reduced at wake onset from non-REM sleep, compared to wake onset from REM, because only from non-REM are such large LC discharges consistently linked to the point of awakening (111).

The less consistent effects of awakening from REM sleep on sensory modulation of startle responses may have simply resulted from the increased variability of responses (131) similar to that observed in many physiological phenomena during REM sleep (16,18). However, it may also have resulted from a prime functional objective of awakening from REM being the facilitation of motor output from a state in which this was previously inhibited. Given the DR neurons are involved in facilitation of gross motor output (116,117), the large transient increases in discharge of these neurons at spontaneous awakening from REM sleep (109,112) (Fig. 11) fit with this notion. Moreover, since the startle reflex is largely attenuated during REM sleep (138), its immediate recovery upon awakening (Fig. 14) may be the result of this DR activation. The inhibitory interaction between LC and DR neurons (Fig. 10) may also reflect the balance upon awakening from REM sleep of a requirement to increase vigilance and sensory responsiveness (a function of the LC) and a requirement to restore motor output (a function of the DR). The prevailing balance between the activity of these two modulating systems may be responsible for the intermediate effect of wake onset from REM sleep on sensory responsiveness, but the immediate facilitation of motor output from a previously inhibited state (131). Indeed, as many of the neurophysiological features of REM sleep are mirrored in the brain during alert wakefulness (151,152), the requirement for immediate recovery of LC activity at awakening from REM may be secondary to the need to restore motor activity via recruitment of DR discharge.

The identified inhibitory interactions of monoaminergic LC and DR neurons with cholinergic LDT/PPT neurons of the reticular activating system (Fig. 15) would predict that a phasic reduction of background discharge would take place in some LDT/PPT neurons at awakening from sleep due to the large firing LC and DR neurons. Although there is evidence that this does occur in a significant percentage of LDT neurons at awakening (106,153), others increase their firing at awakening in keeping with the known discharge profiles of LDT/PPT neurons in wakefulness (105,107,149,150). The mechanisms behind the decreased activity in some LDT neurons at awakening from sleep remains to be determined (153).

At a more global level of neuronal activity, cortical visually responsive neurons have been shown to have smoother, and often reduced, spontaneous firing rates in wakefulness and at arousal compared to the levels observed in sleep (102,129). However, arousal noticeably enhanced the responsiveness of these cortical neurons to optimally orientated visual stimuli (102,129). It has been proposed (102) that awakening increases the ratio of evoked responses to spontaneous discharge in cortical neurons (i.e., the signal-to-noise ratio) and that this effect is mediated by modulatory systems such as the LC. Since LC neurons project widely throughout the central nervous system and enhance synaptic transmission (154) and the signal-to-noise ratio (114,115) in target neurons, the large increase in LC activity at awakening (111) (Fig. 12) would fit with enhanced sensory responsiveness observed at wake onset (131). These considerations have important implications regarding the adequate detection and quantification of arousal phenomena and whether simple measures of changes in EEG activity would be sufficient. Indeed, measurement of gross changes in EEG activity are probably not the best indicators of the neural processes engaged at arousal from sleep if these processes are more relevant to enhancing the responses of cortical neurons to afferent inputs rather than just increasing their discharge per se. Other approaches better suited to detecting changes in ascending arousal systems and responses to afferent inputs, e.g., auditory-evoked cortical responses (for further discussion, see Ref. 155), may be more sensitive and appropriate measures of arousal phenomena.

VI. Summary and Unanswered Questions

This chapter has summarized evidence that suggests that from a standpoint of the neural processes engaged at awakening from sleep, the moments just after awakening are fundamentally different from subsequent periods of established wakefulness that have been the major focus of attention in the past. Indeed, there is also ample evidence to reject the notion that the neural processes engaged at wake onset are simply a reversal of those changes that occur at the onset of sleep. Moreover, it is remarkable that the degree of discharge achieved by certain reticular activating system neurons at spontaneous awakening from sleep are only achieved at other times in wakefulness when external alerting or arousing stimuli are applied (109,111,112). This supports the notion that there is spontaneous activation of a transiently aroused awake state at wake onset. Moreover, this state appears to be associated with enhanced sensorimotor responsiveness (129,131), which from a behavioral perspective may serve a protective function by preparing an animal to respond immediately to sensory stimuli upon awakening (111,112,130). Indeed, taking this suggestion further, it is often recognized that sleep is a state in which mammals are most vulnerable to predation and harm and that sleep onset occurs when there is no perceived threat in the immediate surroundings. However, this latter condition is not guaranteed at awakening from sleep such that the spontaneous generation of a transiently aroused awake state with enhanced sensorimotor responsiveness would be an appropriate and adaptive physiological response. The recognition of this distinct arousal state, spontaneously generated at wake onset, also necessitates important modifications to the current physiological models that are used to explain the cardiorespiratory consequences of awakening from sleep. At present, these models emphasize that the major factor contributing to the large HR, BP, and $\dot{V}$ responses at wake onset is the inappropriate level of the physiological variable at awakening compared to previous sleep (Fig. 9A). However, given the evidence that the ''wakefulness stimulus'' exerts powerful stimulatory effects on respiratory neurons and sympathetic outflow and produces transient vagal withdrawal, it is proposed in this chapter that these models need to include the important contribution of a transiently aroused awake state, which would exert important influences on cardiorespiratory outputs at wake onset (Fig. 9B).

The mechanisms and pathways underlying the influence of this transient arousal state at awakening on cardiorespiratory responses needs to be determined. Indeed, it is a major challenge to uncover the link between the changes in activity of state-dependent neurons (only some of which were discussed in this chapter) with the effects of sleep-wake state on autonomic outputs such as those producing the surges in HR, BP, and $\dot{V}$ at awakening. For example, although changes in LC activity parallel changes in sympathetic tone across sleep-wake states in cats (156), the nature of this association and its relevance to sleep-related cardiovascular control needs to be established. Similar considerations hold for the postulated influences of sleep-wake–related serotonergic neurons on sympathetic output (157). Indeed, it has been shown that serotonergic medullary raphe neurons, like DR neurons, have higher discharge in wakefulness (112,158–161), project to sympathetic preganglionic neurons (157,162,163) where 5-HT depolarizes those neurons and increases BP (164–166). However, although such effects provide appropriate circuitry and an attractive mechanism to explain state-dependent changes in sympathetic outputs, the actual relevance of these mechanisms to the effects of sleep on BP needs to be established. It also remains to be determined if the neuronal systems engaged at awakening from sleep are altered by disturbances in the physiological variables that accompany repetitive apneas, e.g., hypoxia and hypercapnia, and whether these effects can lead to long-term sequelae (e.g., chronic sympathetic activation). Indeed, it is relevant to note that LC discharge is increased by increased Pa_{CO_2} and decreased Pa_{O_2} and that these effects are associated with increased sympathetic output (167,168). Raphe neurons also increase their firing rates with increased levels of inspired CO_2 (161).

Further studies on the basic neuronal mechanisms engaged at awakening from sleep, the modulation of these activities by changes in chemical respiratory stimuli associated with sleep-disordered breathing events, and the role of these central neuronal processes in modulating autonomic outputs will improve understanding of the mechanisms underlying the large HR, BP, and $\dot{V}$ responses at arousal from sleep and the clinical consequences.

Acknowledgments

Professors Adrian Morrison and Allan Pack and Dr. Larry Sanford from The Center for Sleep and Respiratory Neurobiology, University of Pennsylvania, are thanked for helpful discussions. Dr. Dina Brooks from the University of Toronto is thanked for helpful comments on the manuscript. The author is a scholar of the Medical Research Council of Canada.

References

1. Rechtschaffen A, Kales A. A Manual of Standardized Terminology Techniques and Scoring System for Sleep Stages of Human Subjects. Los Angeles: Brain Information Service/Brain Research Institute, University of California, 1968.
2. Ursin R, Sterman MB. A manual for standardized scoring of sleep and waking states in the adult cat. Los Angeles: Brain Information Service/Brain Research Institute, University of California, 1981.
3. Benington JH, Kodali SK, Heller HC. Scoring transitions to REM sleep in rats based on the EEG phenomena of pre-REM sleep: an improved analysis of sleep structure. Sleep 1994; 17:28–36.
4. Gottesmann C. Detection of seven sleep-waking stages in the rat. Neurosci Biobehav Rev 1992; 16:31–38.
5. Phillipson EA, Murphy E, Kozar LF. Regulation of respiration in sleeping dogs. J Appl Physiol 1976; 40:688–693.
6. Carskadon MA, Dement WC. Normal human sleep: an overview. In: Kryger MH, Roth T, Dement WC, eds. Principles and Practice of Sleep Medicine. Philadelphia: WB Saunders, 1994:16–25.
7. American Sleep Disorders. Association EEG arousals: scoring rules and examples. Sleep 1992; 15:173–184.
8. Horner RL, Brooks D, Kozar LF, Tse S, Phillipson EA. Immediate effects of arousal from sleep on cardiac autonomic outflow in the absence of breathing in dogs. J Appl Physiol 1995; 79:151–162.
9. Baust W, Weidinger H, Kirchner F. Sympathetic activity during natural sleep and arousal. Arch Ital Biol 1968; 106:379–390.
10. Davies RJO, Belt PJ, Roberts SJ, Ali NJ, Stradling JR. Arterial blood pressure responses to graded transient arousal from sleep in normal humans. J Appl Physiol 1993; 74:1123–1130.

11. Trinder J, Whitworth F, Kay A, Wilkin P. Respiratory instability during sleep onset. J Appl Physiol 1992; 73:2462–2469.
12. Xie A, Wong B, Phillipson EA, Slutsky AS, Bradley TD. Interaction of hyperventilation and arousal in the pathogenesis of idiopathic central sleep apnea. Am J Respir Crit Care Med 1994; 150:489–495.
13. Shepard JW Jr. Hypertension cardiac arrhythmias myocardial infarction and stroke in relation to obstructive sleep apnea. Clin Chest Med 1992; 13:437–458.
14. Brooks D, Horner RL, Kozar LF, Render-Teixeira CL, Phillipson EA. Obstructive sleep apnea as a cause of systemic hypertension: evidence from a canine model. J Clin Invest 1997; 99:106–109.
15. Ringler J, Basner RC, Shannon R, Schwartzstein R, Manning H, Weinberger SE, Weiss JW. Hypoxemia alone does not explain blood pressure elevations after obstructive apneas. J Appl Physiol 1990; 69:2143–2148.
16. Coote JH. Respiratory and circulatory control during sleep. J Exp Biol 1982; 100:223–244.
17. Remmers JE. Control of breathing during sleep. In: Hornbein TF, ed. Regulation of Breathing. New York: Marcel Dekker, 1981:1197–1249.
18. Phillipson EA, Bowes G. Control of breathing during sleep. In: Cherniack NS, Widdicombe JG, eds. Handbook of Physiology, The Respiratory System, Section 3, Vol. 2, Part 2. Bethesda, MD: American Physiological Society, 1986:649–689.
19. Henke KG, Badr MS, Skatrud JB, Dempsey JA. Load compensation and respiratory muscle function during sleep. J Appl Physiol 1992; 72:1221–1234.
20. Hudgel DW. Role of upper airway anatomy and physiology in obstructive sleep apnea. Clin Chest Med 1992; 13:383–398.
21. Orem J. Respiratory neurons and sleep. In: Kryger MH, Roth T, Dement WC, eds. Principles and Practice of Sleep Medicine. Philadelphia: WB Saunders, 1994:177–193.
22. Lydic R, Baghdoyan HA. The neurobiology of rapid-eye-movement sleep. In: Saunders NA, Sullivan CE, eds. Sleep and Breathing. New York: Marcel Dekker, 1994: 47–77.
23. Pack AI. Changes in respiratory motor activity during rapid eye movement sleep. In: Dempsey JA, Pack AI, eds. Regulation of Breathing. New York: Marcel Dekker, 1995: 983–1010.
24. Mancia G, Zanchetti A. Cardiovascular regulation during sleep In: Orem J, Barnes CD, eds. Physiology in Sleep. New York: Academic Press, 1980:1–55.
25. Phillipson EA. Sleep disorders. In: Murray JF, Nadel JA, eds. Textbook of Respiratory Medicine. Philadelphia: WB Saunders, 1988:1841–1860.
26. Skatrud JB, Dempsey JA. Interaction of sleep state and chemical stimuli in sustaining rhythmic ventilation. J Appl Physiol 1983; 55:813–822.
27. Datta AK, Shea SA, Horner RL, Guz A. The influence of induced hypocapnia and sleep on the endogenous respiratory rhythm in humans. J Physiol 1991; 440:17–33.
28. Douglas NJ, White DP, Weil JV, Pickett CK, Zwillich CW. Hypercapnic ventilatory response in sleeping adults. Am Rev Respir Dis 1982; 126:758–762.
29. Douglas NJ. Control of ventilation during sleep. In: Kryger MH, Roth T, Dement WC, eds. Principles and Practice of Sleep Medicine. Philadelphia: WB Saunders, 1994: 204–211.
30. Skatrud JB, Dempsey JA. Airway resistance and respiratory muscle function in snorers during NREM sleep. J Appl Physiol 1985; 59:328–335.

31. Hudgel DW, Martin RJ, Johnson B, Hill P. Mechanics of the respiratory system and breathing pattern during sleep in normal humans. J Appl Physiol 1984; 56:133–137.
32. Hudgel DW, Mulholland M, Hendricks C. Neuromuscular and mechanical responses to inspiratory resistive loading during sleep. J Appl Physiol 1987; 63:603–608.
33. Orem J, Netick A, Dement WC. Increased upper airway resistance to breathing during sleep in the cat. Electroenceph Clin Neurophysiol 1977; 43:14–22.
34. Weigand L, Zwillich CW, White DP. Sleep and the ventilatory response to resistive loading in normal men. J Appl Physiol 1988; 64:1186–1195.
35. Weigand L, Zwillich CW, White DP. Collapsibility of the human upper airway during normal sleep. J Appl Physiol 1989; 66:1800–1808.
36. Horner RL, Kozar LF, Kimoff RJ, Phillipson EA. Effects of sleep on the tonic drive to respiratory muscle and the threshold for rhythm generation in the dog. J Physiol 1994; 474:525–537.
37. Orem J, Osorio I, Brooks E, Dick T. Activity of respiratory neurons during NREM sleep. J Neurophysiol 1985; 54:1144–1156.
38. Kubin L, Davies RO, Pack AI. Control of upper airway motoneurons during REM sleep. News Physiol Sci 1998; 13:91–97.
39. Baccelli G, Guazzi M, Mancia G, Zanchetti A. Neural and non-neural mechanisms influencing circulation during sleep. Nature 1967; 223:184–185.
40. Baust W, Bohnert B. The regulation of heart rate during sleep. Exp Brain Res 1969; 7:169–180.
41. Hornyak M, Cejnar M, Elam M, Wallin BG. Muscle sympathetic nerve activity during sleep in man. Brain 1991; 114:1281–1295.
42. Okada H, Iwase S, Mano T, Sugiyama Y, Watanabe T. Changes in muscle sympathetic nerve activity during sleep in humans. Neurol 1991; 41:1961–1966.
43. Somers VK, Dyken ME, Mark AL, Abboud FM. Sympathetic-nerve activity during sleep in normal subjects. N Engl J Med 1993; 328:303–307.
44. Morgan BJ, Crabtree DC, Puleo DS, Badr MS, Toiber F, Skatrud JB. Neurocirculatory consequences of abrupt change in sleep-state in humans. J Appl Physiol 1996; 80: 1627–1636.
45. Zemaityte D, Varoneckas G, Sokolov E. Heart rhythm control during sleep. Psychophysiology 1984; 21:279–289.
46. Kirby DA, Verrier RL. Differential effects of sleep stage on coronary hemodynamic function. Am J Physiol 1989; 256:H1378–H1383.
47. Furlan R, Guzzetti S, Crivellaro W, Dassi S, Tinelli M, Baselli G, Cerutti S, Lombardi F, Pagani M, Malliani A. Continuous 24-hour assessment of the neural regulation of systemic arterial pressure and RR variabilities in ambulant subjects. Circulation 1990; 81:537–547.
48. Berlad I, Shlitner A, Ben-Haim S, Lavie P. Power spectrum analysis and heart rate variability in Stage 4 and REM sleep: evidence for state specific changes in autonomic dominance. J Sleep Res 1993; 2:88–90.
49. Futuro-Neto HA, Coote JH. Changes in sympathetic activity to heart and blood vessels during desynchronized sleep. Brain Res 1982; 252:259–268.
50. Mancia G, Baccelli G, Adams DB, Zanchetti A. Vasomotor regulation during sleep in the cat. Am J Physiol 1971; 220:1086–1093.
51. Askelrod S, Gordon D, Madwed JB, Snidman NC, Shannon DC, Cohen RJ. Hemodynamic regulation: investigation by spectral analysis. Am J Physiol 1985; 249:H867–H875.

52. Novak V, Novak P, De Champlain J, Le Blanc AR, Martin R, Nadeau R. Influence of respiration on heart rate and blood pressure fluctuations. J Appl Physiol 1993; 74: 617–626.
53. Kollai M, Koizumi K. Reciprocal and non-reciprocal action of the vagal and sympathetic nerves innervating the heart. J Auton Nerv Syst 1979; 1:33–52.
54. Seals DR, Suwarno NO, Dempsey JA. Influence of lung volume on sympathetic nerve discharge in normal humans. Circ Res 1990; 67:130–141.
55. Somers VK, Mark AL, Zavala DC, Abboud FM. Influence of ventilation and hypocapnia on sympathetic nerve responses to hypoxia in normal humans. J Appl Physiol 1989; 67:2095–2100.
56. Grossman P, Karemaker J, Wieling W. Prediction of tonic parasympathetic cardiac control using respiratory sinus arrhythmia: the need for respiratory control. Psychophysiology 1991; 28:201–216.
57. Halasz P. Arousals without awakening—dynamic aspect of sleep. Physiol Behav 1993; 54:795–802.
58. Parmeggiani PL. The autonomic nervous system in sleep. In: Kryger MH, Roth T, Dement WC, eds. Principles and Practice of Sleep Medicine. Philadelphia: WB Saunders, 1994:194–203.
59. Anrep GV, Pascual W, Rossler R. Respiratory variations of the heart rate. II. The central mechanism of the respiratory arrhythmia and the inter-relations between the central and the reflex mechanisms. Proc R Soc London Ser B 1936; 119:218–230.
60. De Burgh Daly M. Interactions between respiration and circulation. In: Cherniack NS, Widdicombe JG, eds. Handbook of Physiology, The Respiratory System, Section 3, Vol. 2, Part 2. Bethesda, MD: American Physiological Society, 1986:529–594.
61. Shykoff BE, Naqvi SSJ, Menon AS, Slutsky AS. Respiratory sinus arrythmia in dogs: effects of phasic afferents and chemostimulation. J Clin Invest 1991; 87:1621–1627.
62. Horner RL, Brooks D, Kozar LF, Gan K, Phillipson EA. Respiratory-related heart rate variability persists during central apnea in dogs: mechanisms and implications. J Appl Physiol 1995; 78:2003–2013.
63. Hirsch JA, Bishop B. Respiratory sinus arrhythmia in humans: how breathing pattern modulates heart rate. Am J Physiol 1981; 241:H620–H629.
64. Smyth HS, Sleight P, Pickering GW. Reflex regulation of arterial pressure during sleep in man. Circ Res 1969; 24:109–121.
65. Conway J, Boon N, Vann Jones J, Sleight P. Involvement of the baroreceptor reflexes in the changes in blood pressure with sleep and mental arousal. Hypertension 1983; 5:746–748.
66. Bristow JD, Honnour AJ, Pickering TG, Sleight P. Cardiovascular and respiratory changes during sleep in normal and hypertensive subjects. Cardiovasc Res 1969; 3: 476–485.
67. Orem J, Vidruk EH. Activity of medullary respiratory neurons during ventilator-induced apnea in sleep and wakefulness. J Appl Physiol 1998; 84:922–932.
68. Eldridge FL. Subthreshold central neural respiratory activity and afterdischarge. Respir Physiol 1980; 39:327–343.
69. Phillipson EA, Duffin J, Cooper JD. Critical dependence of respiratory rhythmicity on metabolic CO_2 load. J Appl Physiol 1981; 50:45–54.
70. Horner RL, Kozar LF, Phillipson EA. Tonic respiratory drive in the absence of rhythm generation in the conscious dog. J Appl Physiol 1994; 76:671–680.

71. Sears TA. The respiratory motoneuron and apneusis. Fed Proc 1977; 36:2412–2420.
72. Orem J, Lydic R. Upper airway function during sleep and wakefulness: experimental studies on normal and anesthetized cats. Sleep 1978; 1:49–68.
73. Orem J, Lydic R, Norris P. Experimental control of the diaphragm and laryngeal abductor muscles by brain stem arousal systems. Respir Physiol 1979; 38:203–221.
74. St John WM. Influence of reticular mechanisms upon hypoglossal, trigeminal and phrenic activities. Respir Physiol 1986; 66:27–40.
75. Cohen MI, Hugelin, A. Suprapontine reticular control of intrinsic respiratory mechanisms. Arch Ital Biol 1965; 103:317–334.
76. Hugelin A, Cohen MI. The reticular activating system and respiratory regulation in the cat. Ann NY Acad Sci 1963; 109:586–603.
77. Eldridge FL. Central neural respiratory stimulatory effect of active respiration. J Appl Physiol 1974; 37:723–735.
78. Eldridge FL. Central neural stimulation of respiration in unanesthetized decerebrate cats. J Appl Physiol 1976; 40:23–28.
79. Eldridge FL, Millhorn, DE. Oscillation, gating, and memory in the respiratory control system. In: Cherniack NS, Widdicombe JG, eds. Handbook of Physiology, The Respiratory System, Section 3, Vol. 2, Part 1. Bethesda, MD: American Physiological Society, 1986:93–114.
80. Shea SA. Behavioral and arousal-related influences on breathing in humans. Exp Physiol 1996; 81:1–26.
81. Shea SA, Andres LP, Paydarfar D, Banzett RB, Shannon DC. Effect of mental activity on breathing in congenital central hypoventilation syndrome. Respir Physiol 1993; 94: 251–263.
82. Siegel JM. Brainstem mechanisms generating REM sleep. In: Kryger MH, Roth T, Dement WC, eds. Principles and Practice of Sleep Medicine. Philadelphia: WB Saunders, 1994:125–144.
83. McCarley RW, Greene RW, Rainnie D, Portas CM. Brainstem neuromodulation and REM sleep. Semin Neurosci 1995; 7:341–354.
84. Jones BE. Basic mechanisms of sleep-wake states. In:Kryger MH, Roth T, Dement WC, eds. Principles and Practice of Sleep Medicine. Philadelphia: WB Saunders, 1994: 145–162.
85. Kinomura S, Larsson J, Gulyás B, Roland PE. Activation by attention of the human reticular formation and thalamic intralaminar nuclei. Science 1996; 271:512–515.
86. Foutz AS, Boudinot E, Morin-Surun MP, Champagnat J, Gonsalves SF, Denavit-Saubie M. Excitability of 'silent' respiratory neurons during sleep-waking states: an iontophoretic study in undrugged chronic cats. Brain Res 1987; 404:10–20.
87. Orem J. Central respiratory activity in rapid-eye-movement sleep: augmenting and late inspiratory cells. Sleep 1994; 8:665–673.
88. Orem J. Medullary respiratory neuron activity: Relationship to tonic and phasic REM sleep. J Appl Physiol 1980; 48:54–65.
89. Orem J. Neuronal mechanisms of respiration in REM sleep. Sleep 1980; 3:251–267.
90. Morales FR, Engelhardt JK, Soja PJ, Pereda AE, Chase MH. Motoneuron properties during motor inhibition produced by microinjection of carbachol into the pontine reticular formation of the decerebrate cat. J Neurophysiol 1987; 57:1118–1129.
91. Glenn LL, Foutz AS, Dement WC. Membrane potential of spinal motoneurons during natural sleep in cats. Sleep 1978; 1:199–204.
92. Guazzi M, Zanchetti A. Blood pressure and heart rate during natural sleep of the cat

and their regulation by carotid sinus and aortic reflexes. Arch Ital Biol 1965; 103:789–817.

93. Hilton SM. Ways of viewing the central nervous control of the circulation—old and new. Brain Res 1975; 87:213–219.
94. Hilton SM. The defence-arousal system and its relevance for circulatory and respiratory control. J Exp Biol 1982; 100:159–174.
95. Eckberg DL, Sleight P. Human baroreflexes in health and disease. Monogr Physiol Soc 1992; 43:79–119.
96. Moruzzi G, Magoun HW. Brain stem reticular formation and activation of the EEG. Electroencephalogr Clin Neurophysiol 1949; 1:455–473.
97. Marrocco R, Witte EA, Davidson MC. Arousal systems. Curr Opin Neurobiol 1994; 4:166–170.
98. Reiner PB. Are mesopontine cholinergic neurons either necessary or sufficient components of the ascending reticular activating system? Semin Neurosci 1995; 7:355–359.
99. Jones BE. Paradoxical sleep and its chemical/structural substrates in the brain. Neuroscience 1991; 40:637–656.
100. Steriade M, McCarley RW. Brainstem Control of Wakefulness and Sleep. New York: Plenum Press, 1990.
101. Szymusiak R. Magnocellular nuclei of the basal forebrain: substrates of sleep and arousal regulation. Sleep 1995; 18:478–500.
102. Steriade M. Brain electrical activity and sensory processing during waking and sleep states. In: Kryger MH, Roth T, Dement WC, eds. Principles and Practice of Sleep Medicine. Philadelphia: WB Saunders, 1994:105–124.
103. McCormick DA. Neurotransmitter actions in the thalamus and cerebral cortex and their role in neuromodulation of thalamocortical activity. Prog Neurobiol 1992; 39:337–388.
104. Reese NB, Garcia-Rill E, Skinner RD. The pedunculopontine nucleus—auditory input, arousal and pathophysiology. Prog Neurobiol 1995; 42:105–133.
105. El Mansari M, Sakai K, Jouvet M. Unitary characteristics of presumptive cholinergic tegmental neurons during the sleep-waking cycle in freely moving cats. Exp Brain Res 1989; 76:519–529.
106. Kayama Y, Ohta M, Jodo E. Firing of 'possibly' cholinergic neurons in the rat dorsolateral tegmental nucleus during sleep and wakefulness. Brain Res 1992; 569:210–220.
107. Steriade M, Datta S, Paré D, Oakson G, Curro-Dossi RC. Neuronal activities in brainstem cholinergic nuclei related to tonic activation processes in thalamocortical systems. J Neurosci 1990; 10:2541–2559.
108. McGinty D, Harper RM. Dorsal raphe neurons: depression of firing during sleep in cats. Brain Res 1976; 101:569–575.
109. Trulson ME, Jacobs BL. Raphe unit activity in freely moving cats: correlation with level of behavioral arousal. Brain Res 1979; 163:135–150.
110. Cespuglio R, Faradji H, Gomez ME, Jouvet M. Single unit recording in the nuclei raphe dorsalis and magnus during the sleep-waking cycle of semi-chronic prepared cats. Neurosci Lett 1981; 24:133–138.
111. Aston-Jones G, Bloom FE. Activity of norepinephrine-containing locus coeruleus neurons in behaving rats anticipates fluctuations in the sleep-waking cycle. J Neurosci 1981; 1:876–886.

112. Jacobs BL, Azmitia EC. Structure and function of the brain serotonin system. Phys Rev 1992; 72:165–229.
113. Williams JA, Comisarow J, Day J, Fibiger HC, Reiner PB. State-dependent release of acetylcholine in rat thalamus measured by in vivo microdialysis. J Neurosci 1994; 14:5236–5342.
114. Foote SL, Bloom FE, Aston-Jones G. Nucleus locus coeruleus: new evidence of anatomical and physiological specificity. Phys Rev 1983; 63:844–914.
115. Foote SL, Berridge CW, Adams LM, Pineda JA. Electrophysiological evidence for the involvement of the locus coeruleus in alerting orienting and attending. In: Barnes CD, Pompeiano O, eds. Progress in Brain Research. Vol. 88. Amsterdam: Elsevier, 1991:521–532.
116. Jacobs BL, Fornal CA. Serotonin and behavior. A general hypothesis. In: Bloom FE, Kupfer DJ, eds. Psychopharmacology: The Fourth Generation of Progress. New York: Raven Press, 1995:461–470.
117. Jacobs BL, Fornal CA. Activation of 5-HT neuronal activity during motor behavior. Semin Neurosci 1995; 7:401–408.
118. Honda T, Semba K. Serotonergic synaptic input to cholinergic neurons in the rat mesopontine tegmentum. Brain Res 1994; 647:299–306.
119. Leubke JI, Greene RW, Semba K, Kamondi A, McCarley RW, Reiner PB. Serotonin hyperpolarizes cholinergic low threshold burst neurons in the rat laterodorsal tegmental nucleus in vitro. Proc Natl Acad Sci USA 1992; 89:743–747.
120. Leonard CS, Llinas R. Serotonergic and cholinergic inhibition of mesopontine cholinergic neurons controlling REM sleep: an in-vitro electrophysiological study. Neuroscience 1994; 59:309–330.
121. Sanford LD, Ross RJ, Seggos AE, Morrison AR, Ball WA, Mann GL. Central administration of two 5-HT receptor agonists: effect on REM sleep initiation and PGO waves. Pharmacol Biochem Behav 1994; 49:93–100.
122. Horner RL, Sanford LD, Annis D, Pack AI, Morrison AR. Serotonin at the laterodorsal tegmental nucleus suppresses rapid-eye-movement sleep in freely behaving rats. J Neurosci 1997; 17:7541–7552.
123. Williams JA, Reiner PB. Noradrenaline hyperpolarizes identified rat mesopontine cholinergic neurons in vitro. J Neurosci 1993; 13:3878–3883.
124. Koyama K, Kayama Y. Mutual interactions among cholinergic noradrenergic and serotonergic neurons studied by iontophoresis of these transmitters in rat brainstem nuclei. Neuroscience 1993; 55:1117–1126.
125. Adams LM, Foote SL. Effects of locally infused pharmacological agents on spontaneous and sensory-evoked activity of locus coeruleus neurons. Brain Res Bull 1988; 21: 395–400.
126. Egan TM, North RA. Acetylcholine acts on m_2-muscarinic receptors to excite rat locus coeruleus neurones. Br J Pharmacol 1985; 85:733–735.
127. Egan TM, North RA. Actions of acetylcholine and nicotine on rat locus coeruleus neurons in vitro. Neuroscience 1986; 19:565–571.
128. Ennis M, Shipley MT. Tonic activation of locus coeruleus neurons by systemic or intracoerulear microinjection of an irreversible acetylcholinesterase inhibitor: increased discharge rate and induction of C-fos. Exp Neurol 1992; 118:164–177.
129. Livingstone MS, Hubel DH. Effects of sleep and arousal on the processing of visual information in the cat. Nature 1981; 291:554–561.

130. Horner RL. Autonomic consequences of arousal from sleep: mechanisms and implications. Sleep 1996; 19:S193–195.
131. Horner RL, Sanford LD, Pack AI, Morrison AR. Activation of a distinct arousal state immediately after spontaneous awakening from sleep. Brain Res 1997; 778:127–134.
132. Davis M. The mammalian startle response. In: Eaton RC, ed. Neural Mechanisms of Startle Behavior. New York: Plenum Press, 1984:287–351.
133. Davis M, Gendelman DS, Tischler MD, Gendelman PM. A primary acoustic startle circuit: lesion and stimulation studies. J Neurosci 1982; 2:791–805.
134. Lingenhöhl K, Friauf E. Giant neurons in the rat reticular formation: a sensorimotor interface in the elementary acoustic startle circuit? J Neurosci 1994; 14:1176–1194.
135. Hammond GR, McAdams DW, Ison JR. Effects of prestimulation on the electromyographic response associated with the acoustic startle reaction in rats. Physiol Behav 1972; 8:535–537.
136. Geyer MA, Swerdlow NR, Mansbach RS, Braff DL. Startle response models of sensorimotor gating and habituation deficits in schizophrenia. Brain Res Bull 1990; 25:485–498.
137. Swerdlow NR, Caine SB, Braff DL, Geyer MA. The neural substrates of sensorimotor gating of the startle reflex: a review of recent findings and their implications. J Psychopharmacol 1992; 6:176–190.
138. Wu M-F, Mallick BN, Siegel JM. Lateral geniculate spikes muscle atonia and startle response elicited by auditory stimuli as a function of stimulus parameters and arousal state. Brain Res 1989; 499:7–17.
139. Wu M-F, Suzuki SS, Siegel JM. Anatomical distribution and response patterns of reticular neurons active in relation to acoustic startle. Brain Res 1988; 457:399–406.
140. Koch M, Lingenhöhl K, Pilz PKD. Loss of the acoustic startle response following neurotoxic lesions of the caudal pontine reticular formation: possible role of giant neurons. Neuroscience 1992; 49:617–625.
141. Lingenhöhl K, Friauf E. Giant neurons in the caudal pontine reticular formation receive short latency acoustic input: an intracellular recording and HRP-study in the rat. J Comp Neurol 1992; 325:473–492.
142. Yeomans JS, Hempel CME, Chapman CA. Axons and synapses mediating startle-like responses evoked by electrical stimulation of the reticular formation in rats: symmetric and asymmetric collision effects. Brain Res 1993; 617:309–319.
143. Bubser M, Koch M. Prepulse inhibition of the acoustic startle response of rats is reduced by 6-hydroxydopamine lesions of the medial frontal cortex. Psychopharmacology 1994; 113:487–492.
144. Caine SB, Geyer MA, Swerdlow NR. Hippocampal modulation of acoustic startle and prepulse inhibition in the rat. Pharmacol Biochem Behav 1992; 43:1201–1208.
145. Leitner DS, Cohen ME. Role of the inferior colliculus in the inhibition of acoustic startle in the rat. Physiol Behav 1985; 34:65–70.
146. Koch M, Kungel M, Herbert H. Cholinergic neurons in the pedunculopontine tegmental nucleus are involved in the mediation of prepulse inhibition of the acoustic startle response in the rat. Exp Brain Res 1993; 97:71–82.
147. Swerdlow NR, Geyer MA. Prepulse inhibition of acoustic startle in rats after lesions of the pedunculopontine tegmental nucleus. Behav Neurosci 1993; 107:104–117.
148. Reese NB, Garcia-Rill E, Skinner RD. Auditory input to the pedunculopontine nucleus: II. Unit responses. Brain Res Bull 1995; 37:265–273.
149. McCarley RW, Nelson JP, Hobson JA. Ponto-geniculo-occipital PGO burst neurons:

correlative evidence for neuronal generators of PGO waves. Science 1978; 201:269–272.

150. Steriade M, Paré D, Datta S, Oakson G, Curro-Dossi R. Different cellular types in mesopontine cholinergic nuclei related to ponto-geniculo-occipital waves. J Neurosci 1990; 10:2560–2579.
151. Morrison AR. Brainstem regulation of behavior during sleep and wakefulness. In: Sprague JM, Epstein AW, eds. Progress in Psychobiology and Physiological Psychology. Vol 8. New York: Academic Press, 1979:91–131.
152. Llinas RR, Paré D. Of dreaming and wakefulness. Neuroscience 1991; 44:521–535.
153. Koyama Y, Jodo E, Kayama Y. Sensory responsiveness of "broad-spike" neurons in the laterodorsal tegmental nucleus, locus coeruleus and dorsal raphe of awake rats: implications for cholinergic and monoaminergic neuron-specific responses. Neuroscience 1994; 63:1021–1031.
154. Woodward DJ, Moises HC, Waterhouse BD, Hoffer BJ, Freedman R. Modulatory actions of norepinephrine in the central nervous system. Fed Proc 1979; 38:2109–2116.
155. Rye DB. Contribution of the pedunculopontine region to normal and altered REM sleep. Sleep 1997; 20:757–788.
156. Reiner PB. Correlational analysis of central noradrenergic neuronal activity and sympathetic tone in behaving cats. Brain Res 1986; 378:86–96.
157. Guyenet PG. Role of the ventral medulla oblongata in blood pressure regulation. In: Loewy AD, Spyer KM, eds. Central Regulation of Autonomic Functions. Oxford: Oxford University Press, 1990:145–167.
158. Heym J, Steinfels GF, Jacobs BL. Activity of serotonin-containing neurons in the nucleus raphe pallidus of freely moving cats. Brain Res 1982; 251:259–276.
159. Trulson ME, Trulson VM. Activity of nucleus raphe pallidus neurons across the sleep-waking cycle in freely moving cats. Brain Res 1982; 237:232–237.
160. Fornal C, Auerbach S, Jacobs BL. Activity of serotonin-containing neurons in nucleus raphe magnus in freely moving cats. Exp Neurol 1985; 88:590–608.
161. Veasey SG, Fornal CA, Metzler CW, Jacobs BL. Response of serotonergic caudal raphe neurons in relation to specific motor activities in freely moving cats. J Neurosci 1995; 15:5346–5359.
162. Loewy AD. Raphe pallidus and raphe obscurus projections to the intermediolateral cell column in the rat. Brain Res 1981; 211:146–152.
163. Coote JH. Bulbospinal serotonergic pathways in the control of blood pressure. J Cardiovasc Pharmacol 1990; 15(S7):S35–S41.
164. McCall RB. Evidence for a serotonergically mediated sympathoexcitatory response to stimulation of medullary raphe nuclei. Brain Res 1984; 311:131–139.
165. Pilowsky PM, Kapoor V, Minson JB, West MJ, Chalmers JP. Spinal cord serotonin release and raised blood pressure after brainstem kainic acid injection. Brain Res 1986; 366:354–357.
166. Pickering AE, Spanswick D, Logan SD. 5-Hydroxytryptamine evokes depolarizations and membrane potential oscillations in rat sympathetic preganglionic neurons. J Physiol 1994; 480:109–121.
167. Elam M, Yao T, Thorén P, Svensson TH. Hypercapnia and hypoxia: chemoreceptor-mediated control of locus coeruleus neurons and splanchnic sympathetic nerves. Brain Res 1981; 222:373–381.

168. Guyenet PG, Koshiya N, Huangfu D, Verberne AJM, Riley TA. Central respiratory control of A5 and A6 pontine noradrenergic neurons. Am J Physiol 1993; 264:R1035–R1044.
169. Gothe B, Altose MD, Goldman MD, Cherniack NS. Effect of quiet sleep on resting and CO_2-stimulated breathing in humans. J Appl Physiol 1981; 50:724–730.

7

Muscle Factors in Obstructive Sleep Apnea

BASIL J. PETROF

McGill University Health Centre
Montreal, Quebec, Canada

JOAN C. HENDRICKS

School of Veterinary Medicine
University of Pennsylvania
Philadelphia, Pennsylvania

I. Introduction

Obstructive sleep apnea (OSA) is a condition characterized by repeated episodes of pharyngeal closure during sleep. The purpose of this chapter is to provide a general overview of the histological, biochemical, and physiological features of upper airway muscle function in OSA. Because of their importance in upper airway obstructive syndromes, most notably OSA, upper airway muscle physiology has received considerable attention during the last 20 years, and several excellent reviews have been published. The reader is referred to these for detailed discussions of sleep-related changes in muscle activity patterns and neural control (1) and the potential role of such changes in OSA (1,2). In this chapter we will review accumulating evidence that pharyngeal dilator muscle hyperactivity in OSA may lead to adaptive remodeling as well as potentially injurious alterations in the intrinsic properties of these muscles.

II. Normal Structure and Function of Upper Airway Dilator Muscles

OSA patients suffer from collapse of the pharynx during sleep (1). Muscles of the pharynx can act to counteract the collapsing force of inspiratory thoracoabdominal muscle contractions by dilating the lumen or by stiffening the pharyngeal walls. Anatomically, the pharyngeal dilating muscles have been categorized into those affecting the tongue (genioglossus, styloglossus, hyoglossus) and those related to the hyoid (geniohyoid, mylohyoid, stylohyoid, thyrohyoid, sternohyoid, sternothyroid) (1,2). In addition, muscles that elevate or tense the palate (levator palatini, tensor palatini) have been studied in some detail (2). We will not discuss here the muscles that control the larynx and the nares, as these regions are not the primary site of the collapse in OSA.

Skeletal muscles have traditionally been categorized according to their twitch kinetics (i.e., relatively slow versus fast twitch) and the histochemical properties (particularly the ATPase staining) of their individual fibers. The upper airway muscles that facilitate normal respiratory function by dilating the upper airway or preventing its collapse share a number of features. Histochemical studies in experimental animals, and limited studies on humans, have shown that pharyngeal dilators are predominately composed of type II fibers with relatively high ATPase activity, whereas the diaphragm has a significantly lower proportion of such fibers (3). Accordingly, the in vitro contractile kinetic properties of upper airway muscles exhibit the expected characteristics, i.e., upper airway dilator muscles generally demonstrate faster twitch contraction and half-relaxation times than the diaphragm. Interestingly, they also demonstrate a relatively high level of resistance to induction of muscle fatigue in vitro (3). As a group, upper airway muscles are also more sensitive than the diaphragm to the effects of anesthetics, muscle relaxants, and alcohol (1).

A number of factors that predispose individuals to sleep apnea have been studied with regard to their effect on upper airway muscle physiology. These include studies of aging (4) and obesity (5) in rats and of gender and female hormones in humans (6,7). In aging rats, the sternohyoid and geniohyoid muscles exhibited an increase in fast glycolytic over fast oxidative glycolytic fibers. Endurance properties also declined in the upper airway muscles but not in the diaphragms from the same aging animals (4). Obesity, on the other hand, was not found to have any significant effect on in vitro physiology (5) of upper airway muscles in rats. In normal female subjects without sleep apnea, the genioglossus exhibited greater increases in electromyogram (EMG) responses to inspiratory loading during waking (7) as compared to normal men, and these differences may be mediated at least in part by progesterone (6).

III. Function of Upper Airway Dilator Muscles in OSA

It is generally believed that pharyngeal collapse is precipitated by a sleep-induced fall in pharyngeal dilator muscle activity (8,9). This relative decline in pharyngeal dilator muscle activity at sleep onset occurs in both normal individuals and patients with OSA but is felt to have clinical consequences only in the latter group because of a smaller and more anatomically compromised upper airway (10,11). As an apparent compensatory mechanism to counteract small upper airway size, patients with OSA demonstrate abnormally high levels of pharyngeal dilator muscle activity during wakefulness (12,13). Whereas obstructive events are characterized by a transient loss of this compensatory hyperactivity, termination of airway occlusive events in OSA is achieved through massive increases in pharyngeal dilator muscle activity (8,9), which can occur hundreds of times per night in patients with severe disease. Heightened levels of pharyngeal muscle activity are also observed during stable nonobstructed sleep in individuals with OSA (14,15). Therefore, current evidence indicates that the overall level of pharyngeal dilator muscle activity is substantially greater than normal in patients with OSA.

IV. Potential Sources of Upper Airway Muscle Remodeling or Injury in OSA

Given the above evidence for heightened activation of upper airway dilators in OSA, it is reasonable to speculate that these muscles could undergo secondary changes as a direct consequence of their increased activity level. Skeletal muscle is an extremely versatile tissue with the ability to substantially alter its phenotype in order to adapt to the prevailing demands placed upon it. A number of properties such as muscle fiber size, contractile protein isoform profile, and metabolic enzyme content can be readily modified, with attendant changes in muscle performance. In general, these phenotypic transformations allow the muscle to match its shortening velocity profile to the imposed activation history, thereby maximizing muscle efficiency (defined as work/energy utilization). High-repetition, low-load exercise or sustained low-frequency electrical stimulation tend to elicit a fast (type II fibers) to slow (type I fibers) transformation, whereas low-repetition and high-load exercise or intermittent high-frequency electrical stimulation may produce a slow-to-fast transition (16–18). Therefore, an isolated augmentation of tonic (i.e., continuous, low-frequency) activation of upper airway dilator muscles in OSA would be predicted to lead to an increase in slow-twitch type I fibers, whereas a predominant influence of more phasic (i.e., intermittent, high-frequency) activation would be expected to favor transition toward fast-twitch type II fibers. In addition, repeated contractions against a high mechanical load in the upper airway could lead to increases in muscle mass through either hypertrophy or hyperplasia (19).

On the other hand, increased muscle activity could also lead to adverse effects on muscle structure and function. In this regard, considerable mechanical stresses are placed on muscle fibers during muscle contraction, and this has necessitated the evolution of a large array of cytoskeletal proteins whose function is to serve as a supportive network (20). Nonetheless, under conditions of strenuous muscle activity, the structural integrity of the muscle cell can be physically disrupted by the forces engendered during muscle contraction (20). Thus, activity-induced muscle injury has been documented by numerous studies in humans as well as animal models (20–25).

Most forms of exercise involve some combination of *concentric* (active shortening), *isometric* (activation with no change in muscle length), and *eccentric* (active lengthening) muscle contractions. Very intense exercise and that involving eccentric contractions, where the muscle is stretched during its activation, are most likely to produce muscle damage (26,27). Frank muscle fiber necrosis and inflammatory cell infiltrates have been observed after running and with various experimental models of eccentric contraction in animals (21–28). Muscle inflammation has also been demonstrated in the hamster diaphragm after one week of continuous resistive loading of the respiratory system (29), and various morphological abnormalities have been reported in the intercostal muscles of humans suffering from chronic obstructive pulmonary disease (30,31). Muscle biopsies from marathon runners (24) and patients with chronic myalgias due to repetitive limb movements [so-called overuse syndrome (32)] have also been found to exhibit abnormal histological changes. Increased connective tissue, edema, and evidence of muscle regeneration have been described (21,28). At the ultrastructural level, disruptions of sarcomere structure (e.g., loss of sarcomere registry, focal disruptions of the A-band, Z-band dissolution) are observed (26,27). In addition, a prolonged (days to weeks) loss of force-generating capacity can be seen after prolonged or intense exercise, particularly following bouts of eccentric contraction (33–35). The decrease in force-generating capacity is most evident at low stimulation frequencies (33,34) and has also been referred to as low-frequency fatigue. However, the lengthy time course of recovery as well as the dissociation between high-energy phosphate metabolism and recuperation of force generation in this situation is most consistent with the presence of muscle injury rather than metabolic fatigue related to purely energetic considerations (35–37).

Interestingly, eccentric contractions of upper airway dilator muscles have been demonstrated during airway occlusion and progressive hypercapnia in anesthetized cats (37,38). Because similar mechanical and chemical abnormalities of the respiratory system are associated with OSA, it is conceivable that eccentric contractions also occur in the pharyngeal dilator muscles of patients with OSA. In this regard, at least two potential mechanisms could lead to pharyngeal dilators being forcibly lengthened during their activation: (1) muscles that are mechanically linked could contract against one another, as has been demonstrated for the sternohyoid and geniohyoid muscles during airway occlusion in anesthetized animals (37), and (2) large negative intraluminal pressures associated with pharyngeal obstruction could act to forcibly lengthen the opposing dilator muscles.

Finally, an additional potential source of upper airway muscle remodeling or injury in OSA is vibratory trauma to either muscles or nerves present within the upper airway. Vibratory trauma is the presumed mechanism for peripheral nerve injuries observed after chronic exposure to low-frequency vibration (39–41). Therefore, to the extent that severe snoring constitutes a form of sustained exposure of upper airway structures to low-frequency vibration, this could potentially result in denervating effects on the upper airway musculature. Indirect evidence in support of this idea is provided by reports of impaired ability to detect sensory input in the upper airway of OSA patients (42) as well as histological signs of nerve damage (43).

V. Evidence for Remodeling and Injury of Upper Airway Muscles in OSA

A. Animal Studies

The question of whether OSA induces changes in upper airway dilator muscle structure has been addressed in an animal model of the disease, the English bulldog. These dogs have an anatomically compromised upper airway and demonstrate pathological sleep-disordered breathing that occurs primarily during REM sleep (44). As in humans with OSA, a relative decline in pharyngeal dilator muscle activity occurs at the onset of obstructive breathing events, which are then terminated by a large burst of upper airway dilator muscle activity (45). In addition, an abnormally high level of pharyngeal dilator muscle activation is found during stable non-REM sleep (14), a period when obstructive events are rarely observed in the bulldog. Therefore, this animal provides a useful model for studying the effects of muscle hyperactivity on pharyngeal dilator muscle structure in the setting of OSA.

In the bulldog sternohyoid muscle, an upper airway dilator whose changes in activity level correlate with the onset and reversal of obstructive breathing events, Petrof et al. (46) reported an increase in the proportion of fast-twitch (type II) fibers compared to that in control dogs without OSA (46). In addition to differences in fiber type, the bulldog sternohyoid muscle also demonstrated changes consistent with activity-induced muscle injury, consisting of abnormal fiber morphology (central nucleation, fissured and moth-eaten appearance), inflammatory cell infiltrates, and increased connective tissue (Fig. 1). Muscle injury was also found in another bulldog pharyngeal dilator, the geniohyoid muscle (Fig. 2). Importantly, no differences between bulldogs and control dogs were observed in limb musculature, suggesting that the above changes in bulldog pharyngeal dilator muscles were indeed related to the presence of OSA.

In a subsequent study in the bulldog model of OSA, Schotland et al. (47) surveyed a large number of upper airway muscles by magnetic resonance imaging (MRI). Using quantitative measurements of transverse (T2) relaxation times (a physical property that varies with alterations in tissue structure and chemical content), these authors were able to demonstrate changes consistent with muscle edema or fibrosis in four out of five pharyngeal muscles examined in the bulldog (Fig. 3), whereas no such changes were found in control dogs without sleep-disordered breathing. Importantly, limb muscle properties did not differ between bulldogs and controls, and the degree of upper airway muscle abnormality observed in bulldogs was significantly correlated with the sleep-disordered breathing index (47). Therefore, there is compelling evidence, based upon both direct histological (46) and noninvasive imaging (47) studies, to support the presence of altered upper airway muscle structure in an animal model of OSA.

B. Human Studies

There is accumulating evidence that similar changes may also occur in the upper airway muscles of humans with OSA. Stauffer et al. (48) were the first to compare

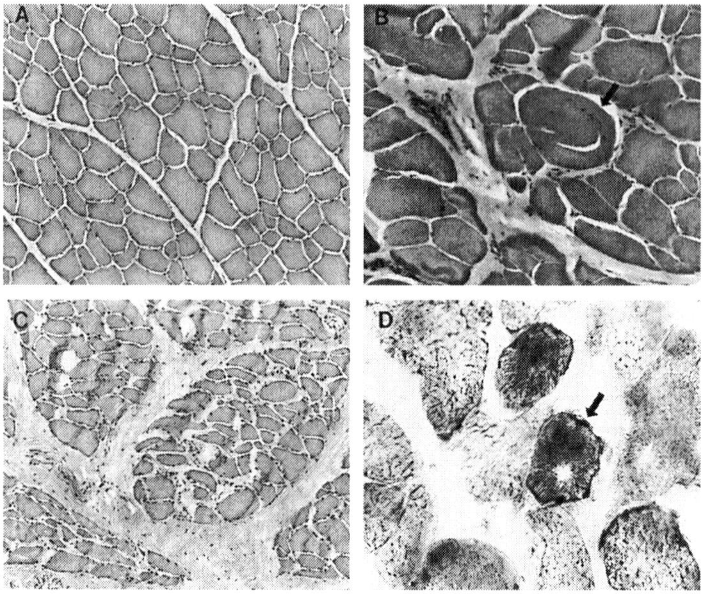

Figure 1 Representative tissue sections from the sternohyoid (SH) muscle of bulldogs and controls. (A) H & E stained control dog SH demonstrating normal skeletal muscle architecture. (B) H & E stained bulldog SH with damaged fiber (arrow) showing fissures or ''splitting'' as well as central nuclei. (C) H & E stained bulldog SH showing a marked increase in connective tissue elements suggestive of fibrosis. (D) Moth-eaten fiber (arrow) in a bulldog SH stained for NADH-TR exhibiting a focal loss of enzyme activity. (From Ref. 46.)

uvula tissue obtained by uvulopalatopharyngoplasty (UPPP) from patients with OSA (mean apnea/hypopnea index = 44/hour) and cadaveric controls. Using morphometric techniques, these authors found that specimens from OSA patients contained more muscle and fat (~twofold increase for both) than control specimens. While the observed increase in muscle content suggested muscle fiber hypertrophy (increased volume) and/or hyperplasia (increased number) in OSA patients, the precise nature of the increase in muscle content was not determined. The increased fat content could theoretically have been related to greater obesity in the OSA group or to muscle injury, since fatty infiltration of muscle is also seen in some other myopathic conditions (49).

Using a similar experimental design, Woodson et al. (43) examined UPPP specimens in a smaller group of OSA patients with more severe disease (n = 4; mean apnea index = 81/hour) and in snorers (n = 4; mean apnea index = 15/hour) and again compared them to cadaveric controls without any history of snoring (n = 4). These investigators described a number of histopathological changes in both the OSA and snorer groups, including atrophy as well as hypertrophy of fibers, edema, tissue fibrosis, and focal degeneration of myelinated nerves (Fig. 4). Although no

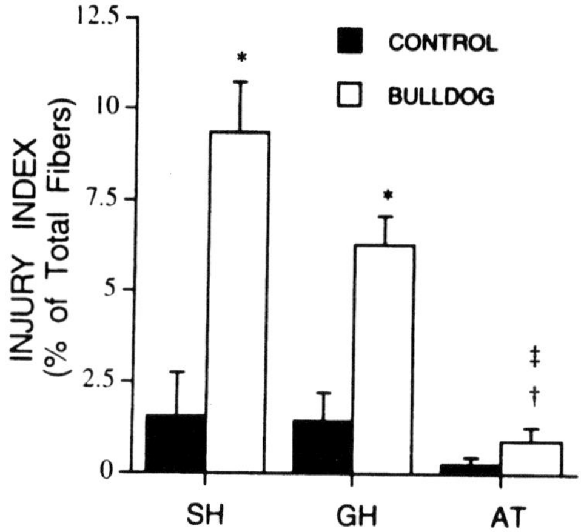

Figure 2 Proportion of abnormal muscle fibers in bulldog and control dog muscles. The two pharyngeal dilator muscles, sternohyoid (SH) and geniohyoid (GH), had a significantly higher injury index (defined as the proportion of morphologically abnormal fibers) in the bulldog as compared to controls. In contrast, there were no significant differences between the two groups of dogs for the limb muscle (AT, anterior tibial) examined. All values are means ± SE. $*p < 0.05$, between group comparisons (control dogs vs. bulldogs); $^{\dagger}p < 0.05$, within group comparisons (SH vs. AT); $^{\ddagger}p < 0.05$, within group comparisons (GH vs. AT). (From Ref. 46.)

quantitative analysis was performed, these abnormalities appeared to be somewhat more pronounced in the severe OSA group than in the snorers. The authors speculated that the histopathological changes observed in both snorers and OSA patients might be due to tissue damage induced by vibratory trauma and large negative pressure swings in the upper airway.

Edstrom and coworkers (50) compared palatopharyngeal muscle biopsies obtained during UPPP from OSA patients (mean number of O_2 desaturations ≥ 4% per hour of 39/hour) to specimens obtained from normal controls without any history of snoring who were undergoing tonsillectomy. Although little quantitative data were provided, the OSA group was reported to exhibit histopathological changes not seen in the control group, consisting of atrophic and hypertrophic fibers, fiber-type grouping, and a number of other morphological abnormalities of muscle fibers (e.g., moth-eaten appearance, core fibers, target fibers, myofibrillar loss, etc.). In a recent follow-up study (51) using semi-quantitative histological methods, comparisons were made of palatopharyngeal muscle biopsies obtained from OSA patients (median number of O_2 desaturations ≥ 4% per hour of 32/hour), habitual snorers (median number of O_2 desaturations ≥ 4% per hour of 0–3/hour), and nonsnoring (by history) control subjects undergoing tonsillectomy or exploratory surgery. Once again, it was reported that OSA patients and habitual snorers had an abnormally high prevalence of atrophic and/or hypertrophic fibers. Although these abnormalities

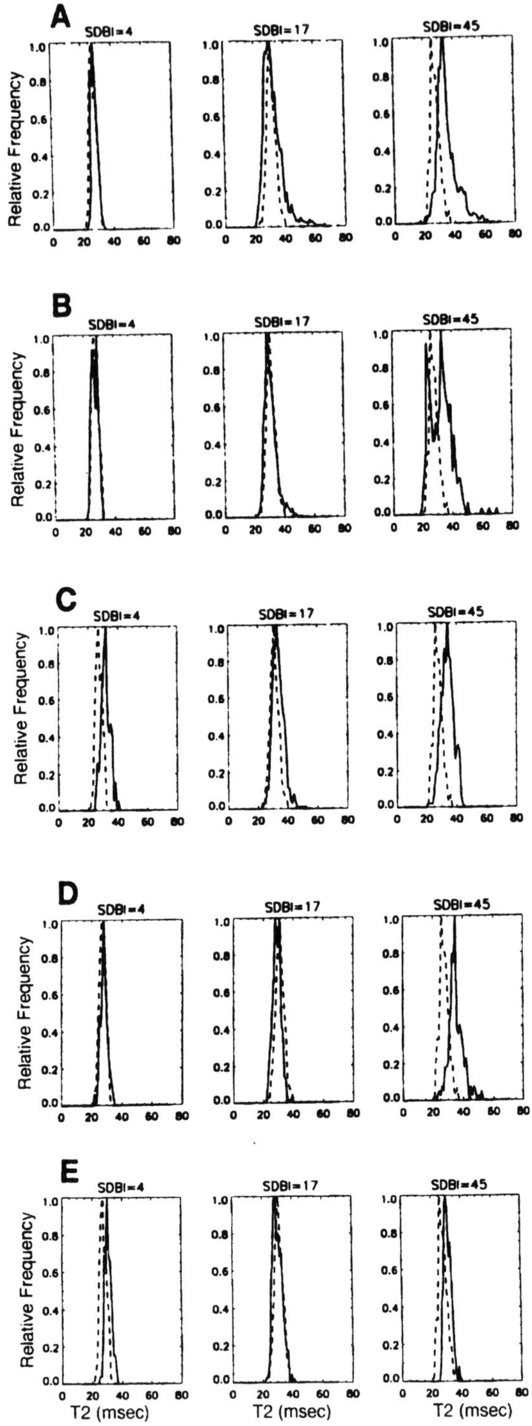
A
B
C
D
E
SDBI=4
SDBI=17
SDBI=45
Relative Frequency
T2 (msec)
0.0
0.2
0.4
0.6
0.8
1.0
0
20
40
60
80

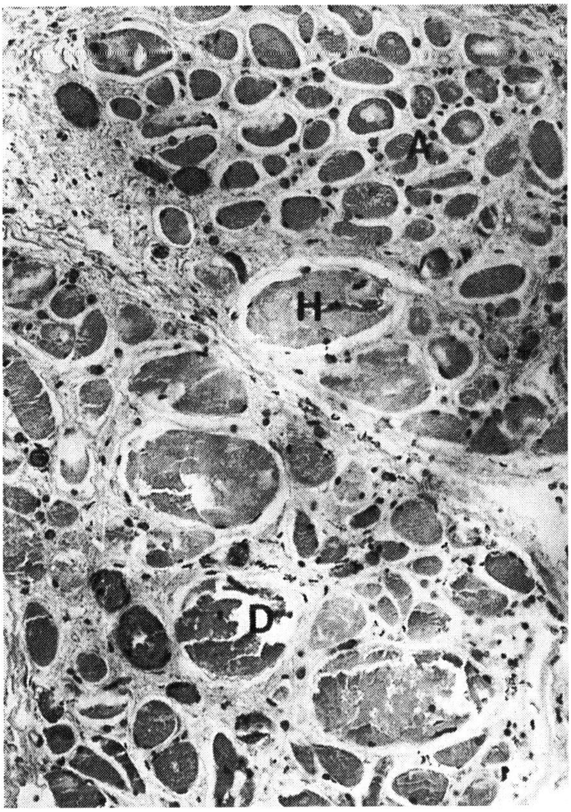

Figure 4 Micrograph of uvula tissue obtained from a patient with severe obstructive sleep apnea. Note the presence of widespread tissue fibrosis along with muscle fibers demonstrating atrophy (A), hypertrophy (H), and focal degeneration (D). (From Ref. 43.)

Figure 3 Histograms of T2 relaxation times in multiple upper airway muscles from three bulldogs with sleep-disordered breathing indices (SDBI) of varying severity (minimal to severe). (A) Geniohyoid; (B) sternohyoid; (C) thyropharyngeus; (D) hypopharyngeus; (E) sternothyroid. Dashed line, control (nonairway) muscle; solid line, airway muscle. Note the greater median values for T2 distributions in upper airway muscles from the most severely affected animal, consistent with the presence of structural alterations of these muscles. (From Ref. 47.)

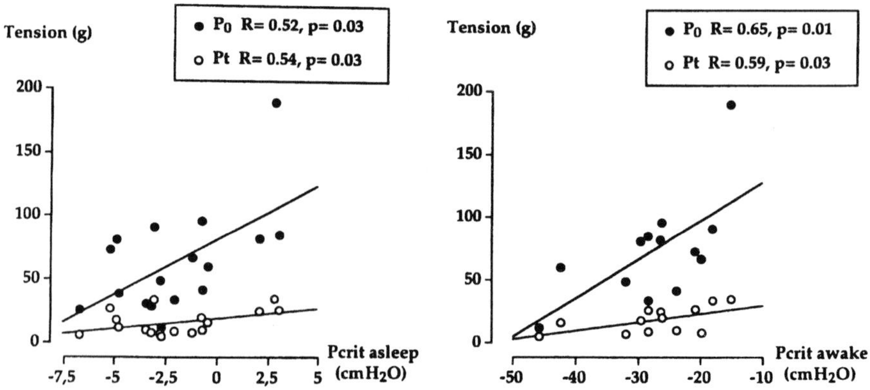

Figure 5 Relationship between maximum twitch (Pt) and tetanic (Po) force production by the musculus uvulae muscle, and critical closing pressure (Pcrit) of the pharynx, measured during wakefulness as well as sleep. There was a significant positive correlation between force-generating capacity and Pcrit values. (From Ref. 55.)

were present for both type I and type IIa fibers, the relative percentage of different fiber types in the palatopharyngeal muscle did not differ among the three groups studied.

Smirne et al. (52), on the other hand, reported a significant increase in the proportion and size of fast-twitch type IIa fibers in upper airway muscle obtained

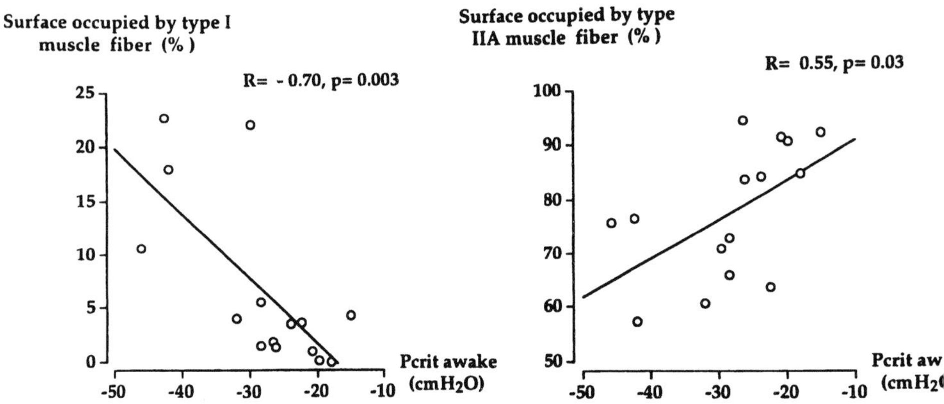

Figure 6 Relationship between the percentage of musculus uvulae cross-sectional area occupied by type I (slow-twitch) and type IIAa (fast-twitch) fibers, and critical closing pressure (Pcrit) of the pharynx measured during wakefulness. There were significant negative and positive correlations, respectively, for type I and type IIA fiber contribution to cross-sectional area as a function of waking Pcrit values. (From Ref. 55.)

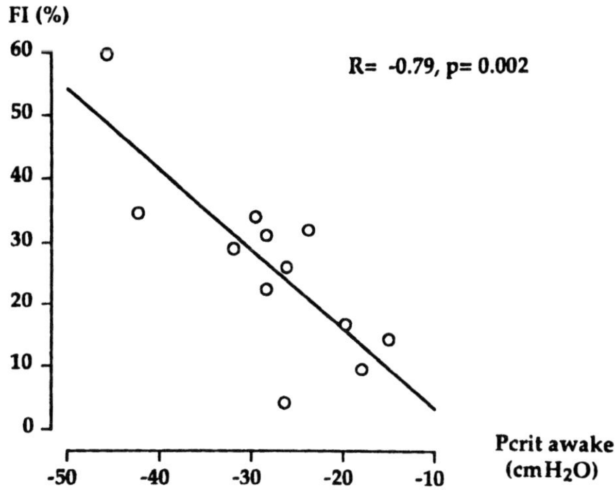

Figure 7 Relationship between the fatigue index (FI) of the musculus uvulae and critical closing pressure (Pcrit) of the pharynx measured during wakefulness. There was a significant relationship between pharyngeal collapsibility during wakefulness, as indicated by less negative Pcrit values, and increased fatiguability of the muscle (lower FI values). (From Ref. 55.)

from habitual snorers as compared to nonsnorers undergoing total laryngectomy for carcinoma in situ. While the precise actions of the upper airway muscle examined (medium pharyngeal constrictor) and consequent effects on upper airway patency are unclear, the authors suggested that the changes could be related to either an inherent or adaptive change in neural output to the muscle in snorers. It should be noted that no form of polysomnography was performed in any of the patients to rule out the presence of concomitant sleep-disordered breathing.

Finally, Sériès et al. (53–55) have performed a series of elegant studies comparing histological, biochemical, and contractile properties of the musculus uvulae muscle in OSA patients (apnea/hypopnea index $>$ 15/h) with those in snorers. Consistent with the findings of Stauffer et al. (48), an increase in total muscle fiber cross-sectional area was found in the OSA group, which appeared to be due to hyperplasia rather than hypertrophy (53). In contrast to the previous studies of UPPP tissue from OSA patients, no myopathic changes were detected. There was an increase in the proportion of fast-twitch (type IIa) fibers and the activity of enzymes of anaerobic metabolism in the OSA group, whereas no differences in oxidative enzyme activity were observed. Although absolute force-generating capacity of the muscle was greater in the OSA group due to the larger muscle mass, isometric force production did not differ between snorers and OSA patients after correcting for differences in muscle cross-sectional area. An increase in type IIa fiber prevalence was also found in the genioglossus muscle of OSA patients (54). Interestingly, there was no apparent relationship between the biochemical or physiological alterations and the frequency or severity of sleep-disordered breathing events (46). However, in a subsequent study, Sériès et al. (53) demonstrated that changes in the musculus uvulae did correlate with collapsibility of the upper airway, as indicated by measurements of the critical closing pressure (Pcrit) during wakefulness. Thus, patients with the most easily collapsible upper airway also showed the greatest increases in force production, type IIa fiber prevalence, anaerobic metabolism, and susceptibility to muscle fatigue (Figs. 5–7).

VI. Perspective on the Potential Importance of Upper Airway Muscle Remodeling and Injury in the Pathogenesis of OSA

The investigations to date in both the bulldog model and human OSA patients strongly favor the occurrence of secondary changes in the upper airway dilator muscles of individuals with OSA. Potentially adaptive responses, consisting of changes in muscle mass and/or fiber type, were found in both the bulldog model and human OSA patients. It seems likely that these changes are the result of alterations in the pattern and magnitude of pharyngeal dilator muscle activation in OSA. This is in keeping with the fact that transformations between slow- and fast-twitch fiber types can occur in response to changes in the pattern and/or level of muscle activation (18). A relatively consistent finding in the different studies was that an increase in fast-twitch fibers was observed in the group with increased upper airway load (46,52–55). This suggests that phasic activations of pharyngeal dilator muscles, which may be most marked at the termination of apneic events, could be an important stimulus for fiber type transitions in these muscles. In addition, the studies by Stauffer et al. (48) and Sériès et al. (53) demonstrated increased upper airway muscle mass in OSA patients, which is also consistent with forceful contractions of the pharyngeal muscles against the elevated load. These changes would be predicted to increase both muscle efficiency and force-generating capacity during the sudden bursts of massive pharyngeal dilator muscle recruitment required to open the collapsed airway during sleep. In addition, given the evidence for heightened pharyngeal dilator muscle activation during wakefulness (12,13), as well as the fact that phenotypic alterations in the musculus uvulae appeared to correlate most closely with waking Pcrit values (55), altered neural input to upper airway muscles during the waking state in OSA may be of even greater importance in providing the stimulus for these changes.

While the above changes in fiber type and muscle mass can be considered adaptive in nature, clearly pathological changes were also found in the bulldog model (46) and in several studies where such changes were sought in human OSA patients (43,48,50). Given the presence of upper airway muscle hyperactivity in OSA and other changes pointing to activity-induced remodeling such as altered fiber type and increased muscle mass, it is plausible that the observed pathological changes are also manifestations of increased muscle activity. Activity-induced muscle injury would be particularly likely to occur if upper airway dilator muscles undergo eccentric contractions in OSA. Furthermore, the continuous nature of the load with consequent hyperactivity during both wakefulness and sleep may lead to a situation in which upper airway dilator muscles are not allowed sufficient rest periods for normal reparative processes to take place (46). In this regard, it may appear somewhat paradoxical that the musculus uvulae muscle of OSA patients takes on a less fatigue-resistant profile with greater reliance on anaerobic metabolism (53). This raises the possibility that upper airway muscle remodeling may be adaptive with respect to certain activities such as the phasic bursts of contraction needed to open the airway but ill-suited to the continuous tonic activation required to stably maintain airway patency at a normal level and thereby prevent obstruction from occurring in the first place.

These considerations lead us to propose a model for the possible role of activity-induced upper airway muscle remodeling and injury in the pathogenesis of OSA (Fig. 8). According to this model, an anatomically small pharynx causes a predisposition to upper airway collapse, which must then be opposed by hyperactivation of pharyngeal dilator muscles. The increased activity level of these muscles can lead

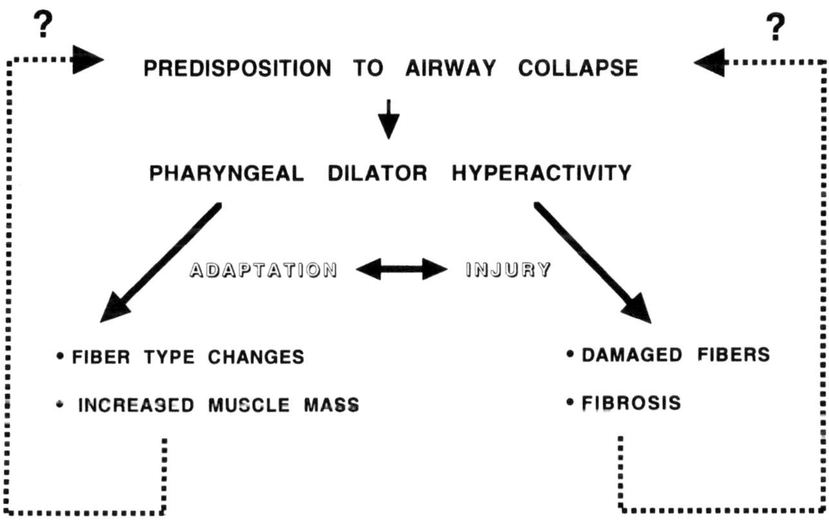

Figure 8 Proposed model for the possible role of activity-induced upper airway muscle remodeling and injury in the pathogenesis of OSA. Anatomical predisposition to upper airway collapse leads to compensatory hyperactivation of upper airway dilator muscles during both wakefulness and sleep. This hyperactivation causes changes in muscle structure, which may be adaptive (i.e., designed to increase muscle efficiency and strength) or injurious. A vicious cycle may be produced if an initially ''adaptive'' change such as increased upper airway muscle mass or increased reliance on anaerobic metabolism (with reduced fatigue resistance) causes further pharyngeal narrowing, or if muscle injury impairs the ability of the pharyngeal dilators to effectively maintain upper airway patency. (From Ref. 62.)

to adaptive changes such as switches in fiber type, altered metabolic enzyme levels, and increased muscle mass. These alterations would generally be expected to augment muscle efficiency and increase absolute force-generating capacity during airway opening and should generally aid in the maintenance of upper airway patency. However, it is also conceivable that an ''adaptive'' increase in pharyngeal muscle mass could ultimately cause further encroachment upon an already narrowed upper airway. If this were to occur, increasing pharyngeal muscle size or bulk could actually have counterproductive effects on upper airway patency and could thus be considered ''maladaptive'' in nature. In addition, a switch in fiber type and energetic metabolism toward a less fatigue-resistant profile could also compromise airway patency under certain conditions. Activity-induced muscle injury consisting of fiber injury, edema, and eventual fibrosis would also be expected to result in a decreased ability to maintain pharyngeal patency. Thus, both ''adaptive'' and frankly injurious changes could lead to a downward spiral in the course of the disease, characterized by a vicious cycle in which pharyngeal dilator muscle hyperactivity promoted further compromise of the upper airway via secondary effects on muscle structure and function. This could subsequently provoke even greater upper airway dilator muscle hyperactivity in an attempt to compensate for the loss of pharyngeal patency, thereby completing a deleterious positive feedback loop.

If the above hypothesis is correct, one would expect OSA to be a progressively worsening condition. Although no long-term prospective studies are available, retrospective analyses suggest that many patients do progress over time from snoring and mild OSA to more severe levels of disease (56–58). In this regard, Lugaresi and colleagues (58) found that most individuals with severe OSA were asymptomatic snorers at an earlier age and that they had developed progressive worsening of snoring and associated symptoms of excessive daytime sleepiness over a period of several years. Kales et al. (56) also described a very similar course of events in OSA patients. On the other hand, Sforza et al. (59) did not find a change in overall disease severity after a follow-up period of at least 5 years in 58 patients with untreated OSA. However, a subgroup ($n = 7$) of patients with initially milder disease demonstrated a significant increase in apnea/hypopnea index (from 14 to 51 events/h) during this period. Finally, although full polysomnography was not performed at the time of the initial overnight evaluation, Svanborg and Larsson (57) reported a significant increase in the number of oxyhemoglobin desaturations per hour following a mean interval of 15.6 months in 42 patients with OSA.

Further studies are needed to ascertain the true prevalence of upper airway muscle adaptation and injury in OSA patients. Studies to date in humans have focused primarily on palatal muscles for practical reasons of tissue availability, and in these muscles vibratory trauma from snoring to muscle and/or nerve structures could also play a role. However, data from the bulldog animal model suggest that the changes are more widespread and involve muscles for which snoring-related trauma is less plausible (46,47). It is also likely that there is considerable heterogeneity in the level of adaptation and/or injury in these muscles due to a number of factors such as disease duration, muscle location and activity level, the presence or absence of eccentric contractions, etc. This is supported by the MRI studies performed in the bulldog model (47) as well as the fact that evidence of muscle injury was not found in all human studies (53). In addition, the use of snorers as a control group in some studies could have underestimated differences between normal individuals and those with OSA, since it is likely that snorers and OSA patients represent a continuum of the same basic underlying pathophysiological process.

VII. Implications for Treatment

It must be emphasized that the role of upper airway remodeling and injury in the pathogenesis of OSA remains speculative at the present time, and additional studies are needed. However, confirmation of the proposed hypothesis in humans would have important implications for the pathogenesis and treatment of OSA, since the scenario outlined predicts a progressive deterioration of upper airway muscle function over time in the absence of therapeutic interventions to interrupt the cycle. It would also be extremely important to determine the reversibility of the changes such as muscle fibrosis after instituting therapy, since a lack of reversibility would point to a need for earlier and more aggressive treatment of the disease. Finally, pending further studies in this area of investigation, it would seem advisable to proceed cautiously with therapies designed to augment upper airway dilator activity in OSA patients such as pharmacological agents or direct electrical stimulation (60,61), since there is at least a theoretical risk of exacerbating adverse effects on muscle structure and function with these interventions.

Acknowledgments

Supported by the Medical Research Council of Canada, the Muscular Dystrophy Association of Canada, and a SCOR grant (HL42236) from NIH.

References

1. Horner RL. Motor control of the pharyngeal musculature and implications for the pathogenesis of obstructive sleep apnea. Sleep 1996; 19:827–853.
2. White, DP. Pathophysiology of sleep apnoea. Thorax 1995; 50:797–804.
3. van Lunteren E, Dick TE. Intrinsic properties of pharyngeal and diaphragmatic respiratory motoneurons. J Appl Physiol 1992; 73:787–800.
4. van Lunteren E, Vafale H, Salomone RJ. Comparative effects of aging on pharyngeal and diaphragm muscles. Respir Physiol 1995; 99:13–25.
5. van Lunteren E. Effects of genetic obesity on rat upper airway muscle and diaphragm contractile properties. Eur Respir J 1996; 9:39–44.
6. Popovic RM, White DP. Upper airway muscle activity in normal women: influence of hormonal status. J Appl Physiol 1998; 84:1055–1062.

7. Popovic RM, White DP. Influence of gender on waking genioglossus electromyogram and upper airway resistance. Am J Respir Crit Care Med 1995; 152:725–731.
8. Onal E, Lopata M, O'Connor T. Pathogenesis of apneas in hypersomnia-sleep apnea syndrome. Am Rev Respir Dis 1982; 125:167–174.
9. Remmers JE, DeGroot WJ, Sauerland EK, Anch AM. Pathogenesis of upper airway occlusion during sleep. J Appl Physiol 1978; 44:931–938.
10. Haponick EF, Smith PL, Bohlman ME, Allen RP, Goldman SM, Bleecker ER. Computerized tomography in obstructive sleep apnea: correlation of airway size with physiology during sleep and wakefulness. Am Rev Respir Dis 1983; 127:221–226.
11. Schwab RJ, Gefter WB, Hoffman EA, Gupta KB, Pack AI. Dynamic upper airway imaging during awake respiration in normal subjects and patients with sleep disordered breathing. Am Rev Respir Dis 1993; 148:1385–1400.
12. Mezzanotte WS, Tangel DJ, White DP. Waking genioglossal EMG in sleep apnea patients versus normal controls (a neuromuscular compensatory mechanism). J Clin Invest 1992; 89:1571–1579.
13. Mezzanotte WS, Tangel DJ, White DP. Influence of sleep onset on upper-airway muscle activity in apnea patients versus normal controls. Am J Respir Crit Care Med 1996; 153:1880–1887.
14. Hendricks JC, Petrof BJ, Panckeri K, Pack AI. Compensatory hyperactivity of an upper airway dilator in bulldogs. Am Rev Respir Dis 1993; 148:185–194.
15. Suratt PM, McTier RF, Wilhoit SC. Upper airway muscle activation is augmented in patients with obstructive sleep apnea compared with that in normal subjects. Am Rev Respir Dis 1988; 137:889–894.
16. Yarasheski KE, Lemon PWR, Gilloteaux J. Effect of heavy-resistance exercise training on muscle fiber composition in young rats. J Appl Physiol 1990; 69:434–437.
17. Fitzsimons DP, Diffee GM, Herrick RE, Baldwin KM. Effects of endurance exercise on isomyosin patterns in fast- and slow-twitch skeletal muscles. J Appl Physiol 1990; 68:1950–1955.
18. Westgaard RH, Lomo T. Control of contractile properties within adaptive ranges by patterns of impulse activity in the rat. J Neurosci 1988; 8:4415–4426.
19. Russell B, Dix DJ, Haller L, Jacobs-El J. Repair of injured skeletal muscle: a molecular approach. Med Sci Sports Exerc 1992; 24:189–196.
20. Waterman-Storer CM. The cytoskeleton of skeletal muscle: is it affected by exercise? A brief review. Med Sci Sports Exerc 1991; 23:1240–1249.
21. McCully KK, Faulkner JA. Injury to skeletal muscle fibers of mice following lengthening contractions. J Appl Physiol 1985; 59:119–126.
22. McCully KK, Faulkner JA. Characteristics of lengthening contractions associated with injury to skeletal muscle fibers. J Appl Physiol 1986; 61:293–299.
23. Armstrong RB. Initial events in exercise-induced muscular injury. Med Sci Sports Exerc 1990; 22:429–435.
24. Hikida RS, Staron RS, Hagerman FC, Sherman WM, Costill DL. Muscle fiber necrosis associated with human marathon runners. J Neurol Sci 1983; 59:185–203.
25. Jones DA, Newham DJ, Round JM, Tolfree SEJ. Experimental human muscle damage: morphological changes in relation to other indices of damage. J Physiol 1986; 375: 435–448.
26. Newham DJ, McPhail G, Mills KR, Edwards RHT. Ultrastructural changes after concentric and eccentric contractions of human muscle. J Neurol Sci 1983; 61:109–122.

27. Ogilvie RW, Armstrong RB, Baird KE, Bottoms CL. Lesions in the rat soleus muscle following eccentrically biased exercise. Am J Anat 1988; 182:335–346.
28. Stauber WT, Clarkson PM, Fritz VK, Evans WJ. Extracellular matrix disruption and pain after eccentric muscle action. J Appl Physiol 1990; 69:868–874.
29. Reid WD, Huang J, Bryson S, Walker DC, Belcastro AN. Diaphragm injury and myofibrillar structure induced by resistive loading. J Appl Physiol 1994; 76:176–184.
30. Campbell JA, Hughes RL, Sahgal V, Frederiksen J, Shields TW. Alterations in intercostal muscle morphology and biochemistry in patients with obstructive lung disease. Am Rev Respir Dis 1980; 122:679–686.
31. Hards JM, Reid WD, Pardy RL, Pare PD. Respiratory muscle morphometry: correlation with lung function and nutrition. Chest 1990; 97:1037–1044.
32. Dennett X, Fry HJH. Overuse syndrome: a muscle biopsy study. Lancet 1988; II:905–908.
33. Edwards RHT, Hill DK, Jones DA, Merton PA. Fatigue of long duration in human skeletal muscle after exercise. J Physiol 1977; 272:769–778.
34. Faulkner JA, Jones DA, Round JM. Injury to skeletal muscles of mice by forced lengthening during contractions. Q J Exp Physiol 1989; 74:661–670.
35. Brooks SV, Faulkner JA. Contraction-induced injury: recovery of skeletal muscles in young and old mice. Am J Physiol 1990; 258:C436–C442.
36. Vollestad NK, Sejerstaed OM. Biochemical correlates of fatigue. A brief review. Eur J Appl Physiol 1988; 57:336–347.
37. van Lunteren E, Haxhiu MA, Cherniack NS. Effects of tracheal airway occlusion on hyoid muscle length and upper airway volume. J Appl Physiol 1989; 67:2296–2302.
38. van Lunteren E, Haxhiu MA, Cherniack NS. Mechanical function of hyoid muscles during spontaneous breathing in cats. J Appl Physiol 1987; 62:582–590.
39. Ekenvall L, Nilsson BY, Gustavsson P. Temperature and vibration thresholds in vibration syndrome. Br J Ind Med 1986; 43:825–829.
40. Lundborg G, Dahlin L, Hansson HA, Kanje M, Necking LE. Vibration exposure and peripheral nerve fiber damage. J Hand Surg 1990; 15A:346–351.
41. Takeuchi T, Futatsuka M, Imanishi H, Yamada S. Pathological changes observed in the finger biopsy of patients with vibration-induced white finger. Scand J Work Environ Health 1986; 12:280–283.
42. Larsson H, Carlsson-Nordlander B, Linblad LE, Norbeck O, Svanborg E. Temperature thresholds in the oropharynx of patients with obstructive sleep apnea syndrome. Am Rev Respir Dis 1992; 146:1246–1249.
43. Woodson BT, Garancis JC, Toohill RJ. Histopathologic changes in snoring and obstructive sleep apnea syndrome. Laryngoscope 1991; 101:1318–1322.
44. Hendricks JC, Kline LR, Kovalski RJ, O'Brien JA, Morrison AR, Pack AI. The English bulldog: a natural model of sleep-disordered breathing. J Appl Physiol 1987; 63:1344–1350.
45. Hendricks JC, Kovalski RJ, Kline LR. Phasic respiratory muscle patterns and sleep-disordered breathing during rapid eye movement sleep in the English bulldog. Am Rev Respir Dis 1991; 144:1112–1120.
46. Petrof BJ, Pack AI, Kelly AM, Eby J, Hendricks JC. Pharyngeal myopathy of loaded upper airway in dogs with sleep apnea. J Appl Physiol 1994; 76:1746–1752.
47. Schotland HM, Insko EK, Panckeri KA, Leigh JS, Pack AI, Hendricks JC. Quantitative magnetic resonance imaging of upper airway musculature in an animal model of sleep apnea. J Appl Physiol 1996; 81:1339–1346.

48. Stauffer JI, Buick MK, Bixler EO, Sharkey FE, Abt AB, Manders EK, et al. Morphology of the uvula in obstructive sleep apnea. Am Rev Respir Dis 1989; 140:724–728.
49. Carpenter S, Karpati G. Pathology of Skeletal Muscle. New York: Churchill Livingstone Inc., 1984.
50. Edstrom L, Larsson H, Larsson L. Neurogenic effects on the palatopharyngeal muscle in patients with obstructive sleep apnoea: a muscle biopsy study. J Neurol Neurosurg Psychiatry 1992; 55:916–920.
51. Friberg D, Ansved T, Borg K, Carlsson-Nordlander B, Larsson H, Svanborg E. Histological indications of a progressive snorers disease in an upper airway muscle. Am J Respir Crit Care Med 1998; 157:586–593.
52. Smirne S, Iannaccone S, Ferini-Strambi L, Comola M, Colombo E, Nemni R. Muscle fibre type and habitual snoring. Lancet 1991; 337:597–599.
53. Sériès F, Cote C, Simoneau J-A, Gelinas Y, St. Pierre S, Leclerc J, et al. Physiologic, metabolic, and muscle fiber type characteristics of musculus uvulae in sleep apnea hypopnea syndrome and in snorers. J Clin Invest 1995; 95:20–25.
54. Sériès F, Simoneau J-A, St. Pierre S, Marc I. Characteristics of the genioglossus and musculus uvulae in sleep apnea hypopnea syndrome and in snorers. Am J Respir Crit Care Med 1996; 153:1870–1874.
55. Sériès F, Cote C, Simoneau J-A, St. Pierre S, Marc I. Upper airway collapsibility, and contractile and metabolic characteristics of musculus uvulae. FASEB J 1996; 10:897–904.
56. Kales A, Cadieux RJ, Bixler EO, Soldatos CR, Vela-Bueno EO, Misoul CA, et al. Severe obstructive sleep apnea-I: Onset, clinical course and characteristics. J Chron Dis 1985; 5:419–425.
57. Svanborg E, Larsson H. Development of nocturnal respiratory disturbance in untreated patients with obstructive sleep apnea syndrome. Chest 1993; 104:340–343.
58. Lugaresi E, Cirignotta F, Gerardi R, Montagna P. Snoring and sleep apnea: natural history of heavy snorers disease. In: Guilleminault C, Partinen M, eds. Obstructive Sleep Apnea Syndrome: Clinical Research and Treatment. New York: Raven Press, 1990: 25–36.
59. Sforza E, Addati G, Cirignotta F, Lugaresi E. Natural evolution of sleep apnea syndrome: a five year longitudinal study. Eur Respir J 1994; 7:1765–1770.
60. Schwartz AR, Eisele DW, Hari A, Testerman R, Erickson D, Smith PL. Electrical stimulation of the lingual musculature in obstructive sleep apnea. J Appl Physiol 1996; 81: 643–652.
61. Guilleminault C, Powell N, Bowman B, Stoohs R. The effect of electrical stimulation on obstructive sleep apnea syndrome. Chest 1995; 107:67–73.
62. Petrof BJ, Hendricks JC, Pack AI. Does upper airway muscle injury trigger a vicious cycle in obstructive sleep apnea? A hypothesis. Sleep 1996; 19(6):465–471.

8

The Genetics of the Obstructive Sleep Apnea Hypopnea Syndrome

SUSAN REDLINE

Rainbow Babies and Children's Hospital
and Case Western Reserve University
Cleveland, Ohio

PETER V. TISHLER

VA Boston Healthcare System
and Harvard Medical School
Boston, Massachusetts

KINGMAN P. STROHL

Case Western Reserve University
Cleveland, Ohio

I. Introduction

The development of increasingly powerful molecular and statistical methods for dissecting the genetic bases of complex diseases has encouraged studies of a number of chronic diseases. Many of these are of major economic and societal importance, as they are responsible for increasing illness with age. One of these is obstructive sleep apnea hypopnea syndrome (OSAHS), a syndrome likely determined by multigenic factors, environmental exposures, and their interactions. The evidence for a genetic basis for OSAHS has been developed from the application of progressively more quantitative methods to the study of this disorder. These have included, in roughly chronological order, descriptive studies of families with multiply affected members; studies of OSAHS prevalence among relatives of affected probands; quantification of the familial aggregation of OSAHS by comparing the prevalence of OSAHS among relatives of affected probands with that in control samples; and segregation analysis. Information from these studies has been useful in establishing a likely role for inheritance apart from familial influences related to obesity and for suggesting ways to characterize the phenotype of the disorder, an important prerequisite for linkage analysis. In parallel with human studies has been the development of rodent models to identify genes that influence the expression of traits that may underlie OSAHS. It is anticipated that the successful iteration of information gleaned from human and animal work will lead to the mapping of genes for traits that substantially influence the expression of OSAHS in humans.

This chapter will review the data that suggest the operation of familial factors in influencing disease expression, the potential genetic bases for OSAHS, and animal work and human data that implicate specific genetic systems in the expression of the disorder. When read in the context of our earlier review of this subject in 1994, this review points out the remarkable progress that has been made in establishing the biological basis of OSAHS (1). Even so, the material comprising this review constitutes a very early, rudimentary step along the path to the complete journey.

II. Studies of the Familial Aggregation of Obstructive Sleep Apnea

A. Reports of Affected Families

There have been at least four reports of multigenerational families with multiple members with OSAHS. The first report identified three brothers (ages 39–44 years) with OSAHS documented by polysomnography. Their deceased father was described as a restless sleeper with nighttime apneas and daytime sleepiness (2). The proband, who was the most severely affected subject, was obese; no other risk factors for OSAHS were identified. This family has been reinvestigated recently, and additional members, involving a third generation, have been identified. In the second report, OSAHS was demonstrated in a father and son who also suffered from a seizure disorder and anosmia (3). The authors suggested that the association of OSAHS, seizures, and anosmia may have represented an inherited syndrome. The association with anosmia is provocative, and studies of sleep in other anosmic syndromes, such as Kallmann syndrome, would be of interest. Four siblings (three males) aged 5–15 years with OSAHS were described in the third report; these children appeared to be predisposed to OSAHS because of their obesity and the presence of upper airway congestion (4). The last report describes a family with OSAHS in nonobese members of three generations (eight males, one female, aged 7–64 years) (5). Cephalometry and tests of ventilatory responses to chemical loading were performed in five affected subjects. These studies demonstrated blunted ventilatory responses to progressive eucapneic hypoxia in all subjects; the two subjects with the most severe sleep disorders also had the longest soft palates and most inferiorly displaced hyoids. Together, the case studies suggest that certain families are especially predisposed to OSAHS. The findings of El-Bayadi et al. also suggest that familial OSAHS may be associated with abnormalities in the control of ventilation and that the expression and severity of sleep apnea may result from interactions of physiological and anatomical abnormalities (5).

B. Clustering of Symptoms

The aforementioned reports of pedigrees do not indicate the overall degree to which OSAHS is a familial or inherited disorder, however. Four systematic population studies have examined the familial aggregation of symptoms of OSAHS. Kaprio et al., in their study of sleep in >4000 Finnish twins, found that the concordance for snoring among monozygotic (MZ) twins was greater than among dizygotic (DZ) twins, suggesting a role for inheritance (6). Among 776 twin pairs, Ferini-Strambi and associates showed stronger associations between known risk factors and snoring in DZ twin pairs discordant for snoring than in MZ discordant twin pairs, which also was interpreted as evidence that genetic factors predispose to snoring (7). Redline et al. estimated the degree of familial aggregation of several symptoms of OSAHS in families of probands with polysomnographically proven OSAHS and in control families (8). Habitual snoring, excessive daytime sleepiness, and snorting, gasping, or apneas were reported more frequently among the first-degree relatives of patients with OSAHS than among control subjects. Moreover, odds ratios for the likelihood of manifesting symptoms increased progressively for subjects with increasing number of symptomatic relatives. These findings were independent of familial similarities in weight, smoking, and alcohol consumption, as well as age and gender. Among 3308 men aged 54–74 years of age who participated in the Copenhagen Male Study, a prospective cardiovascular cohort study, a significant relationship was demonstrated between family history of snoring and self-reported snoring (9). Risk of snoring was increased approximately threefold when at least one first-degree relative was reported to be a snorer and increased fourfold when both parents were reportedly snorers (9). These relationships were independent of age, body mass index (BMI), blood pressure levels, and cardiovascular risk factors (including smoking, lipid levels, and physical activity levels). Thus, symptoms associated with OSAHS aggregate significantly within families and are not fully explained by other risk factors.

C. Familial Clustering of AHI Levels

Significant family clustering of apneic-hypopneic activity, demonstrated by objective monitoring, has been demonstrated in four distinct populations, including samples from Israel, the United Kingdom, northern California, and Cleveland, OH (10–13) (Table 1). The prevalence of increased apneic hypopneic indices (AHIs) among first-degree relatives of probands with OSAHS has varied from 21% (in the Cleveland Family Study) (12) to as high as 84% (in the California sample) (13). Likewise, among the studies that included control samples, the odds ratios, relating the likely existence of an individual with sleep-disordered breathing in a family with affected relatives to the likelihood for someone without an affected relative, have varied from 2 to 46 (11–13) (Table 1). Thus, the available data are consistent in demonstrating familial aggregation for OSAHS; however, the magnitude of increased risk attributable to family membership is not clear.

Differences in the estimates of relative risk are due to several factors, including

Table 1 Prevalence of Sleep-Disordered Breathing Among First-Degree Relatives of Probands with Obstructive Sleep Apnea

Sample	Probands/ Relatives	Controls	Phenotype	% Affected	Odds ratio
Israel (10) unselected probands and offspring	45/108	—	AHI > 20, by lab PSG	33	—
United Kingdom (14) probands <30 kg/m^2 and offspring	20/40	—	AHI > 15, by lab PSG	25	—
United Kingdom (11) offspring of probands <30 kg/m^2	0/51	51	AHI > 15, by lab PSG	45	20
California (13) probands and first-degree relatives	157/166	69	AHI > 5, by home PSG, EDS, ≥ 1 symptom	84	46
			AHI > 5, by home PSG, EDS, abnormal hard palate	68	11
Cleveland (12) probands, spouses, first-degree relatives	47/219	223	AHI > age-specific threshold, by home PSG	21	2
			AHI > 15+ Sleepiness	13	5

AHI = Apnea hypopnea index; lab = laboratory; PSG = polysomnograph; EDS = excessive daytime sleepiness.

differences in the samples and different characterizations of phenotype. For example, whereas probands identified for the United Kingdom studies all had BMIs of <30 kg/m^2 (11,14), the other studies enrolled subjects with laboratory-confirmed OSAHS, regardless of associated obesity. Estimates of genetic risk could be lower or higher among nonobese than obese subjects, according to the extent to which obesity directly or interactively contributes to the genetic predisposition. The Israel and United Kingdom samples both restricted studies of relatives to adult offspring of affected probands (10,11); the U.S. studies included all first-degree relatives (12), and the Cleveland study also assessed spouses. The analysis of data from a wide range of ages, as done in the latter two studies, requires consideration of the age dependency of the AHI, and potential differences in penetrance, which may vary as a function of age as well as be influenced by age and gender interactions. Additionally, some of the differences in the strength of the associations among studies may be explained by chance (as evidenced by the nearly twofold difference in prevalence among relatives studied by the same U.K. investigators one year apart), and/or by sampling biases, associated with differential participation rates of symptomatic cases and controls.

D. Defining the Phenotype and Impact on Analyses

Definitions of affection status have been based on threshold levels of the AHI, with and without associated symptoms and/or other findings. In the California study, when affection was defined by an AHI > 5 occurring with daytime tiredness or sleepiness and one other symptom, prevalence among first-degree relatives was 84% (13). When also requiring the finding of a high, narrow hard palate (by physical examination) to define affection, prevalence dropped to 68% and the odds ratio fell from 46 to 11. In the Cleveland sample, use of an age-dependent AHI threshold level resulted in identification of 21% of all first-degree relatives as ''affected'' (12). Changing the definition of affection to require an AHI > 15 and the occurrence of daytime sleepiness reduced the prevalence to 13% and increased the odds ratio to 5. Thus, these studies suggest the importance of careful consideration of characterization of the OSAHS phenotype.

Since AHI is a continuous trait that varies with age and gender, age- and gender-specific threshold levels may be most useful to identify polysomnographically defined levels of abnormality. Use of multiple measurements of AHI may be useful to minimize the effects of night-to-night variation in severity of sleep-disordered breathing and any attendant misclassification. Alternatively, combining polysomnography data with other information (e.g., symptoms, anthropometry, etc.) may improve the ability to accurately classify individuals. As one example, in the Cleveland Family Study a stronger relationship between familial risk and OSAHS was observed when OSAHS was defined by an AHI > 15 level and reported sleepiness than when disease was defined by AHI level alone. In the study of the genetics of psychiatric bipolar disease, where similar problems in defining phenotype arise, use of a relatively broad definition of affection status results in stronger genetic associations than more restrictive definitions (16). It is possible that stronger genetic associations for OSAHS also will emerge with approaches that consider a phenotype of intermediate severity, using criteria that clearly identify individuals with values beyond what may be observed commonly with increasing age or obesity level, but are not so rigid that very few relatives meet the criteria.

Assessment of the genetics of OSAHS also may be improved by analyses that utilize continuous measures of disease, with no attempt to define threshold levels. This is analogous to the use of measured levels of methacholine responsiveness to study the genetics of airway hyperresponsiveness or of blood pressure levels to focus on the genetics of hypertension. It has improved statistical efficiency over approaches that rely on analyses of binary or categorical traits. Quantification of the extent to which the AHI *level* is explained by familial factors was performed only in the Cleveland Family Study (12). Parent-offspring and sib-sib correlations for

Table 2 Familial Correlations for AHI, Cleveland Family Data, 1990–1995 ($n = 561$)

	Partially adjusted correlation[a]	p-value	BMI-adjusted correlation[a]	p-value
Parent-offspring	0.21	0.002	0.17	0.017
Sib-sib	0.21	0.003	0.18	0.008

[a] Adjusted for age, race, and gender.

AHI, log transformed and adjusted for age, sex, and BMI, are shown in Table 2. An empirical estimate of heritability was calculated to be 0.42. While the heritability (h^2) is a crude statistic, this level does suggest that a substantial proportion of the variability in AHI levels may be explained by familial factors.

In ongoing work, multivariate models are being employed to more fully describe OSAHS as a phenotype composed of a number of related traits. Preliminary analyses suggest that multivariate analysis of several polysomnography measures, measures of body habitus, and symptoms, analyzed jointly, may provide stronger measures of aggregation than analyses that attempt to characterize the population and familial distributions of single characteristics.

E. Identification of Mode of Inheritance

In the Cleveland Family Study, OSAHS appeared as a familial disorder affecting ≥2 members in 114 of 175 families with an affected proband (65%) and as a ''sporadic'' disorder in 61 families (35%). This suggests that familial OSAHS occurs more frequently than the ''sporadic'' form, although other explanations are possible. Mode of inheritance may be inferred from examination of pedigrees of affected families. Inspection of the pedigrees from the Cleveland families has identified a number of families in which the segregation of OSAHS is consistent with an autosomal dominant mode of inheritance. One example is provided in Figure 1. In this family, OSAHS (AHI > 15) was demonstrated in both siblings of the proband (generation II) and their father (generation I). Three of the five members of the third generation, all aged <25 years, also had levels of AHI considered elevated for their age (17).

A more formal approach to identifying mode of inheritance is the use of segregation analysis, which provides rigorous tests of the likelihood of the observed phenotypes based on specified genetic hypotheses. Parameters are estimated by maximum likelihood, and tests of hypotheses are performed via likelihood ratio tests. The methodology, originally developed by Elston and Stewart (18), and its extensions can examine genetic models such as those specifying a single major gene effect, two linked genes, polygenic inheritances, and environmental effects. The phenotype of interest may be described by multivariate outcomes that incorporate information from measures such as the AHI and desaturation profile and physical traits such as obesity and craniofacial structure.

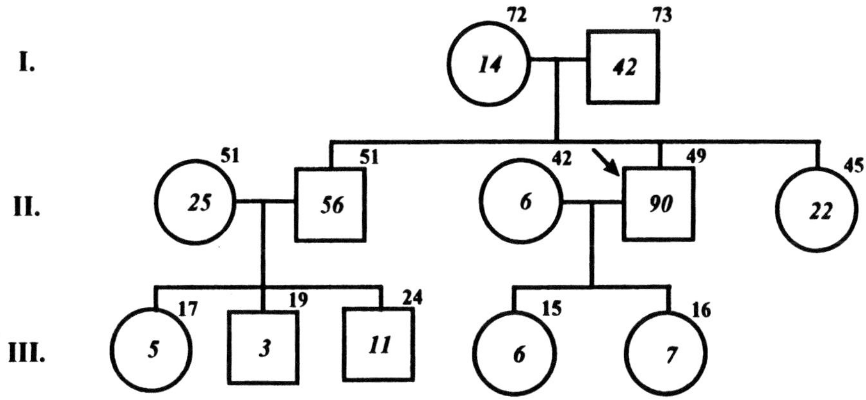

Figure 1 Pedigree of one family studied in the Cleveland Family Study. Values for AHI are shown in the interior in the squares (males) and circles (females). The index proband is identified by an arrow. Ages of each family member are shown outside the upper righthand corner of each symbol.

Work to date that has employed segregation analyses to assess the genetics of OSAHS is still preliminary. Segregation analyses of self-reported snoring in 584 pedigrees assembled as part of the Tucson Epidemiologic Survey of Obstructive Airways Disease suggested a major gene effect; however, the evidence for this weakened after adjustments were made for obesity and sex (19). Segregation analyses are underway using data from the Cleveland Family Study. Preliminary analyses suggest that the use of multivariate outcomes may be more informative than modeling the AHI alone.

III. Risk Factors for Obstructive Sleep Apnea and Their Genetic Bases

Risk factors for OSAHS include factors that are largely determined by genes and those that appear due to environmental influences (Table 3). The expression of many traits associated with OSAHS also may be influenced by developmental exposures, which may affect the development of craniofacial structure and central and peripheral nervous system function. Obesity, craniofacial structure, and ventilatory control, three areas that appear to be substantially influenced by genetic factors and may influence the expression of OSAHS, are reviewed below.

A. Obesity

Obesity is one of the most commonly recognized risk factors for OSAHS. Approximately two thirds of patients with documented sleep apnea are obese (>120% ideal

Table 3 Risk Factors for OSAHS: Relative Contribution of Genetic, Developmental, and Environmental Influences

	Genetic	Developmental	Environmental
Obesity/Central obesity	+++	?	++
Craniofacial dysmorphisms	+++	+	+
Ventilatory control abnormalities			
Chemoregulation	++	+	++
Load compensation	?	?	++
Rhythmogenesis	++	++	+
Neuromuscular abnormalities			
Muscle weakness/fatigability	+++/−	?	+++/−
Other	?	?	?
Connective tissue abnormalities			
Laxity	++++	−	+
Fibrosis	+	−	++++
Sleep homeostasis			
Sleep deprivation	−	−	+++++
Tolerance to sleep restriction	++	?	++
Alcohol/Stimulant/Hormone/Sedative use	+/−	−	+++++
Irritant exposures (tobacco)	−	−	+++++

body weight) (20). In one study of elderly subjects, obesity was found to be the strongest predictor of the number of respiratory disturbances measured during sleep (21); the effect of obesity was estimated to be approximately fourfold stronger than the influence of age and twice as strong as the influence of male gender in predicting sleep-related respiratory disturbances. A predisposition to OSAHS in obese subjects may result from reduction in nasopharyngeal caliber secondary to fat deposition in upper airway tissues and/or from hypoventilation occurring in association with reduced chest wall compliance. Alternatively, it is possible that the association between obesity and OSAHS may be partly based on pleiotropic effects, as may occur if the same gene or set of genes influences both body mass and ventilatory control and/or craniofacial morphology. The expression of certain candidate genes for obesity (e.g., leptin, adenosine deaminase, and melanocortin-3 receptor) in a variety of tissues and brain sites important in breathing regulation suggests the plausibility of this notion (22).

The results of twin studies suggest that approximately 70% of the variance in obesity within the population may be attributed to genetic factors (23,24). Several studies have suggested that the inheritance of obesity follows a recessive Mendelian model (25,26). However, multigenic effects, with codominance and age- and sex-specific effects, were suggested by analyses of 220 families studied in France (27). Genetic factors that influence metabolic rate, thermogenesis, fat storage, and eating behavior and that are associated with abnormalities in autonomic, endocrinological, and hypothalamic functions are thought to contribute significantly to the development of obesity (24,28 31). Efforts in recent years to identify genes involved in body fat distribution and somatotype have been intense. Currently, possible or probable candidate genes lie on chromosome 2p21 (possible candidates are glucokinase regulatory protein, pro-opiomelanocortin genes) (32), 6p21.3 (possibly tumor necrosis factor-α gene) (34), 7q31 (?OB gene?) (22), and 20q12-q13.3 [adenosine deaminase, melanocortin-3 receptor, human agouti homolog genes (35)]. Candidate loci, for which specific candidate genes are not identified, include 1p32-p22, 3p24.2-p22, and 11q21-q22 (22,23). Genetic factors may be particularly important in influencing regional body fat distribution and may account for as much as 25% of the intersubject variability in this trait (36). This may be of particular relevance to the pathogenesis of OSAHS, in which upper body obesity may be a relatively greater risk factor than is total body fat mass. Even relatively nonobese individuals with OSAHS may have regional excess fat deposition, especially in the anterior-lateral upper airway (37). Data from several populations that have demonstrated that genetic effects may be different for men and women (25,27,38) are also interesting because of the predisposition of males to OSAHS. This raises the possibility that sex-specific genes for obesity may, in part, account for sex differences in OSAHS.

The extent to which genetically determined levels of obesity account for the familiarity of OSAHS is not completely clear. However, adjustments for familial similarities in body mass index in the Cleveland Family Study did not appreciably reduce the estimates of familial aggregation of the AHI, suggesting the importance of other inherited factors (12).

B. Craniofacial Morphology

Various craniofacial morphological features, affecting both bony and soft tissues, are thought to predispose to OSAHS by reducing the size of the upper airway, thus predisposing to collapse of the upper airway during sleep (39). Indeed, Jamieson et al. have indicated that abnormalities in craniomandibular morphology are almost universal in subjects with OSAHS (40). Reduced pharyngeal dimensions in this patient population are associated with posterior facial compression and facial elongation (41). Structural abnormalities that have been described commonly in subjects with OSAHS include reduction of the anterior-posterior dimension of the cranial base (41), a reduced nasion-sella-basion angle (40), reduction of the size of the posterior and superior airway spaces (41), inferior displacement of the hyoid (42), elongation of the soft palate (43), macroglossia, adenoidotonsillar hypertrophy, and increased vertical facial dimension, with a disproportionate increase in the lower facial height (41). Retrognathia, micrognathia, and type II malocclusions have been reported, albeit less consistently, among patients with OSAHS (39).

A genetic basis for craniofacial morphology is suggested by twin and family studies. Osborne and De George (44), in a study of a series of approximately 60 MZ and 40 DZ twins, estimated the heritability of a number of morphological variables. The heritability of one of these, cephalic index (head breadth/head length), was extremely high (0.90 in males, 0.70 in females) (44). Heredity appeared to account for 40% of the variability of dental and facial characteristics associated with malocclusions according to a review by Lundstrom (45). Nance et al. applied multivariate analytic techniques to the analysis of cephalometric data from 24 MZ and 21 DZ twin pairs of the same gender, aged 10–17 years (46). A high heritability estimate (>0.59) was found for all eight cephalometric parameters, including several measures that were abnormal in studies of OSAHS [the distance between basion and nasion; the overall length of the cranial base, which was reduced in length in the study of Bacon et al. (41) and the nasion-sella-basion angle, which was reduced in the study of Jamieson et al. (40)]. Further statistical analysis indicated that at least four significant independent dimensions of hereditary variation contributed to the overall variation in these measurements: the first influenced primarily two horizontal mandibular measurements; the second, the horizontal cranial base measurements and the mandibular gonial angle; the third, the nasion-sella-basion angle; and the fourth, the posterior cranial base and the mandibular ramus. All of these factors may influence the relative patency of nasopharynx.

Mouse models suggest that a number of different genes may influence craniofacial development. Craniofacial defects, including retrognathia and micrognathia, have been described in mice deficient in the growth and differentiating factor transforming growth factor-β2 (47). Similar defects have been described in mice deficient for the retinoic acid receptor-αγ (48) and endothelin-1 (49). It is likely that a further understanding of homeobox genes and genes controlling growth factors will illuminate the origins of craniofacial dysmorphisms found in OSAHS.

Inherited abnormalities of craniofacial structure appear to explain at least a portion of the familial clustering of OSAHS. In the U.K. family study, a comparison of upper airway dimensions between relatives of OSAHS probands and controls, by acoustic reflectometry and cephalometry, demonstrated relatives to have decreased total pharyngeal volumes and glottic cross-sectional areas, retropositioned maxillae and mandibles, and longer soft palates (11). In the northern California study, relatives of patients with OSAHS were shown by cephalometry to have a more retropositioned mandible and smaller posterior superior airway space as compared to normative data (13). In the Cleveland Family Study, both hard tissue (e.g., head form, intermaxillary length) and soft tissue factors (e.g., soft palate length, tongue volume) that influence airway patency were noted to be risk factors for OSAHS in Caucasian families; however, hard tissue anatomical features appeared to play a smaller role in the pathogenesis of OSAHS in black families (50). The latter data suggest that the anatomical underpinnings for OSAHS may differ among racial groups. Thus, a large source of heterogeneity in genetic studies of OSAHS may relate to the racial composition of the sample under investigation.

C. Control of Ventilation

The pathogenesis of OSAHS may relate not only to anatomical risk factors but also to abnormalities in the neural mechanisms for activation of respiratory muscles.

Potentially inherited abnormalities of ventilatory control may predispose to obstructive or central sleep apnea or both by several different mechanisms. Central ventila tory drive is depressed during sleep, but the level of activation of upper airway muscles is reduced to a greater degree than that of chest wall muscles. An imbalance between the dilating effect of upper airway muscle contraction and the constricting effect of negative intrathoracic pressure can lead to upper airway collapse (51). Altered ventilatory drive also may precipitate apnea by promoting respiratory control instability and, subsequently, periodic breathing (52). In this regard, ventilatory control instability could result from either blunted or augmented sensitivity to hypercapnia or hypoxia (52–54). Additionally, reductions in respiratory responsiveness to chemical or mechanical stimulation may prolong the duration of apneas by impairment of the arousal response to the obstructive episode. This notion is supported by the demonstration that the degree of oxygen desaturation is the greatest and the duration of apneas the longest in subjects with OSAHS in whom ventilation in response to hypoxia during wakefulness is the most blunted (55).

An inherited basis for ventilatory responsiveness to hypoxemia or hypercapnia has been suggested by the findings from several human studies. Abnormalities in ventilatory responsiveness to hypoxia and/or hypercapnia have been described in the first-degree relatives of probands with various pulmonary diseases or syndromes, including unexplained respiratory failure (56,57), chronic obstructive pulmonary disease (58–60), and asthma (61). A genetic basis for the peripheral chemoresponse to blood oxygen saturation is suggested by several twin studies that have demonstrated similarities in ventilatory responses to hypoxia or hyperoxia to be greater in MZ than in DZ twins (62–65). Thomas and colleagues, in their study of infants tested during sleep, estimated that approximately 75% of the variance in the peripheral chemoresponse to hyperoxia in MZ twins could be accounted for by genetic factors (64). A recent study of an isolated Tibetan population living at high altitude, studied with a modified rebreathing technique, demonstrated that 34% of the variance in the hypoxic ventilatory response was attributable to genetic factors (66). A similar study performed in a high-altitude Bolivian sample also suggested a significant, but lesser, role for inheritance in the hypoxic ventilatory response (66).

Evidence for a role of genetics in the ventilatory response to hypercapnia in humans is less consistent than the data regarding hypoxic responses. Steady-state ventilatory responses to carbon dioxide have been demonstrated to be lower in 12 New Guinea subjects when compared to responses in Australian city dwellers; these racial differences could have been partly based on genetic factors (67). Heritability also has been suggested to influence ventilatory responses to hypercapnia among endurance athletes, in whom similarities among siblings in ventilatory responses to hypercapnia have been demonstrated (68). In contrast, twin studies have shown that in the absence of hypoxia, intrapair differences in ventilation in response to hypercapnia are comparable for MZ and DZ twins, suggesting that this trait may be determined largely by nongenetic factors (62,64,65,69). Greater similarities in MZ than in DZ twins, however, have been demonstrated for hypercapnic responses when measured during normoxia or hypoxia (rather than hyperoxia) (63,65). Changes in tidal volume, but not in frequency, with progressive hypercapnia also have been shown to be more similar in MZ than DZ twins, suggesting that genetic control may vary for different components of the ventilatory response to hypercapnia (69).

Abnormalities in ventilatory control in patients with OSAHS have not been demonstrated consistently, however. Thus, the extent to which acquired rather than genetic abnormalities of ventilatory control increase susceptibility to OSAHS is unclear. Studies of ventilatory control in OSAHS have been difficult to interpret secondary to patient heterogeneity in regard to age, race, gender, and comorbidity. Assessments may have been limited by difficulties in the measurement of ventilatory responses in subjects in whom breathing may be impaired mechanically because of obesity or airway obstruction. Also, abnormalities in ventilatory responses in subjects with OSAHS may be observed as secondary effects of chronic hypoxemia or sleep fragmentation associated with recurrent apneas (70,71). The importance of acquired factors is suggested by improvement in the hypercapnic ventilatory response and load compensation with treatment of upper airway obstruction in patients with OSAHS (72–75). Despite these limitations, the potential importance in OSAHS of inherited impairments of ventilatory control, including abnormalities in chemoregulation as well as in load compensation, has been suggested by several studies of carefully characterized families. The importance of genetically determined levels of hypoxic responsiveness in OSAHS is suggested by our studies with familial sleep apnea. In one family with 9 affected members, we demonstrated depressed hypoxic responses in all 5 affected members in whom this was assessed (5). We recently extended this work by assessing respiratory responses to hypoxia, hypercapnia, and ventilatory loading in 22 subjects from 13 well-defined families in which multiple members had OSAHS and in a control sample derived from 9 families with no member with OSAHS (76). Members of OSAHS families demonstrated significantly lower ventilatory responses to progressive eucapnic hypoxia measured during wakefulness as compared to members of control families. Additionally, impairment in load compensation was suggested by the finding of a significantly greater increase in ventilatory impedance with inspiratory resistive loading in OSAHS family members as compared to control subjects. This finding is consistent with the observations made by Lavie and colleagues, who described increased apneic activity following nasal occlusion and impaired load compensation during sleep in family members of OSAHS patients as compared to controls (77,78). These data suggest that the familial aggregation of OSAHS is in some instances based on inherited abnormalities in respiratory control, perhaps related to chemoregulation (specifically, the hypoxic response) and/or load compensation. The upper airway of genetically susceptible individuals appears vulnerable to excessive collapsibility during conditions of mild inspiratory loading. This may occur especially during sleep as the balance between upper airway and chest wall activation changes or intrathoracic airway pressure during inspiration becomes more subatmospheric. Further investigation of ventilatory control in carefully characterized subjects with OSAHS and their family members is needed to better understand the roles of peripheral and central chemoreceptors and of the central nervous ventilatory control system in the pathogenesis of

OSAHS. Although the specific bases for these deficits are not clear, further studies should considcr thc rolc of inhcritcd physiological factors that influence airway pa tency.

IV. Insights from Associations of OSAHS with Other Disorders

Considering the relationship of OSAHS to disorders with known genetic causes or known physiological bases may provide important insights into the genetic bases of OSAHS.

A. Congenital Disorders Associated with Abnormal Upper Airway Anatomy or Function

There are at least 50 syndromes in which congenital malformations of mandibular and maxillary structure occur. These entities include Pierre Robin syndrome, a rare congenital disorder that results in mandibular hypoplasia and in which sudden death due to respiratory impairment occurs commonly, and Treacher Collins syndrome, a rare autosomal dominant disorder also associated with upper airway obstruction.

Down syndrome may predispose to upper airway collapse because of a number of factors that predispose to pharyngeal crowding, including macroglossia, brachycephaly, tonsillar hypertrophy, and obesity. Individuals with Down syndrome appear particularly predisposed to OSAHS.

Marfan syndrome is characterized by generalized connective tissue laxity. Its pathogenesis appears to relate to a decrease in the normal and/or presence of an abnormal form of the connective tissue microfibrillar protein fibrillin, encoded by a gene at the locus 15q21 (79,80). Studies by Cistulli et al., yet unconfirmed by others, indicate that as many as 64% of patients with Marfan syndrome have AHIs > 5 (81). The pathogenesis of apnea in these individuals is thought to be due to excessive upper airway collapsibility associated with the connective tissue abnormality (82). Since maxillary arch constriction is also common in this syndrome, it contributes to the liability for apnea by the reduced upper airway dimensions and the increased nasal rcsistancc (83).

Patients with the Prader-Willi syndrome, characterized by neonatal hypotonia, obesity, mental retardation, hypogonadism, and short stature, are often sleepy and demonstrate sleep-related hypoventilation and OSAHS (84–87). Sleep-related respiratory disturbances may occur independently of the obesity (84). Absent or markedly reduced ventilatory response to isocapnic hypoxia and to hypercapnea has been described in both obese and nonobese subjects with Prader-Willi syndrome (88–90). In one morbidly obese female, ventilatory response to hypercarbia improved dramatically after tracheostomy, although mean resting minute ventilation and end-tidal carbon dioxide tension remained elevated many weeks later (91). The pathogenesis of the breathing disorder in this syndrome probably involves additional factors, including hypothalamic dysfunction, facial dysmorphism, obesity, and adenotonsillar hypertrophy. Prader-Willi syndrome is usually associated with a small deletion in paternal chromosome 15q11–q13. The gene that is responsible for this syndrome has not been identified, but several are under active investigation: SNRPN, a gene for small nuclear ribonucleoprotein-associated polypeptide that is expressed in neural tissue; IPW, a gene whose paternal copy only is expressed (imprinted); and NDN, the necdin-encoding gene, a gene that may govern the permanent arrest of cell growth of postmitotic cells, particularly in the nervous system (92,93).

Individuals with Tourette's syndrome and/or attention-deficit hyperactivity disorder (ADHD) appear to have an increased liability for sleep disorders and OSAHS (94,95). This intriguing finding deserves further examination.

B. Associations with Neurological or Neuromuscular Disease

OSAHS has been reported in numerous neurological and neuromuscular disorders, including Duchenne muscular dystrophy, amyotrophic lateral sclerosis, myotonic dystrophy, myasthenia gravis, Parkinson's disease, and various encephalopathies. The pathogenesis of the sleep-related breathing disorder in these conditions appears to relate to either upper airway muscular dysfunction or to disorders of ventilatory control. Many times, however, it is difficult to distinguish the relative contributions of peripheral muscle dysfunction from dysfunctional ventilatory control mechanisms in disease pathogenesis. An example of this problem was highlighted in a report of a family with congenital myopathy in which members had both impaired ventilatory drive and reduced muscle strength (as well as abnormal facial features) (96).

C. Sudden Infant Death Syndrome and OSAHS

Sudden infant death syndrome (SIDS) and near-miss SIDS or acute life-threatening events (ALTEs) probably are related entities in which apneas present as life-threatening events during the first year of life (97). Both entities appear to be more common in males and in children born prematurely and/or small for gestational age (98). These syndromes likely include heterogeneous subgroups, including a subgroup at risk due to neglect or abuse. However, there are likely subgroups predisposed to these conditions because of inherited risk factors. Siblings of SIDS cases appear to be at 3- to 10-fold increased risk of experiencing either SIDS or ALTEs, and subjects with two affected siblings appear to be at even greater risk (99,100). Abnormalities of ventilatory control, including abnormalities in arousal responses to hypoxia, hypercapnia, and inspiratory resistive loading (101,102), as well as anatomical risk factors that compromise the posterior airway space (103), have been postulated to be potentially important in the pathogenesis of SIDS and ALTEs. As previously discussed, abnormalities of ventilatory control and craniofacial morphology have a familial basis, and they also are thought to be risk factors for OSAHS in adults.

Several studies suggest that SIDS, ALTEs, and OSAHS may aggregate within the same families. Guilleminault and colleagues observed an elevated AHI and excessive daytime sleepiness among parents or grandparents in three of five families with children with SIDS or near-miss SIDS (103). The seven children with near-miss SIDS all had OSAHS when studied at age 12 months. Risk appeared to relate to the presence of a small posterior airway space and mandibular malocclusion. In a subsequent study, Guilleminault et al. identified 25 of a series of 700 infants with ALTE at ages up to 4.5 months (104). These individuals required polygraphic monitoring for periods in excess of one year. All 25 infants developed OSAHS by age 5. Kahn et al. (105,106) reviewed the polygraphs of 30 infants who ultimately died of SIDS. Obstructed breathing events were observed in 23 of the SIDS victims, but in only 9 of the 60 tracings from controls, who survived the first year of life (105,106). Sequeiros and Martins da Silva described a family that included six siblings with SIDS, one sibling with near-miss SIDS who had central sleep apnea at age 3.5 months, and two first-cousins with near-miss SIDS who had central sleep apnea at ages 3 and 5 years (107). Deray et al. found that the frequency of loud snoring in fathers of infants with SIDS or near-miss SIDS was more than twofold greater than that in fathers of control infants (108). On the other hand, Acres and associates were unable to find strict polysomnographic evidence of OSAHS in any of 12 parents of SIDS victims, although the number of apneic episodes in 2 of these parents was distinctly greater than those of all other parents (109). Mathur and Douglas, using a mail questionnaire survey, found 8 unexplained infant deaths among 29 families with a member with OSAHS, as compared to no infant deaths in 35 control families (15). In the Cleveland Family Study, 18 cases of sudden unexpected infant death or ALTEs were reported in 14 of 175 families that were recruited through an affected proband with laboratory confirmed OSAHS (case families). Two of 70 control families also had infants who died suddenly (3 cases) (110; Redline et al., unpublished data). All cases, in both case and control families, were in families where at least one member had polysomnography-confirmed OSAHS (16 of 205 families with OSAHS vs. 0 of 40 families without OSAHS). Members of families in which an aggregation of OSAHS, SIDS, and/or ALTEs were observed also tended to be brachycephalic (i.e., have a head form characterized by a width:anterior-posterior dimension >0.81) and had relatively smaller airway spaces and greater blunting of the hypoxic ventilatory response as compared to families without aggregation of these disorders (110). A recent survey of families identified through The Massachusetts Center for SIDS identified snoring or other sleep-related breathing problems in the parents of 10 of 25 SIDS victims (P. Tishler, M. Corwin, and M. McClain, unpublished data). In toto, the finding of an association between OSAHS and SIDS strongly suggests that there is a subset of families at risk for both disorders, perhaps because of the operation of common inherited anatomical and/or physiological risk factors.

D. Central Hypoventilation Syndromes and Lethal Infantile Apnea

The literature abounds with case reports and short series of patients with central hypoventilation syndromes, many manifest at or shortly after birth and some associated with early death (96,111–113). Many of the cases are due to severe chemoregulatory dysfunction, manifest as profound blunting of the hypercapnic and hypoxic ventilatory responses (112). Some are associated with marked developmental abnormalities of the brainstem or cerebral cortex. In the absence of frank neuromuscular or lung disease, such cases are labeled as idiopathic congenital central hypoventilation (CCH). Familiality in CCH has been described (114–117), and complex segregation analyses suggest that the disorder can be explained by either multifactoral threshold or major locus models (118). Interestingly, Hirschsprung's disease (HSCR), a congenital disorder characterized by intestinal dysmotility and absence of myenteric and submucosal ganglia in the distal bowel (119), occurs in approximately 20% of cases of CCH (120). Defects in genes for the receptor tyrosine kinase ret, endothelin-b receptor, and endothelin-3 have been described in subjects with HSCR (121). A mutation in endothelin-3 also has been identified in a case of CCH occurring in the absence of frank HSCR (121). This, together with the aforementioned co-occurrence of two rare diseases, has suggested that CCH and HSCR may share common pathogenetic etiologies related to disorders of neural crest development and migration, influencing central ventilatory control and colonic motility, respectively (122). Thus, identification of genes important for breathing may be facilitated by further understanding the pathogenesis and genetic bases for Hirschsprung's disease.

V. Approaches to the Identification of Genes Underlying OSAHS

A. Use of Intermediate Phenotypes

The multiplicity of potential etiologies for OSAHS and the likelihood that disease expression may be influenced by a number of factors, each of small to modest influence, augment the difficulties in identifying specific causal genes. The potential complexity of dissecting the genetic bases for OSAHS is shown in Figure 2, a model used by Schork to describe general approaches to the analysis of the genetics of complex diseases (123). A complex disease, or high-level phenotype, may be considered to be determined by a number of intermediate phenotypes, which in turn are determined by a number of lower-level phenotypes. Lower-level phenotypes may be more directly influenced by specific gene products than higher-level phenotypes, which often result as an expression of the operation of a number of factors, including lower-level phenotypes and environmental influences.

As seen in Figure 2 and summarized in Table 4, traits such as chemosensitivity, load compensation, connective tissue laxity, muscle fatigability, and central obesity may be considered intermediate phenotypes for OSAHS. In other words, these are traits that may be measured and defined more easily than a "complex" disease or syndrome; identification of genes for these traits may be easier than identifying genes for the higher-level phenotype. Genetic analyses of families with multiple affected members in whom disease etiology appears related to one of these risk factors may provide important insights into the genetic basis of traits associated with the complex phenotype. Examples of this approach are the choice of studying the genetics of atopy and bronchial responsiveness in asthmatic families (rather than "asthma") or of glucose intolerance and insulin resistance in diabetes. The utility of these approaches rests, in part, on the strength of the association between the

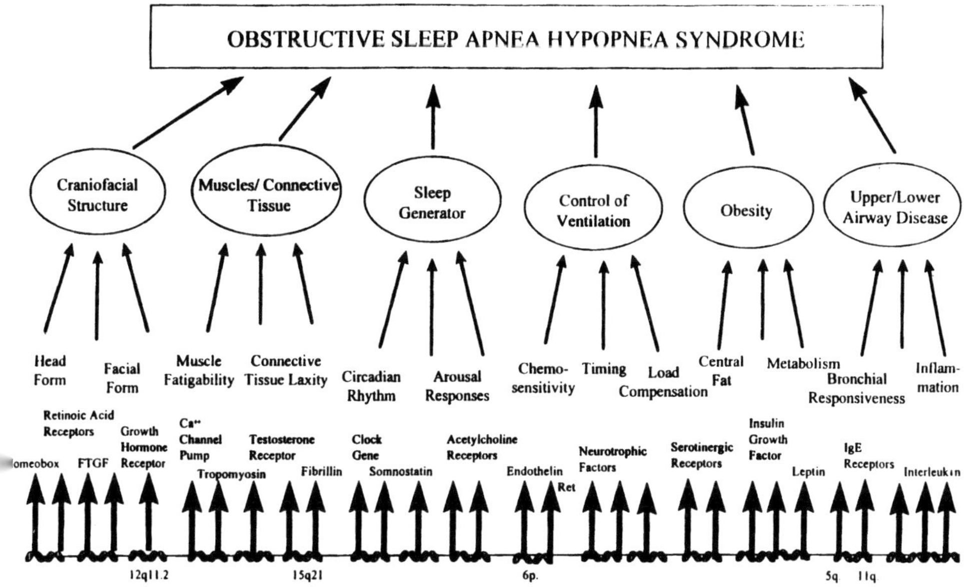

Figure 2 Theoretical schema showing the interrelationships among genes, low-level phenotypes, intermediate phenotypes, and high-level phenotypes (OSAHS).

trait and the complex phenotype, as well as the intrinsic interest in understanding the genetic bases for the given trait.

B. Studies of Biochemical and Genetic Markers

Studies of intermediate phenotypes for OSAHS would be greatly enhanced by identification of good biochemical markers of normal physiological or disease processes. The distribution of various biochemical markers in samples of OSAHS patients has been examined to understand how end-organ effects of OSAHS, such as sleepiness or hypertension, may be mediated. Two recent controlled studies in OSAHS subjects demonstrated elevations in levels of circulating endothelin-1 (124), a peptide with vasoconstrictor effects, and in the inflammatory cytokines tumor necrosis factor and interleukin (125). These elevations were thought to be secondary effects resulting from apnea-mediated hypoxia or adrenergic stimulation or from the obesity of the OSAHS subjects, rather than from primarily genetically aberrant physiological systems. A number of studies also have examined catecholamine and sex and growth hormone levels in OSAHS. However, data from these studies have not been used for phenotypic characterization of groups of subjects with OSAHS. Analyses also have not addressed the extent to which the biochemical perturbation was a primary or secondary phenomenon. Studies of the genetics of OSAHS may be greatly enhanced by the identification of serum markers associated inherently with disease

Table 4 Some Candidate Genes for OSAHS

Intermediate phenotypes	Candidate genes
Ventilatory control	RET-proto-oncogene
	Neurotrophic growth factors (BDNF, GDNF)
	Endothelin-1
	Endothelin-3
	Krox-20
	Retinoic acid receptor $\alpha\gamma$
Craniofacial structure	Homeobox genes
	TGF $\beta 2$
	Growth hormone receptors
	Growth factor receptors
	Retinoic acid receptor $\alpha\gamma$
	Endothelin-1
Obesity	Leptin
	Insulin growth factor
	Glucokinase
	Adenosine deaminase
	Melanocortin-3 receptor
	Tumor necrosis factor α
	Glucose regulatory protein
	Pro-opiomelanocortin
	Agouti homolog
Connective tissue	Fibrillin
	Testosterone receptors
Muscle function	Ca^{+}-K^{+} pump
	Tropomyosin

pathogenesis. In this regard, markers associated with derangements in neurotransmitters involved with central ventilatory control or with sleep homeostasis should be explored for their utility in better describing the OSAHS phenotype.

There has been minimal investigation of genetic markers in OSAHS. An approximately twofold increase in the HLA-A2 antigen was demonstrated in a sample of Japanese subjects with OSAHS as compared to age-matched controls (126). HLA-A2–positive subjects with OSAHS were more obese than OSA patients negative for this antigen, suggesting a relationship between this genetic marker and obesity. However, other phenotypic differences were not examined. HLA-DR2, which is strongly associated with narcolepsy, has not been found to be associated with OSAHS (127). A higher prevalence of the Lewis blood group phenotype Le(a + b−) was found in those who reported very disruptive snoring as compared to other snorers that comprised a subsample of Danish subjects with habitual snoring (9). The implication of this observation, which has not been confirmed, is not clear.

C. Animal Models of Disease

Animal models of disease could provide a broad, initial perspective toward identifying gene loci involved in the physiological underpinnings for traits such as ventilatory patterns, chemoregulation, fat distribution, and facial dysmorphisms. Selective breeding may create animals that model human illness or animals with a spectrum of traits, which, through quantitative trait linkage, allow identification of gene loci. Once loci are shown to have a significant correlation with a trait value, one can proceed to determine gene homologs and, then, proteins and structures that influence physiological variation or pathology in humans. The utility of these approaches is somewhat dependent on the appropriateness of the animal model to human physiological and pathological responses. The development of transgenic and knock-out animal models provides powerful means for identifying the physiological actions of genes of interest. However, even data from these highly sophisticated experiments require cautious extrapolation to humans, where physiological correlates may differ, or the expression of the trait may vary because of the operation of other genetic or environmental factors.

Animal Models of OSAHS

OSAHS animal models are few. Hendricks and associates have investigated respiration during wakefulness and sleep in the English bulldog, a highly inbred dog with daytime somnolence and sleep-disordered breathing (128). The dogs appear predisposed to OSA because of an abnormal upper airway anatomy, with brachycephaly, enlargement of the soft palate, and narrowing of the oropharynx. Myopathic changes, present in their upper airway muscles, possibly a secondary response to chronic loading, may contribute to pharyngeal obstruction (129). OSAHS in these dogs also appears related to abnormalities in central drive, as evidenced by experiments demonstrating exacerbations of OSA during rapid eye movement (REM) sleep, an association of apneic events with suppression of drive to both the diaphragm and upper airway muscles, and modulation of such responses by serotoninergic mediators (130,131). Thus, this animal model may simulate human disease well because the disorder appears to involve interactions between abnormal ventilatory physiology and abnormal upper airway anatomy. However, this same complexity may hinder identification of etiological genes.

Remarkable advances from the Human Genome Project make it possible to use rodent models for identifying genes that control specific physiological processes. Unfortunately, in mice, for which the most genetic data exist, physiological studies of sleep and breathing are limited by their small size. Neurophysiological and cardiopulmonary measurements are more easily made in rats, in which there is a limited but growing genetic data base. The upper airway anatomy and function of both the rat and the mouse is distinctly different from that of the human. Nevertheless, these animals may be useful and have been used for the study of ventilation and chemoregulation.

The traits of relevance to OSAHS that have been studied most in rodents are ventilatory patterns and chemoregulation. These traits have numerous biochemical, physiological, environmental, and genetic determinants and can be measured quantitatively. Like blood pressure and airway responses, variability in trait values is derived from a number of peripheral and central anatomical structures linked by an integrated control system.

Ventilatory Pattern and Chemoregulation

Tankersley and associates have used a mouse intercross strategy to study the inherited basis for respiratory frequency at rest (132). They observed significant interstrain differences in respiratory pattern (frequency and tidal volume) (133); inheritance pattern was most consistent with the operation of a small number of genes. Recently, this group reported linkage between phenotypic differences in inspiratory timing and two putative quantitative trait loci on mouse chromosome 3 (134). Candidate genes include a family of genes that encode neuroreceptors thought to be important in neural regulation of breathing (e.g., glycine receptor, glutamate receptor) and other genes that influence the postnatal development of the lung (e.g., basic fibroblast growth factor, bFGF). Strohl et al. reported measurements of ventilation and metabolism in four inbred strains of rats chosen for a wide variation in body weight and/or blood pressure regulation (135). Significant differences in the pattern of breathing persisted when animals were exposed to 100% oxygen, an observation that suggests genetic differences in the central regulation of breathing pattern. This group is exploring quantitative trait loci that influence these traits.

An inherited basis for ventilatory responsiveness to hypoxemia or hypercapnia is supported by a limited number of observations in animals. In 1984, Ou et al. reported that differences in resting ventilation and ventilatory responses to hypoxia differed between two lines of Sprague-Dawley rats obtained from different vendors (136). These differences in ventilatory responsiveness correlated with differences in erythropoietic and pulmonary vascular pressor responses to chronic hypobaric hypoxia (137). Tankersley et al. demonstrated significant interstrain differences in hypoxic responsiveness and hypercapnic responsiveness (133). Comparing differences in breathing among different rat strains, Strohl and associates showed that tidal volume and minute ventilation in response to inhalation of 7% CO_2 differed between rat strains (138). Heritability estimates (h^2) for frequency and minute ventilation during hypercapnia were >0.50. The findings of both Tankersley and Strohl suggest that a substantial proportion of the variation in ventilation during chemical loading may be explained by genetic rather than environmental factors.

Knock-out and transgenic mouse models have been used to identify genes potentially important in the control of ventilation. A European group has identified the zinc finger protein Krox-20, which affects the development of the hindbrain. When it is deleted by homologous recombination, mice demonstrate slow respiratory frequencies and long apneas (139). Katz and coworkers have shown in a knock-out mouse model that loss of brain-derived neurotrophic factor (BDNF) results in reduced survival of neurons in the nodose-petrosal ganglion (140). Homozygous mice demonstrated irregular and depressed ventilation, including spontaneous apneas, and abnormalities in chemoregulation, specifically related to hyperoxia but not to hypercapnia. Heterozygous mice demonstrated ventilatory responses intermediate to those of wild-type and homozygous mice, suggesting that nonlethal alterations in the genetic control of neural growth factors may contribute to phenotypic variations in ventilatory traits (140). The RET proto-oncogene, which has been implicated in HSCR (141,142), also modulates ventilatory responses to carbon dioxide, as shown by the demonstration of progressive reductions in the hypercapnic ventilatory responses of heterozygous and homozygous RET knock-out mice (122). As noted previously, CCH also is associated with HSCR, thus providing support in humans for this evidence in mice of the importance of RET in ventilatory control. Endothelin-1 (ET-1) (6p24-p23), a potent vasoactive peptide, may also participate in control of ventilation. In a knock-out mouse model, absence of ET-1 results in respiratory failure, ventilatory control abnormalities, craniofacial abnormalities, and hypertension, characteristics remarkably similar to traits found in OSAHS (49). Mutant mice deficient in ET-1 have impaired ventilatory responses to both hypoxia and hypercapnia (143). The findings of reductions in both responses suggest impairment of central control mechanisms.

Models of Spontaneous Apneas

The occurrence of spontaneous apneas during sleep may be examined to provide insight into aspects of ventilatory control that may be relevant to OSAHS. The rat can exhibit spontaneous apneas during sleep. Carley and associates have observed the occurrence of spontaneous apneas to differ among rat strains, in particular between hypertensive and nonhypertensive strains (144). The extent to which the apneas were secondary to blood pressure changes rather than represent primary genetic differences is under active investigation.

Obesity

A number of single gene mutations have been implicated in obesity in mice, involving chromosomes 4 (*db*), 6 (*ob*), 7 (*tub* and *Ad*), 8 (*fat*), and 2 (agouti) (145). Mutations have been associated with a variety of protein abnormalities leading to neuroendocrine disturbances, including hyperinsulinemia (145).

There is growing interest in studying ventilation in genetically obese rodents as a means for both understanding the physiological correlates of obesity and exploring the effects of pleiotropy; i.e., the extent to which one gene or set of genes may influence a number of related traits. For example, in OSAHS, genes that influence body fat distribution also may influence insulin resistance, chest wall mechanics, upper airway patency, and ventilatory responses. In this regard, the Zucker obese rat, homozygous at the *fatty* locus (146), shows impaired chest wall mechanics, insulin resistance, and metabolic and ventilatory differences that model the obese state in humans (147). Recently, the *ob/ob* mouse has been shown to have blunted ventilatory responses to hypercapnia, suggesting that leptin may influence the control of breathing (148). Animal models like this may be increasingly useful to elucidate the role of specific genetic aberrations in producing complex phenotypes. The potential for pleiotropic effects to explain the co-occurrence of OSAHS, central obesity, and hyperinsulinemia provides intriguing avenues to pursue parallel studies of the biochemical linkages among these disorders and of their genetic bases.

VI. Finding the Genes for OSAHS

Table 4 summarizes a number of specific potential candidate genes for the intermediate phenotypes associated with OSAHS, most of which were discussed in previous sections. Factors that influence hindbrain, cervical spinal cord, and nodose-petrosal ganglionic development may be anticipated to influence the control of breathing as well as craniofacial structure. These broadly include the family of homeobox genes (Hox), zinc finger genes (139), genes involved in neural crest differentiation and development (48,49), and neuronal growth factors [glial-derived neurotrophic factor, GDNF, and BDNF (140)], members of the transforming growth factor-β family (47), and their respective receptors. Other candidate genes may influence several traits relevant to OSAHS. Fibrillin (15q21.1), when abnormal, contributes to both craniofacial dysmorphism and upper airway connective tissue laxity (149). Other loci of interest may be elsewhere on chromosome 15, mutations of which may result in a number of somatic abnormalities (e.g., Prader-Willi syndrome) as well as OSAHS.

VII. Summary

OSAHS is a classic complex disorder, influenced almost certainly by multiple factors, including multiple genes, environmental influences, and developmental factors. Its etiology and perhaps its clinical manifestations also are probably heterogeneous. Describing samples with more homogeneous characteristics is often difficult because it appears that disease occurs because of the interaction among a number of risk factors, with the overall import of any one unclear, and because there are few biochemical ''markers'' to improve disease classification. Despite these challenges, there is growing evidence from clinical and epidemiological studies that genetic influences importantly influence the expression of OSAHS. The overall magnitude of the effect that may be attributable to genetic factors, and whether the disorder is due to genes of large effect requires, further definition. Recent animal work and studies in humans have provided intriguing clues to the possibilities of a number of candidate genes related to growth factor regulation, neural development, and other areas influencing ventilatory control and craniofacial structure. Further understanding of the actions of these genes will provide insight into the development of neuroanatomic interconnections needed for normal physiology and may also shed light on pathogenetic processes influential in OSAHS.

Acknowledgment

This work was supported by the NIH NHLBI, HL 46380.

References

1. Redline S, Tishler PV. Familial influences on sleep apnea. In: Saunders NA, Sullivan CE, eds. Sleep and Breathing Disturbances. 2d ed. New York: Marcel Dekker, 1994: 363–377.
2. Strohl KP, Saunders NA, Feldman NT, Hallett M. Obstructive sleep apnea in family members. N Engl J Med 1978; 299:969–973.
3. Manon-Espaillat R, Gothe B, Adams N, Newman C, Ruff R. Familial 'sleep apnea plus' syndrome. Report of a family. Neurology 1988; 38:190–193.
4. Wittig RM, Zorick FJ, Roehrs TA, Sicklesteel JM, Roth T. Familial childhood sleep apnea. Henry Ford Hosp Med J 1988; 36:13–15.
5. El-Bayadi S, Millman RP, Tishler PV, Rosenberg C, Boucher MA, Redline S. A family study of sleep apnea: anatomic and physiologic interactions. Chest 1990; 98:554–559.
6. Kaprio J, Koskenvuo M, Partinen M, Telakivi I. A twin study of snoring (abstr). Sleep Res 1988; 17:365.
7. Ferini-Strambi L, Calori G, Oldani A, et al. Snoring in twins. Respir Med 1995; 89: 337–340.
8. Redline S, Tosteson T, Tishler PV, Carskadon MA, Millman R. Studies of the genetics of obstructive sleep apnea: familial aggregation of symptoms associated with sleep related breathing disturbances. Am Rev Respir Dis 1992; 145:440–444.
9. Jennum P, Hein HO, Suadicani P, Sorensen H, Gyntelberg F. Snoring, family history, and genetic markers in men: The Copenhagen Male Study. Chest 1995; 107:1289–1293.
10. Pillar G, Lavie P. Assessment of the role of inheritance in sleep apnea syndrome. Am J Respir Crit Care Med 1995; 151:688–691.
11. Mathur R, Douglas NJ. Family studies in patients with the sleep apnea-hypopnea syndrome. Ann Intern Med 1995; 122:174–178.
12. Redline S, Tishler PV, Tosteson TD, et al. The familial aggregation of obstructive sleep apnea. Am J Respir Crit Care Med 1995; 151:682–687.
13. Guilleminault C, Partinen M, Hollman K, Powell N, Stoohs R. Familial aggregates in obstructive sleep apnea syndrome. Chest 1995; 107:1545–1551.
14. Douglas NJ, Luke M, Mathur R. Is the sleep apnoea/hypopnoea syndrome inherited? Thorax 1993; 48:719–721.
15. Mathur R, Douglas NJ. Relation between sudden infant death syndrome and adult-sleep apnoea/hypopnoea syndrome. Lancet 1994; 344:819–820.
16. Collins JS, Go RCP. Disease classification and transmission effects on linkage analysis in the NIMH1 bipolar disorder pedigrees. Genetic Epidemiol 1997; 14:587–592.
17. Redline S, Briones B, Spry K, Tishler PV, Dockery DW. What is a 'normal' Respiratory Disturbance Index? Am J Respir Crit Care Med 1995; 151:A104.
18. Elston RC, Stewart J. A general model for the genetic analysis of pedigree data. Hum Hered 1971; 21:523–542.
19. Holberg CJ, Natrajan S, Cline MG, Quan SF. Family aggregation and segregation analysis of snoring. Am J Respir Crit Care Med 1997; 155:A844.

20. Guilleminault C. Clinical features and evaluation of obstructive sleep apnea. In: Kryger MH, Roth T, Dement WC, eds. Principles and Practice of Sleep Medicine. Philadelphia: Saunders, 1989:552–558.
21. Bliwise DL, Feldman DE, Bliwise NE, et al.. Risk factors for sleep disordered breathing in heterogeneous geriatric populations. J Am Geriatr Soc 1987; 35:132–141.
22. Bray G, Bouchard C. Genetics of human obesity: research directions. FASEB J 1997; 11:937–945.
23. Strunkard AJ, Harris JR, Pedersen NL, McClearn GE. The body-mass index of twins who have been reared apart. N Engl J Med 1990; 322:1483–1487.
24. Bodurtha JN, Mosteller M, Hewitt JK, et al. Genetic analysis of anthropometric measures in 11-year-old twins: the Medical College of Virginia Twin Study. Pediatr Res 1990; 28:1–4.
25. Comuzzie AG, Blangero J, Mahaney MC, et al. Major gene with sex-specific effects influences fat mass in Mexican Americans. Genet Epidemiol 1995; 12:475–488.
26. Rice T, Borecki IB, Bouchard C, Rao DC. Segregation analysis of body mass index in an unselected French-Canadian sample: The Quebec family study. Obesity Res 1993; 1:288–294.
27. Lecomte E, Herbeth B, Nicaud V, Rakotovao R, Artur Y, Tiret L. Segregation analysis of fat mass and fat-free mass with age- and sex-dependent effects: The Stanislas Family Study. Genet Epidem 1997; 14:51–62.
28. Trayhurn P. The development of obesity in animals: the role of genetic susceptibility. Clin Endocrinol Metab 1984; 13:451–474.
29. Van Itallie TB. Obesity, genetics and ponderal set point. Clin Neuropharmacol 1988; 11 (suppl 1):S1–7.
30. Bray GA. Genetic and hypothalamic mechanisms for obesity—finding the needle in the haystack. Am J Clin Nutr 1989; 50:891–902.
31. Ravussin E, Bogardus C. Energy expenditure in the obese: is there a thrifty gene? Infusionstherapie 1990; 17:108–112.
32. Comuzzie AG, Hixson JE, Almasy L, et al. A major quantitative trait locus determining serum leptin levels and fat mass is located on human chromosome 2. Nature Genetics 1997; 15:273–276.
33. Norman RA, Thompson DB, Foroud T, et al. Genome-wide search for genes influencing percent body fat in Pima Indians: suggestive linkage at chromosome 11q21-q22. Am J Hum Genet 1997; 60:166–173.
34. Norman RA, Bogardus C, Ravussin E. Linkage between obesity and a marker near the tumor necrosis factor locus in Pima Indians. J Clin Invest 1995; 96:158–162.
35. Lembertas AV, Perusse L, Chagnon YC, et al. Identification of an obesity quantitative trait locus on mouse chromosome 2 and evidence of linkage to body fat and insulin on the human homologous region 20q. J Clin Invest 1997; 100:1240–1247.
36. Bouchard C. Genetic factors in obesity. Med Clin North Am 1989; 73:67–81.
37. Mortimore IL, Marshall I, Wraith PK, Sellar RJ, Douglas NJ. Neck and total body fat deposition in nonobese and obese patients with sleep apnea compared to that in control subjects. Am J Respir Crit Care Med 1998; 157:280–283.
38. Harris JR, Tambs K, Magnus P. Sex-specific effects for body mass index in the new Norwegian twin panel. Genet Epidem 1995; 12:251–265.
39. Lowe AA, Santamaria JD, Fleetham JA, Price C. Facial morphology and obstructive sleep apnea. Am J Orthod Dentofacial Orthop 1986; 90:484–91.

40. Jamieson A, Guilleminault C, Partinen M. Obstructive sleep apnea patients have craniomandibular abnormalities. Sleep 1986; 9:469–477.
41. Bacon WH, Krieger J, Turlot J-C, Stierle JL. Craniofacial characteristics in patients with obstructive sleep apneas syndrome. Cleft Palate J 1988; 25:374–378.
42. Guilleminault C, Riley R, Powell N. Obstructive sleep apnea and abnormal cephalometric measurements. Implications for treatment. Chest 1984; 86:793–794.
43. Riley R, Guilleminault C, Herran J, Powell N. Cephalometric analyses and flow-volume loops in obstructive sleep apnea patients. Sleep 1983; 6:303–311.
44. Osborne RH, De George FV. Genetic Basis of Morphologic Variation; An Evaluation and Application of the Twin Study Method. Cambridge MA: Harvard University Press, 1959.
45. Lundstrom A. Nature versus nurture in dentofacial variation. Eur J Orthod 1984; 6: 77–91.
46. Nance WE, Nakata M, Paul TD, Yu PI. The use of twin studies in the analysis of phenotypic traits in man. In: Janerich DT, Skalko RG, Porter IH, eds. Congential Defects. New Directions in Research. New York: Academic Press, 1974:23–49.
47. Sanford LP, Ormsby I, Gittenberger-de Groot AC, et al. TGF Beta-2 knockout mice have multiple developmental defects that are non-overlapping with other TGF beta knockout phenotypes. Development 1997; 124:2659–2670.
48. Lohnes D, Mark M, Mendelsohn C, et al. Function of the retinoic acid receptors (RARs) during development. (I) Craniofacial and skeletal abnormalities in RAR double mutants. Development 1994; 120:2723–2748.
49. Kurihara Y, Kurihara H, Suzuki H, et al. Elevated blood pressure and craniofacial abnormalities in mice deficient in endothelin-1. Nature 1994; 368:703–710.
50. Redline S, Tishler PV, Hans MG, Tosteson TD, Strohl KP, Spry K. Racial differences in sleep-disordered breathing in African Americans and Caucasians. Am J Respir Crit Care Med 1997; 155:186–192.
51. Strohl KP, Cherniack NS, Gothe B. Physiologic basis of therapy for sleep apnea. Am Rev Respir Dis 1986; 134:791–802.
52. Cherniack NS. Respiratory dysrhythmias during sleep. N Engl J Med 1981; 305:325–330.
53. Dempsey JA, Skatrud JB. A sleep-induced apneic threshold and its consequences. Am Rev Respir Dis 1986; 133:1163–1170.
54. Gleeson K, Zwillich CW, White DP. Chemosensitivity and the ventilatory response to airflow obstruction during sleep. J Appl Physiol 1989; 67:1630 1637.
55. Kunitomo F, Kimura H, Tatsumi K, et al. Abnormal breathing during sleep and chemical control of breathing during wakefulness in patients with sleep apnea syndrome. Am Rev Respir Dis 1989; 139:164–169.
56. Martin RJ, Ballard RD, Hudgel DW, Hill PL. The effects of weight and chemosensitivity on respiratory sleep abnormalities: A family study. Int J Obesity 1986; 10:283–292.
57. Moore GC, Zwillich CW, Battaglia JD, Cotton EK, Weil JV. Respiratory failure associated with familial depression of ventilatory response to hypoxia and hypercapnia. N Engl J Med 1976; 295:861–865.
58. Fleetham JA, Arnup ME, Anthonisen NR. Familial aspects of ventilatory control in patients with chronic obstructive pulmonary disease. Am Rev Respir Dis 1984; 129: 3–7.

59. Kawakami Y, Irie T, Shida A, Yoshikawa T. Familial factors affecting arterial blood gas values and respiratory chemosensitivity in chronic obstructive pulmonary disease. Am Rev Respir Dis 1982; 125:420–425.
60. Mountain R, Zwillich C, Weil J. Hypoventilation in obstructive lung disease: the role of familial factors. N Engl J Med 1978; 298:521–525.
61. Hudgel DW, Weil JV. Asthma associated with decreased hypoxic ventilatory drive: a family study. Ann Intern Med 1974; 80:622–625.
62. Collins DD, Scoggin CH, Zwillich CW, Weil JV. Hereditary aspects of decreased hypoxic response. J Clin Invest 1978; 62:105–110.
63. Kawakami Y, Yamamoto H, Yoshikawa T, Shida A. Chemical and behavioral control of breathing in adult twins. Am Rev Respir Dis 1984; 129:703–707.
64. Thomas DA, Swaminathan S, Beardsmore CS, et al. Comparison of peripheral chemoreceptor responses in monozygotic and dizygotic twin infants. Am Rev Respir Dis 1993; 148:1605–1609.
65. Kobayashi S, Nishimura M, Yamamoto M, Akiyama Y, Kishi F, Kawakami Y. Dyspnea sensation and chemical control of breathing in adult twins. Am Rev Respir Dis 1993; 147:1192–1198.
66. Beall CM, Strohl KP, Blangero J, et al. Ventilation and hypoxic ventilatory response of Tibetan and Aymara high altitude natives. Am J Phys Anthropol 1997; 104:427–444.
67. Beral V, Read DJC. Insensitivity of respiratory center to carbon dioxide in the Enga people of New Guinea. Lancet 1971; 2:1290–1294.
68. Saunders NA, Leeder SR, Rebuck AS. Ventilatory response to carbon dioxide in young athletes: a family study. Am Rev Respir Dis 1976; 113:497–502.
69. Arkinstall WW, Nirmel K, Kilssouras V, Milic-Emili J. Genetic differences in the ventilatory response to inhaled CO_2. J Appl Physiol 1974; 36:6–11.
70. Santiago TV, Scardella AT, Edelman NH. Determinants of the ventilatory responses to hypoxia during sleep. Am Rev Respir Dis 1984; 130:179–182.
71. Phillipson EA, Bowes G, Sullivan CE, Woolf GM. The influence of sleep fragmentation on arousal and ventilatory responses to respiratory stimuli. Sleep 1980; 3:281–288.
72. Gislason T, Tammivaara R. Airway obstruction, obesity and CO_2 ventilatory responsiveness in the sleep apnea syndrome. Upsala J Med Sci 1992; 97:141–148.
73. Guilleminault C, Cummiskey J. Progressive improvement of apnea index and ventilatory response to CO_2 after tracheostomy in obstructive sleep apnea syndrome. Am Rev Respir Dis 1982; 126:14–20.
74. Berthon-Jones M, Sullivan CE. Time course of change in ventilatory response to CO_2 with long-term CPAP therapy for obstructive sleep apnea. Am Rev Respir Dis 1987; 135:144–147.
75. Greenberg HE, Scharf SM. Depressed ventilatory load compensation in sleep apnea: Reversal by nasal CPAP. Am Rev Respir Dis 1993; 148:1610–1615.
76. Redline S, Leitner J, Arnold J, Tishler PV, Altose MD. Ventilatory control abnormalities in familial sleep apnea. Am J Respir Crit Care Med 1997; 156:155–160.
77. Lavie P, Rubin AE. Effects of nasal occlusion on respiration in sleep. Evidence of the inheritability of sleep apnea proneness. Acta Otolaryngol 1984; 97:127–130.
78. Pillar G, Schnall RP, Peled NIR, Oliven A, Lavie P. Impaired respiratory response to resistive loading during sleep in healthy offspring of patients with obstructive sleep apnea. Am J Respir Crit Care Med 1997; 155:1602–1608.

79. Lee B, Godfrey M, Vitale E, et al. Linkage of Marfan syndrome and a phenotypically related disorder to two different fibrillin genes. Nature 1991; 352:330–334.
80. Dietz HC, McIntosh I, Sakai LY, et al. Four novel FBN1 mutations: significance for mutant transcript level and EGF-like domain calcium binding in the pathogenesis of Marfan syndrome. Genomics 1993; 17:468–475.
81. Cistulli PA, Sullivan CE. Sleep-disordered breathing in Marfan's syndrome. Am Rev Respir Dis 1993; 147:645–648.
82. Cistulli PA, Sullivan CE. Sleep apnea in Marfan's syndrome: Increased upper-airway collapsibility during sleep. Chest 1995; 108:631–635.
83. Cistulli PA, Richards GN, Palmisano RG, Unger G, Berthon-Jones M, Sullivan CE. Influence of maxillary constriction on nasal resistance and sleep apnea severity in patients with Marfan's syndrome. Chest 1996; 110:1184–1188.
84. Clarke DJ, Waters J, Corbett JA. Adults with Prader-Willi syndrome: abnormalities of sleep and behavior. J Roy Soc Med 1989; 82:21–24.
85. Cassidy SB, McKillop JA, Morgan WJ. Sleep disorders in Prader-Willi syndrome. Dysmorphol Clin Genet 1990; 4:13–17.
86. Hertz G, Cataletto M, Feinsilver SH, Angulo M. Developmental trends of sleep-disordered breathing in Prader-Willi syndrome: the role of obesity. Am J Med Genet 1995; 56:188–190.
87. Velo-Bueno A, Kales A, Soldatos CR, et al. Sleep in the Prader-Willi syndrome. Clinical and polygraphic findings. Arch Neurol 1984; 41:294–296.
88. Arens R, Gozal D, Omlin KJ, et al. Hypoxic and hypercapnic ventilatory responses in Prader-Willi syndrome. J Appl Physiol 1994; 77:2224–2230.
89. Gozal D, Arens R, Omlin KJ, Ward SL, Keens TG. Absent peripheral chemosensitivity in Prader-Willi syndrome. J Appl Physiol 1994; 77:2231–2236.
90. Schluter B, Buschatz D, Trowitzsch E, Aksu F, Andler W. Respiratory control in children with Prader-Willi syndrome. Eur J Pediatr 1997; 156:65–68.
91. Gozal D, Torres JE, Menendez AA. Longitudinal assessment of hypercapnic ventilatory drive after tracheotomy in a patient with the Prader-Willi syndrome. Eur Respir J 1996; 9:1565–1568.
92. Yang T, Adamson T, Wevrick R, Francke U, Brannan CI. A mouse model for Prader-Willi syndrome. Am J Hum Genet 1997; 61:A39.
93. MacDonal HR, Wevrick R. The necdin gene is deleted in Prader-Willi syndrome and is imprinted in human and mouse. Hum Mol Genet 1997; 6:1873–1878.
94. Allen RP, Singer HS, Brown JE, Salam MM. Sleep disorders in Tourette syndrome: a primary or unrelated problem? Pediat Neurol 1992; 8:275–280.
95. Sverd J, Montero G. Is Tourette syndrome a cause of sudden infant death syndrome and childhood obstructive sleep apnea? Am J Med Genet 1993; 46:494–496.
96. Wilson DO, Sanders MH, Dauber JH. Abnormal ventilatory chemosensitivity and congenital myopathy. Arch Intern Med 1987; 147:1773–1777.
97. Wennergren G, Milerad J, Lagercrantz H, et al. The epidemiology of sudden infant death syndrome and attacks of lifelessness in Sweden. Acta Paediatr Scand 1987; 76: 898–906.
98. Buck GM, Cookfair DL, Michalek AM, et al. Intrauterine growth retardation and risk of sudden infant death syndrome (SIDS). Am J Epidemiol 1989; 129:874–884.
99. Beal SM, Blundell HM. Recurrence incidence of sudden infant death syndrome. Arch Dis Child 1988; 63:924–930.

100. Oren J, Kelley DH, Shannon DC. Familial occurrence of sudden infant death syndrome and apnea of infancy. Pediatrics 1987; 80:355–358.
101. Schulte FJ, Albani M, Schnizer H, Bentele K. Neuronal control of neonatal respiration—sleep apnea and the sudden infant death syndrome. Neuropediatrics 1982; 13(suppl):3–14.
102. Schiffman PL, Friedman B, Santiago TV, Edelman NA. Effect of naloxone on ventilatory control in parents of victims of sudden infant death syndrome. Am Rev Respir Dis 1984; 130:964–968.
103. Guilleminault C, Heldt G, Powell N, Riley R. Small upper airway in near-miss sudden infant death syndrome infants and their families. Lancet 1986; 1:402–407.
104. Guilleminault C, Stoohs R. From apnea of infancy to obstructive sleep apnea syndrome in the young child. Chest 1992; 102:1065–1071.
105. Kahn A, Blum D, Rebuffat E, et al. Polysomnographic studies of infants who subsequently died of sudden infant death syndrome. Pediatrics 1988; 82:721–727.
106. Kahn A, Grosswasser J, Rebuffat E, et al. Sleep and cardiorespiratory characteristics of infant victims of sudden death: a prospective case-control study. Sleep 1992; 15: 287–292.
107. Sequeiros J, Martins da Silva A. Autosomal dominant central sleep apnea: the sudden infant death syndrome (SIDS), infantile sleep apnea (''near-miss SIDS''), and asymptomatic carriers in two generations of a large family. Am J Hum Genet 1988; 43 (suppl):A70.
108. Deray MJ, Duchowny MS, Resnick T. Snoring in fathers of infants with SIDS and apnea (abstr). Sleep Res 1987; 16:176.
109. Acres JC, Sweatman P, West P, Brownell L, Kryger MH. Breathing during sleep in parents of sudden infant death syndrome victims. Am Rev Respir Dis 1982; 125:163–166.
110. Tishler PV, Redline S, Ferrette V, Hans M, Altose MD. The associations of sudden unexpected infant death with obstructive sleep apnea. Am J Respir Crit Care Med 1996; 153:1857–1863.
111. Perry TL, Wright JM, Berry K, Hansen S, Perry TL, Jr. Dominantly inherited apathy, central hypoventilation, and Parkinson's syndrome: clinical, biochemical, and neuropathologic studies of 2 new cases. Neurology 1990; 40:1882–1887.
112. Paton JY, Swaminathan S, Sargent CW, Keens TG. Hypoxic and hypercapnic ventilatory responses in awake children with congenital central hypoventilation syndrome. Am Rev Respir Dis 1989; 140:368–372.
113. Adickes ED, Buehler BA, Sanger WG. Familial lethal sleep apnea. Hum Genet 1986; 73:39–43.
114. Kerbl R, Litscher H, Grubbauer H, et al. Congenital central hypoventilation syndrome (Ondine's curse syndrome) in two siblings: delayed diagnosis and successful noninvasive treatment. Eur J Pediatr 1996; 155:977–980.
115. Whyte KF, Gugger M, Gould GA, Molloy J, Wraith PK, Douglas NJ. Accuracy of respiratory inductive plethysmograph in measuring tidal volume during sleep. J Appl Physiol 1991; 71:1866–1871.
116. Khalifa MM, Flavin MA, Wherrett BA. Congenital central hypoventilation syndrome in monozygotic twins. J Pediatr 1988; 113:853–855.
117. Haddad GG, Mazza NM, Defendini R, et al. Congenital failure of automatic control of ventilation, gastrointestinal motility and heart rate. Medicine 1978; 57:517–526.
118. Weese-Mayer DE, Silvestri JM, Marazita ML, Hoo JT. Congenital central hypoventila-

tion syndrome: inheritance and relation to sudden infant death syndrome. Am J Med Genet 1993; 47:360–367.

119. Kapur RP. Contemporary approaches toward understanding the pathogenesis of Hirschsprung disease. Pediatr Pathol 1993; 13:83–100.
120. Minutillo C, Pemberton PJ, Goldblatt J. Hirschsprung's disease and Ondine's curse: further evidence for a distinct syndrome. Clin Genet 1989; 36:200–203.
121. Bolk S, Angrist M, Schwartz S, Silvestri JM, Weese-Mayer DE, Chakravarti A. Congenital central hypoventilation syndrome: mutation analysis of the receptor tyrosine kinase RET. Am J Med Genet 1996; 63:603–609.
122. Burton MD, Kawashima A, Brayer JA, et al. RET proto-oncogene is important for the development of respiratory CO_2 sensitivity. J Auton Nerv Sys 1997; 63:137–143.
123. Ghosh S, Schork NJ. Genetic analysis of NIDDM: the study of quantitative traits. Diabetes 1996; 45:1–14.
124. Saarelainen S, Seppala E, Laasonen K, Hasan J. Circulating endothelin-1 in obstructive sleep apnea. Endothelium 1997; 5:115–118.
125. Vgontzas AN, Papanicolaou DA, Bixler EO, Kales A, Tyson K, Chrousos GP. Elevation of plasma cytokines in disorders of excessive daytime sleepiness: role of sleep disturbance and obesity. J Clin Endocrinol Metab 1997; 82:1313–1316.
126. Yoshizawa T, Akashiba T, Kurashina K, Otsuka K, Horie T. Genetics and obstructive sleep apnea syndrome: a study of human leukocyte antigen (HLA) typing. Int Med 1993; 32:94–97.
127. Rubin RL, Hajdukovich RM, Mitler MM. HLA-DR2 association with excessive somnolence in narcolepsy does not generalize to sleep apnea and is not accompanied by systemic autoimmune abnormalities. Clin Immunol Immunopathol 1988; 49:149–158.
128. Hendricks JC, Kline LR, Kovalski RJ, O'Brien JA, Morrison AR, Pack AI. The English bulldog: a natural model of sleep-disordered breathing. J Appl Physiol 1987; 63:1344–1350.
129. Schotland HM, Insko EK, Panckeri KA, Leigh JS, Pack AI, Hendricks JC. Quantitative magnetic resonance imaging of upper airways musculature in an animal model of sleep apnea. J Appl Physiol 1996; 81:1339–1346.
130. Hendricks JC, Kovalski RJ, Kline LR. Phasic respiratory muscle patterns and sleep-disordered breathing during rapid eye movement sleep in the English bulldog. Am Rev Respir Dis 1991; 144:1112–1120.
131. Veasey SC, Panckeri KA, Hoffman EA, Pack AI, Hendricks JC. The effects of serotonin antagonists in an animal model of sleep-disordered breathing. Am J Respir Crit Care Med 1996; 153:776–786.
132. Tankersley CG, Fitzgerald RS, Mitzner WA, Kleeberger SR. Hypercapnic ventilatory responses in mice differentially susceptible to acute ozone exposure. J Appl Physiol 1993; 75:2613–2619.
133. Tankersley CG, Fitzgerald RS, Kleeberger SR. Differential control of ventilation among inbred strains of mice. Am J Physiol 1994; 267:R1371–R1377.
134. Tankersley CG, Fitzgerald RS, Levitt RC, Mitzner WA, Ewart SL, Kleeberger SR. Genetic control of differential baseline breathing pattern. J Appl Physiol 1997; 82: 874–881.
135. Strohl KP, Thomas AJ, St. Jean P, Schlenker EH, Koletsky RJ, Schork NJ. Ventilation and metabolism among rat strains. J Appl Physiol 1997; 82:317–323.
136. Ou LC, Hill NS, Tenney SM. Ventilatory responses and blood gases in susceptible and resistant rats to high altitude. Respir Physiol 1984; 58:161–170.

137. Ou LC, Smith RP. Probable strain differences of rats in susceptibilities and cardiopulmonary responses to chronic hypoxia. Respir Physiol 1983; 53:367–377.
138. Strohl KP, Thomas AJ, St. Jean P, Schlenker EH, Schork N. Estimates of heritability for ventilatory traits from a rat intercross. Am J Respir Crit Care 1997; 155:A444.
139. Jacquin TD, Borday Y, Schneider-Maundury S, et al. Reorganization of pontine rhythmogenic neuronal networks in Krox-20 knockout mice. Neuron 1996; 17:747–758.
140. Erickson JT, Conover JC, Borday V, et al. Mice lacking brain-derived neurotrophic factor exhibit visceral sensory neuron losses distinct from mice lacking NT4 and display a severe developmental deficit in control of breathing. J Neurosci 1996; 16:5361–5371.
141. Edery P, Lyonnet S, Mulligan LM, et al. Mutations of the RET proto-oncogene in Hirschsprung's disease. Nature 1994; 367:378–380.
142. Romeo G, Ronchetto P, Luo Y, et al. Point mutations affecting the tyrosine kinase domain of the RET proto-oncogene in Hirschsprung's disease. Nature 1994; 367:377–378.
143. Kuwaki T, Cao W-H, Kurihara Y, et al. Impaired ventilatory responses to hypoxia and hypercapnia in mutant mice deficient in endothelin-1. Am J Physiol 1996; 270: R1279–R1286.
144. Carley DW, Trbovic SM, Radulovacki M. Hydralazine reduces elevated sleep apnea index in spontaneously hypertensive (SHR) rats to equivalence with normotensive Wistar-Kyoto rats. Sleep 1996; 19:363–366.
145. Naggert JK, Fricker LD, Varlamov O, et al. Hyperproinsulinaemia in obese *fat/fat* mice associated with a carboxypeptidase E mutation which reduces enzyme activity. Nat Genet 1995; 10:135–142.
146. Kershaw EE, Chua SC, Williams JA, Murphy EH, Leibel RL. Molecular mapping of SSRs for Pgm1 and C8b in the vicinity of the rat fatty locus. Genomics 1995; 27: 149–154.
147. Farkas GA, Schlenker EH. Pulmonary ventilation and mechanics in morbidly obese Zucker rats. Am J Respir Crit Care Med 1994; 150:356–362.
148. Schaub CD, Tankersley C, Schwartz AR, Smith PL, Robothham JL, O'Donnell CP. Blunted hypercapnic ventilatory sensitivity and elevated $PaCO_2$ in the genetically obese (ob/ob) mouse. Proceedings of the 5th International Symposium on Sleep and Breathing Symposium, Edinburgh, October 5–7, 1997.
149. Hollister DW, Godfrey M, Sakai LY, Pyeritz RE. Immunohistologic abnormalities of the microfibrillar-fiber system in the Marfan syndrome. N Engl J Med 1990; 323:152–159.

9

Mechanisms of Sleepiness in Obstructive Sleep Apnea

DEEPAK K. CHUGH

MCP Hahnemann University Hospital
Philadelphia, Pennsylvania

DAVID F. DINGES

University of Pennsylvania School of Medicine
Philadelphia, Pennsylvania

Sleepiness is a major problem for many patients with obstructive sleep apnea syndrome (OSAS). In fact, daytime sleepiness and tiredness are the most commonly reported presenting complaints of OSAS patients (1). Young and colleagues (2) reported that 2% of women and 4% of men in a middle-aged population had an apnea-hypopnea score of 5 or higher along with self-reported hypersomnolence. Lavie (3), in a survey of industrial workers in Israel, found that 40% of the subjects who reported daytime sleepiness had more than 5 apneas per sleep hour and 52% of respondents with daytime sleepiness had a history of work-related accidents as compared to 36% of respondents without self-reported daytime hypersomnolence. Findley and colleagues (4) estimated that patients with severe sleep apnea may have a sevenfold greater rate of driving accidents than subjects without sleep apnea.

I. Mechanisms of Sleepiness in OSAS

Depending on the severity of OSAS, the sleep of patients with OSAS is subject to repeated arousals and oxygen desaturations. The frequent disruptions of sleep caused by apneic airway obstruction result in an elevated homeostatic sleep drive as expressed in pathological sleepiness, which not only increases the frequency of sleep onsets but also enhances the rate of sleep onset. Because apnea tends to occur whenever the patient sleeps, the disorder is characterized by an elevated biological drive for sleep no matter how much sleep the untreated patient obtains. Many OSAS patients, therefore, continue to function in a sleep-deprived state in terms of neurobehavioral performance and increased sleep propensity.

Neurobehavioral functioning in patients severely afflicted with OSAS often involves increasing fluctuation among alertness, lowered vigilance, drowsiness, and microsleeps, which results in a pressure for rapid transition from wake to sleep (5). In this regard untreated OSAS shares many characteristics with the hypovigilance, uncontrolled sleepiness, and labile waking state found in healthy individuals who are subjected to experimental sleep deprivation. This labile waking state is the result of sleep loss engendered through a number of mechanisms.

A. Arousal from Sleep

Obstructive apneas are characterized by progressively increasing hypoxemia and hypercapnia. There is also an associated gradual increase in intrathoracic and transdiaphragmatic pressure during efforts against the closed airway (6,7). The arousal and the increase in upper airway muscle activity that mark the end of obstructive apneas could be mediated by central or peripheral chemoreceptor stimuli, mechanoreceptor stimuli arising in the respiratory system, or the interaction of both chemoreceptor and mechanoreceptor stimuli (8). The input from chemoreceptor and/or respiratory mechanoreceptors leads to activation of the reticular activating system. This activation of the reticular activating system is in opposition to the physiological state of sleep in the patients with OSAS. Therefore, the sleep system is subjected to an induced countervailing activation during each apneic event. The frequency with which this activation occurs is thought to be an index of severity of sleep disturbance and therefore is a reflection of the severity of increased sleep propensity. This assumption has only been recently tested.

Krieger and colleagues (9) have shown that sleep propensity in a group of 44 untreated patients with OSAS correlated with the increase in esophageal pressure swings during obstructive apneas, indicating that the increased respiratory effort against the occluded upper airway was part of the pathophysiology of daytime sleepiness in these patients. The role of respiratory effort is further illustrated by the findings of Gleeson and coworkers (10), who observed that arousal tended to occur at the same level of respiratory effort, as indicated by similar peak negative esophageal pressure (during the breath preceding the arousal), in a given subject whether hypoxia, hypercapnia, or addition of a resistive load is used as a mechanism of respiratory stimulation during NREM sleep in normal healthy men. Gleeson and Zwillich (11) also showed that the minute ventilation of breathing (13 ± 1.4 L/m) preceding arousal from sleep in association with adenosine infusion (a respiratory stimulant) was similar to the ventilation preceding arousal produced by hypercapnia (12.9 ± 1.1 L/m). This suggests that increased ventilation (irrespective of the stimulus responsible for it) induces arousal. Kimoff and colleagues (12) also showed that the mean maximal end-apneic diaphragmatic tension time index during obstructive sleep apnea on room air (0.12 ± 0.01) was significantly altered neither by O_2 (0.12 ± 0.01) nor by CO_2 (0.11 ± 0.01) administration. The consistency of the end-apneic diaphragmatic tension-time index, despite the varying chemical drive, supports the concept that apnea termination in OSAS is mediated by respiratory effort.

The increased respiratory effort that produces arousal and sleep fragmentation is not consistent across a night of sleep. Montserrat and colleagues (13) have shown that there is a blunting over the night of the arousal response to neural stimuli produced by obstructed inspiratory effort. This plays a role in mediating apnea lengthening across the night in patients with OSAS. They reported that both transdiaphragmatic pressure and the diaphragm tension-time index at end-apnea just prior to arousal increased significantly from the beginning to the end of the night (e.g., transdiaphragmatic pressure increased from 41.0 ± 4.9 to 49.9 ± 7.9 cmH_2O; $p < 0.05$).

There is also a relatively poor understanding of what criteria define an arousal that might be significant from the standpoint of daytime sleepiness. Not all apneas and hypopneas terminate in awakenings or arousals. Rechtschaffen and Kales (14) have defined awakenings as any stage shift to wakefulness >15 s. Other definitions of sleep fragmentation have more recently been proffered. All of the following definitions of arousals require 10 s of sleep prior to scoring the arousal. A working group of the American Sleep Disorders Association (ASDA) has defined an arousal as a return to alpha or theta on the EEG channels for a minimum of 3 s during non–rapid eye movement (NREM) sleep with the addition of a concurrent minimum 3-s rise in submental EMG tone during REM sleep (15). A modification of the ASDA definition was proposed by Mathur and Douglas (16), i.e., with a duration criteria of 1.5 s. Cheshire and colleagues (17) have defined an arousal as a return to alpha or theta on the EEG channels for a minimum of 1.5 s accompanied by any increase in EMG tone, however brief. Consequently, many definitions of arousals are currently used, and only recently have studies begun to document the nature of arousals during apnea.

In a study on 63 patients of sleep apnea, Martin and colleagues (18) reported that more apneas and hypopneas were terminated by 1.5-s arousals than by ASDA-defined (15) arousals ($p < 0.001$) or Rechtschaffen and Kales (14) arousals ($p < 0.001$). They also reported that even using the more liberal 1.5-s arousal definition of 18 = 4% of apneas and hypopneas did not terminate in arousals. Rees and colleagues (19) also reported that not all apneas and hypopneas were terminated by arousals. Failure to observe EEG arousal activity could, however, be due to only using the conventional central/occipital montage for EEG recordings in polysomnography (PSG). For example, using 21 channel EEG recordings in three patients, O'Malley and colleagues (20) reported that 14.4% of apneas and hypopneas have only frontal arousals, which would have been missed using conventional PSG. Martin and colleagues (21) reported that even those arousals that were defined by autonomic nervous system changes alone, such as transient increase in blood pressure or heart rate, had a significant positive relationship to level of daytime sleepiness. However, it remains uncertain whether the occurrence of autonomic nervous system activation during apneic episodes has any relation to reports that many patients with OSAS have hypertension (22–24) or to the recent report that there is a linear increase in the risk of hypertension with an increasing apnea-hypopnea index (25). Whether or not arousals are involved in an elevated risk for hypertension for patients with untreated OSAS, their frequency, timing, and duration are likely to have key roles in determining the severity of sleep loss.

B. Sleep Fragmentation

Frequent arousals from sleep inhibit sleep consolidation and progression from lighter to deeper stages of sleep. Bonnet and colleagues (26) observed that patients with mild OSAS (apnea/hypopnea index = 5–20) had relatively long periods of consolidated sleep (20–90 min) between bursts of apnea, while patients with severe sleep apnea (apnea/hypopnea index > 45) essentially never slept as long as 10 min without an apneic event. A significant negative correlation was observed between sleepiness ratings and the period of consolidated sleep as measured by the median of the longest undisrupted sleep period between every 100 apnea periods ($r = -0.68$; $p < 0.02$). Experimental sleep disruption alone, in the absence of a loss of total sleep time, has also been demonstrated to result in sleepiness (27,28).

Sleep apnea is also often associated with selective sleep stage deprivation. Sleep fragmentation results in increased light sleep (NREM stage 1 sleep) while reducing deeper stages of sleep (slow-wave sleep and REM sleep) and total sleep duration. There is a relationship between total number of arousals, sleepiness (as measured by multiple sleep latency test, MSLT), and percentage of stage 1 sleep. In a study involving 15 OSAS patients with excessive daytime sleepiness, 15 patients with periodic leg movements disorder and excessive daytime sleepiness, 15 patients with insomnia, and 10 healthy controls, Stepanski and colleagues (29) observed a significant increase in stage 1 sleep percentage in patients having OSAS relative to patients having periodic leg movements, normals, and insomniacs. This paralleled the pattern of total arousals as well as sleepiness indices in these conditions. Percentage of stage 1 sleep was correlated with sleepiness as observed on the MSLT across groups ($r = -0.48$; $p = 0.0002$). Total number of arousals also correlated with MSLT across groups ($r = -0.48$; $p = 0.0002$). Arousals, but not awakenings, were observed to be far more common in patients with sleep apnea as compared to other groups. In a study by Vgontzas and colleagues (30) comparing patients with OSAS, narcolepsy, idiopathic hypersomnia, and controls, it was observed that patients with sleep apnea had significantly higher percentage of stage 1 sleep (62.7 ± 7.2, 17.2 ± 3.5, 11.6 ± 1.2, and 7.9 ± 2.0, respectively) and significantly lower slow-wave sleep (0.0 ± 0.0, 4.5 ± 1.6, 3.4 ± 1.4, and 4.3 ± 1.5, respectively) and REM sleep (12.7 ± 2.1, 20.6 ± 1.3, 19.7 ± 1.9, and 24.1 ± 1.8, respectively) as compared to controls. In fact, patients with OSAS had no measurable slow wave sleep (SWS) as compared to healthy controls.

Therefore, high rates of arousals that are associated with apneic and hypopneic events during sleep result in a cascade of effects including sleep fragmentation, failure to progress to deeper stages of sleep, and selective sleep stage deprivation. Any of these factors alone or in combination can produce daytime sleepiness and neurobehavioral dysfunction. In addition, and somewhat surprisingly, this sleep disruption syndrome also includes a reduction in total sleep time, despite the elevated homeostatic pressure for sleep engendered by OSAS. Figure 1 illustrates these points. Polysomnographic data were evaluated from 1521 patients diagnosed with OSAS at the University of Pennsylvania Sleep Disorders Center. As apnea-hypopnea index (RDI) increased, PSG scoring revealed that patients had not only increased numbers of arousals during sleep but also a marked reduction in total sleep time and elevation in stage 1 sleep (5).

Consequently excessive daytime sleepiness reported in sleep apnea seems to be associated with increasing frequency of arousals, increased sleep fragmentation, loss of sleep continuity, and simultaneous increase in stage 1 sleep, decrease in both slow-wave sleep and REM sleep, and decrease in total sleep time.

C. Hypoxia During Sleep

Hypoxia has long been associated with sleep apnea, but not all apneic events involve oxygen desaturations. The rate of desaturations as well as the lowest Sa_{O_2} vary markedly among patients and are poorly correlated with apnea rate. However, there is recent limited evidence that cerebral hypoxia does occur during apneic events. Using near-infrared spectroscopy simultaneously with PSG in five patients of OSAS, Hayakawa and colleagues (31) demonstrated that there is a consistent decrease of cerebral oxyhemoglobin and increases in levels of deoxyhemoglobin and total hemoglobin (total hemoglobin = oxyhemoglobin + deoxyhemoglobin and represents the relative tissue blood volume) during apneas in the dominant frontal region up to a depth of 4 cm from surface. Thus, cerebral tissue hypoxia may occur during apnea associated with low Sa_{O_2}. The relationship between hypoxia and neuropsychological performance is, however, not clear, and it is not known whether hypoxic events are sufficient to directly produce the neuropsychological and neurobehavioral disturbances in OSAS patients.

D. Chronic Sleep Restriction

The final mechanism by which sleep disruption from OSAS may lead to daytime sleepiness and neurobehavioral deficits is associated with the chronicity of the disruption and sleep loss (5). A recent experiment suggests that waking neurobehavioral deficits accumulate when sleep loss is chronic. In a study by Dinges and colleagues (32), 16 healthy adults had their sleep restricted to 33% below habitual sleep duration, to an average 4.98 (SD = 0.57) h per night for seven consecutive nights. Sleep restriction resulted in statistically robust cumulative effects on waking function. Stanford Sleepiness Scale (SSS) ratings, subscale scores for fatigue, confusion, tension, and total mood disturbance from the profile of mood states (POMS), and visual analog scales (VAS) ratings of mental exhaustion and stress were significantly ($p \leq 0.009$) elevated across days of sleep restriction. Frequency and duration of lapses

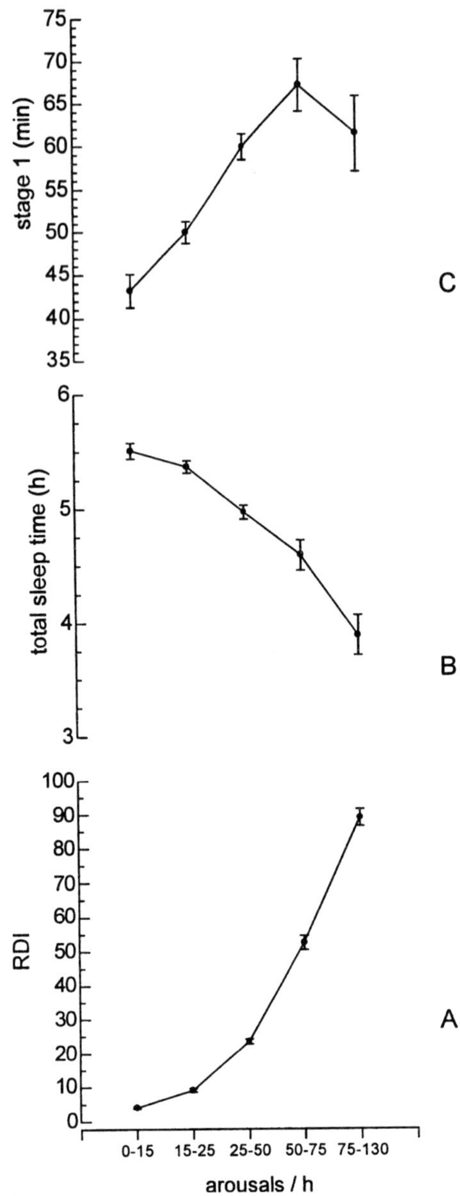

Figure 1 Sleep characteristics of 1521 OSAS patients grouped according to arousal index (5). With increasing arousals there is increased RDI (apnea + hypopneas per hour), increased stage 1 sleep, and diminished total sleep time: (A) the RDI as it increases with increasing arousals per hour; (B) diminishing total sleep time in hours with increasing arousal index; (C) increasing stage 1 sleep time in minutes as the number of arousals/h increase.

on psychomotor vigilance test performance were also significantly increased by restriction ($p \leq 0.018$). Remarkably, the profile of cumulative vigilance lapses during sleep restriction in this experiment on healthy adults correlated highly ($r = -0.957$) with the profile of decreasing MSLT scores from a comparable experiment performed 17 years earlier by Carskadon and Dement (33). Although these two laboratory experiments were performed on healthy adults, they suggest that chronic sleep restriction even without sleep fragmentation or selective sleep stage loss can lead to daytime sleepiness impairments in patients with OSAS. What is not understood is why patients with severe untreated OSAS have such a reduced time in bed in the face of elevated sleep pressure (see Fig. 1).

II. The Neurobehavioral Expression of Sleepiness

Just as there has been an expanding body of knowledge about the mechanisms that result in sleepiness in untreated OSAS, there has been a growing effort to measure the nature and severity of sleepiness and its waking neurobehavioral sequelae. In this section we will review some of the primary categories by which sleepiness has been defined, evaluated, and quantified.

A. Subjective Sleepiness

The assessment of sleepiness through introspective self-report has proved to be one of the most challenging and inconsistent outcomes in sleep apnea research. A large number of subjective scales have been used to assess subjective sleepiness in patients with sleep apnea. For example, the Stanford Sleepiness Scale (34) asks respondents to choose one of seven statements describing their state of sleepiness from the following range: (1) feeling active and vital, alert, wide awake to (7) almost in reverie, sleep onset soon, lost struggle to remain awake. While not isolated to SSS as a measurement tool, untreated sleep apnea patients sometimes report SSS ratings indicative of alertness (i.e., little or no sleepiness) while they appear to be behaviorally very sleepy. This paradoxical self-report of alertness in the face of behavioral sleepiness appears to be the result of chronic sleep disruption from untreated sleep apnea, that is, the patient loses a frame of reference with regard to what "normal alertness" feels like and therefore no longer reports the experience as sleepiness. For this reason subjective sleepiness ratings based on psychometric scales are often not valid or reliable indicators of sleepiness when administered pretreatment to chronically and extremely sleepy patients with apnea (35). This problem applies to nearly all sleepiness scales regardless of their psychometric properties (i.e., Likert type, visual analog, adjective checklist, etc.). However, those subjective sleepiness scales predicated on asking subjects about sleepy behaviors can often more accurately identify chronically sleepy patients who might otherwise deny being sleepy. A popular example of such a scale is the Epworth Sleepiness Scale (ESS) (36). The ESS asks respondents to choose a number from 0 to 3 corresponding to the likelihood (never, slight, moderate, and high) that they would doze in eight situations: (1) sitting and reading,

(2) watching TV, etc. An ESS score can range between 0 and 24. Another type of self-report scale that appears to accurately reflect the behavioral consequences of sleepiness is the Functional Outcomes of Sleep Questionnaire (FOSQ) developed by Weaver and colleagues (37).

All subjective scales have some degree of limitation when it comes to estimating the severity of sleepiness. In addition to their potential report bias due to age, sex, education, and background, subjective reports of sleepiness often do not correlate highly with apnea severity as assessed by RDI or with objective tests of sleepiness, such as MSLT or with performance tests of alertness/sleepiness. A recent study by Redline and colleagues (38) has also shown that ESS scores between patients with mild OSAS and controls were not significantly different (OSAS patients with RDI = 17.01 ± 4.95 had ESS scores of 9.84 ± 4.55; ESS scores for controls were 8.95 ± 4.14; $p = 0.26$). However, subjective sleepiness scales are particularly useful to give change scores in comparing outcome evaluations, the effect of therapy and other remedial interventions over time in patients.

B. Performance Effects of Sleepiness

Elsewhere we have reviewed the performance effects of experimentally induced sleep loss and have identified a taxonomy of effects on basic cognitive processes (39–41). Here we have organized these effects into those associated with lapses, vigilance decrement, and more complex neuropsychological functioning.

Attentional Lapses and State Instability

Increased lapsing is the best known effect of sleep loss. Attentional lapses refer to a period of response delay or of nonresponding (often from microsleeps), resulting in progressive unevenness in the performance of a sleepy subject (39). Both the number and duration of lapses can increase dramatically with induced impairment as a result of increasing sleepiness. Lapsing is particularly likely to occur when sleepy persons, including untreated patients with sleep apnea (42), perform a task requiring sustained attention, such as a psychomotor vigilance task (41,43).

Using a high-signal-rate psychomotor vigilance task (PVT) (44), which requires simple sustained attention, we have been able to demonstrate the instability of waking state that characterizes the performance of sleepy subjects (44). The frequency and duration of lapses (defined as a reaction time more than twice the duration of the average mean reaction time or ≥ 500 ms) during PVT performance reveals that a profoundly sleepy individual who is motivated and attempting to perform at an optimum level is capable of doing so only for brief periods of time. Waking performance is punctuated in such an individual by uncontrollable loss of alertness for brief moments of time, as reflected in attentional lapses. Figure 2 illustrates this inherent instability of alertness in a patient with OSAS prior to treatment (RDI = 73.4) compared to an age-matched control subject. While the visual reaction times on this simple vigilance task for the control subject are consistently below 1 s

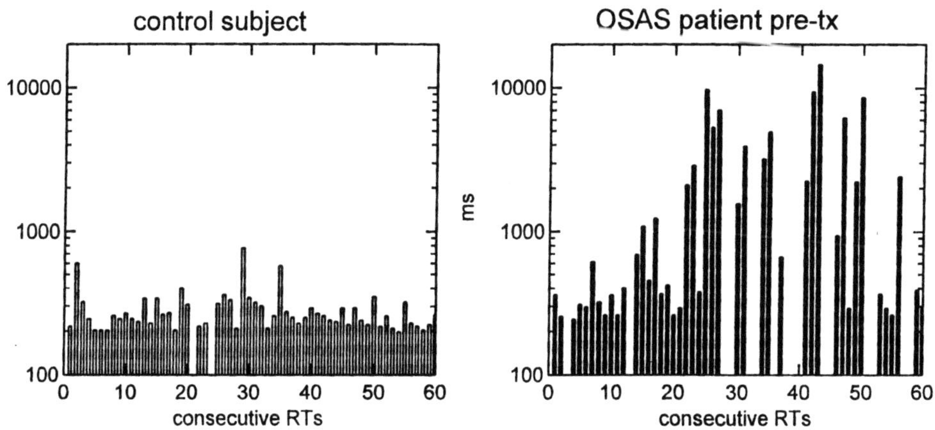

Figure 2 Consecutive reaction times for first 60 visual stimuli during psychomotor vigilance task performance for an untreated female OSAS patient (apneas + hypopneas/h = 73.4) and a male age-matched control subject. For the control subject the reaction times are consistently less than 1000 ms (mean ± SD = 278.8 = 101.0), while for the untreated patient with OSAS, after the initial dozen responses with normal reaction times (i.e., <500 ms), prolonged lapses (reaction times >1000 ms) predominate and are interspersed with false responses. Both false responses and prolonged reaction times highlight wake state instability in the untreated OSAS patient.

(1000 ms) and often below 300 ms (mean ± SD = 278.8 ± 101.0), which is the normal range for a healthy alert individual, the reaction times of the untreated OSAS patient are much more variable as the task progresses. Like the control, the patient manages relatively normal rapid reaction times (i.e., below 500 ms) for the first dozen responses. Averages for the first dozen reaction times for the OSAS patient and the control subject were 334.9 ms (SD = 106.4 ms) and 272.7 ms (SD = 109.6 ms), respectively (which were not significantly different, $p = 0.2$). After this apparently normal beginning, lasting only 70 seconds, the OSAS patient begins to experience an instability of wakefulness reflected in difficulty in avoiding lapses, and after the first 20 responses (≅2 min) lapses predominate along with false responses.

False responses are reflected in the graph of Figure 2 as zero reaction time or the blanks in the histogram sequence. They occur when the patient presses the response button in the absence of a stimulus and often reflect an increased motivation to respond accurately in the face of an inability to do so. While the control subject shows only two such false responses, the patient with OSAS has nine such responses, many of which occur in alternation with prolonged lapses (i.e., reaction time ≥ 1000 ms). Consequently, while the control subject's PVT performance is characterized by relatively stable, fast reaction times with few lapses and few false responses, the patient with untreated OSAS has many lapses and many false responses, reflecting a progressive lability of alertness, and instability of waking state despite repeated attempts to produce motivated performance. In another experiment involving 88 h of total sleep deprivation in normal healthy males, Doran and colleagues (45) observed that fast, stable responding was possible for the first 10 PVT reaction times (i.e., approximately the first minute of responding) of all the test bouts irrespective of the duration of sleep deprivation (in a representative single subject). After 84 h without sleep, the number of false starts and long duration lapses increased following the initial 12 fast reaction times. During the performance of a 60-min driving simulation task, Risser and colleagues (46) observed that ''crashes'' in the apnea group increased significantly over time (as compared to controls) and peak crash frequency occurred in the fifth 10-min block ($\chi^2 = 35.56$; $p < 0.0001$).

It is this instability of state, as reflected in attentional lapses, that is the hallmark of performance in sleepy subjects. It accounts for many of the cognitive and higher-order executive deficits described in both experimentally sleep-deprived subjects and pathologically sleepy patients. That is, many of the cognitive and neuropsychological deficits measurable in sleepy individuals come about through an inability of sleepy subjects to sustain attention to salient information, even when highly motivated. The salient information may be stimuli for a working memory task, key criteria to apply to an executive function task, or routine visual information in a driving task. Performance in all of these tasks can be eroded by lability in alertness and instability of wakefulness caused by elevated homeostatic drive for sleep. However, lapses do not account for all the effects of sleepy performance (39). For example, sleepiness is also associated with significant decreases in the fastest reaction times on sustained attention tasks that are not attributable to lapses (47).

Vigilance and Time on Task Decrements

Another major effect of sleep loss on performance is associated with task duration. Sleepiness accentuates the classic vigilance decrement function. Time-on-task decrements are observed in sleepy subjects (including untreated patients with apnea) performing different types of cognitive tasks (41). They appear to be a direct reflection of the inability of the individual to sustain attention to tasks (39). This has also been described as a ''fatigability function'' (41). This is illustrated in Figure 3, in which the mean reaction times on a 10-min PVT given to 18 OSAS patients before starting treatment with continuous positive airway pressure (CPAP) and 9 control subjects are shown. After the initial 2 min the mean response time increases with every passing minute in pretreatment sleep apnea patients as compared to controls. Using ''Steer Clear,'' a computerized simple reaction time driving simulation task, Findley and colleagues (48) also observed that the performance of patients with narcolepsy showed a clear decrement with time during the 30-min duration of the task (adjusted $R^2 = 0.87$; $F_{1,4} = 34.63$; $p = 0.004$). The performance of sleep apnea patients in the same task exhibited a trend toward a vigilance decrement (adjusted $R^2 = 0.42$; $F_{1,4} = 4.65$; $p = 0.097$), while control subjects showed no significant increase in collision errors with time-on-task (adjusted $R^2 = 0.22$; $F_{1,4} < 1$) (48). Consequently,

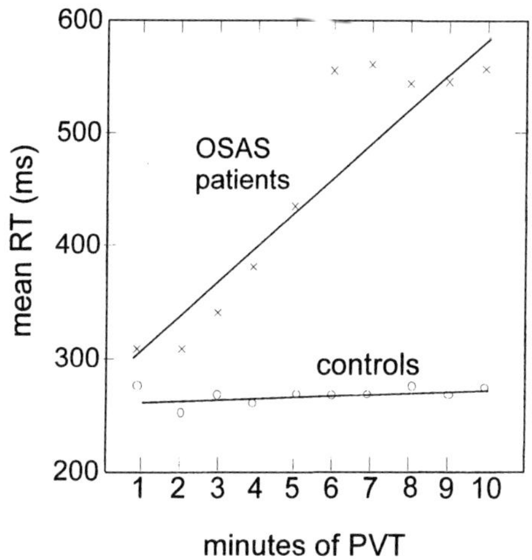

Figure 3 Changes in mean response time over 10-min PVT trials for 9 control subjects and 18 untreated patients with OSAS. Untreated OSAS patients show the classic decrement function in vigilance as the mean response time increases with each passing minute on the test after the initial 2 min.

sleepy subjects may begin a test doing well, but their ability to sustain a high level of output is often markedly impaired relative to when they are not sleepy.

Neuropsychological Deficits

Cognitive Slowing and Working Memory

Sleepiness is also associated with a number of deficits in fundamental cognitive processes. As sleepiness increases, performance on ''subject-paced'' cognitive tasks (e.g., mental arithmetic, logical reasoning, symbol substitution) begins to show reductions in the number of correct responses per unit time. This is referred to as a ''throughput'' decrement. If the subject is not permitted to slow down to maintain accuracy because the task is ''work-paced,'' then errors increase. Thus, the choice of whether to measure speed or errors on a cognitive performance probe of sleepiness is determined by how the task is paced, moreso than by the type of task (40).

Reductions in working memory have also been shown to occur in sleepy subjects (39), even when it is verified that the to-be-remembered material was perceived by the subject. Long-term recall does not appear to be impaired (or as impaired as short-term recall) if the stimulus information is taken in prior to sleep loss (49). Williams and colleagues (49) observed that both immediate and delayed recall were impaired for information acquired after a night without sleep. Cognitive slowing, increased errors, and working memory deficits have been observed in patients with untreated OSAS (38,41,50–54).

Complex Cognitive Deficits

More complex cognitive deficits also occur in sleepy persons. A recent study by Feuerstein and colleagues (55) compared frontal lobe function in 10 patients with OSAS aged 44.8 ± 2.5 (mean ± SEM) years complaining of daytime sleepiness and age-matched normal controls. OSAS patients had significant impairments on the Modified Wisconsin Card Sorting Test (55) relative to controls, with OSAS patients having more total number of errors ($p < 0.04$) and an increased percentage of perseverative errors ($p < 0.04$). On a reevaluation after 6.5 ± 1.28 months of CPAP treatment, significant improvements were observed in the OSAS patients compared to pretreatment state ($p < 0.014$ and $p < 0.05$, respectively). These findings support the hypothesis put forward by Horne (57) that sleep deprivation results in dysfunction of prefrontal cortex. It remains to be determined, however, whether the deficits seen on more complex cognitive tasks are the product of the more basic cognitive deficits ubiquitously observed in sleepy individuals, some of which are mediated in the frontal lobe of the cerebral cortex.

C. Physiological Markers of Sleepiness

The most widely used physiological markers of sleepiness are measures of the latency from wakefulness to various stages of sleep, especially wakefulness to stage 1 NREM sleep and wakefulness to stage 2 NREM sleep. It has been argued that reduction in such latencies, regardless of whether sleep was voluntary or involuntary, reflect an increased propensity for sleep (i.e., sleep drive). This conceptualization of sleep latency tests fits nicely with concepts of state instability and time-on-task decrements discussed in earlier sections of this chapter. But perhaps the strongest case for validity of sleep latency tests as measures of sleepiness derives from experimental sleep deprivation, where it has been shown that not only the latency to stage 1 sleep is shortened in a sleep-deprived subject but also the latency to stage 2 sleep, as well as the latency from stage 2 sleep to SWS sleep. Thus, with escalating sleep pressure comes a simultaneous shortening of all NREM sleep latencies—a phenomenon that has been characterized as an accelerated EEG hypersynchrony. Figure 4 illustrates these decreased latencies between wake and NREM sleep stages as prior wake time increased from 6 to 54 h in healthy human subjects (58). As can be seen in the figure, that latency from wake to stage 1 sleep dropped from 9 min to near zero after a night without sleep, consistent with the original finding by Carskadon and Dement (59). There was an even more dramatic decline of latency to stage 2 sleep across a single sleepless night. Similarly, slow-wave sleep occurred much sooner in the NREM cycle as prior wakefulness increased. These data suggest that elevation of homeostatic sleep drive, as occurs in untreated sleep apnea, can result in reduced latencies to all NREM sleep stages. However, in pathological conditions, such as sleep apnea, the progression to SWS does not occur due to interruption by an apneic and or hypopneic events. This sets up an alternation between disruption of sleep with a rapid return to sleep (5).

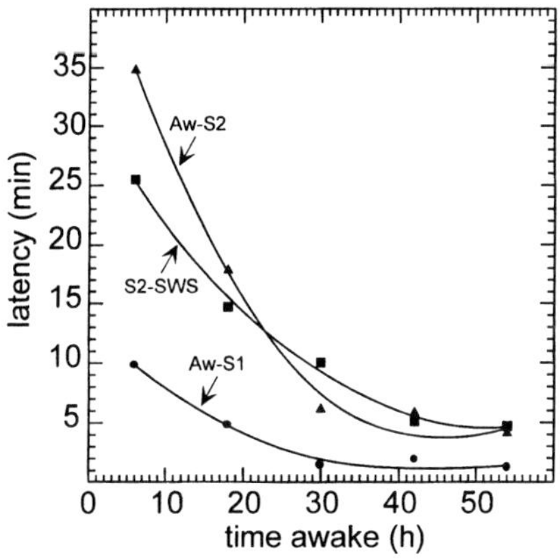

Figure 4 Latencies from wake (Aw) to Stage 1 sleep (S1), from awake (Aw) to Stage 2 NREM sleep (S2) and from Stage 2 to SWS in healthy adults with gradually increasing prior wake time from 6 to 54 hours (58).

Sleep Latency Tests

The Multiple Sleep Latency Test

The objective assessment of sleepiness using the multiple sleep latency test (60,61) measures sleep tendency or the rate at which patients can fall asleep voluntarily (i.e., in the absence of alerting factors). It is an electroencephalographically based method in which, after an overnight sleep study, the subject is permitted four to six daytime sleep opportunities of 20-min duration at 2-h intervals after getting up in the morning. The time between the point at which lights are turned out and the first evidence of EEG sleep is the sleep latency. This test has been used to aid in the differential diagnoses of disorders of excessive somnolence, especially OSAS and narcolepsy, by measuring latencies to sleep and to REM onset (35,62,63). Normal adult mean MSLT latencies range from 10 to 20 min, and latencies of 5 min or less are considered in the pathological zone (61). The scores ranging from 6 to 10 min are in the diagnostic gray area (61,64). If the patient falls asleep within the 20-min nap opportunity period, he is permitted to continue sleep for 15 more min, allowing a possible REM onset, which is used in the diagnosis of narcolepsy (61,65). The tendency to fall asleep when presented an opportunity in a quiet environment is considered a measure of physiological sleepiness (59). Mean latencies in most apnea patients with RDI $\geq$ 30 have been found to be in the pathological zone (<5 min) and are significantly different from those of normals (66).

The MSLT has been widely used in research on sleepiness. However, its clinical utility in sleep apnea diagnosis and treatment has been under question. It does provide an objective measure of sleepiness and can be useful in the diagnosis of narcolepsy, which can coexist with sleep apnea syndrome (67). Some sources recommend the MSLT in the routine evaluation of sleep apnea syndrome. For example, the Diagnostic and Coding Manual of the American Sleep Disorders Association (68) does recommend, although it does not require, an MSLT in evaluating sleep apnea, especially when excessive daytime sleepiness is the presenting complaint.

One of the paradoxes of the MSLT is the consistent finding that, although statistically significant improvement in MSLT values occur following OSAS treatment with CPAP, the posttreatment level of sleepiness as reflected in the MSLT is not normal. Pathological sleepiness may persist, indicated by a mean sleep latency in the "gray area" levels or low level of normal sleep propensity (69–72). Thus, the MSLT does not fully normalize following successful elimination of sleep-disordered breathing. It is not certain what significance should be attached to a failure of the MSLT to normalize following treatment for OSAS: Are patients still physiologically sleepy, or is the MSLT slow to adjust to therapeutic gains, and, if so, why? Similarly, it is not clear why some healthy individuals have short sleep latencies while others do not (73). Although sleep extension (up to 12 h in bed) can lengthen MSLT values in such individuals, the effect is often modest. Hence, the "resistance" of the MSLT to large acute effects suggests that the measure is either responsive to chronic elevated sleep propensity or that, if it does reflect sleep propensity, there can be a dissociation between sleep propensity and the frank expression of sleepiness in performance and other neurobehavioral variables.

Maintenance of Wakefulness Test

One of the instructional variants of the MSLT is the Maintenance of Wakefulness Test (MWT) (74). Also named by Hartse and colleagues (75) as the Repeated Test of Sustained Wakefulness, the MWT is considered by some to be more practical in its clinical application, as it measures the amount of time a patient is able to remain awake in a quiet environment. It is considered by some to be a more ecologically valid index of sleepiness since it measures the propensity for wakefulness rather than the tendency to fall asleep (74). Though not widely used, single-nap measures of sleepiness have also been proposed and shown to be helpful in distinguishing among the various forms of hypersomnia (76). It has been argued that although the MWT indicates the ability of an individual to stay awake, it is strongly influenced by individual differences in motivation. The MSLT maximizes the likelihood of sleep by removing all competing factors, therefore reflecting the degree to which an individual is prone to fall asleep (61). It appears that MWT is comparable and correlated to the MSLT in the information about sleepiness that it provides (43).

Other Psychophysiological Markers

In the past 100 years since the seminal study of human sleep deprivation by Patrick and Gilbert (77), there has been a bewildering array of putative physiological markers of sleepiness including measurement of blood, urine, saliva, cerebrospinal fluid, eye blinks, pupillary responses, heart rate responses, hemodynamic responses, temperature responses, neurovestibular responses, sensorimotor responses, electrodermal responses, electromyographic responses, and electroencephalographic responses. Within each of these areas there have been many different measurement strategies. However, it remains a fair generalization to state that none of these approaches have thus far consistently led to scientifically valid, reliable, and practical measures of sleepiness. Perhaps the most extensive area has been measurement of EEG and its evoked components since its original description. These efforts have ranged from the identification of ''microsleeps'' underlying performance lapses (see Ref. 39 for review) to more recent efforts to quantify subtle shifts in alertness (78,79).

Space limitations preclude review of the various central nervous system and autonomic nervous system physiological tests for sleepiness. There has been renewed interest in physiological markers of sleepiness with the advent of miniaturized technology for online monitoring of drowsiness and alertness in safety-sensitive occupations (e.g., truck driving) (see Ref. 80). Unfortunately, the development of such technology often does not involve careful scientific validation of the devices. Consequently, while there is merit to preventing sleepiness in safety-sensitive activities through monitoring, the use of sleepiness-monitoring technologies requires that scientific implementation and legal standards be met to insure that such devices do not do more harm than good (80).

III. Sleepiness Impairment Versus Alcohol Impairment

In recent years there has been an effort to equate the levels of sedation and neurobehavioral impairment produced by sleepiness with the levels produced by alcohol, because the latter is widely regarded in public policy debates as a scale for determining unacceptable levels of dysfunction. Recently Dawson and Reid (81) quantified performance impairment due to sleeplessness by expressing it in terms of its equivalence to varying levels of alcohol intoxication. They studied the same 40 subjects (21.1 ± 3.7 years; 27 M, 13 F) 1 week apart for alcohol condition [maximum blood alcohol concentration (BAC) of 0.1%] and for 28 hours of wakefulness. It was observed that cognitive psychomotor performance levels decreased significantly in both the alcohol and sleep-deprived conditions. For each hour of wakefulness after the initial 13 h, a relative performance decrement equivalent to the performance decrement observed with a 0.04% rise in BAC was recorded. After 24 h of wakefulness, performance decreased to a level equivalent to the performance observed at a BAC of 0.096%. The cognitive psychomotor performance showed a strong linear decline between the 10th and 26th hours of wakefulness as compared to mean baseline performance (significant linear correlation between mean relative performance and hours of wakefulness; $R^2 = 0.92$; $p < 0.05$). These observations suggest that between 0300 and 0800 h on the first night of wakefulness, a shift worker (or an automobile driver) would show a cognitive psychomotor performance impairment similar to or greater than the legally proscribed BAC.

Powell and colleagues (56) compared the psychometer vigilance performance of untreated patients with OSAS to the performance of healthy subjects with various blood alcohol levels. They found that the performance of mild-to-moderate OSAS patients was worse than that of healthy adults with alcohol levels of 0.08 g/dL (56).

There have also been studies demonstrating a synergy between alcohol and sleep loss in terms of sedating effects (82). This may suggest a mechanism by which sleepiness is also a cofactor in many alcohol-related accidents (83,84). A moderate dose of alcohol ingested at 2130 hours increases physiological sleepiness from 0100 to 0500 h, even when the alcohol has been eliminated from the blood (85). Roehrs and colleagues (82) have also shown that sleepiness and low-dose ethanol combine to impair simulated automobile driving.

IV. Conclusion

Sleepiness is a frequent and serious consequence of sleep apnea and many other life style–related and medical conditions. There are a number of mechanisms by which sleep apnea may produce sleepiness and waking neurobehavioral dysfunction. These include frequent brain oxygen desaturations and repeatedly occurring apneas (and hypopneas), leading to arousals, sleep fragmentation, selective sleep stage loss, and diminished total sleep time. The chronicity of sleep apnea further compounds these effects cumulatively. Performance impairment, as a result of sleepiness, is characterized by attentional lapses (both increased lapses and longer duration lapses), state instability (uncontrollable sleep/microsleep attacks), time-on-task decrements, cognitive and motor slowing with impairment, i.e., short-term recall, and performance on tasks such as mental arithmetic, logical reasoning, etc., as well as complex cognitive deficits. Various objective and subjective sleepiness measures have been developed that vary greatly in sensitivity and reliability. Subjective measures are useful for monitoring outcomes of remedial interventions. Sleep latency tests are useful to diagnose narcolepsy, which may coexist along with sleep apnea, but often sleep latencies persist in the gray zone in sleep apneics despite treatment. There is a very well-recognized need for developing and scientifically validating a miniaturized technology for online monitoring of sleepiness in occupations requiring constant vigilance and immediate response.

Acknowledgments

Support for this research was provided by grants from the National Institutes of Health (HL42236, HL07713, NR04281, RR00040), U.S. Public Health Service, and the Institute for Experimental Psychiatry Research Foundation.

References

1. Kribbs NB, Getsy J, Dinges DF. Investigation and management of daytime sleepiness in sleep apnea. In: Saunders NA, Sullivan CE, eds. Sleep and Breathing. Vol. 2. New York: Marcel Dekker, 1994:575–604.

2. Young T, Palta M, Dempsey J, Skatrud J, Weber S, Badr S. The occurrence of sleep-disordered breathing among middle-aged adults. N Engl J Med 1993; 328:1230–1235.
3. Lavie P. Sleep habits and sleep disturbances in industrial workers in Israel. Sleep 1981; 4:147–158.
4. Findley LJ, Unverzagt ME, Suratt R. Automobile accident involving patients with obstructive sleep apnea. Am Rev Respir Dis 1988; 138:337–340.
5. Chugh DC, Weaver TE, Dinges DF. Neurobehavioral consequences of arousals. Sleep 1996; 19:S198–S201.
6. Sullivan CE, Issa FG. Pathophysiologic mechanisms in obstructive sleep apnea. Sleep 1980; 3:235–246.
7. Vincken W, Guilleminault C, Silvestri L, Cosio M, Grasino A. Inspiratory muscle activity as a trigger causing the airways to open in obstructive sleep apnea. Am Rev Respir Dis 1987; 135:372–377.
8. Bowes G, Phillipson EA. Arousal responses to respiratory stimuli during sleep. In: Saunders NC, Sullivan CE, eds. Sleep and Breathing. New York: Marcel Dekker, 1984: 137–161.
9. Krieger J, Zamagni M, Sforza E, Petiau C, Trautmann D. Propensity for sleep and diurnal somnolence in the course of sleep apnea syndrome. Neurophysiol Clin 1996; 26:131–137.
10. Gleeson K, Zwillich CW, White DP. The influence of increasing ventilatory effort on arousal from sleep. Am Rev Respir Dis 1990; 142:295–300.
11. Gleeson K, Zwillich CW. Adenosine stimulation, ventilation, and arousal from sleep. Am Rev Respir Dis 1992; 145:453–457.
12. Kimoff RJ, Cheong TH, Olha AE, Charbonneau M, Levy RD, Cosio MG, Gottfried SB. Mechanisms of apnea termination in obstructive sleep apnea: role of chemoreceptor and mechanoreceptor stimuli. Am J Respir Crit Care Med 1994; 149:707–714.
13. Montserrat JM, Kosmas EN, Cosio M, Kimoff RJ. Mechanism of apnea lengthening across the night in obstructive sleep apnea. Am J Respir Crit Care Med 1996; 154:988–993.
14. Rechtschaffen A, Kales A. A Manual of Standardized Terminology and Scoring System for Sleep Stages of Human Subjects. Los Angeles: BIS/BRI, UCLA, 1968.
15. Atlas Task Force of the American Sleep Disorders Association. EEG arousals: scoring rules and examples a preliminary report. Sleep 1992; 15:174–184.
16. Mathur R, Douglas NJ. Frequency of EEG arousals from nocturnal sleep in normal subjects. Sleep 1995; 18:330–333.
17. Cheshire K, Engleman HM, Deary IJ, Saphiro C, Douglas NJ. Factors impairing daytime performance in patients with sleep apnoea/hypoapnoea syndrome. Arch Int Med 1992; 152:538–541.
18. Martin SE, Engleman HM, Kingshott RN, Douglas NJ. Microarousals in patients with sleep apnoea/hypoapnoea syndrome. J Sleep Res 1997; 6:276–280.
19. Rees K, Spence DPS, Earis JE, Calverley PMA. Arousal responses from apneic events during non-rapid-eye-movement sleep. Am J Respir Crit Care Med 1995; 152:1016–1021.
20. O'Malley EB, Norman RG, Walsleben JA, Rapoport DM. Upper airway obstructive events and location of EEG arousal activity. Sleep Res 1996; 25:321.
21. Martin SE, Wraith PK, Deary IJ, Douglas NJ. The effect of non-visible sleep fragmentation on daytime function. Am J Respir Crit Care Med 1997; 155:1596–1601.
22. Guilleminault C, Tilkian A, Dement WC. The sleep apnea syndrome. Ann Rev Med 1976; 27:465–484.

23. Williams A, Houston D, Finberg S, Lam C, Kinney J, Santiage S. Sleep apnea syndrome and essential hypertension. Am J Cardiol 1985; 55:1019–1022.
24. Fletcher EC, DeBehnke RD, Lovoi MS, Gorin AB. Undiagnosed sleep apnea in patients with essential hypertension. Ann Intern Med 1985; 103:190–195.
25. Nieto FJ, Young TB, Lind BK, Shahar E, Samet JM, Redline S, D'Agostino RB, Newman AB, Lebowitz MD, Pickering TG. Association of sleep-disordered breathing, sleep apnea, and hypertension in a large community-based study. JAMA 2000; 14:1829–1836.
26. Bonnet MH, Downey R, Wilms D, Dexter J. Sleep continuity theory as a predictor of EDS in sleep apneics. Sleep Res 1986; 15:105.
27. Bonnet MH. Performance and sleepiness as a function of frequency and placement of sleep disruption. Psychophysiology 1986; 23:263–271.
28. Stepanski E, Lamphere J, Roehrs T, Zorick F, Roth T. Experimental sleep fragmentation in normal subjects. Int J Neurosci 1987; 33:207–214.
29. Stepanski J, Lamphere J, Badia P, Zorick F, Roth T. Sleep fragmentation and daytime sleepiness. Sleep 1984; 1:18–26.
30. Vgontzas AN, Papanicolaou DA, Bixler EO, Kales A, Tyson K, Chrousos GP. Elevation of plasma cytokines in disorders of excessive daytime sleepiness: role of sleep disturbance and obesity. J Clin Endocrinol Metab 1997; 82:1313–1316.
31. Hayakawa T, Terashima M, Kayukawa Y, Ohta T, Okada T. Changes in cerebral oxygenation and hemodynamics during obstructive sleep apneas. Chest 1996; 109:916–921.
32. Dinges DF, Pack F, Williams K, Gillen KA, Powell JW, Ott GE, Aptowicz C, Pack AI. Cumulative sleepiness, mood disturbance, and psychomotor vigilance performance decrements during a week of sleep restricted to 4–5 hours per night. Sleep 1997; 20: 267–277.
33. Carskadon MA, Dement WC. Cumulative effects of sleep restriction on daytime sleepiness. Psychophysiology 1981; 18:107–113.
34. Hoddes E, Zarcone V, Smythe H, Phillips R, Dement WC. Quantification of sleepiness: a new approach. Psychophysiology 1973; 10:431–436.
35. Dement WC, Carskadon MA, Richardson G. Excessive daytime sleepiness in the sleep apnea syndrome. In: Guilleminault C, Dement WC, eds. Sleep Apnea Syndromes. New York: Liss, 1978:23–46.
36. Johns MW. A new method for measuring daytime sleepiness: the Epworth sleepiness scale. Sleep 1991; 6:540–545.
37. Weaver TE, Laizner AM, Evans LK, Maislin G, Chugh DK, Lyon K, Smith PL, Schwartz AR, Redline S, Pack AI, Dinges DF. An instrument to measure functional status outcomes for disorders of excessive sleepiness. Sleep 1997; 10:835–843.
38. Redline S, Strauss ME, Adams N, Winters M, Roebuck T, Spry K, Rosenberg C, Adams K. Neuropsychological function in mild sleep-disordered breathing. Sleep 1997; 20: 160–167.
39. Dinges DF, Kribbs NB. Performing while sleepy: effects of experimentally induced sleepiness. In: Monk TH, ed. Sleep, Sleepiness and Performance. Philadelphia: Wiley & Sons, 1991:97–128.
40. Dinges DF. Probing the limits of functional capability: the effects of sleep loss on short duration tasks. In: Broughton RJ, Ogilvie RD, eds. Sleep, Arousal and Performance. Boston: Birkhauser, 1992:176–188.

41. Kribbs NB, Dinges DF. Vigilance decrement and sleepiness. In: Harsh JR, Ogilvie RD, eds. Sleep Onset Mechanisms. Washington, DC: American Psychological Association, 1994:113–125.
42. Kribbs NB, Pack AI, Kline LR, Getsy JE, Schuett JS, Henry JN, Dinges DF. The effects of one night without nasal CPAP treatment on sleep and sleepiness in patients with obstructive sleep apnea syndrome. Am Rev Respir Dis 1993; 147:1162–1168.
43. Dinges DF. The nature of sleepiness: causes, contexts, and consequences. In: Stunkard AJ, Baum A, eds. Perspectives in Behavioral Medicine: Eating, Sleeping, and Sex. Hillsdale, NJ: Lawrence Erlbaum Associates, 1989:147–179.
44. Dinges DF, Powell JW. Microcomputer analyses of performance on a portable, simple visual RT task during sustained operations. Behav Res Methods Instruments Computers 1985; 17:652–655.
45. Doran SM, Van Dongen HPA, Dinges DF. Sustained attention performance during sleep deprivation: evidence of state instability. Arch Ital Biol 2001; 139:253–267.
46. Risser MR, Ware JC, Freeman FG. Driving simulation with EEG monitoring in normal and obstructive sleep apnea patients. Sleep 2000; 23:393–398.
47. Dinges DF, Powell JW. Sleepiness is more than lapsing. Sleep Res 1988; 17:84.
48. Findley LJ, Suratt PM, Dinges DF. Time-on-task decrements in "Steer Clear" performance of patients with sleep apnea and narcolepsy. Sleep 1999; 22:804–809.
49. Williams HL, Gieseking CF, Lubin A. Some effects of sleep loss on memory. Percept Mot Skills 1966; 23:1287–1293.
50. Engleman HM, Martin SE, Deary IJ, Douglas NJ. Effect of continuous positive airway pressure treatment on daytime function in sleep apnea/hypopnea syndrome. Lancet 1994; 343:572–575.
51. Engleman HM, Martin SE, Deary IJ, Douglas NJ. Effect of CPAP therapy on daytime function in patients with mild sleep apnoea/hypopnoea syndrome. Thorax 1997; 52: 114–119.
52. George CF, Boudreau AC, Smiley A. Effects of nasal CPAP on simulated driving performance in patients with obstructive sleep apnoea. Thorax 1997; 52:648–653.
53. Schulz H, Wilde-Frenz J, Grabietz-Kurfurst U. Cognitive deficits in patients with daytime sleepiness. Acta Neurol Belg 1997; 97:108–112.
54. Kotterba S, Widdig W, Duscha C, Rasche K. Event related potentials and neuropsychological studies in sleep apnea patients. Pneumologie 1997; 51(suppl 3):712–715.
55. Feuerstein C, Naegele B, Pepin JL, Levy P. Frontal lobe-related cognitive functions in patients with sleep apnea syndrome before and after treatment. Acta Neurol Belg 1997; 97(2):96–107.
56. Powell NB, Riley RW, Schechtman KB, Blumen MB, Dinges DF, Guilleminault C. A comparative model: reaction time performance in sleep-disordered breathing versus alcohol-impaired controls. Laryngoscope 1999; 109:1648–1654.
57. Horne JA. Human sleep, sleep loss and behavior. Implications for the prefrontal cortex and psychiatric disorder. Br J Psychiatry 1993; 162:413–419.
58. Dinges DF. Differential effects of prior wakefulness and circadian phase on nap sleep. Electroencephalogr Clin Neurophysiol 1986; 64:224–227.
59. Carskadon MA, Dement WC. Sleep tendency: an objective measure of sleep loss. Sleep Res 1977; 6:200.
60. Carskadon MA, Dement WC. Effects of total sleep loss on sleep tendency. Percept Mot Skills 1979; 48:495–506.
61. Carskadon MA, Dement WC, Mitler MM, Roth T, Westbrook PR, Keenan S. Guidelines

for the Multiple Sleep Latency Test (MSLT): a standard measure of sleepiness. Sleep 1986; 9:519–524.
62. Zorick F, Roehrs T, Koshorek G, Sicklesteel J, Hartse K, Wittig R, Roth T. Patterns of sleepiness in various disorders of excessive daytime somnolence. Sleep 1982; 5: S165–S174.
63. Reynolds CF III, Coble PA, Kupfer DJ, Holzer BC. Application of the multiple sleep latency test in disorders of excessive sleepiness. Electroencephalogr Clin Neurophysiol 1982; 53:443–452.
64. van den Hoed J, Kraemer H, Guilleminault C, Zarcone VP Jr, Miles LE, Dement WC, Mitler MM. Disorders of excessive daytime somnolence: polygraphic and clinical data for 100 patients. Sleep 1981; 4:23–37.
65. Guilleminault C. Narcolepsy syndrome. In: Kryger MH, Roth T, Dement WC, eds. Principles and Practice of Sleep Medicine. Philadelphia: WB Saunders Company, 1989: 338–346.
66. Roth T, Hartse KM, Zorick F, Conway W. Multiple naps and the evaluation of daytime sleepiness in patients with upper airway sleep apnea. Sleep 1980; 3:425–439.
67. Reimao R, Lemmi H. Concomitant narcolepsy and sleep apnea: report of a case. Arq Neuropsiquiatr 1986; 44:73–77.
68. American Sleep Disorders Association. ICSD–International classification of Sleep Disorders, Revised: Diagnostic and Coding Manual. Rochester, MN: American Sleep Disorders Association, 1997.
69. Wittig RM, Zorick FJ, Conway WA, Ward J, Roth T. Normalization of the MSLT after six weeks of CPAP for sleep apnea syndrome. Sleep Res 1986; 15:185.
70. DiPhillipo MA, Fry JM, Pressman MR. Objective measurement of daytime sleepiness following treatment of obstructive sleep apnea with nasal CPAP. Sleep Res 1988; 17: 167.
71. Lamphere J, Roehrs T, Wittig R, Zorick F, Conway WA, Roth T. Recovery of alertness after CPAP in apnea. Chest 1989; 96:1364–1367.
72. Kribbs NB, Dinges DF, Schuett JS, Pack AI, Kline LR. Prevalence and effects of intermittent CPAP use in obstructive sleep apnea. Sleep Res 1989; 18:251.
73. Roehrs T, Shore E, Papineau K, Rosenthal L, Roth T. A two-week sleep extension in sleepy normals. Sleep 1996; 19:576–582.
74. Mitler MM, Gujavarty KS, Browman CP. Maintenance of wakefulness test: a polysomnographic technique for evaluating treatment in patients with excessive somnolence. EEG Clin Neurophysiol 1982; 53:658–661.
75. Hartse KM, Roth T, Zorick FJ. Daytime sleepiness and daytime wakefulness: the effect of instruction. Sleep 1982; 5:S107–S118.
76. Roth B, Nevsimalova S, Sonka K, Docekal P. A quantitative polygraphic study of daytime somnolence and sleep in patients with excessive diurnal sleepiness. Schweiz Arch Neurol Neurochir Psychiatr 1984; 135:265–272.
77. Patrick GT, Gilbert JA. On the effects of loss of sleep. Psychological Rev 1896; 3: 469–483.
78. Makeig S, Jung T-P. Changes in alertness are a principal component of variance in the EEG spectrum. NeuroReport 1995; 7:213–216.
79. Stampi C, Stone P, Michimori A. A new quantitative method for assessing sleepiness: the Alpha Attenuation Test. Work Stress 1995; 9:368–376.
80. Dinges DF, Mallis MM. Managing fatigue by drowsiness detection: can technological promises be realized? In: Hartley L, ed. Coping with the 24 Hour Society: Fatigue

Management Alternatives to Prescriptive Hours of Service. From the Proceedings of the 3rd International Conference on Fatigue in Transportation. Bristol, PA: Taylor & Francis, in press.

81. Dawson D, Reid K. Fatigue, alcohol and performance impairment. Nature, 1997; 388: 235.
82. Roehrs T, Beare D, Zorick F, Roth T. Sleepiness and ethanol effects on simulated driving. Alcohol Clin Exp Res 1994; 1:154–158.
83. Horne JA, Baumber CJ. Time-of-day effects of alcohol intake on simulated driving performance in women. Ergonomics 1991; 34:1377–1383.
84. Horne JA, Gibbons H. Effects on vigilance performance and sleepiness of alcohol given in the early afternoon (''post lunch'') vs. early evening. Ergonomics 1991; 34:67–77.
85. Walsh JK, Humm T, Muelbach MJ, Sugerman JL, Schweitzer PK. Sedative effects of ethanol at night. J Stud Alcohol 1991; 52:597–600.

10

Functional Brain Imaging During Sleep and Sleep Deprivation in Health and Disease

J. CHRISTIAN GILLIN, CAMELLIA P. CLARK, SEAN P.A. DRUMMOND, and GREGORY G. BROWN

University of California, San Diego
and VA San Diego Healthcare System
San Diego, California

JOSEPH WU, LOUIS A. GOTTSCHALK, and WILLIAM E. BUNNEY, Jr.

University of California College of Medicine
Irvine, California

MONTE S. BUCHSBAUM

Mount Sinai School of Medicine
New York, New York

CHARLES HONG

Johns Hopkins University School of Medicine
Baltimore, Maryland

I. Introduction

The workings and purpose of sleep and dreaming have long been shrouded in mystery. A major scientific goal is to shed the light of modern neurobiology on the inner mechanisms of the brain during sleep and wakefulness. In recent years, new methods of functional brain imaging have made it possible to literally see what happens in the living brain, particularly in people, as they sleep and dream or deal with sleep deprivation. The emerging technologies of functional brain imaging include positron emission tomography (PET), functional magnetic resonance imaging (FMRI), magnetic resonance spectroscopy (MRS), and older methods such as xenon-133 (^{133}Xenon), single photon emission computerized tomography (SPECT), and Doppler measures of arterial blood flow. These brain-imaging methods can be associated, in some conditions, with topographic EEG, magneto-encephalography (MEG), or other ways of assessing localized cerebral activity.

Measurements of brain metabolism traditionally assumed that cerebral neuronal activity was tightly coupled to both energy metabolism and blood flow (1–3). Thus, in theory, the rates of cerebral glucose metabolism, of cerebral oxygen metabolism, or of cerebral blood flow (CBF) have been equated with neuronal activity. Energy is needed to maintain cell membrane potentials, to drive glycolysis, and to synthesize neurotransmitters.

Changes in blood flow associated with altered behavioral or cognitive states presumably reflect changes in synaptic activity. Local increases in both excitatory and inhibitory electrical neuronal activity lead to increased consumption of glucose and oxygen, increased CBF and velocity, increased local blood volume, and decreased oxygen extraction fraction. Since glucose and oxygen are necessary for aerobic metabolism in the brain, and since neither is stored in appreciable amounts in the brain, the brain depends upon cerebral blood flow for a moment-to-moment delivery of these substrates. The coupling between glucose metabolism, oxygen utilization, and cerebral blood flow is still poorly understood. According to the diffusion limit model of Buxton and Frank (4), oxygen consumption and flow are coupled, although flow increases more. The local capillary response to neural activity is extremely rapid, on the order of 0.2–2 s (4). Local capillary blood flow appears to increase before, rather than after, changes in local pH, Pa_{O_2}, Pa_{CO_2}, or the ratio of oxyhemoglobin (hemoglobin with oxygen) to deoxyhemoglobin (hemoglobin that has given up its oxygen) (4). Although ATP can be partially synthesized without oxygen in the glycolytic pathway, the amount of ATP produced from a molecule of glucose is about 16 times greater during oxidative metabolism than during anaerobic glycolysis.

Since sleep has traditionally been considered to be a period of "rest" or "restoration" (5–9) the study of whole brain metabolic rate is relevant to understanding the functions of sleep. Furthermore, because recent functional brain-imaging techniques have better temporal and anatomical resolution than previously, these methods also reveal local brain mechanisms involved in the regulation of sleep and wakefulness.

The physiological interpretation of functional brain images is fraught with difficulties, some of which will be briefly reviewed here. Interestingly, however, spike activity of neurons has little effect per se on brain glucose metabolism; rather, nerve terminals are more metabolically active than cell bodies (2,4). Therefore, changes in local metabolism and blood flow may reflect neurophil activity at some distance removed from the cell bodies, even though the latter show little or no metabolic change despite increased cell-firing rates. Furthermore, FMRI primarily records changes in the local hemodynamic response to local activation of nerve terminals. FMRI using the blood oxygen level–dependent (BOLD) method, however, measures changes in the ratio of oxygenated to deoxygenated hemoglobin in veins draining a significant area of neuronal activation rather than in veins in a small area of activation. Therefore, because of the time delay associated with draining the general area, the signal may be delayed and dispersed by as much as 2–14 s after a stimulus and be a maximum of several millimeters away from the initial site of neuronal activation (10).

In this chapter we will review selected studies of functional brain imaging of cerebral metabolism in sleep and sleep deprivation in normal adult subjects and depressed patients. These studies have implications not only for normal function and basic mechanisms of sleep and dreaming but also for the pathophysiology and treatment of depression. The interested reader may wish to consult other references on functional imaging during sleep in human stable premature infants (11), fetal lambs (12), piglets (13), and children with Landau-Kleffner syndrome (14,15).

II. An Overview of Selected Functional Brain-Imaging Methods

Early attempts to measure functional brain activity included urinary phosphorylated compounds, presumably reflecting metabolic energy turnover, and ausculation of arterio-venous malformations since the noise of cerebral blood flow increased with cerebral activity (2). With regard to sleep, early philosophers thought that sleep and wakefulness might be connected to blood flow. Nathaniel Kleitman, in his classic book, *Sleep and Wakefulness* (16), credited Croton, a contemporary of Pythagorus, with the first theory of sleep. Croton proposed that sleep resulted from a retreat of the blood to the veins; wakening followed venous disgorgement. In the last century and the first half of this century, many investigators sought evidence that sleep resulted from either ''cerebral anemia'' or peripheral congestion. Disputes raged about whether or not the surface blood vessels in puppies blanched as they slept or brain volume decreased during sleep in individuals with cranial defects. In the mid-1930s, Gibbs and coworkers attempted to measure cerebral circulation during sleep with thermo-electrode blood-flow recorders inserted in the juggler vein but concluded that blood flow did not change when subjects either fell asleep or woke up. In the 1940s Seymour Kety and others developed quantitative measures of global cerebral blood flow and oxygen consumption. The Kety-Schmidt method determined the timed difference between arterial and jugular venous concentrations of oxygen and the tracer gas, such as nitrous oxide (N_2O), with which CBF can be measured. Perhaps the first quantitative study of cerebral metabolism during sleep was conducted by Mangold et al. (1) even before rapid eye movement (REM) sleep was discovered. Using the N_2O method, they reported that cerebral blood flow increased during sleep. [The investigators excluded data with an ''activated'' low-voltage, fast-frequency EEG since they thought the subjects were awake. In retrospect, they regretted that they missed the opportunity to discover REM sleep before its discovery in 1953 by Aserinsky and Kleitman (17) (L. Sokoloff, personal communication).]

One of the next great advances was the development of quantitative measures of cerebral glucose metabolism, the 2-deoxyglucose (2DG) autoradiographic technique by Sokoloff and colleagues in 1977 (3). This method was soon married with computerized tomography to measure local cerebral glucose metabolic rate (LCGMR) in humans with PET. A fluorinated analog of glucose, deoxyglucose, was linked with ^{18}Fluorine to form ^{18}F-deoxyglucose (FDG). Both 2DG and FDG are analogs of glucose, which are transported like glucose from blood into brain parenchyma at a rate proportional to local metabolic rate. Either radiolabeled compound can be administered as a bolus intravenously, while arterial or arterialized blood samples are taken rapidly to measure plasma concentrations of 2DG or FDG. The model for determining absolute rates of cerebral glucose metabolism depends upon the individual pharmacokinetics of the 2DG or FDG. The radioactive label, ^{18}F, has a half-life of 108 min. Once 2DG or FDG enter brain parenchyma, they are phosphorylated by hexokinase to the 6-phosphate products. These phosphorylated compounds of 2DG or FDG are essentially trapped intracellularly; they are not permeable across the cell membrane, not capable of proceeding down the anaerobic pathway, and not susceptible to dephosphorylation within the timeframe of the study. A period of about 30–45 min in a constant state is needed for uptake of 2DG or FDG into brain tissue. After this time, the 2DG is stable and the tissue can be frozen and examined at a later time. In the case of FDG, the brain must be scanned immediately because of the short half-life of ^{18}F; the scanning period takes about 20–40 min. The radioactive label of the FDG-6-phosphate, ^{18}F, emits positrons, which collide with electrons after traveling about 1–2 mm. The two particles are annihilated, producing two annihilation photons, traveling at 180° from each other. These are recognized by an array of multiple radiation detectors, which are connected by coincidence circuits and arranged about the subject's head. A quantitative map of the concentration of the radioactive tracer is obtained by the scanner and its program. Based upon a mathematical model and the individual pharmacokinetics of FDG, the absolute and relative (region of interest divided by, e.g., whole brain) rates of glucose metabolism can then be estimated for each subject. Because of its radioactivity and 2-h half-life, FDG cannot be readministered more than two or three times in normal controls, or less than about 2 hours apart (18).

Cerebral blood flow has been measured during sleep with inert gases, such as nitrous oxide or ^{133}xenon, or, more commonly in recent years, with radiopharmaceutical compounds, such as $H_2{}^{15}O$, using PET. Compared with FDG, $H_2{}^{15}O$ has a very short half-life. It can be administered two to six times at 10-min intervals in one session while maintaining equivalent radiation doses. It provides a rapid, quantitative measurement of CBF over relatively short periods of time (<1 min). PET has also been used to measure the $CMRO_2$ but, to our knowledge, not in relationship to sleep or sleep deprivation. SPECT studies, with a radioactively labeled compound technetium-99-hexamethyl propyleneamine oxime (^{99m}Te-HMPAO or HMPAO), have usually been regarded as a measure of cerebral blood flow. HMPAO rapidly binds to areas of the brain at a rate that is probably proportional, but not precisely related to, CBF (19). A more conservative term—HMPAO uptake—is probably more accurate than CBF in describing the HMPAO method. The anatomical resolution is not as good as some of the other methods mentioned above.

The FDG method with PET and the HMPAO methods with SPECT have an advantage for studying cerebral metabolism during sleep compared with the $H_2{}^{15}O$ method and FMRI. During the FDG and HMPAO uptake period, the subject can sleep in a comfortable bed with EEG recordings without disturbance. Following the intravenous administration of the FDG or HMPAO while the subject slept, he or she can be awakened and taken to the scanner. In contrast, because of the 2-min half-life of the ^{15}O-labeled water, the PET with the $H_2{}^{15}O$ method requires the subject to sleep in an uncomfortable scanner when the tracer is administered and CBF is simultaneously measured. The CBF and, in theory, the FMRI methods have the advantage over FDG that the subject can undergo repeated measures within a single session. Understandably, many of the CBF studies with $H_2{}^{15}O$ have used subjects who were sleep deprived in order to insure sleep during the metabolic measures.

Both the PET and the SPECT methods have been wedded with labeled pharmaceutical agents to study specific neurotransmitter systems. With dopaminergic systems, for example, it is possible to measure turnover of the presynaptic dopamine transporter and postsynaptic D_1 or D_2 receptors.

FMRI is a relatively new, exciting method for assessing local cerebral activity. In its most common application, FMRI can detect small changes in the magnetic properties between oxyhemoglobin and deoxyhemoglobin (20). The ratio of these two compounds apparently changes as blood flow overperfuses the local area of neuronal activation and oxygen is given up for local oxidative metabolism. Many different applications of FMRI are available. Each are suited to different requirements of a specific research design. New methods are being developed as experience grows and new needs emerge. For example, methods are developing for quantitative blood flow studies.

Studying sleep in the FMRI environment or PET scanner is difficult. The scanner is uncomfortable and claustrophobic for many subjects. The FMRI scanner is extremely noisy (about 110 dB). To minimize movement artifacts, the head is encased and virtually immobilized in a head coil or head holder. Despite these physical constraints, head movement is almost unavoidable. Unfortunately, even submillimeter movements can obscure the BOLD signal. Acquiring EEG signals in a high-intensity, rapidly changing magnetic field poses formidable challenges. At the time of writing this review, few publications have used FMRI to study sleep (21,22). Nevertheless, FMRI has contributed significantly to understanding basic localized hemodynamic changes associated with neural activation during wakefulness. In addition, unlike either the LCGMR or regional CBF methods, FMRI can image local hemodynamic changes over long periods of time rather than as a one-time snapshot of brain activity.

Another new method, which has apparently not been used very much in sleep studies, is near-infrared spectroscopy (NIRS), which can measure CBF, oxygen consumption, and concentrations of oxygenated and deoxygenated hemoglobin (23–25). This interesting new brain-imaging method will only be mentioned in passing in this chapter.

Once functional images of the brain are acquired, the quantitative and anatomical analysis of functional activity poses another set of methodological challenges. Increasingly, structural brain images are also taken so that the functional images can be analyzed against the template of the subject's own anatomy. Alternatively, the functional or structural images can be transformed into standardized, stereotaxic space, such as the system of Talairach and Tournoux (26). While this approach blurs the boundaries of true functional anatomy, it allows statistical analysis of groups of individual subjects. In addition, because of the large number of voxels or pixels in the brain, special approaches are necessary to avoid Type I and Type II statistical errors when identifying the important, relevant clusters of anatomical units of interest. Functional brain-mapping studies usually use some form of statistical parametric mapping (SPM). SPM refers to the construction of spatially extended statistical processes to test hypotheses about regionally specific effects.

Rates of regional cerebral glucose metabolism, CBF, or oxygen utilization can be measured in either absolute units or relative units. For example, LCGMR in an anatomical region of interest could be presented as either mmol of glucose/100 g of brain tissue/min or as a ratio of activity within the region of interest compared with metabolic activity for the entire brain or a specific slice. Each approach has its advantages and disadvantages. In the case of sleep, and particularly non-REM sleep, however, as will be discussed later, overall rates of whole brain metabolism or CBF typically falls by 20–30% compared with wakefulness or REM sleep. Therefore, since the absolute value of the denominator is significantly reduced in the non-REM state compared with the wakefulness, the relative change in an area of interest, for example, the occipital lobe, would be increased in non-REM sleep compared with wakefulness, even if the absolute rate of CBF in the occipital lobe was significantly reduced, but to a lesser degree than whole brain CBF. Unless these issues are clearly clarified, the unwary could falsely conclude that the occipital lobe is ''activated'' during non-REM sleep compared with wakefulness.

To summarize some of the advantages and disadvantages of functional mapping tools, EEG and MEG have good temporal resolution (ms to s) but poor spatial resolution. Metabolic measures include FDG with PET, which has poor temporal (20–45 min) and fair anatomical resolution. HMPAO SPECT has fair temporal (several minutes) and poor anatomical resolution. For hemodynamic measures, $H_2{}^{15}O$ PET has moderate temporal (<1 min) and fair spatial resolution. NIRS has fair temporal resolution (s) and fair spatial resolution. FMRI has relatively good temporal (s) and spatial resolution.

III. An Overview of Sleep

Sleep is characterized by two major states—REM sleep and non-REM sleep. Non-REM sleep in humans is divided into four stages, based primarily on EEG characteristics. Stage 1 is a brief transitional state between wakefulness and sleep, typically about 1–5% of total sleep time; the EEG is typically low voltage, mixed frequency. Stage 2, characterized by sleep spindles and K complexes, occupies about 40–60% of total sleep time. Stages 3 and 4 are defined by the proportion of an epoch occupied by delta waves [high-amplitude (>75 μV), slow waves (>0.5 s)]: 20–50% for Stage 3 and >50% for Stage 4. Stages 3 and 4 sleep are sometimes referred to as delta sleep or slow-wave sleep. Delta sleep is strongly influenced by age, with maximum percentages in the preadolescent period, gradually falling to near zero in late middle age. It also increases during recovery sleep after sleep deprivation. REM sleep is defined by a relatively activated EEG (low voltage, mixed frequency), bursts of rapid eye movements, and atonia of the antigravity muscles, such as the submental muscles. REM sleep typically occupies about 20–25% of total sleep time. In addition, the amount of ocular activity during an epoch of REM sleep is usually called REM density; while no standardized method exists for the measurement of REM density, it is often scored visually on a scale of 0–8 per minute of REM sleep.

REM sleep is more activated psychologically and physiologically than non-REM sleep. Non-REM sleep is associated with decreased brain temperature; diminished and steady autonomic activity; increased release of growth hormone, aldosterone, testosterone, prolactin, and insulin; and reduced release of ACTH, cortisol, and thyrotropin near sleep onset. During non-REM sleep, dreams are relatively rare, except perhaps during the initial Stage 1 period in the transition from wakefulness into sleep. Otherwise, mentation during non-REM sleep is usually conceptual or abstract. In contrast, REM sleep is associated with increased brain temperature compared with non-REM sleep; variable autonomic function; penile erections (in males); active motor inhibition of the antigravity muscles; a tendency to poikilothermia; reduced ventilatory response to CO_2; and increased whole body metabolic rate compared with non-REM sleep. Mentation during REM sleep is usually perceptual with dreaming; furthermore, reality testing and reflective thought are diminished or suspended.

The physiological basis for sleep remains largely unknown. No specific anatomical center has been identified for sleep or wakefulness or for either non-REM sleep or REM sleep. REM sleep can be generated from the brainstem. After transaction about the level of the colliculi, REM-like physiological activity continues in the brainstem. Cholinergic neurons originating in the lateral dorsal tegmental (LDT) and pedunculopontine tegmental (PPT) nuclei appear to facilitate REM sleep and cortical arousal, in the latter case, mediated through their effects on the nucleus reticularis in the thalamus. These cholinergic neurons are inhibited by noradrenergic and serotonergic neurons in the locus coeruleus and dorsal raphe nucleus. Histaminergic neurons in the posterior hypothalamus also mediate arousal. As for non-REM sleep, facilitory neurons have been implicated in the nucleus of the solitary tract, anterior hypothalamus, and basal forebrain. During non-REM sleep, as cholinergic input to the nucleus reticularis is reduced, thalamocortical neurons become progressively hyperpolarized. As they do so, their firing patterns become more synchronized, first in the spindle frequency range (12–14 Hz) and later in the delta frequency range (0.5–2 Hz). The thalamocortical cells synchronize the rhythmicity of cortical neurons, thereby producing EEG patterns that define sleep Stages 2–4 (27). There is also evidence of an inherent slow wave generated in the cortical mantel (28).

Finally, it should be emphasized that sleep and wakefulness are regulated by at least three processes:

1. A *homeostatic process*: the longer the wake period, the greater the propensity to sleep. Furthermore, the amount of slow wave sleep (SWS) increases with duration of wakefulness and declines over the sleep period.

These changes in delta sleep may be consistent with the homeostatic functions of sleep; thus, delta sleep has been hypothesized to reverse the effects of wakefulness (8).

2. A *circadian process*: the propensity to be asleep or to be awake at any time over the 24-h day is influenced by an endogenous pacemaker, the suprachiasmatic nucleus (SCN), in the anterior hypothalamus. For most persons whose endogenous rest-activity cycle is synchronized with the light-dark cycle, sleep is most likely at night and at midday (siesta period). The phase position of coordinated cellular activity in the SCN is normally synchronized by the ambient light-dark cycle.
3. An *ultradian process*: non-REM and REM sleep alternate with one another, with a cycle length (time between onsets of REM sleep) of about 90 min.

Like the basic mechanisms of sleep, the basic functions of sleep remain largely unknown (9). Many of the proposed functions, however, are directly related to functional metabolic changes that occur during sleep. For instance, among the most widely quoted functions of sleep are energy conservation, thermoregulation of the brain and body, restoration of tissue integrity, maintenance of neural plasticity, and memory. In this context it is interesting that we have preliminary data that the greater the CBF is in the midafternoon, as assessed by HMPAO uptake with SPECT, the faster the onset of sleep, the greater the amount of delta sleep, and the lesser the amount of Stage 2 sleep that night (29).

Benington and Heller have proposed that the restoration of brain energy metabolism is a primary function of sleep, especially delta sleep (7,30). Specifically, they postulate that the concentration of high-energy phosphorylated compounds, such as ATP, decrease during wakefulness relative to adenosinediphosphate (ADP) and adenosine. Adenosine promotes sleep, especially delta sleep (31,32). Furthermore, they postulate that high-energy phosphate bonds are restored during sleep.

IV. Functional Imaging Demonstrates Reduced Rates of Cerebral Metabolism During Delta Sleep

Based upon the brief overview of non-REM and REM sleep, it should be no surprise that recent studies have usually reported that global and local measures of cerebral metabolism and blood flow are significantly reduced during non-REM sleep (especially Stages 3 and 4 sleep, delta sleep, or slow-wave activity) compared with either REM sleep or wakefulness (33–35). Earlier studies, however, using older methods had sometimes reported increased cerebral metabolism during non-REM sleep (36). Metabolic rate is particularly reduced during Stages 3 and 4 (slow-wave) sleep rather than Stage 2 sleep (37,38). To briefly summarize, decreased whole brain metabolic rate during non-REM sleep has been reported with cerebral glucose utilization in the monkey (39,40), cat (41), rat (42,43), and normal human subjects (35,37,44–46), with decreased regional and global cerebral blood flow (38,47–51) and decreased middle cerebral arterial blood flow velocity (52–54) in normal human subjects, and with decreased whole brain cerebral oxygen consumption in humans (48,49). The changes in whole brain metabolism during non-REM sleep are usually in the order of 20–35% compared with either the waking resting brain or REM sleep (35,35a,39), although considerable variation has been reported in some studies.

The changes during non-REM sleep compared with wakefulness are not uniform throughout the brain. In our original 2DG study in monkeys, the areas showing the greatest reduction during non-REM sleep compared to drowsy animals awake in the dark were auditory cortex (−44%), lateral geniculate (−41%), reticular nucleus of the thalamus (−40%), inferior parietal cortex (−38%), corona radiata (−38%), and mesencephalic reticular formation (−36%) (39,40). In human studies, the greatest metabolic reductions were in medial prefrontal cortex, corpus callosum and frontal white matter, and thalamus (35,37,45). In a similar fashion, reduced CBF has been reported in basal forebrain/hypothalamus, orbitofrontal cortex, anterior cingulate, thalamus, basal ganglia, as well as pons and mesencephalon (38,50).

In a more recent study, spectral activity of the EEG was correlated with normalized CBF measured with PET and the $H_2{}^{15}O$ method in normal volunteers (38). EEG in the delta frequency bands [slow-wave activity (SWA)] correlated negatively with CBF in the thalamus, brainstem reticular formation, cerebellum, anterior cingulate, basal ganglia, and orbitofrontal cortex. After controlling for delta frequency activity, the residual regional CBF in the medial thalamus correlated negatively with spindle activity. The authors suggest that these may reflect the disfacilitation and active inhibition of thalamocortical relay neurons in association with delta and spindles. This would be consistent with the work of Steriade and colleagues, which suggests that progressive hyperpolarization of the reticular nucleus and other thalamic nuclei is associated with, first, sleep spindles, and, later, with delta EEG waves (27,55).

In a recent study, using near-infrared spectroscopy in the transitions between wakefulness and napping sleep, synchronized, parallel, and short-duration (~3–5 s) changes in concentrations of oxyhemoglobin and deoxyhemoglobin in frontal cortex were observed (25). The two light-absorbing molecules decreased at sleep onset and increased at sleep offset. These findings are consistent with other methods of measuring cerebral metabolism in the transitions between sleep and wakefulness.

V. Is Cerebral Protein Synthesis Enhanced During Delta Sleep?

If sleep, and especially delta sleep, are associated with restorative physiological processes, the reduced metabolic demands during sleep could free up resources for cerebral anabolic processes and protein synthesis. While protein synthesis requires relatively little energy, it is sensitive to the cellular energy charge, which may be increased in the brain during delta sleep (5,6).

To investigate the relationship between sleep and cerebral protein synthesis, two groups have measured the local cerebral protein synthesis (LCPS), as assayed by the autoradiographic A[1-^{14}C] leucine uptake method, in rats (56) and monkeys (57). Both studies suggest that protein synthesis is correlated with duration of delta sleep. In the monkey study, after controlling for weighted time in delta sleep with integrated specific activity of leucine in grey matter, LCPS was positively correlated with the amount of delta sleep in all 57 regions of interest (ROIs) and to a statistically significant extent ($p < 05$) in 18 areas. The correlations were strongest in the limbic system (lateral septum, basal forebrain), basal ganglia (caudate nucleus, global pallidus, putamen), ventral posterior lateral nucleus of the thalamus, white matter (optic chiasm), hypothalamus (preoptic area, arcuate nucleus, suprachiasmatic nucleus, supraoptic nucleus, posterior nucleus), and brainstem (ventral raphe nucleus, ventral tegmental nucleus, dorsal motor nucleus of the vagus, and solitary nucleus). Correlations between ''light'' sleep and LCPS were either infrequent or negative (9 ROIs). The possibility that protein synthesis takes place during REM sleep has not been investigated with the leucine uptake method, which requires a long period of incubation.

These findings of decreased cerebral metabolism (glucose metabolic rates, CBF, and oxygen consumption) and increased protein synthesis during delta sleep may be consistent with the conventional wisdom that sleep has a restorative function, replenishing energy stores and promoting protein synthesis. We must recognize, however, that these findings are preliminary, especially the data on protein synthesis. We also note that local areas with the highest metabolic rates during wakefulness do not necessarily show the greatest reduction in metabolic rate during non-REM sleep.

VI. Functional Brain Imaging Demonstrates Localized Cerebral Metabolic Changes During Normal REM Sleep

Most studies indicate that rates of global cerebral metabolic rate and cerebral blood flow are similar during REM sleep and wakefulness (34–36,53,54,58–60). Nevertheless, the metabolic patterns throughout the brain are dissimilar during REM sleep compared with wakefulness. For example, limbic structures, including the cingulate gyrus, may be more active metabolically during REM sleep than during wakefulness, whereas higher-order association areas, such as the orbital and dorsolateral frontal and inferior parietal cortices, may be relatively deactivated (35,60–62).

In recent studies of CBF, utilizing $H_2{}^{15}O$ with PET, sleep-deprived normal subjects were studied during wakefulness and different stages of sleep in a within subjects experiment (38,61). These studies reported increased CBF in limbic structures, including anterior cingulate, during REM sleep compared with wakefulness or NonREM sleep. In addition, these studies also suggested that REM sleep was characterized by generalized activation of the brain (particularly pons, midbrain, caudate, paralimbic-limbic structures) without participation of regions in the fronto-parietal areas, which are normally involved in higher-order analysis and integration of neural information. Maquet et al. (61) particularly emphasized the activation of the amygdala during REM sleep in humans. With its interactions with the anterior cingulate and posterior cortices, the amygdala might reactivate affective components of memories, bringing about the consolidation of memory traces during REM sleep. In a similar fashion, Nofzinger et al. (62), emphasizing the widespread activation of midline limbic and paralimbic structures, temporal and insular cortex, and enterorhinal cortex in REM sleep, compared with quiet presleep wakefulness, suggest that one function of REM sleep is the integration of neocortical activity with hypothalamic-basal forebrain regulatory and motivational mechanisms.

In a discussion of their $H_2{}^{15}O$ CBF study in normal subjects, Braun et al. (50) noted that centrencephalic regions, including brainstem, thalamus, and basal forebrain, are deactivated during slow-wave sleep compared with presleep wakefulness and reactivated during REM sleep. Similar changes were observed in anterior insula, anterior cingulate, and mesial temporal cortex. In contrast, dorsolateral and orbital prefrontal cortices were deactivated during both slow-wave sleep and REM sleep compared with wakefulness.

Braun et al. (50) proposed that sleep can be defined by the sleep-related deactivation of the dorsolateral and prefrontal cortices, which are the only anatomical areas showing decreased CBF during both non-REM and REM sleep compared with wakefulness. Furthermore, they suggested that the psychological characteristics of dreaming are accounted for by the relative deactivation of prefrontal cortex (which normally maintains ''reality testing'' during the waking state), the activated limbic system (which is responsible for the emotionality of dreams), and the activation of the hippocampal and parahippocampal system (which may recall the memory elements on which dreams are built).

As an illustration of a dream, a former World War II prisoner of war suffering from posttraumatic stress disorder (PTSD) recently described to one of the authors (JCG) a frightening nightmare in which he was chased by tigers dressed in the uniforms of his former prison guards. During the nightmare he fully believed the scene to be real, and he awoke sweating and shaking with fear. The terror he experienced may reflect an overactive limbic system, the tiger and the uniforms may recall the prison camp in which he was held, and the suspension of reality testing and the acceptance of this bizarre scene may reflect an underactive rationale, analytic system located in the prefrontal cortices.

Braun et al. (60) also found that cerebral blood flow increased during REM sleep in extrastriate visual cortices but not in the primary striate visual cortex. This finding is interesting since it has never been clear if the primary visual cortex (V1 or BA 17) was necessary for the experience of a visual dream. This observation suggests that the visual experience of dreaming is not associated with primary visual sensory areas. Furthermore, activity in extrastriate cortex correlated positively with activity in limbic and paralimbic regions and negatively with lateral orbital and dorsolateral prefrontal cortices.

In a follow-up to our original PET study comparing REM sleep and waking in normal controls, we investigated the neural substrates for rapid eye movements specifically by correlating the LCGMR in oculomotor areas with the number of rapid eye movements during a 30-min period during wakefulness and REM sleep

(63). We found significant positive correlations between the number of eye movements during REM sleep and rate of glucose metabolism in neuroanatomical areas corresponding to (1) the saccadic eye movement system (frontal eye field and the right dorsolateral prefrontal cortex), (2) midline attentional system (cingulate and medial frontal cortex, precuneus), and (3) parietal visual spatial attentional system (bilateral superior parietal lobules, right inferior parietal lobule); in addition, the number of eye movements correlated negatively with the left inferior parietal lobule. In general, similar correlations were found during wakefulness, with some exceptions. These results suggest that some of the same neural mechanisms may be involved in eye movements during REM sleep and wakefulness and that the cortex may play an important role in initiating eye movements in REM sleep, as in wakefulness.

In their more recent studies, Braun et al. (60) found similar relationships between REM density and local cerebral activation. They reported that REM density during 90-second epochs was positively correlated with regional CBF in extrastriate cortex, hippocampus, and parahippocampus and was negatively correlated with regional CBF in lateral orbital cortex, dorsolateral prefrontal cortex, and striate cortex. The relationship to cortical oculomotor areas was not examined.

Since some but not all studies suggest that eye movements ''scan'' the subjective dream during REM sleep, these results may further our basic understanding of the neurobiology of dreaming (63,64). Moreover, REM density (a measure of average amount of eye movement activity/min during REM sleep) is elevated in depression, schizophrenia, and some alcoholics (65–67) and decreased in Alzheimer's disease (68). These results also have implications for understanding the pathophysiology of the physiological sleep abnormalities associated with these disorders. Furthermore, the presence of functionally significant local cortical deactivation during REM sleep may be inconsistent with dream theories, which appear to suggest widespread cortical activation (64,69).

VII. Is the Dream Content Associated with Localized Changes in Cerebral Metabolism?

The discovery that REM sleep is associated with dreaming provided relatively easy access to dream reports by awakening subjects from REM sleep during the night. Furthermore, investigators found that some dreaming or at least some type of conceptual thinking probably occurs during non-REM sleep, perhaps at lower rates than during REM sleep. It also stimulated new interest in the nature and neural basis of dreaming. For example, what neural systems are necessary or involved in specific characteristics of dreaming?

As Maquet et al. (61), Braun et al. (60), and Nofzinger et al. (62) have speculated, functional imaging studies of REM sleep may contribute to understanding the neuropsychology of dreaming. Braun et al. for example, suggested that cholinergic activation of basal forebrain favored the ventral rather than the dorsal cholinergic pathways from the brainstem. We previously showed that double-blind infusion of physostigmine, a cholinesterase inhibitor, during non-REM sleep initiated REM sleep and dreaming in normal volunteers (71). Likewise, Braun et al. suggested that dreaming might be facilitated by activation of the unimodal association visual and auditory cortices at the same time that heteromodal association areas in frontal cortex and parietal cortex were deactivated.

In our PET with FDG study during REM sleep (35), we initiated an exploratory analysis linking LCGMR in specific brain regions with measures of emotion and anxiety, based on verbal reports from subjects awakened from sleep about 32 min after receiving FDG intravenously while they were asleep. The transcripts of the verbal reports were scored blindly on the Gottschalk-Gleser Content Analysis Scales for total anxiety and six anxiety scales and measures of hostility (72,73). The scales and subscales were correlated with LCGMR in cortical and subcortical areas. To give selected examples, ratings for shame, guilt, anxiety, and covert hostility toward others during REM sleep correlated positively and significantly with LCGMR in bilateral anterior cingulate gyrus but negatively in the left midcingulum. Likewise, anxiety scores and hostility correlated negatively and significantly with the left temporal lobe. In addition, this study suggested that dreaming and waking mentation involve not only neural systems associated with language (temporal lobes) but also those involved with intellect and reasoning (frontal lobes) and primary visual imagery (occipital lobes). Further studies of this sort, with more attention to other limbic-paralimbic systems, might be informative about the basic neural mechanisms underlying dream production and experience.

It should be noted, in passing, that Solms has recently proposed a neuropsychological model for dreaming based on autopsy and neuropsychological studies of patients with neurological lesions (74). For example, total cessation of dreaming (‘‘global anoneria’’) is associated with either posterial cortical or deep bilateral frontal lesions. He also noted that increased frequency and vivacity of dreaming is associated with anterior limbic lesions. The combination of localization of lesions affecting dreaming and functional imaging opens new opportunities to study the neural basis of dreaming.

VIII. How Does a Sleeping Pill Affect LCGMR During Non-REM Sleep in Normal Controls?

In an effort to better understand the mechanisms by which sleeping pills promote sleep, we compared the effects of zolpidem (Ambien 10 mg), an imidazopyridine hypnotic that is relatively selective for BZ_1 receptors, and placebo on LCGMR during the first non-REM period in 12 normal young volunteers (75). As before, subjects maintained a normal sleep-wake schedule and were adapted to sleeping in the sleep laboratory and to the conditions of the study before participating in the study. They received active or placebo pills in a random, double-blind fashion about 20 min before lights out. FDG was infused about 10 min after sleep onset each night. The effects of zolpidem on LCGMR varied directly with the plasma concentration of zolpidem. The higher the mean concentration of plasma zolpidem during the 90 min after oral administration, the greater the reduction of LCGMR on the active drug night compared with the placebo last night in medial frontal cortex, cingulate gyrus, putamen, thalamus, and hippocampus. A limitation of this study was that the plasma concentrations of zolpidem were considerably lower and more variable than expected on the basis of previous studies. While zolpidem decreased metabolic rates in cingulate and cerebellum, which are known to have high concentrations of BZ_1 receptors, these effects were not observed in other areas that have high densities of the BZ_1 receptor, such as frontal-parietal and sensorimotor cortex. Areas low in BZ_1 receptors, such as the hippocampus, did not show decreased CGMR. The biggest increases were in occipital cortex.

In a more recent study, Finelli et al. (76) compared the effects of zolpidem (20 mg) and placebo in 8 healthy men with the $H_2{}^{15}O$ method. Subjects were sleep deprived for 40 h on two occasions in order to promote sleep about 4 h each time (23:00–03:00) in the PET scanner. Plasma zolpidem concentrations were not reported. During sleep (Stages 2, 4, and REM), relative regional CBF was lower after zolpidem than placebo in the basal ganglia and insula, but higher in the parietal cortex. These findings suggest that zolpidem intensified the normal reduction in regional CBF associated with non-REM sleep compared with presleep wakefulness. During REM sleep, CBF in the anterior cingulate was reduced after zolpidem compared to placebo. Interestingly, the typical EEG patterns associated with sleep did not have counterparts with the regional CBF changes, another example of a dissociation between states of consciousness and cerebral metabolism. A limitation of the present study was the small sample size available for a within subject comparison in specific states of sleep.

Previous studies with benzodiazepines in anxiety patients during wakefulness also found elevated LCGMR in occipital cortex (77).

IX. How Well Coupled Is CBF to Neural and EEG Activity?

CBF is regulated in part by two needs: as a buffer against the effects of systemic changes in blood pressure, heart rate, Pa_{O_2}, Pa_{CO_2}, and pH and as a response to local metabolic demands. In recent years, new information from PET studies, Doppler measures of middle arterial blood flow, and FMRI have challenged the assumption that regional cerebral blood flow is always tightly coupled to glucose and oxygen metabolism during wakefulness (4,78). These concerns have also emerged from some sleep studies. For example, during a study of REM sleep in goats, (1) the brain was ''overperfused'' compared with arterial CO_2 tension or cerebral oxidative metabolism, (2) CBF varied with Pa_{CO_2} tension during non-REM sleep and with diaphragmatic movement in REM sleep, and (3) localized cerebral hypocapnia sometimes occurred during sleep (79,80).

In a study of mean flow velocity in the middle cerebral arteries in normal subjects using Doppler ultrasonography, Hajak et al. (52) noted that spontaneous or evoked awakenings from non-REM sleep were not associated with increased blood flow. Furthermore, flow rates were uncoupled with EEG activity, for example, they were lower during stage 2 sleep than the preceding stage 4 sleep. The authors suggested that cerebral perfusion is not solely regulated by the cerebral metabolic rate.

Buxton and Frank (4) have argued that the dominant factor influencing local blood flow during neural stimulation is the need to deliver oxygen to the involved tissue. They suggest that a large change in CBF is necessary to produce a small increase in oxygen delivery and to increase oxidative metabolism of glucose. Unlike oxygen, which is nearly 100% metabolized into brain tissue, only about 50% of the glucose in tissue is metabolized; unlike oxygen, which is ''bound'' to hemoglobin in blood, glucose is free to move back and forth across capillary walls. In principle, therefore, CGMR can be increased during neural activity without dramatically increasing blood flow. The increase in blood flow associated with neuronal activity apparently results from increased flow velocity through capillaries rather than recruitment of more dormant capillaries. Studies of regional cerebral blood flow in rats, cats, rabbits, and piglets during sleep basically support this hypothesis: the number of capillaries recruited for perfusion does not change during the transition from non-REM sleep to REM sleep even though blood flow increased (81). Thus, increased local CBF may result from increased flow velocity rather than increased number of vessels. A better understanding of local cerebral vascular response to neuronal activity would be helpful in the physiological interpretation of studies of cerebral blood flow and of FMRI.

X. Changes in Cerebral Blood Flow as Subjects Wake Up

Several studies suggest that cerebral metabolism does not return immediately to presleep values upon awakening. One of these observations came from the work of Hajak et al. (52), mentioned above, who noted that mean flow velocity in the middle cerebral artery in the morning after awakening required several minutes to half an hour to reach levels corresponding to the waking state of the previous evening. Braun et al. (50) reported similar findings in their studies with $H_2{}^{15}O$ CBF in normal controls. Both absolute and normalized CBF were reduced in hippocampus, dorsolateral prefrontal cortex, temporal cortex, occipital, angular cortex, and striate cortex after sleep compared with presleep values. In a recent abstract, Balkin et al. (82) reported that it took about 20 min to ''wipe the cobwebs out'' in the morning, that is, the time required before CBF returned to normal.

These observations not only demonstrate the uncoupling between CBF, EEG, and behavioral state but may help explain ''sleep inertia,'' the well-known timelag that many persons experience in fully waking up after sleep.

XI. Summary of Functional Cerebral Metabolism During Wakefulness, REM Sleep, and Non-REM Sleep in Normal Humans

At one level, the functional imaging studies of sleep are, in general, consistent with the widely held concept that we live our lives in three major states of consciousness: wakefulness, REM sleep, and non-REM sleep. One caveat here is that we restrict non-REM sleep to ''deep'' sleep (delta sleep, Stages 3 and 4, or slow-wave sleep). Stage 2 sleep appears to be an intermediate state of non-REM sleep, less ''deep'' than delta sleep, but equal to or slightly lower than presleep wakefulness. With few exceptions, the current studies indicate that whole brain metabolic rate can be ranked as follows: pre-sleep wakefulness $=$ REM sleep $\geq$ Stage 2 $\gg$ delta sleep.

In greater anatomical detail, the majority of studies indicate the metabolic rate during presleep wakefulness or REM sleep, compared with delta sleep, is significantly greater in brainstem (pontine tegmentum, midbrain, and mesencephalon), diencephalon (thalamus, hypothalamus, basal forebrain), the limbic system (amygdala, septal nuclei, hippocampus, anterior cingulate, infralimbic, parahippocampal, interhinal cortex), basal ganglia and striatum (caudata, putamen), cerebellum, and temporal area.

Although mean whole brain metabolic rate is about the same during REM compared with wakefulness, localized rates of metabolism may distinguish the two states. For instance, Braun et al. (50) and Maquet et al. (61) reported decreased CBF in dorsal lateral prefrontal cortex during REM sleep compared with wakefulness. Likewise, Braun et al. reported decreased CBF in posterior insula and striate cortex. Braun et al. (50) have gone so far as to suggest that the defining characteristics of sleep (both SWS and REM sleep) may be reduced metabolic rate in the orbital, dorsolateral prefrontal cortex, and inferior parietal cortex compared with wakefulness. It should be noted, however, that dorsal lateral prefrontal cortex was not different during REM sleep compared to wakefulness in the PET/FDG study of Nofzinger et al. (62).

In contrast to the concept that the three states of consciousness (wakefulness, non-REM sleep, and REM sleep) are distinct entities, some data from functional brain image studies suggest that the boundaries between the three states are less distinct. For instance, the ''normal'' coupling between state CGMR, CBF, and EEG may be unhinged in each of these states. An example is sleep inertia after sleep.

XII. How Does Sleep Deprivation Affect Normal Brain Metabolism?

Acute or chronic sleep deprivation is a common complaint in our 24-h-a-day society. It has been said that Thomas Edison was the ''enemy of sleep.'' Aside from promoting himself as an extremely ''short sleeper,'' he invented the electric light bulb, which enabled wakefulness to invade one of the last frontiers of human activity, namely, night. School and work schedules, the demands of family, the lure of television and nocturnal recreational activities, and travel across time zones all compete with sleep. The negative consequences include daytime sleepiness, fatigue, impaired performance, accidents, and dysphoria.

The effects of sleep deprivation on basic neural mechanisms underlying behavior are only poorly understood. In an effort to improve this knowledge, we studied cerebral glucose metabolic rates with PET during wakefulness in the afternoon in eight normal controls before and after a night of total deprivation (83). During the FDG uptake period, subjects performed a visual continuous performance task (CPT), which required them to press a button in response to selected visual stimuli. Absolute LCGMR in thalamus and cerebellum decreased significantly during vigilance testing after sleep deprivation compared with the rested state. Whole brain metabolic rate did not change significantly (~14%). Relative LCGMR analysis showed significant reductions in the temporal lobe, right cerebellum, and left thalamus; in contrast, relative LCGMR increased significantly in the occipital lobe. Furthermore, statistically significant cortical lobe by condition effects were noted for both absolute and relative LCGMR measures: frontal and temporal lobes decreased following sleep deprivation, whereas parietal lobes increased. These findings in sleep-deprived normal subjects were somewhat similar to our earlier study in monkeys in which we compared drowsy and alert animals; LCGMR was not statistically different, although it was 18% higher in the lateral habenula ($p < 0.01$) and 17% lower in the hippocampus in the drowsy animals compared with the alert animals (40).

Not surprisingly, vigilance performance on the CPT declined significantly after sleep deprivation. Moreover, the greater the impairment of performance, the greater the reduction in absolute LCGMR in amygdala, thalamus, caudate, and putamen. No significant correlations were found between LCGMR in cortical lobes and performance measures, suggesting that the attention and performance deficits associated with sleep deprivation result from subcortical rather than primary cortical dysfunction.

More recently, Portas et al. (84) investigated the interaction of selective attention and arousal in five normal experimental subjects and two controls. Using FMRI blood oxygen level–dependent (BOLD) methods, they reported that the ventrolateral thalamus was activated during a visual attentional task in a low arousal state (24 h of sleep deprivation) compared with either the control state or a high arousal state (caffeine 5 mg/kg by mouth). Other areas were activated by the attentional task but did not vary with level of arousal: intraparietal sulcus, superior parietal gyrus, middle frontal gyrus, superior and anterior portions of the precentral gyrus, and a small area of the cerebellum. Levels of performance did not change with the three levels of arousal. They suggest that the thalamus represents a functional interface between cortical attentional areas and subcortical arousal systems.

Sleep deprivation also affects cognitive performance as well as attention. Drummond et al. (85,86) studied the effects of total sleep deprivation for 35 h in 13 healthy young adults on serial subtraction and verbal learning while their hemodynamic response was assessed by the FMRI BOLD technique. Following sleep deprivation, performance measures fell significantly: serial subtraction (from 89% to 82% correct answers; missed attempts increased from 2% to 8%). The number of words correctly recalled fell by 40%. The effects of sleep deprivation on cerebral activation varied with the two tasks. During serial subtraction in the rested state, widespread prefrontal and parietal cortical areas were activated; after sleep deprivation, however, virtually no areas were activated by subtraction compared with the control state. During verbal learning, prefrontal and left temporal areas were activated in the rested state. After sleep deprivation, however, activation of the prefrontal cortex was increased. This was unexpected based on the work of Harrison and Horne (87). We had actually hypothesized that PFC would be less activated. Instead, the sleepier the subjects were, the greater the activation of the PFC. Second, the temporal lobe was no longer activated. Instead, the parietal lobe was activated. In fact, the better the subjects performed on the verbal learning task, the greater the activation of the parietal lobe during the sleep-deprived state. These results of the Drummond et al. studies (85,86) suggest that the effects of sleep deprivation on cortical activation are dynamic, complex, and task-dependent. In some conditions, sleep deprivation may be associated with neural compensatory mechanisms as other areas faltered.

The effect of chronic experimental sleep deprivation on cerebral metabolism has not been studied in normal human subjects. Everson et al. (88), however, conducted a study of quantitative LCGMR with 2DG comparing six rats who had been sleep deprived for 11–12 days with six yoked controls. Both experimental and control animals lived on separate sides of a disc over a shallow water pan. Whenever the experimental animal entered sleep, as detected by an on-line computer that continuously recorded the EEG, the disc rotated, thereby keeping the experimental animal moving and awake. The yoked animals had to move the same amount as the experimental animals but could sleep while the experimental animals were resting and awake. Despite significantly increased deep brain temperature, increased systemic hypermetabolism, and sympathetic activation, the experimental animals did not show a change in whole brain absolute glucose utilization. Compared with the yoked controls, however, the sleep-deprived animals showed significantly reduced LCGMR in hypothalamus, thalamus, and limbic system. Thus, the results from both the acute human study and the more chronic rodent study suggest that sleep deprivation probably affects subcortical regions to a greater extent than cortical regions. In particular, sleep deprivation seems to affect areas of the brain traditionally thought to regulate emotions and arousal. Not surprisingly, the conventional wisdom is that sleep deprivation interferes with attention, motivation, spontaneity, and initiative.

To determine the effects of REM sleep deprivation on LCGMR with the 2DG method, Peder et al. (89) compared three rats who were REM deprived for 5 days with three rats who were not. REM deprivation was achieved by the small platform method, which prevents REM sleep because rats fall into a water bath during the muscle atonia of REM sleep. Control rats also lived on small platforms but were allowed to have REM sleep because of supporting cuffs on the platform. In the 60 anatomical areas examined, the only statistically significant changes were increased

LCGMR in the lateral habenula, in the REM-deprived rats the caudal and middle parts of the limbic system, and corpus collosum. Since the lateral habenula was activated in sleepy monkeys (40) and REM-deprived rats, its role in sleep deprivation deserves more attention.

Having reviewed some of the findings relating functional brain imaging to normal sleep and sleep deprivation, we will now turn to clinical studies in patients with sleep disorders and depression.

XIII. Functional Brain-Imaging Studies in Patients with Obstructive Sleep Apnea

Sleep apnea is a disorder characterized by repetitive episodes of apnea (lasting 10 seconds or more) and hypopnea (decrement in airflow with a drop in oxyhemoglobin saturation of at least 4%) during sleep (90). Episodes of apnea are central if respiratory effort ceases for the duration of the apneic episode and obstructive if ventilatory efforts continue in the absence of effective airflow because of a transient obstruction in the upper airway. Episodes are classified as mixed if ventilatory effort is absent before the onset of obstruction. Most patients with obstructive sleep apnea (OSA) or mixed apnea are middle-aged, obese men. They typically have hypertension, excessive daytime sleepiness, morning headaches and sluggishness, cognitive impairment, personality changes, erythrocytosis, and increased risk for strokes and cardiovascular disease. During the episodes of apnea, these patients display dramatic changes in autonomic function, including tachy- and bradycardia, cardiac arrhythmia, changes in blood gas concentrations, snoring and gasping, frequent body movements, and hundreds of brief interruptions of sleep.

During the last 20 years or so, functional brain-imaging studies have been used to investigate cerebral functioning during sleep and wakefulness in patients with OSA. In early studies using the xenon method in patients with OSA, Meyer and colleagues (47,91) demonstrated significant reductions of CBF at the onset of sleep compared with normal controls. Since then, several detailed studies have used doppler techniques to measure cerebral blood flow in the middle cerebral arteries during and after sleep. They have revealed a constellation of abnormalities, including periods of cerebral hypoxemia, and both diminished and highly variable rates of CBF and cerebral blood flow velocity (CBFV) during apneic episodes during sleep (92,92). Netzer et al. (94) reported significant reductions in CBF during 76% of obstructive hypopneas, 80% of obstructive apneas, and 14% of central apneas. The reduction of CBF was related to the duration of and the decrease in arterial oxygen saturation of the hypopneic episode.

The Doppler method only measures CBF in the middle cerebral artery and, therefore, does not provide a full picture of the whole brain. Ficker et al. (95) administered HMPAO with the SPECT method during sleep in 14 patients with severe OSA. Five of the patients showed significant hyperperfusion in the frontal lobes, possibly related to repetitive episodes of arousal. Overall, however, the left parietal area was significantly underperfused. These abnormalities were completely reversed with adequate nasal continuous positive airway pressure (nasal CPAP), a treatment that helps maintain airway patency during sleep.

The safety of nasal CPAP in patients with sleep apnea has been questioned, however, in part because of concerns that patients with OSA might have a higher cerebrovascular reactivity to changes in end-tidal pCO_2. To investigate these worries, Droste et al. (96) studied patients with OSA and normal controls with the doppler method during normal breathing with and without nasal CPAP. They reported that nasal CPAP was safe at a pressure of 9 cm of water and that the cerebrovascular response to end-tidal pCO_2 was normal in patients with OSA.

In a challenge study, however, patients with OSA showed a diminished cerebral vascular response to hypercapnia in the morning compared with the evening. Qureshi et al. (97) measured cerebral blood flow velocity (CBFV) in the middle cerebral arteries with the Doppler method in 30 patients with OSA while breathing either room air or 5% CO_2. A diminished hypercapnic vasomotor response in the morning was related to fragmented sleep and greater CO_2 retention during sleep. Sleep fragmentation during the night predicted approximately twice the variance in morning hyercapnic vasomotor reactivity relative to overnight CO_2 retention.

Rehan et al. (98) studied cyclic variations in CBF and CBFV in the middle cerebral arteries with the Doppler method in "healthy" preterm babies during quiet sleep and REM sleep. They found that the variability of CBFV was greater in REM sleep than in quiet sleep and that it varied with periodic and apneic breathing rather than regular or irregular respiration.

In a study of eight men with moderate to severe OSA, Hayakawa et al. (99) used NIRS simultaneously with polysomnography during nocturnal sleep (five patients) and daytime naps (three patients). They reported a consistent reduction in concentrations of oxyhemoglobin and increases in deoxyhemoglobin and total hemoglobin during apnea. Changes were greater during REM sleep than during non-REM sleep and varied directly with the duration of the apneic period. In contrast to other studies, they concluded that CBF increased during apnea. This discrepancy could reflect differences in methodology.

To test the hypothesis that repeated apneic episodes during sleep may lead to cerebral damage in patients with OSA, Kamba et al. (100) performed proton magnetic resonance (MR) spectroscopic studies in 15 healthy subjects and 23 patients with OSA who displayed no anatomical abnormalities on MR imaging. The *N*-acetylaspartate (NAA)/choline (Cho), NAA/creatine (Cre), and Cho/Cre ratios for cerebral cortex and white matter were calculated. The OSA patients had significantly lower NAA/Cho ratios in cerebral white matter. This ratio was significantly lower in patients with moderate to severe OSA than in patients with mild OSA ($p < 0.01$) and healthy subjects ($p < 0.01$). These results indicate that cerebral metabolic changes occur in normal-appearing brain tissue in patients with moderate to severe OSA. The reduced NAA/Cho ratio in the presence of cerebral damage was probably caused by repeated apneic episodes.

These functional imaging studies clearly indicate that OSA is significantly associated with dramatic and variable changes in spontaneous CBF and CBFV during apneic episodes and after sleep, as well as, perhaps, to hypercapneic challenges. The MRS study suggests that repeated apneic episodes causes cerebral white matter damage. Further studies will be needed to determine whether the changes in CBF are associated with greater risk for cerebral vascular accidents, white matter damage, cognitive impairment, personality changes, daytime sleepiness, morning headaches, and so forth. Patients with sleep apnea frequently have other risk factors for CNS, cardiovascular, arteriosclerosis, and pulmonary disorders, such as smoking, platelet activation and aggregation, obesity, and so forth. Sleep apnea probably diminishes the normal restorative functions of sleep and may be especially detrimental in patients who have had head injuries, stroke, increased intracranial pressure, or other CNS disorders. If the nasal CPAP reverses the abnormalities in global and regional CBF, as suggested by Ficker et al. (95), there may be opportunities to test the causal link between CBF abnormalities and these unfortunate consequences on the brain and function. Prevention may be possible.

XIV. Functional Brain Imaging in Narcolepsy

Narcolepsy is characterized by excessive daytime sleepiness, "attacks" of sleepiness, cataplexy, sleep paralysis, and hypnogogic hallucinations (90). It normally begins in the teenage years or young adulthood. A genetic predisposition has been known for some time. Recently, a peptide (called either hypocretin or orexin) in the hypothalamus has been implicated in the disorder. Treatment usually includes stimulants, such as amphetamines, methylphenidate, or modafinil, to combat sleepiness, and tricyclic antidepressants or selective serotonin reuptake inhibitors to prevent cataplexy.

In an early study of cerebral blood flow using the xenon method, Meyer and colleagues (47) reported increased CBF from wakefulness to sleep in narcoleptics; in contrast, normal controls showed a significant decrease in that transition. These results suggested that sleep onset was regulated in an abnormal manner in narcoleptic patients compared with normal controls, perhaps more of an active rather than a passive process.

Asenbaum et al. (101), using HMPAO uptake with SPECT, compared unmedicated narcoleptic patients during wakefulness and sleep-onset REM periods. In contrast to the finding of Meyer et al. (47), they found no suggestion of increased global CBF during sleep onset. Instead, they observed significantly greater HMPAO uptake in the right hemisphere than the left, which might be associated with the involvement of the right hemisphere in visual-spatial perceptions, such as visual hypnogogic hallucinations. They also found increased HMPAO uptake in superior parietal regions during sleep, which could be linked to an activation of associative cortical areas. Finally, HMPAO uptake in thalamic regions tended to be decreased during sleep, suggesting dysfunction or diminished activation of arousal systems during sleep in the thalamus.

In part based upon an autopsy study suggesting increased dopamine receptors in the brain of narcoleptic patients, several groups of investigators have used functional brain-imaging methods to measure dopamine receptor concentrations in the brains of living narcoleptic patients. Hublin et al. (102) used SPECT with ^{123}I-iodobenzamide (IBZM) to measure D_2 receptor density in six unmedicated narcoleptic patients compared with eight unmedicated Parkinsonian patients with unilateral symptoms. No differences were found.

Khan et al. (103) measured D_2 receptor binding using C-11-raclopride and PET in the striatum of 17 patients with the narcoleptic syndrome. Although C-11-raclopride uptake was increased in the putamen of narcoleptic subjects older than 31 years ($n = 11$) when compared with age-matched controls ($n = 15$), the authors concluded that the striatal D_2 dopaminergic neurotransmitter system was not involved in the basic pathophysiology of the narcolepsy. Using the same methodology, Rinne et al. (104) also found no difference in D_2 receptor binding between seven narcoleptic patients and seven controls in either caudate nucleus or putamen.

Cholinergic neurotransmission has been implicated in the onset of some narcoleptic symptoms, such as cataplexy, short REM latency, and hypnogogic hallucinations. Nevertheless, Sudo et al. (105) found no difference between unmedicated patients with narcolepsy and normal controls in the concentration of muscarinic receptors in pons, thalamus, striatum, and cerebral cortex in 11 drug-naive/free patients with narcolepsy and 21 normal controls. They used PET with [^{11}C]*N*-methyl-4-piperidylbenzilate ([^{11}C]NMPB). In addition, 7 of the 11 patients were studied with and without medication therapy. [^{11}C]NMPB binding was slightly reduced in thalamus during medication administration of anticholinergic drugs.

Parks et al. (106) conducted two studies with FMRI on the effects of stimulants in narcoleptic patients and normal controls. In the first study, amphetamine was administered to two narcoleptic patients and three normal controls while subjects responded to visual and auditory stimuli. Amphetamine decreased cortical areas of activation in normal controls but increased activation of the hemodynamic response in narcoleptic patients (106). Likewise, when modafanil (400 mg) was administered to eight normal subjects and eight subjects with narcolepsy, low cortical activation levels in both normal and narcoleptic subjects were increased following the administration of modafinil. These observations suggest that stimulants might have greater effects in subjects whose cortical regions were less activated compared with those whose regions were more activated.

XV. Functional Brain Imaging in Patients with Restless Legs Syndrome and Periodic Limb Movements of Sleep

Restless legs syndrome (RLS) is ''characterized by disagreeable leg sensations, usually at sleep onset, that cause an almost irresistible urge to move the legs'' (90). In contrast, periodic limb movements of sleep (PLMS) is characterized by ''periodic episodes of repetitive and highly stereotyped limb movements that occur during sleep'' (90). The two disorders often occur together. Central dopaminergic abnormalities have been postulated in the pathophysiology of these two syndromes, and dopaminergic agonists have been used as treatment. Brain-imaging studies with two D_2 receptor ligands—^{123}IBZM (107,108) and [^{11}C] raclopride (109)—revealed decreased concentrations of D_2 receptors in striatum. In addition, Ruottinen et al. (110) reported reduced dopamine turnover, using 6-[^{18}F]-fluoro-L-dopa (FLDOPA), in caudate nucleus and putamen in 9 drug-free patients with RLS or PLMS compared with 27 drug-free normal controls. Furthermore, Staedt et al. (111) also measured the effect of dopamine replacement on D_2 receptor occupancy in four patients suffering from severe insomnia as associated with nocturnal myoclonus (PLMS). They found that improvement in sleep quality was accompanied by increased binding of ^{123}IBZM in striatum.

XVI. Sleep: A Neurobiological Window in Depression

Insomnia and hypersomnia are among the most common diagnostic symptoms for major depression. Based upon dozens of sleep laboratory studies involving thousands of patients around the world, there is general agreement that 40–60% of unmedicated patients with a major depressive disorder show a constellation of sleep abnormalities, more often insomnia than hypersomnia (65,66,112). Frequent EEG sleep abnormalities include prolonged sleep latency, reduced total sleep time and sleep efficiency, loss of delta sleep, short REM latency, and increased REM density. The first REM period of the night is typically longer and has more ocular activity per minute of REM sleep (increased REM density) in depressed patients compared with normal controls. Other sleep-related abnormalities include the ''microarchitecture'' sleep EEG (113), increased core body temperature (114), abnormal neuroendocrine secretion (increased cortisol and decreased testosterone, growth hormone, prolactin, and, possibly, melatonin secretion) (115–119). Loss of non-REM sleep and Stage 4 sleep are correlated with reduced natural killer cell activity in normal controls and depressed patients (120). The objective sleep abnormalities generally ameliorate with clinical improvement in depression. Nevertheless, certain abnormalities may persist during remission, for example, loss of delta sleep, short REM latency, and loss of sleep-related growth hormone secretion (118,121). Whether these enduring sleep-related abnormalities reflect genetic risk factors, subsyndromal disorders, dysthymia, minor depression, ''scars,'' or state-independent traits remains to be determined.

In hopes of better understanding the basic and pathophysiological mechanisms of sleep and sleep deprivation, we have undertaken a series of studies using functional brain imaging to measure both global and LCGMR in patients with unipolar depression. Since physiological, and especially synaptic, activity within a region of interest of the brain is apparently directly related to local glucose utilization, we anticipated that we would be able to identify some of the specific brain circuitry involved in normal physiological and pathophysiological mechanisms related to sleep and sleep deprivation.

At this time, only two functional brain-imaging studies have been reported in depressed patients while they were asleep: one in non-REM sleep (122), the other in REM sleep (123).

XVII. The First Non-REM Sleep Period in Depression Is Characterized by Both Increased Global Metabolic Rate and Localized Changes in CGMR

Based on the premise that depressed patients are overaroused, we hypothesized that the patients would show increased whole brain absolute CGMR, as well as hypofrontality, and increased absolute activity within limbic structures and cortex. Using PET with FDG, we compared 10 unmedicated men with unipolar depression with 12 normal controls during the first non-REM period of the night (122). Even though these patients were only mildly depressed (HRSD-17 item = 17 ± 9) and had fairly normal polygraphic sleep measures, such as REM latency and Stages 3 and 4 sleep, whole brain absolute glucose metabolism was 47% higher in the patients than in the controls. Mean absolute LCGMR was higher in every brain region examined in patients compared with controls, especially in limbic structures (posterior cingulate, amygdala), hippocampus, occipital and temporal cortex, and pons. Interestingly, more anterior and medial areas showed significantly reduced relative CGMR, e.g., medio-orbital frontal cortex (hypofrontality), anterior cingulate, caudate, and medial thalamus. Absolute thalamic CGMR was not significantly different in patients compared with controls. Whole brain CGMR was negatively correlated with percent of the FDG uptake time spent in delta sleep to a significant degree in depressed patients and at trend levels in controls.

Although hypermetabolism during non-REM sleep characterized the mildly depressed patients compared with normal controls, it was not uniform throughout the brain. Indeed, relative hypometabolism was found in medial orbital-prefrontal cortex and anterior cingulate compared with the whole brain. Hypofrontality during daytime waking scans in depressed patients has been reported by several investigators (124–127).

Does the hypermetabolic GMR we observed during non-REM sleep in depression represent a failure to reduce metabolism during non-REM sleep compared with wakefulness? In an earlier study of cerebral blood flow with the xenon techniques, Meyer et al. (47) reported that CBF was increased in narcoleptics and decreased in normal controls as subjects transitioned from wakefulness into Stages 1 and 2 sleep. Comparisons of cerebral metabolism before and after sleep onset in depressed patients and normal controls would be informative.

XVIII. Changes in Forebrain Function from Waking to REM Sleep in Depressed Patients

Nofzinger et al. (123) recently compared six unipolar depressed patients and eight normal controls who underwent relative FDG measures during wakefulness in the morning and during REM sleep that night. The major focus was the examination of groups (depressed versus controls) versus state (waking versus REM) interactions. Perhaps the most interesting findings were that the depressed patients failed to activate the anterior paralimbic structures (anterior cingulate, right parahippocampal gyrus, right insular cortex), whereas normal controls did. These areas, ventral to genu of the corpus callosum, had previously been shown to be hypoactive during the waking state by Drevets et al. (128). (As we shall review in the following sections, this area has been implicated in the antidepressant effects of sleep deprivation.) An area, probably superior to Drevet's area, was hypoactive during wakefulness in the Nofzinger et al. study and failed to activate with REM sleep. Another finding of interest was greater activation of the tectal area and left hemisphere areas from wakefulness to REM sleep in depressed patients compared to normal controls. The authors speculate that this area could be associated with increased ocular activity (REM density) during REM sleep in depression.

XIX. Sleep Deprivation Has a Paradoxical Antidepressant Effect in Many Patients with Depression

Sleep deprivation for a night or for half a night has dramatic and paradoxical antidepressant benefits in about 40–60% of depressed patients (129–132). The clinical improvement can be striking, with responders often showing reductions of 50% or more in depression rating scales within a period of 4–12 h. Unfortunately, the antidepressant effects often disappear after sleep. Although sleep deprivation has not found its way into the clinical armamentarium, it remains a powerful research tool. Sleep deprivation and recovery sleep are the only experimental manipulations that consistently turn depression ''off and on,'' respectively.

XX. The Antidepressant Effects of Sleep Deprivation May Involve the Anterior Cingulate and Medial Prefrontal Cortex

In order to better understand the mechanism of sleep deprivation's antidepressant effects, five different research groups have by now published nine reports using functional brain-imaging methods to investigate the cerebral mechanisms of sleep deprivation in patients with depression (see Table 1). Two groups used PET with FDG—Wu et al. (133,134) and Smith et al. (135); three groups used SPECT with HMPAO—Ebert et al. (136,137), Volk et al. (138,139), and Holthoff et al. (140); and one group used SPECT with IZBM, a dopamine receptor (D_2) ligand—Ebert et al. (141). Preliminary findings have also been reported using quantitative perfusion with FMRI (141a).

The overall results suggest two major findings with regard to cerebral metabolism before and after sleep deprivation. First, all studies that measured localized cerebral metabolism or perfusion in cortical and subcortical areas at baseline reported that responders had increased localized metabolic activity in the general area

Table 1 PET and SPECT Studies of Sleep Deprivation in Depression (134a,b)

Author (Ref.)	Subjects/Method	Pre–sleep deprivation baseline	Sleep deprivation–induced changes within groups	Comments
Wu et al. (133,134)	36 MDD patients 24 controls Age ~ 30 years Unmedicated > 2 weeks HRSD-24 items > 16 Baseline means HRSD ~ 23–24 TSD: awake ~ 32–36 hours Responder: >40% ↓ HRSD 12 responders 24 nonresponders 26 controls FDG/PET: relative LCGMR Subjects performed a visual continuous performance task (CPT)	Responders vs nonresponders: ↑ Bilateral ventral anterior cingulate (BA 24), MPFC (BA 32), and posterior subcallosal cortex (BA 25) ↑ Left superior and inferior temporal cortex (BA 38, 21) ↓ Midbrain and hippocampus Responders vs controls: ↑ Bilateral ventral anterior cingulate (BA 24), MPFC (BA 32), and posterior subcallosal cortex (BA 25) ↓ Putamen and superior temporal gyrus (BA 37) ↓ Midbrain ↑ Occipital cortex and inferior temporal cortex (BA 38,21) Nonresponders vs controls: ↓ Right interior cingulate and MPFC (BA 24, 25, 32) ↓ Putamen, striatum, inferior temporal cortex (BA 21,38) ↑ Frontal pole (BA 10) and MPFC (BA 47), occipital cortex	Responders: ↓ Left anterior MPFC (BA 32) and frontal pole (BA 32) ↑ Right lateral prefrontal cortex (BA 45) and right insula (BA 52) Nonresponders: None Controls: ↓ Right lateral PFC (BA 46), mid-temporal gyrus (BA 21), caudate putamen ↑ Occipital cortex (BA 19) hippocampus Nonresponders and controls showed significant ↓ performance in CPT	The greater the reduction in the modified Hamilton Rating Scale for Depression, the greater the reduction of relative LCGMR in left medial prefrontal cortex and the greater the increase in the left temporal cortex The area in the PFC that correlated with clinical improvement is slightly anterior to the area at baseline which differed in responders compared with nonresponders and controls. It centered in the medial prefrontal BA 32.

Volk et al. (139)	13 MDD, 2 BP depressed: age 55 years Rx: tricyclic antidepressants (TCAs) Baseline mean HRSD ~ 21 PSD: Up at 2:30 am, ~5 hours awake Responder: ↓30% modified HRSD 9 responders 6 nonresponders SPECT/HMPAO	Responders vs nonresponders: ↑ Relative perfusion in right orbital/basal cingulate complex	Responders: ↓ Relative perfusion in orbitofrontal cortex	Multiple regression analysis shows that pre-PSD perfusion in right orbitofrontal/cingulate complex and post-PSD perfusion in left inferior temporal cortex correlated with improvement The pre-PSD measure of strain correlated significantly with a decrease in orbitofrontal perfusion
Volk et al. (138)	15 MDD, 2 BP depressed, 3 dysthymic RX: TCAs Age ~ 49 years Baseline mean HRSD ~ 23 TSD ~ 26 hours Responder: ↓30% modified HRSD 11 responders 9 nonresponders SPECT/HMPAO	Responders vs nonresponders: No difference	Responders: ↑ Relative perfusion in the left temporal region and right parietal region	The higher the perfusion in the occipital regions, orbitofrontal region, and left temporal region, the greater the improvement with TSD The focus of the study was on the neocortical regions. The limbic structures were not examined.
Ebert et al. (136)	20 MDD, melancholic Age ~ 39 years 11 patients Rx: with amitriptyline; 9 no Rx TSD ~ 26 hours Responders: ↓40% HRSD 11 responders 9 nonresponders SPECT/HMPAO	Responders vs nonresponders: ↑ Perfusion in right anterior cingulate gyrus and bilateral fronto-orbital region with basal cingulate gyrus	Not reported	7 of 11 responders and 2 of 9 nonresponders have a brief hypomanic episode after TSD Using a 50% threshold to define response, ↑ perfusion in right hippocampus was observed in addition to the other areas

Table 1 Continued

Author (Ref.)	Subjects/Method	Pre–sleep deprivation baseline	Sleep deprivation–induced changes within groups	Comments
Ebert et al. (137)	10 MDD with melancholia Age ~ 42 years Unmedicated HRSD > 19 8 controls, age ~ 42 TSD ~ 26 hours Responder: ↓50% HRSD 5 responders 5 nonresponders SPECT/HMPAO	Responders vs nonresponders: ↑ Perfusion in bilateral fronto-orbital cortex with lower parts of the cingulate gyrus, right hippocampus, parahippocampus, amygdala, and bilateral infratemporal neocortical lobe Responders and nonresponders vs controls: ↓ Perfusion before and after TSD in the lower parts of the anterior lateral prefrontal cortex Responders vs controls: ↓ Perfusion in upper parts of anterolateral prefrontal cortex	Responders: ↓ Perfusion in bilateral fronto-orbital cortex with lower parts of the cingulate gyrus, right hippocampus, parahippocampus, amygdala, and bilateral infratemporal neocortical lobe Nonresponders: ↓ Perfusion in left anterolateral PFC Controls did not undergo TSD or second scan	Both responders and nonresponders showed hypoperfusion in the left anterolateral PFC before and after TSD
Ebert et al. (141)	10 BP II, melancholic Age ~ 33 years Rx: amitriptyline 5 controls TSD ~ 26 hours Responder: ↓40% HRSD 5 responders 5 nonresponders IBZM/SPECT (dopamine D2 receptor ligand)	Responders vs nonresponders vs controls: D_2 receptor in striatum occupancy similar at baseline	Responders: ↓ Relative activity in right basal ganglia Nonresponders: No significant change Controls did undergo TSD or second scan	Post-TSD, responders had significantly less activity on the right basal ganglia and trend decrease on the left compared with nonresponders Authors conclude that the antidepressant effect of TSD was associated with increased endogenous dopamine release post-TSD. IBZM competes with endogenous dopamine for the D_2 receptor

Smith et al. (135)	6 elderly MDD 6 elderly normals Age ~ 71 years TSD ~ 26 hours PET/FDG Patients 4 scans: baseline, post-TSD, postrecovery, post 12 weeks Rx paroxetine, which started on recovery night Controls: 1rst scans	Patients vs controls: Not reported	Patients: From baseline to post-TSD, ↓ LCGMR in right anterior cingulate (BA 24) and right MFC (BA 47); after recovery sleep, compared with baseline, ↓ right middle frontal gyrus (BA 47), right and left inferior frontal gyrus, left anterior cingulate (BA 24), ↑ right post central gyrus Comparison, normal controls: From baseline to post-TSD, no change. After recovery night, ↓ right middle frontal gyrus (BA 8,9) and right anterior cingulate (BA 24)	Patients improved as a group after TSD and throughout the 12 week paroxetine treatment period, when 5 of 6 were responders LCGMR in anterior cingulate increased from baseline to postrecovery sleep in controls but not in patients
Holthoff et al. (140)	12 MDD, 2 BP Age ~ 53 years Rx: various medications HRSD ~ 31 TSD Responder ≥ ↓ 40% in HRSD 8 responders 6 nonresponders HMPAD/SPECT	Responder (n = 8) vs nonresponder (n = 6): ↑ Perfusion in anterior cingulate gyru All patients (n = 14): Both patient groups showed significantly greater perfusion on the right side compared to the left side in the prefrontal cortex	Responders: ↓ Perfusion in anterior cingulate Nonresponders: No significant change All patients: PFC did not change in either group	In three patients followed to remission, prefrontal hypoperfusion remitted

Source: Refs. 134a,b.

of the anterior cingulate/prefrontal cortex compared with nonresponders or controls—Wu et al. (133,134), Ebert et al. (136,137), Volk et al. (139), and Holthoff et al. (140). [Volk et al. (138) did not examine baseline subcortical areas in their 1992 study.] Second, all studies that have compared patients both pre–and post–sleep deprivation have reported that clinical improvement is associated with normalization of the increased metabolic activity in the general area of the anterior cingulate/prefrontal regions—Wu et al. (133,134), Ebert et al. (136), Volk et al. (139), Smith et al. (135), and Holthoff et al. (140).

The similarity of the results in these studies is all the more remarkable since the methods varied between groups: PET with FDG or SPECT with HMPAO, different definitions for a clinical response (30–50% reduction in a modified HRSD), medicated or unmedicated patients, inpatients versus outpatients, melancholic versus nonmelancholic, young versus geriatric patients, with and without a cognitive or attentional task during the uptake process, and total sleep deprivation versus partial sleep deprivation.

Reduced activity in nonresponders compared with normals at baseline was also reported in right anterior cingulate and medial prefrontal cortex (134). Furthermore, the areas of activation at baseline in responders did not overlap exactly with the areas correlated with clinical improvement after sleep deprivation. For instance, Wu et al. (134) reported that sleep deprivation benefits were located in Brodmann (BA) area 32 rather than the baseline areas of elevation in Brodmann 24 and 25.

Nevertheless, functional imaging has contributed new insights into the neural circuitry of a well-established antidepressant intervention. Whether the same areas are involved in the mechanisms of antidepressant medications, cognitive behavioral psychotherapy, electroconvulsive treatment, or other antidepressant treatments remain to be determined. These findings with sleep deprivation are consistent in some respects with a reciprocal limbic-cortical model of depression and normal sadness proposed by Mayberg et al. (142,143).

The basic mechanisms of the antidepressant effects of sleep deprivation remain uncertain, despite many thoughtful efforts to understand them (144). Among the more commonly discussed theories are the two-process model of sleep regulation and its implications for depression (145), circadian dysregulation models (146), overarousal (147), and the role of serotonin (148). Of particular interest, the beneficial effects of sleep deprivation may be attributed to enhanced neurotransmission of dopamine. It has been reported, for example, that sleep deprivation improves mood and motor activity in patients with Parkinson's disease, which is associated with deficient dopamine activity (149). These results are consistent with a previous study that responders showed increased concentrations of homovanillic acid (HVA), a metabolite of dopamine, in spinal fluid after sleep deprivation than before (150). Ebert et al. (141) also investigated the role of dopamine in the antidepressant effects of sleep deprivation in depression. Utilizing a specific D_2 radioligand, ^{123}I-3-iodomethoxybenzamide (IBZM) with SPECT, they concluded that the antidepressant effects of sleep deprivation were associated with decreased relative occupancy of the dopamine receptor after sleep deprivation, whereas nonresponders showed an increase. They interpreted these results as indicating enhanced dopamine release following TSD.

XXI. Summary

Functional brain imaging provides new insights into the basic normal physiology and pathophysiology associated with the three major states of consciousness: wakefulness, non-REM sleep, and REM sleep. Cerebral metabolic activity clearly differs between sleep and wakefulness in the whole brain and regionally. In general, whole brain metabolism appears to be reduced during slow-wave sleep compared with both wakefulness and REM sleep.

Although cerebral glucose metabolism, oxygen utilization, regional CBF, and behavior appear to be closely coupled much of the time, they also appear to be dissociated at times, during sleep and the transition from sleep to wakefulness. For example, the brain may be overperfused during REM sleep relative to oxygen or glucose utilization. Likewise, the brain appears to be underperfused during the period of sleep inertia as people wake up. These observations highlight difficult unanswered questions about how the brain works. What are the basic relationships between neuronal activity, global and regional glucose metabolism, regional and local CBS and oxygen utilization, behavioral state (wakefulness, non-REM sleep, and REM sleep) behavior and mentation, and effect? Further studies are needed at the basic level to understand these relationships and to interpret functional brain imaging observations during sleep and wakefulness in normal and clinical populations.

Functional brain-imaging studies may also shed light on the functions of sleep. While the amount of delta sleep appears to be negatively correlated with whole brain metabolic rate, preliminary results suggest that it is positively correlated with protein synthesis. If further studies confirm this finding, it will have significant implications for the functions of sleep and, especially, the relationship between delta sleep, sleep deprivation, clinical disorders, such as sleep apnea, periodic limb movements of sleep, restless legs syndrome, narcolepsy, aging, depression, insomnia, schizophrenia, and dementia, and with certain medications, including benzodiazepines, which suppress delta sleep.

For the clinician, functional brain imaging in association with sleep and sleep deprivation provides a unique window through which to see the workings of the brain during psychopathology and during clinical response. For instance, the functional brain-imaging studies of sleep deprivation therapy have stimulated the studies of localized metabolic activity within the anterior cingulate and medial prefrontal cortex, which may be associated with antidepressant clinical improvement. Furthermore, preliminary studies comparing depressed patients and normal controls during non-REM sleep provide a physiological basis for the "overarousal hypothesis" related to sleep in depression. Moreover, the presence of relative hypometabolism in ventral medial prefrontal cortex and anterior cingulate in depressed patients during non-REM sleep suggests that state-independent pathophysiological mechanisms are operating during sleep and wakefulness. Future studies with functional brain imaging during sleep and sleep deprivation offer new opportunities for the mutual enrichment of basic neuroscience and clinical science.

Acknowledgments

This publication was supported by grants from the Mental Health Clinical Research Center's Program, MH30914, and 5-R01-MH57134, of the National Institutes of Health, and by the Department of Veterans Affairs.

References

1. Mangold R, Sokoloff L, Conner E, Kleinerman J, Therman POJ, Kety SS. The effects of sleep and lack of sleep on the cerebral circulation and metabolism of normal young men. J Clin Invest 1995; 34:1092–1100.
2. Raichle ME. Circulatory and metabolic correlates of brain function in normal humans. In: Plum F, ed. Handbook of Physiology: The Nervous System V. Higher Functions of the Brain. Bethesda, MD: American Physiological Society, 1987:643–674.
3. Sokoloff L, Reivich M, Kennedy C, DesRosiers MH, Patlak CS, Pettigrew KD, et al. The (^{14}C Deoxyglucose method for the measurement of local cerebral glucose utilization: theory, procedure, and normal values in the conscious and anesthetized albino rat. J Neurochem 1977; 28:897–916.
4. Buxton RB, Frank LR. A model for the coupling between cerebral blood flow and oxygen metabolism during neural stimulation. J Cerebral Blood Flow and Metabolism 1997; 17:64–72.
5. Adam K, Oswald I. Sleep is for tissue restoration. J R Coll Physicians 1977; 11:376–388.
6. Adam K, Oswald I. Protein synthesis, bodily renewal, and sleep-wake cycle. Clin Sci 1983; 65:561–571.
7. Benington JH, Heller HC. Restoration of brain energy metabolism as the function of sleep. Prog Neurobiol 1995; 45:347–360.
8. Borbely AA. A two process model of sleep regulation. Hum Neurobiol 1982; 1:195–204.
9. Rechtschaffen A. Current perspectives on the function of sleep. Perspect Biol Med 1998; 41:359–390.
10. Lee AT, Glover GH, Meyer CH. Discrimination of large venous vessels in time-course spiral blood-oxygen-level-dependent magnetic-resonance functional neuroimaging. Magn Reson Med 1995; 33:745–754.
11. Greisen G, Hellstrom-Vestas L, Lou H, Rosen I, Svenningsen N. Sleep-waking shifts and cerebral blood flow in stable preterm infants. Pediatr Res 1875; 19:1156–1159.
12. Day MA, Darby P, Hagin S. Autoradiographic analysis of regional brain glucose utilization in chronically monitored unanesthetized fetal sleep. Dev Brain Res 1983; 11: 133–136.

13. Cote A, Haddad GG. Effects of sleep on regional blood flow distribution in piglets. Pediatr Res 1990; 28:218–222.
14. Gaggero R, Caputo M, Fiorio P, Pessagno A, Baglietto MG, Muttini P, et al. SPECT and epilepsy with continuous spike waves during slow-wave sleep. Childs Nerv Syst 1995; 11:154–160.
15. Rintahaka PJ, Chugani HT, Sankar R. Landau-Kleffner syndrome with continuous spikes and waves during slow-wave sleep. J Child Neurol 1995; 10:127–133.
16. Kleitman N. Sleep and Wakefulness. Chicago: The University of Chicago Press, 1963.
17. Aserinsky E, Kleitman N. Regularly occurring periods of eye motility and concomitant phenomenon during sleep. Science 1953; 118:273–274.
18. Murase K, Kuwabara H, Yashuhara Y, Evans AC. Mapping of change in cerebral glucose utilization using fluorine-18 fluorodeoxyglucose double injections and the contrained weighted-integration method. IEEE Trans Med Imag 1996; 15:824–835.
19. Lamoureux G, Dupont RM, Ashburn WL, Halpern SE. "CORT-EX:" a program for quantitative analysis of brain SPECT data. J Nucl Med 1990; 31:1862–1871.
20. Ogawa S, Lee TM, Nayak AS, Glynn P. Oxygenation sensitive contrast in magnetic resonance image of rodent in high magnetic fields. Magn Reson Med 1990; 14:68–78.
21. Sutton JR, Holmes J., Caplan J, Rudnick L, Kwong KK, Breiter HC, et al. Investigation of human sleep using simultaneous fMRI and polysomnography. Sleep 1998; 21 (suppl):271.
22. Lovblad KO, Thomas R, Jacob P, Scammell T, Griswold M, Ives J, et al. Silent functional magnetic resonance imaging demonstrates focal activation in rapid eye movement sleep. Neurology 2000; 53:2193–2195.
23. Hoshi Y, Mizukami S, Tamura M. Dynamic features of hemodynamic and metabolic changes in the human brain during all-night sleep as revealed by near-infrared spectroscopy. Brain Res 1994; 652:257–262.
24. Onoe H, Watanabe Y, Tamura M, Hayaishi O. REM sleep-associated hemoglobin oxygenation in the monkey forebrain studied using near-infrared spectrophotometry. Neurosci Lett 1991; 129:209–213.
25. Spielman AJ, Zhang G, Yang CM, D'Ambrosio PD, Serizawa S, Nagata M, et al. Intracerebral hemodynamics probed by near infrared spectroscopy in the transition between wakefulness and sleep. Brain Res Interact 2000; 866:313–325.
26. Talairach J, Tournoux P. Co-Planar Stereotaxic Altas of the Human Brain. New York: Thieme Medical Publishers, 1988.
27. Steriade M, McCormick DA, Sejnowski TJ. Thalamocortical oscillations in the sleeping and aroused brain. Science 1993; 262:679–685.
28. Steriade M, Nuñez A, Amzica F. A novel slow (<1 Hz) oscillation of neocortical neurons in vivo: depolarizing and hyperpolarizing components. J Neurosci 1993; 13: 3252–3265.
29. Clark C, Dupont R, Lehr P, Yeung D, Halpern S, Golshan S, et al. Is there a relationship between delta sleep at night and afternoon cerebral blood flow, assessed by HMPAO-SPECT, in depressed patients and normal controls? Preliminary data. Psychiatr Res 1998; 84:89–99.
30. Benington JH, Heller HC. Does the function of REM sleep concern non-REM sleep or waking? Prog Neurobiol 1994; 44:433–449.
31. Radulovacki M, Virus RM, Djuricic-Nedelson M, Green RD. Adenosine analogs and sleep in rats. J Pharmacol Exp Ther 1984; 228:268–274.

32. Porkka-Heiskanen T, Strecker RE, Thakker M, Bjorklund A, Greene RW, McCarley RW. Adenosine: a mediator of the sleep-inducing effects of prolonged wakefulness. Science 1997; 276:1268.
33. Greenberg JH. Sleep and the cerebral circulation. In: Orem J, Barnes CD, eds. Physiology in Sleep. New York: Academic Press, 1980:57–95.
34. Madsen PL. Blood flow and oxygen uptake in the human brain during various states of sleep and wakefulness. Acta Neurol Scand 1993; 88(suppl 148):5–25.
35. Buchsbaum MS, Gillin JC, Wu J, Haslett E, Sicotte N, Dupont R, et al. Regional cerebral glucose metabolic rate in human sleep assessed by positron emission tomography. Life Sci 1989; 45:1349–1356.
35a. Buchsbaum MS, Hazlett EA, Wu J, Bunney WE Jr. Positron-emission tomography with deoxyglucose-F18 imaging of sleep. Neuropsychopharmacology 2001; 25:S50–S56.
36. Franzini C. Brain metabolism and blood flow during sleep. J Sleep Res 1992; 1:3–16.
37. Maquet P, Dive D, Salmon E, Sadzot B, Franco G, Poirrier R, et al. Cerebral glucose utilization during stage 2 sleep in man. Brain Res 1992; 571:149–153.
38. Hofle N, Paus T, Reutens D, Fiset P, Gotman J, Evans AC, et al. Regional cerebral blood flow changes as a function of delta and spindle activity during slow wave sleep in humans. J Neurosci 1997; 17:4800–4808.
39. Kennedy C, Gillin JC, Mendelson WB, Suda S, Miyaoka M, Ito M, et al. Local cerebral glucose utilization in non-REM sleep. Nature 1982; 297:325–327.
40. Nakamura R, Kennedy C, Gillin JC, Suda S, Ito M, Storch FI, et al. Hypnogenic center theory of sleep: No support from metabolic mapping in monkeys. Brain Res 1983; 268:372–376.
41. Ramm P, Frost BJ. Cerebral and local glucose cerebral metabolism in the cat during slow wave and REM sleep. Brain Res 1986; 365:112–124.
42. Ramm P, Frost BJ. Regional metabolic activity in the rat brain during sleep-wake activity. Sleep 1983; 6:196–216.
43. Pavlides C, Aoki V, Chen J-S, Bailey WH, Winson J. Differential glucose utilization in the parafascicular region during slow-wave sleep, the still-alert state and locomotion. Brain Res 1987; 423:399–402.
44. Heiss WD, Pawlik G, Herholtz K, Wagner R, Wienhard K. Regional cerebral glucose metabolism in man during wakefulness, sleep, and dreaming. Brain Res 1985; 327: 362–366.
45. Maquet P, Dive D, Salmon E, Sadzot B, Franco G, Poirrier R, et al. Cerebral glucose utilization during sleep wake cycle in man determined by positron tomography and 18F-2-fluoro-2-deoxy-D-glucose method. Brain Res 1990; 513:136–143.
46. Franck G, Salmon E, Poirrier E, Sadozt B, Franco G. Etude du metabolism glucidique cerebral regional chez l'homme au cours de l'eveli et du sommeil par tomographie a emission de positrons. Rev EEG Neurophysiol Clin 1987; 17:71–77.
47. Meyer JS, Ishikawa Y, Hata T, Karacan I. Cerebral blood flow in normal and abnormal sleep and dreaming. Brain Cogn 1987; 6:266–294.
48. Madsen PL, Schmidt JF, Wildschiodtz G, Friberg L, Holm S, Vorstrup S, et al. Cerebral oxygen metabolism and cerebral blood flow in humans during deep sleep and rapid-eye-movement sleep. J Appl Physiol 1991; 70:2597–2601.
49. Boyle PJ, Scott JC, Krentz AJ, Nagy RJ, Comstock E, Hoffman C. Diminished brain

glucose metabolism is a significant determinant for falling rates of systemic glucose utilization during sleep in normal humans. J Clin Invest 1994; 93:529–535.

50. Braun AR, Balkin TJ, Wesenten NJ, Carson RE, Varga M, Baldwin P, et al. Regional cerebral blood flow throughout the sleep-wake cycle. An H2(15)O PET study. Brain 1997; 520:1173–1197.
51. Townsend RE, Prinz PN, Obrist WD. Human cerebral blood flow during sleep and waking. J Appl Physiol 1973; 35:620–625.
52. Hajak G, Klingelhöfer J, Schulz-Varszegi M, Matzander G, Sander D, Conrad B, et al. Relationship between cerebral blood flow velocities and cerebral electrical activity in sleep. Sleep 1994; 17:11–19.
53. Droste DW, Berger W, Schuler E, Krauss JK. Middle cerebral artery blood flow velocity in healthy persons during wakefulness and sleep: a transcranial Doppler study. Sleep 1993; 16:603–609.
54. Kuboyama T, Hori A, Sato T, Mikami T, Yamaki T, Ueda S. Changes in cerebral blood flow velocity in healthy young men during overnight sleep and while awake. Electroencephalogr Clin Neurophysiol 1997; 102:125–131.
55. Steriade M, Contreras D, Amzica F. Synchronized sleep oscillations and their paroxysmal developments. Trends Neurosci 1994; 17:199–208.
56. Ramm P, Smith CT. Rates of cerebral protein synthesis are linked to slow wave sleep in the rat. Physiol Behav 1990; 48:753.
57. Nakanishi H, Sun Y, Nakamura RK, Mori K, Ito M, Suda S, et al. Positive correlations between cerebral protein synthesis rates and deep sleep in Macaca mulatta. Eur J Neurosci 1997; 9:271–279.
58. Madsen PL, Holm S, Vorstrup S, Friberg L, Lassen NA, Wildschiodtz G. Human regional cerebral blood flow during rapid-eye-movement sleep. J Cereb Blood Flow Metab 1991; 11:502–507.
59. Lydic R, Baghdoyan HA, Hibbard L, Bonyak EV, DeJoseph MR, Hawkins RA. Regional brain glucose metabolism is altered during rapid eye movement sleep in the cat: A preliminary study. J Comp Neurol 1991; 304:517–529.
60. Braun AR, Balkin TJ, Wesensten FG, Carson RE, Varga M, Baldwin P, et al. Dissociated pattern of activity in visual cortices and their projections during human rapid eye movement sleep. Science 1998; 279:91–95.
61. Maquet P, Peters JM, Aerts J, Delfiore G, Dequeldres C, Luxen A, et al. Functional neuroanatomy of human rapid eye movement sleep and dreaming. Nature 1996; 383: 163–165.
62. Nofzinger EA, Mintun MA, Wiseman MB, Kupfer DJ, Moore RY. Forebrain activation in REM sleep: an FDG PET study. Brain Res 1997; 770:192–201.
63. Hong CC, Gillin JC, Dow BM, Wu J, Buchsbaum MS. Localized and lateralized cerebral glucose metabolism associated with eye movements during REM sleep and wakefulness: a position emission tomography (PET) study. Sleep 1995; 18:570–580.
64. Hobson JA. The Dreaming Brain. New York: Basic Books, 1988.
65. Benca RM, Obermeyer WH, Thisted RA, Gillin JC. Sleep and psychiatric disorders: a meta-analysis. Arch Gen Psychiatry 1992; 49:651–668.
66. Gillin JC, Dow BM, Thompson P, Parry B, Tandon R, Benca RM. Sleep in depression and other psychiatric disorders. Clin Neurosci 1993; 1:90–96.
67. Gillin JC, Smith TL, Irwin M, Butters N, Demodena A, Schuckit M. Increased pressure for rapid eye movement sleep at time of hospital admission predicts relapse in nonde-

pressed patients with primary alcoholism at 3-month follow-up. Arch Gen Psychiatry 1994; 51:189–197.
68. Bahro M, Riemann D, Stadtmüller G, Berger M, Gattaz WF. REM sleep parameters in the discrimination of probable Alzheimer's disease from old-age depression. Biol Psychiatry 1993; 34:482–486.
69. Crick F, Mitchinson G. The function of dreaming sleep. Nature 1983; 304:111–114.
70. Giles DE, Jarrett RB, Roffwarg HP, Rush AJ. Reduced REM latency: A predictor of recurrence in depression. Neuropsychopharmacology 1988; 1:33–39.
71. Sitaram N, Moore AM, Gillin JC. The effect of physostigmine on normal human sleep and dreaming. Arch Gen Psychiatry 1978; 35:1239–1243.
72. Gottschalk LA, Buchsbaum MS, Gillin JC, Wu JC, Reynolds CA, Herrera DB. Anxiety levels in dreams: relation to localized cerebral glucose metabolic rate. Brain Res 1991; 538:107–110.
73. Gottschalk LA, Buchsbaum MS, Gillin JC, Wu JC, Reynolds CA, Herrera DB. Positron emission tomographic studies of the relationship of cerebral glucose metabolism and the magnitude of anxiety and hostility experienced during dreaming and waking. J Neuropsychiatry Clin Neurosci 1991; 3(2):131–142.
74. Solms M. The Neuropsychology of Dreams: A Clinico-anatomical Study. Hillsdale, NJ: Lawrence Erlbaum Associates, 1997.
75. Gillin JC, Buchsbaum MS, Valladares-Neto DC, Hong CC, Hazlett E, Langer SZ, et al. Effects of zolpidem on local cerebral glucose metabolism during non-REM sleep in normal volunteers: a positron emission tomography study. Neuropsychopharmacology 1996; 15:302–313.
76. Finelli LA, Landolt HP, Buck A, Roth C, Berthold T, Borbely AA, et al. Functional neuroanatomy of human sleep states after zolpidem and placebo: a H215O-PET study. J Sleep Res 2000; 9:161–172.
77. Buchsbaum MS, Wu J, Haier R, Hazlett E, Ball R, Katz M, et al. Positron emission tomography assessment of effects of benzodiazepines on regional glucose metabolic rate in patients with anxiety disorder. Life Sci 1987; 40:2393–2400.
78. Fox PT, Raichle ME, Mintun MA, Dence C. Nonoxidative glucose consumption during focal physiologic neural activity. Science 1988; 241:462–464.
79. Parisi RA, Neubauer JA, Frank MM, Santiago TV, Edelman NH. Linkage between brain blood flow and respiratory drive during rapid-eye-movement sleep. Am J Physiol 1988; 1457–1465.
80. Santiago TV, Guerra E, Neubauer JA, Edelman NH. Correlation between ventilation and brain blood flow during sleep. J Clin Invest 1984; 73:497–506.
81. Franzini C, Zoccoli G, Cianci T, Lenzi P. Sleep-dependent changes in regional circulations. News Physiol Sci 1996; 11:274–280.
82. Balkin TJ, Wesenten NJ, Braun AR, Varga M, Baldwin P, Carson RE, et al. Shaking out the cobwebs: Changes in regional cerebral blood flow (rCBF) across the first 20 minutes of wakefulness. Sleep 1998; 21(suppl):271.
83. Wu JC, Gillin JC, Buchsbaum MS, Hazlett E, Sicotte N, Bunney WE Jr. The effect of sleep deprivation on cerebral glucose metabolic rate in normal humans assessed with positron emission tomography. Sleep 1991; 14:155–162.
84. Portas CM, Rees G, Howseman AM, Josephs O, Turner R, Frith CD. A specific role for the thalamus in mediating the interaction of attention and arousal in humans. J Neurosci 1998; 18:8979–8989.
85. Drummond SPA, Brown GG, Stricker JL, Buxton RB, Wong EC, Gillin JC. Sleep

deprivation-induced reduction in cortical functional response to serial subtraction. NeuroReport 1999; 10:3745–3748.
86. Drummond SPA, Brown GG, Gillin JC, Stricker JL, Wong EC, Buxton RB. Altered brain response to verbal learning following sleep deprivation. Nature 2000; 403:605–657.
87. Harrison Y, Horne JA. Sleep loss impairs short and novel language tasks having a prefrontal focus. J Sleep Res 1998; 7:95–100.
88. Everson CA, Smith CB, Sokoloff L. Effects of prolonged sleep deprivation on local rates of cerebral energy metabolism in freely moving rats. J Neurosci 1994; 14:6769–6778.
89. Peder M, Lindroos F, Laakso ML, Porkka-Heiskanen T, Johansson G. Effects of rapid eye movement sleep deprivation on regional brain metabolism as measured by 2-[^{14}C]deoxyglucose autoradiography. Behav Neural Biol 1986; 45:71–80.
90. Thorpy MJ, ed. International Classification of Sleep Disorders: Diagnostic and Coding Manual. Diagnostic Classification Steering Committee. Rochester, MN: American Sleep Disorders Association, 1990.
91. Meyer JS, Sakai F, Karacan I, Derman S, Yamamoto M. Sleep apnea, narcolepsy, and dreaming: Regional cerebral hemodynamics. Ann Neurol 1980; 7:479–485.
92. Hajak G, Klingelheofer J, Schulz-Varszegi M, Sander D, Reuther E. Sleep apnea syndrome and cerebral hemodynamics. Chest 1996; 110:670–679.
93. Balfors EM, Franklin KA. Impairment of cerebral perfusion during obstructive sleep apneas. Am J Respir Crit Care Med 1994; 150:1587–1591.
94. Netzer N, Werner P, Jochums I, Lehmann M, Strohl KP. Blood flow of the middle cerebral artery with sleep-disordered breathing: correlation with obstructive hypopneas [see comments]. Stroke 1998; 29:87–93.
95. Ficker JH, Feistel H, Meoller C, Merkl M, Dertinger S, Siegfried W, et al. Changes in regional CNS perfusion in obstructive sleep apnea syndrome: initial SPECT studies with injected nocturnal 99mTc-HMPAO. Pneumologie 1997; 51:926–930.
96. Droste DW, Leudemann P, Anders F, Kemaeny V, Thomas M, Krauss JK, et al. Middle cerebral artery blood flow velocity, end-tidal pCO_2 and blood pressure in patients with obstructive sleep apnea and in healthy subjects during continuous positive airway pressure breathing. Neurol Res 1999; 21:737–741.
97. Qureshi AI, Christopher W, Bliwise DL. Sleep fragmentation and morning cerebrovasomotor reactivity to hypercapnia. Am J Respir Crit Care Med 1999; 160:1244–1247.
98. Rehan VK, Fajardo CA, Haider AZ, Alvaro RE, Cates DB, Kwiatkowski K, et al. Influence of sleep state and respiratory pattern on cyclical fluctuations of cerebral blood flow velocity in healthy preterm infants. Biol Neonate 1996; 69:357–367.
99. Hayakawa T, Terashima M, Kayukawa Y, Ohta T, Okada T. Changes in cerebral oxygenation and hemodynamics during obstructive sleep apneas. Chest 1996; 109:916–921.
100. Kamba M, Suto Y, Ohta Y, Inoue Y, Matsuda E. Cerebral metabolism in sleep apnea. Evaluation by magnetic resonance spectroscopy. Am J Respir Crit Care Med 1997; 156:296–298.
101. Asenbaum S, Zeithofer J, Saletu B, Frey R, Brucke T, Podreka I, et al. Technetium-99m-HMPAO SPECT imaging of cerebral blood flow during REM sleep in narcoleptics. J Nucl Med 1995; 36:1150–1155.
102. Hublin C, Launes J, Nikkinen P, Partinen M. Dopamine D_2-receptors in human narcolepsy: a SPECT study with 123I-IBZM. Acta Neurol Scand 1994; 90:186–189.
103. Khan N, Antonini A, Parkes D, Dahlitz MJ, Meier-Ewert K, Weindl A, et al. Striatal dopamine D_2 receptors in patients with narcolepsy measured with PET and ^{11}C-raclopride. Neurology 1994; 44:2101–2104.

104. Rinne JO, Hublin C, Partinen M, Ruottinen H, Ruotsalainen U, Neagren K, et al. Positron emission tomography study of human narcolepsy: no increase in striatal dopamine D_2 receptors. Neurology 1995; 45:1735–1738.
105. Sudo Y, Suhara T, Honda Y, Nakajima T, Okubo Y, Suzuki K, et al. Muscarinic cholinergic receptors in human narcolepsy: a PET study. Neurology 1998; 51:1297–1302.
106. Howard RJ, Ellis C, Bullmore ET, Brammer M, Mellers JD, Woodruff PW, et al. Functional echoplanar brain imaging correlates of amphetamine administration to normal subjects and subjects with the narcoleptic syndrome. Magn Reson Imaging 1996; 14:1013–1016.
107. Staedt J, Stoppe G, Kögler A, Munz D, Riemann H, Emrich D, et al. Dopamine D_2 receptor alteration in patients with periodic movements in sleep (nocturnal myoclonus). J Neural Transm 1993; 93:71–74.
108. Staedt J, Stoppe G, Kogler A, Riemann H, Hajak G, Munz DL, et al. Nocturnal myoclonus syndrome (periodic movements in sleep) related to central dopamine D_2-receptor alteration. Eur Arch Psychiatry Clin Neurosci 1995; 245:8–10.
109. Turjanski N, Lees AJ, Brooks DJ. Strial dopaminergic function in restless legs syndrome: ^{18}F-dopa and ^{11}C-raclopride PET studies. Neurology 2000; 52:932–937.
110. Ruottinen HM, Partinen M, Hublin C, Bergman J, Haaparanta M, Solin O, et al. An FDOPA PET study in patients with periodic limb movement disorder and restless legs syndrome. Neurology 2000; 54:502–504.
111. Staedt J, Stoppe G, Kogler A, Riemann H, Hajak G, Munz DL, et al. Single photon emission tomography (SPET) imaging of dopamine D_2 receptors in the course of dopamine replacement therapy in patients with nocturnal myoclonus syndrome (NMS). J Neural Transm Gen Sect 1995; 99:187–193.
112. Nofzinger EA, Buysse DJ, Reynolds CF, III, Kupfer DJ. Sleep disorders related to another mental disorder (nonsubstance/primary): a DSM-IV literature review. J Clin Psychiatry 1993; 54:244–255.
113. Armitage R. Microarchitectural findings in sleep EEG in depression: Diagnostic implications. Biol Psychiatry 1995; 37:72–84.
114. Avery DH, Wildschiodtz G, Smallwood RG, Rafaelson DJ. REM latency and core temperature relationships in primary depression. Acta Psychiatr Scand 1986; 74:269–280.
115. Souêtre E, Wehr TA, Sack DA, Kreb B, Darcourt G. 24-hour profiles of body temperature and plasma TSH in bipolar patients during depression and during remission and in normal controls subjects. Am J Psychiatry 1988; 145:1133–1137.
116. Poland RE, McCracken JT, Luchmansingh P, Tondo L. Relationship between REM sleep latency and nocturnal cortisol concentrations in depressed patients. J Sleep Res 1992; 1:54–57.
117. Steiger A, von Bardeleben U, Guldner J, Lauer C, Rothe B, Holsboer F. The sleep EEG and nocturnal hormonal secretion studies on changes during the course of depression and on effects of CNS-active drugs. Prog Neuro-Pharmacol Biol Psychiatry 1993; 17:125–137.
118. Jarrett DB, Kupfer DJ, Miewald JM, Grochocinski VJ, Franz B. Sleep-related growth hormone secretion is persistently suppressed in women with recurrent depression: a preliminary longitudinal analysis. J Psychiatr Res 1994; 28:211–223.
119. Voderholzer U, Laakmann G, Wittmann R, Daffner-Bujia C, Hinz A, Haag C, et al.

Profiles of spontaneous 24-hour and stimulated growth hormone secretion in male patients with endogenous depression. Psychiatry Res 1993; 47:215–227.
120. Irwin M, McClintick J, Costlow C, Fortner M, White J, Gillin JC. Partial night sleep deprivation reduces natural killer and cellular immune responses in humans. FASEB J 1996; 10:643–653.
121. Giles DE, Jarrett RB, Rush AJ, Biggs MM, Roffwarg HP. Prospective assessment of electroencephalographic sleep in remitted major depression. Psychiatry Res 1993; 46: 269–284.
122. Ho AP, Gillin JC, Buchsbaum MS, Wu JC, Abel L, Bunney WEJ. Brain glucose metabolism during non-rapid eye movement sleep in major depression. A positron emission tomography study. Arch Gen Psychiatry 1996; 53:645–652.
123. Nofzinger EA, Nichols TE, Meltzer CC, Price J, Steppe DA, Miewald JM, et al. Changes in forebrain function from waking to REM sleep in depression: preliminary analyses of [^{18}F]FDG PET studies. Psychiatry Res Neuroimaging 1999; 91:59–78.
124. Buchsbaum MS, Wu J, DeLisi LE, Holcomb H, Kessler R, Johnson J, et al. Frontal cortex and basal ganglia metabolic rates assessed by positron emission tomography with [^{18}F]2-deoxyglucose in affective illness. J Affect Disord 1986; 10:137–152.
125. Baxter LR, Schwartz JM, Phelps ME, Mazziotta JC, Guze BH, Selin CE, et al. Reduction of prefrontal cortex glucose metabolism common to three types of depression. Arch Gen Psychiatry 1989; 46:243–250.
126. Bench CJ, Friston KJ, Brown RG, Scott LC, Frackowiak RSJ, Dolan RJ. The anatomy of melancholia—focal abnormalities of cerebral blood flow in major depression. Psychol Med 1992; 22:607–615.
127. Drevets WC, Videen TO, Price JL, Preskorn SH, Carmichael ST, Raichle ME. A functional anatomical study of unipolar depression. J Neurosci 1992; 12:3628–3641.
128. Drevets WC, Price JL, Simpson JR, Jr., Todd RD, Reich T, Vannier M, et al. Subgenual prefrontal cortex abnormalities in mood disorders. Nature 1997; 386:824–827.
129. Vogel GW, Vogel F, McAbee RS, Thurmond AJ. Improvement of depression by REM sleep deprivation. New findings and a theory to explain why. Arch Gen Psychiatry 1980; 37:247–253.
130. Gillin JC. The sleep therapies of depression. Prog Neuropsychopharmacol Biol Psychiatry 1983; 7:351–364.
131. Wu JC, Bunney WR, Jr. The biological basis of an antidepressant response to sleep deprivation and relapse: review and hypothesis. Am J Psychiatry 1990; 147:14–21.
132. Leibenluft E, Wehr TA. Is sleep deprivation useful in the treatment of depression? Am J Psychiatry 1992; 149:159–168.
133. Wu JC, Gillin JC, Buchsbaum MS, Hershey T, Johnson JC, Bunney WE, Jr. Effect of sleep deprivation on brain metabolism of depressed patients. Am J Psychiatry 1992; 149:538–543.
134. Wu JC, Buchsbaum MS, Gillin JC, Tang JL, Cadwell S, Wiegand M, et al. Prediction of antidepressant effects of sleep deprivation by metabolic rates in the ventral anterior cingulate and medial prefrontal cortex. Am J Psychiatry 1999; 156:1149–1158.
134a. Gillin JC, Buchsbaum M, Wu J, Clark C, Bunney W, Jr. Sleep deprivation as a model experimental antidepressant treatment: findings from functional brain imaging. Depress Anxiety 2001; 14:37–49.
134b. Wu JC, Buchsbaum M, Bunney WE, Jr. Clinical neurochemical implications of sleep deprivation's effects on the anterior cingulate of depressed responders. Neuropsychopharmacology 2001; 25:S74–S78.

135. Smith GS, Reynolds CF, Pollock B, Derbyshire S, Nofzinger E, Dew MA, et al. Cerebral glucose metabolic response to combined total sleep deprivation and antidepressant treatment in geriatric depression. Am J Psychiatry 1999; 156:683–689.
136. Ebert D, Feistel H, Barocka A, Kaschka W. Increased limbic blood flow and total sleep deprivation in major depression with melancholia. Psychiatry Res Neuroimaging 1994; 55:101–109.
137. Ebert D, Feistel H, Barocka A. Effects of sleep deprivation on the limbic system and the frontal lobes in affective disorders: a study with Tc-99m- HMPAO SPECT. Psychiatry Res Neuroimaging 1991; 40:247–251.
138. Volk S, Kaendler SH, Weber R, Georgi K, Maul F, Hertel A, et al. Evaluation of the effects of total sleep deprivation on cerebral blood flow using single photon emission computerized tomography. Acta Psychiatr Scand 1992; 86:478–483.
139. Volk SA, Kaendler SH, Hertel A, Maul FD, Manoocheri R, Weber R, et al. Can response to partial sleep deprivation in depressed patients be predicted by regional changes of cerebral blood flow? Psychiatry Res Neuroimag 1997; 75:67–74.
140. Holthoff VA, Beuthien-Baumann B, Pietrzyk U, Pinkert J, Oehme P, Franke WG, et al. Regionale funktionsstörung bei der Depression. Nervenartz 1999; 70:620–626.
141. Ebert D, Feistel H, Kaschka W, Barocka A, Pirner A. Single photon emission computerized tomography assessment of cerebral dopamine D_2 receptor blockade in depression before and after sleep deprivation—preliminary studies. Biol Psychiatry 1994; 35:880–885.
141a. Clark CP, Frank LR, Brown GG. Sleep deprivation, EEG, and functional MRI in depression: preliminary results. Neuropsychopharmacology 2001; 25:S79–S84.
142. Mayberg HS, Brannan SK, Mahurin RK, Jerabek PA, Brickman JS, Tekell JL, et al. Cingulate function in depression: a potential predictor of treatment response. NeuroReport 1997; 8:1057–1061.
143. Mayberg HS. Limbic-cortical dysregulation: a proposed model of depression. J Neuropsychiatry 1997; 9:1–11.
144. Wirz-Justice A, van den Hoofdakker R. Sleep deprivation in depression: What do we know, where do we go? Biol Psychiatry 1999; 46:445–453.
145. Borbely AA, Wirz-Justice A. Sleep, sleep deprivation and depression: a hypothesis derived from a model of sleep regulation. Hum Neurobiol 1982; 1:205–210.
146. Wehr TA, Wirz-Justice A, Goodwin FK, Duncan W, Gillin JC. Phase advance of the circadian sleep-wake cycle as an antidepressant. Science 1979; 206:210–213.
147. Van Den Burg W, Beersma DGM, Bouhuys AL, Van Den Hoofdakker RH. Self-rated arousal concurrent with the antidepressant response to total sleep deprivation of patients with a major depressive disorder: a disinhibition hypothesis. J Sleep Res 1992; 1:211–222.
148. Praevot E, Maudhuit C, Le Poul E, Hamon M, Adrien J. Sleep deprivation reduces the citalopram-induced inhibition of serotoninergic neuronal firing in the nucleus raphe dorsalis of the rat. J Sleep Res 1996; 5:238–245.
149. Bertolucci PH, Andrade LA, Lima JG, Carlini EA. Total sleep deprivation and Parkinsons disease. Arq Neuro-Psiquiatria (Sao Paulo) 1987; 45:224–230.
150. Gerner TH, Post RM, Gillin JC, Bunney WE Jr. Biological and behavioral effects of one night sleep deprivation in depressed patients and normals. J Psychiatr Res 1979; 15:21–40.

11

Cytokines and Sleep Promotion
A Potential Mechanism for Disorders of Excessive Daytime Sleepiness

MARK R. OPP

University of Michigan
Ann Arbor, Michigan

I. Introduction

The major physiological consequences of sleep apnea include (excessive) daytime sleepiness and effects on the cardiovascular system. Daytime sleepiness is a typical complaint of sleep apnea patients and has generally been thought to result from the repeated arousals during nighttime sleep that are necessary to breathe, i.e., nighttime sleep of apneic patients is fragmented and not refreshing. Although the daytime sleepiness can occur at any time of the day, it most commonly occurs during the afternoon or early evening. The observation that naps do not usually provide relief from feelings of daytime sleepiness suggests that factors other than nighttime sleep fragmentation may be involved. In this chapter, we first briefly review data indicating that cytokines are involved in sleep regulation. We then present evidence that some effects of sleep apnea may include alterations in cytokine profiles. Finally, we conclude by speculating that alterations in cytokine concentrations/profiles may be one of several causal factors of the daytime sleepiness typically associated with sleep apnea.

II. Cytokines and Sleep Promotion

A role for cytokines in the regulation of sleep was anticipated long before empirical evidence supporting such a contention was available. Physicians for millennia have advised their patients to sleep during the course of an illness, and we have all experienced a perception of increased sleep need during mild infections such as ''a cold'' or ''the flu.'' Given this conventional wisdom, it is somewhat surprising that systematic studies of the alterations in sleep throughout the course of an acute infection, or of the interactions of the central nervous system with the immune system as they pertain to sleep, have only recently begun. For a historical overview of the observations that provided the foundation for modern experimentation on the involvement of cytokines in the regulation of sleep, the interested reader is referred to Krueger and Karnovsky (1).

The term ''cytokine'' refers to a large group of low molecular weight proteins that mediate many aspects of immunity, inflammation, tissue remodeling, and embryonic development. Although cytokines were originally described as products of the immune system, we now know that circulating cytokines modulate many central nervous system (CNS) processes, including, among others, sleep, thermoregulation, appetite and feeding, and sexual behavior. Not only does the CNS respond to changes in peripheral cytokine concentrations, but many cytokines are also produced and act within the CNS. Observations that the CNS both responds to and produces cytokines suggest the possibility that cytokines may also play a role in the regulation/modulation of normal physiology in addition to mediating responses to pathology. The evidence that supports this hypothesis, as it pertains to sleep, is briefly reviewed in this chapter. For discussions of more global actions of cytokines within the CNS, the reader is referred to recent volumes devoted to this topic (e.g., Refs. 2,3).

Any discussion of the involvement of cytokines in the regulation of sleep, or any other physiological process, must be prefaced by several caveats. It is important to remember that all cytokines studied to date are pleiotropic, i.e., they have multiple biological actions. Interleukin (IL)-1, for example, via CNS mechanisms induces fever, alters sleep, suppresses feeding and appetite, and reduces social exploration, in addition to its multiple roles in the peripheral immune system. Furthermore, not only are cytokines pleiotropic, but the biological actions of cytokines generally overlap to a large extent, i.e., there is redundancy in the system. For example, IL-1, tumor necrosis factor (TNF), and IL-6 all induce fever, although to date only IL-1 and TNF have been reported to modulate sleep (see later). Another complicating issue is the fact that cytokines also influence each other's synthesis and secretion. IL-1 induces not only its own synthesis, for example (4), but also that of IL-6, the IL-1 receptor antagonist (IL-1ra), and IL-10, to name but a few (5). These actions are generally regulatory in nature and create either feed-forward or feedback loops that normally ensure that the effects of cytokines are moderated before they become detrimental. Similarly, cytokines induce the synthesis/secretion of neurotransmitters, neuropeptides, and hormones, all of which may affect sleep either directly or indirectly (see, e.g., Refs. 6,7 for reviews).

What has emerged is a complex picture in which cytokines interact with multiple systems at multiple levels to alter the precise way in which sleep is manifest. With these caveats in mind, a brief examination of what constitutes a realistic expectation for results of sleep studies in which the cytokine network has been targeted is warranted. First, the redundancy of the cytokine network makes it difficult to attribute specific effects on sleep to individual cytokines. Since there are several cytokines that are well-documented modulators of sleep (see later), and these cytokines interact with a variety of other systems/substances that modulate sleep, the degree to which sleep is altered by targeting a single cytokine may not be large in absolute terms. This is particularly true when considering observations of sleep patterns in transgenic animals in which the gene(s) for specific cytokine(s) have been ''knocked out.'' Given the degree of redundancy in the cytokine network, the loss of one cytokine gene may be compensated by recruitment during development of another cytokine to perform the same function. As such, negative data from knockout animals do not necessarily indicate that the cytokine knocked out is not involved in sleep regulation. The production of inducible knockouts should help address this issue as expression of the gene of interest may be reduced in adult animals that have developed normally. Second, the outcome of acute vs. chronic manipulations of a particular system may differ. As with transgenic animals, the targeted system (cytokine) in animals subjected to chronic administration of a particular antagonist may, over time, compensate. As such, sleep parameters determined at the end of a period of chronic manipulation may not differ greatly from those obtained prior to the manipulation. Under these conditions, a logical conclusion is that the system (cytokine) may not be involved in sleep regulation/modulation, and such a conclusion may well be erroneous. Third, as with other systems, the time at which a cytokine, or the cytokine network, is manipulated will determine to a large extent the specific effects of the manipulation on sleep. This is particularly critical when conducting studies on rodents or other animals that are highly circadian in nature. For example, doses of IL-1 that enhance slow-wave sleep (SWS) when administered to rats during the active (dark) period reduce SWS when administered during the rest (light) period (8) (see later).

Finally, if direct intervention of a particular system alters the expression of sleep, a fundamental functional question remains. What constitutes a biologically relevant change in behavior? If a particular manipulation results in a complete elimination of sleep, most would agree there are likely to be functional consequences. If, on the other hand, sleep is less dramatically altered in response to a well-controlled and carefully planned manipulation (e.g., sleep is reduced or increased by 30 or 60 min across a 24-h period), it is more difficult to ascertain whether or not such an alteration ''means'' anything to the animal, even though a logical conclusion is that the targeted system may be involved in the regulation of sleep. A corollary to this question is whether all alterations in sleep are ''equal.'' Is a reduction in sleep due to antagonism of a cytokine functionally equivalent to that achieved by targeting a neurotransmitter? These questions are rarely addressed and are beyond the scope of this chapter. However, it is important to remember that the absolute magnitude of alterations in sleep following most experimental manipulations that target the cytokine network, or any other system for that matter, is relatively small, and the effects are generally of short duration (i.e., a few to several hours). As previously mentioned, it is difficult at best to assess the biological relevance or functional significance of a change in sleep. The relatively small changes in sleep induced by a particular manipulation reflect not only the complexity of the multiple regulatory mechanisms and systems involved, but also the evolutionary age and significance of this behavior; the brain aggressively protects its ability to sleep. Similarly, cytokines are evolutionarily ancient; they are produced by and are biologically active in phyla ranging from invertebrates to mammals. Given the critical nature of the immune system, it seems logical that a high degree of redundancy and complexity is incorporated into the system.

The first reports of the effects of IL-1 on sleep were published in 1983/1984 (9–11). In the approximately 16–17 years since these first reports, the effects of several other cytokines on sleep have been described. These include IL-2, IL-4, IL-6, IL-10, TNF, fibroblast growth factor (FGF), interferon (IFN), nerve growth factor (NGF), and granulocyte-macrophage colony-stimulating factor (GM-CSF). Cytokine actions within the CNS with regard to sleep have been frequently reviewed in recent years (6,12–16). In this chapter we focus primarily on the effects of IL-1, TNF, and IFN, as these have been the most extensively studied cytokines with regard to sleep.

A. Interleukin-1

IL-1β is a pleiotropic cytokine that belongs to a gene family that also includes IL-1α and the IL-1 receptor antagonist (IL-1ra). IL-1β, IL-1α, and the IL-1ra bind to two IL-1 receptors, the IL-1 type I and type II receptors. The IL-1 type I receptor complexes with an accessory protein to form the unit for signal transduction, whereas the IL-1 type II receptor is nonsignaling. IL-1α and IL-1β are derived from two distinct gene products. IL-1α is generally cell-associated, whereas IL-1β is the predominant form found in tissue fluids and plasma. For more information about the biology of IL-1 and the IL-1 gene family, the reader is referred to several reviews by Dinarello (5,17,18). Although IL-1α is somnogenic (19), almost all sleep studies have used IL-1β, and for the remainder of this chapter we designate IL-1β as simply IL-1.

After more than 15 years of work, Pappenheimer and colleagues identified muramyl peptide as a sleep-promoting factor in the cerebral spinal fluid of sleep-deprived animals (20). Muramyl peptides were known to be immune active substances that induced IL-1 activity (at that time called endogenous pyrogen). Although IL-1 was at that time thought to be a product solely of the immune system, Fontana's observation (21) that astrocytes (neuroglia) produce IL-1 provided a rationale to determine whether IL-1 was somnogenic. In the initial studies of Krueger (9,10), purified human endogenous pyrogen was injected intracerebroventricularly (ICV) into rabbits; SWS was increased. Several important observations of the effects of IL-1 on sleep were made during these studies: (1) the effects of IL-1 on sleep are dose-related; (2) administration of IL-1 increases electroencephalogram (EEG) slow wave activity in the delta frequency band; (3) the effects of IL-1 are specific to the protein as heat-treated preparations do not alter sleep or brain/body temperature; and (4) the enhancement of SWS by IL-1 is not merely a byproduct of fever because pretreatment of animals with anisomycin abolishes IL-1–induced fever but not IL-1–induced SWS. These initial observations of the effects of IL-1 on the sleep of rabbits have been reproduced many times (19,22–28). Although not reported in the initial studies of Krueger, moderate or high doses of IL-1 also suppress rapid-eye movement (REM) sleep, although at low doses SWS may be enhanced without altering REM sleep.

IL-1 has proven to be somnogenic in species other than rabbits, including rats (8,11,29–35), mice (36), cats (37), and monkeys (38,39). The first report of IL-1 effects on sleep in the rat provided an early indication that not all species would respond to IL-1 in the same way as the rabbit. Tobler et al. (11) administered a single dose of astrocyte-derived IL-1 ICV into rats at the beginning of the light period of the light-dark cycle. Although the amount of total sleep time was not altered, REM sleep was reduced, and slow wave activity in the delta frequency band was increased, indicating that this IL-1 preparation was active in the CNS and influenced sleep mechanisms. This first study of IL-1 effects on rat sleep did not address the issue of interactions between IL-1 and circadian regulatory mechanisms, but it provided an indication that circadian influences would be a complicating factor in species that are highly circadian in their sleep-wake activity patterns. Subsequent studies using rats (8,29,32,33,35) have demonstrated that IL-1 also increases SWS duration in addition to enhancing EEG slow wave activity. Low doses of recombinant IL-1 (e.g., 0.5–1.0 ng ICV) increase SWS regardless of whether they are administered during the light period or during the dark period. However, as the dose of IL-1 is increased, the somnogenic responses diverge depending on the timing of administration. Moderate doses (e.g., 2.5–5.0 ng ICV) enhance EEG slow wave activity during the light period with little effect on SWS duration, whereas during the dark period these doses increase SWS duration with little effect on EEG slow wave activity. These circadian-dependent patterns of responses are apparent when IL-1 is administered both centrally (ICV) (8,32) and peripherally (intraperitoneally) (35). At higher doses of IL-1 (e.g., 10–25 ng ICV), SWS in the rat is suppressed for a period of several hours after administration (8,33). Although definitive experiments have not been conducted, it is likely that the status of feedback mechanisms for IL-1 actions at the time of administration and/or the extent to which negative feedback mechanisms for IL-1 actions are stimulated dictate to a great extent the specific behavioral responses that follow. This is due to the fact that corticotropin-releasing hormone (CRH) and the hypothalamic-pituitary-adrenal (HPA) axis constitute the major negative feedback mechanism for IL-1 synthesis and secretion in brain

(40). CRH induces waking and antagonizes IL-1 effects on sleep (25). Therefore, responses to IL-1 administered at a time when CRH/HPA axis activity is high differ from those that follow administration of the same dose when CRH/HPA axis activity is low (8). Similarly, since IL-1 is a potent stimulator of CRH and HPA axis activity, the higher the dose of IL-1 administered, the greater the extent of CRH/HPA axis activation (41). Therefore, initial responses to administration of high doses of IL-1 include reductions in sleep (8). As such, IL-1 per se may be considered sleep-inducing, although at high doses it stimulates systems that at least transiently reduce sleep and increase waking.

The effects of exogenously administered IL-1 are specific for the protein and are receptor mediated. As mentioned above, when IL-1 is heat-treated prior to administration, sleep and thermoregulation are not altered indicating that these responses are not due to contamination during the production of the recombinant product. Furthermore, pretreating experimental animals with the specific IL-1ra results in a complete block of IL-1–induced somnogenic and febrile responses (27,28,42). These types of experiments, in which animals are pretreated with purported IL-1 antagonists, have been repeated several times, with generally similar results. Thus, pretreatment with a soluble IL-1 receptor completely blocks somnogenic and pyrogenic responses to IL-1 (28), whereas an IL-1 receptor fragment (43) blocks completely the somnogenic responses to IL-1 but not IL-1–induced fever.

The observations that sleep is altered in response to exogenous IL-1 does not necessarily implicate IL-1 in sleep regulation. As stated previously, IL-1 and other cytokines stimulate the synthesis/secretion of multiple neurotransmitters, neuropeptides, and hormones that alter sleep. An abbreviated list of neurotransmitters, neuropeptides, and hormones implicated in the regulation/modulation of sleep that are altered by IL-1 and/or other cytokines includes noradrenaline, dopamine, serotonin, acetylcholine, GABA, glutamic acid, histamine, nitric oxide, adenosine, CRH, and growth hormone–releasing hormone (24,44,45). As such, the effects of exogenously administered IL-1 on sleep may be indirect. This possibility has been explored in several studies in which endogenous IL-1, or components of the IL-1 system, have been directly targeted in otherwise normal animals. For example, central administration of the IL-1ra reduces spontaneous SWS in rabbits for about 1 h postinjection (27). The relatively short duration of this effect is likely due to the short (~10 minute in blood) half-life of the IL-1ra. However, central administration of antibodies directed against IL-1 reduces spontaneous SWS for up to 12 h in rats (46), whereas anti-rabbit IL-1 reduces spontaneous SWS of rabbits for about 4 h (47). Furthermore, central administration of an IL-1 receptor fragment also inhibits spontaneous sleep in the rabbit (48). Observations such as these indicate that direct and specific intervention in the binding of IL-1 to its receptor reduces sleep in otherwise normal animals and provide strong supporting evidence for the hypothesis that IL-1 is involved in the regulation of sleep.

Further evidence suggesting that IL-1 is involved in physiological sleep regulation comes from sleep-deprivation studies. Animals respond to periods of sleep deprivation with a rebound in SWS duration and an increase in EEG slow wave activity after the sleep deprivation ends (see, e.g., Refs. 49–51). There is evidence suggesting that IL-1 may be involved in mediating responses to sleep deprivation. For example, plasma concentrations of IL-1 in rabbits (47) and plasma IL-1–like activity in humans (52,53) increase during sleep deprivation. Furthermore, ICV administration into rabbits (47) or rats (46) of antibodies directed against IL-1 attenuates or blocks completely sleep deprivation–induced increases in SWS duration. Similarly, sleep deprivation–induced increases in SWS are attenuated in rabbits pretreated with an IL-1 receptor fragment (48). In addition, IL-1 mRNA expression in the hypothalamus and brain stem of rats increases following sleep deprivation (54). Finally, although IL-1 alters sleep when administered centrally or peripherally, it appears as if central pools, rather than circulating IL-1, are the important mediators of responses to sleep deprivation; an IL-1 receptor fragment attenuates sleep deprivation-induced increases in SWS when administered ICV, but not when administered intravenously (48).

In summary, there is ample evidence supporting the hypothesis that IL-1 is involved in physiological sleep regulation, in addition to the alterations in sleep that occur throughout the course of an acute infection. A great deal of this evidence is indirect. For example, IL-1 enhances SWS in every species thus far examined, whether administered ICV, intravenously, or intraperitoneally. [Anecdotally, humans undergoing IL-1 therapy complain of excessive sleepiness (18).] Furthermore, the machinery for IL-1 to modulate sleep is in place. IL-1 receptors are widespread in the CNS in regions important in the regulation of sleep (55–57), IL-1–containing neurons are located in the hypothalamus (58), and IL-1 mRNA may be detected in many brain regions (59,60). IL-1 mRNA expression in rat brain exhibits diurnal variation with greater levels during the early light (rest/sleep) period than during the dark (active) period (61). IL-1 mRNA expression increases during sleep deprivation (54), and plasma IL-1 protein levels are detected more frequently in samples from sleep-deprived rabbits than in samples from rested rabbits (47). Similarly, IL-1 is detected more frequently in plasma samples taken from humans during sleep than during waking (62). IL-1–like activity in cerebrospinal fluid of cats varies in phase with the sleep-wake cycle (63), and plasma levels in humans peak at sleep onset (52). Stimulated whole blood cell cultures from samples taken during sleep produce more IL-1 than those from cultures taken during waking (64). Substances that induce IL-1 production induce SWS, whereas substances that inhibit IL-1 synthesis or actions inhibit SWS (reviewed in Refs. 13,16). There is also direct evidence that IL-1 is involved in sleep regulation. Interfering with the binding of IL-1 to its receptor by administering the IL-1ra, antibodies directed against IL-1, or a soluble IL-1 receptor fragment reduces spontaneous SWS in otherwise normal animals (27,42,43). Furthermore, sleep deprivation–induced enhancement of SWS is attenuated or blocked when experimental animals are pretreated with anti-IL-1 or with an IL-1 receptor fragment (46–48). Collectively, these data provide strong evidence that IL-1 plays a role in the regulation of physiological sleep.

B. Tumor Necrosis Factor

TNF, like IL-1, is a pleiotropic cytokine that is constitutively expressed in normal brain. There are two forms of TNF. TNF-α (cachectin) is a product primarily of macrophages, whereas TNF-β (lymphotoxin) is a product of lymphocytes. Although TNF-β is somnogenic (65), most sleep studies have used TNF-α, to which we will refer in the remainder of this chapter as simply TNF. These proteins share about 30% amino acid sequence homology and have similar, although not identical, biological activities (reviewed in Ref. 66). TNF is produced by astrocytes, and TNF immunoreactive neurons exist in the CNS (67) TNF receptor mRNA is expressed in normal brain (68), and the soluble TNF receptor occurs normally in cerebrospinal fluid (69). There are two cell surface TNF receptors, designated 55 kDa and 75 kDa TNF receptors (70,71), that mediate distinct actions (72). It appears that the 55 kDa receptor is responsible for mediating the somnogenic effects of TNF (36).

There is a large degree of overlap between the biological actions of IL-1 and TNF. IL-1 and TNF induce each other's synthesis (73,74), and in many instances these two substances are synergistic. The interactions between IL-1 and TNF may also be relevant for sleep regulation. For example, TNF-induced SWS responses are attenuated in animals pretreated with a soluble IL-1 receptor, and TNF antagonists inhibit somnogenic responses to IL-1 (75). As such, the evidence suggesting a role for TNF in sleep regulation follows similar lines as those reviewed previously concerning IL-1. Plasma TNF concentrations exhibit circadian rhythms that correlate with EEG slow wave activity in humans (76). In rat brain, TNF mRNA (77) and TNF protein (78) exhibit a diurnal variation, with peak concentrations occurring during the light (rest) period of the light-dark cycle. Similarly, TNF protein in human plasma (62) exhibits a diurnal variation with peak concentrations detected during sleep. SWS is increased in rabbits (23,65), mice (79), and rats (80) in response to administration of TNF, as are amplitudes of EEG slow waves (23). TNF-induced increases in SWS are generally accompanied by reductions in REM sleep, although low doses that promote SWS in mice do not affect REM sleep (36).

Direct intervention with the TNF system reduces spontaneous SWS in otherwise normal animals. For example, antibodies directed against TNF reduce spontaneous SWS in rats and rabbits (81). Similarly, a fragment of the soluble TNF binding protein and a synthetic TNF receptor fragment also reduce SWS in rabbits (82,83). TNF may also be involved in mediating alterations in sleep that follow changes in ambient temperature. It has long been known that thermoregulation and sleep are tightly coupled (84–87), and most cytokines to which a role in sleep regulation has been attributed also alter thermoregulatory mechanisms (reviewed in Ref. 88). Mild increases in ambient temperature enhance sleep (89). The amount of time rabbits spend in SWS, and EEG slow wave activity during SWS, increase when the ambient temperature is acutely raised from 21 to 27°C. Although the precise mechanisms for these ambient temperature-associated alterations in sleep are not known, the increase in SWS duration and in EEG slow wave activity are blocked when the animals are pretreated with a soluble TNF receptor fragment (90). Finally, the rebound in SWS that characteristically follows periods of sleep deprivation is attenuated by central administration of a soluble TNF receptor fragment (83).

In summary, TNF induces SWS in several species (23,65,79,80,91). TNF mRNA (77) and protein (78) in brain and protein in plasma (62,76) exhibit circadian rhythms that coincide with sleep-wake activity. Direct intervention with the TNF system by the use of antibodies (81), binding proteins (82), or soluble receptors or receptor fragments (82) reduces SWS in otherwise normal animals. Mice that lack the 55 kDa TNF receptor sleep less than background strain controls (79). Increases in SWS following periods of sleep deprivation (83) or mild increases in ambient temperature (90) are attenuated when experimental animals are pretreated with TNF antagonists. Collectively, these data provide support for the hypothesis that TNF is involved in the regulation of sleep.

C. Interferons

Palmblad et al. (92) were the first to demonstrate a link between cytokines and sleep when they reported that sleep deprivation enhanced the ability of leukocytes to produce interferon. Palmblad's study is more than 20 years old, yet the role of IFNs in the regulation of sleep has not been studied to the same extent as IL-1 or TNF. There is limited evidence suggesting a role for IFN in physiological sleep regulation. For example, human recombinant IFN-α induces cortical EEG synchronization in the rat (93–95) increases SWS in rabbits (96,97), and reduces latency to REMS in monkeys (98), and stimulated whole blood cell cultures from samples taken during sleep produce more IFN-γ than those from samples taken during waking (64). [Anecdotally, humans undergoing IFN therapy complain of excessive sleepiness (99).]

IFNs may play a greater role, however, in mediating some of the somnogenic responses to infection, particularly those in which a virus is the etiological agent. IFNs are well documented for their antiviral activity. IFN-α receptors are found in brain (100), and in response to infection almost all nucleated cells produce IFNs (101). Alterations in sleep have been described in response to several viruses, including influenza, human immunodeficiency virus, feline immunodeficiency virus, and Newcastle disease virus (reviewed in Refs. 16,102–104). The degree of somnogenic response to viral infection may depend on the ability of the organism to mount an IFN response. For example, C57BL/6 and Swiss Webster, but not BALB/c, mice exhibit increased SWS in response to influenza infection (105,106). These strains differ in IFN production in response to viral challenge; C57BL/6 mice are high IFN producers, whereas BALB/c are low IFN producers (103,107). Furthermore, viral components that are IFN inducers such as polyinosinic:polycytidilic acid enhance sleep and concurrently increase plasma IFN activity (108). Finally, viral infections have also been linked to chronic fatigue syndrome (109) and have been implicated as an etiological factor in the occurrence of the sudden infant death syndrome (110). Collectively, these observations suggest that IFNs may be important mediators of sleep alterations that occur throughout the course of a viral infection.

D. Other Cytokines

Several other cytokines have been studied with regard to the regulation/modulation of sleep. These include IL-2, IL-4, IL-6, IL-10, fibroblast growth factor, nerve growth factor, and granulocyte-macrophage colony-stimulating factor. In most cases, these cytokines have been the subject of single experiments that generate reports that are often preliminary in nature. In addition, hypotheses that each of these cytokines is involved in sleep regulation are based generally on correlative data, with no evidence that direct intervention alters spontaneous sleep. Criteria have been proposed that define a substance as a ''sleep factor'' and that should be met before a role in sleep regulation is attributed to any factor (see, e.g., Refs. 111–113). As proposed by Krueger (112), these criteria include: (1) the substance should induce physiological sleep; (2) receptors for the substance should be present in brain in regions important for the regulation of sleep; (3) the concentrations of the substance or its receptor should change with sleep-wake activity; (4) increases in concentrations of the substance should increase sleep; (5) inhibition of the substance or its receptor should reduce spontaneous sleep; (6) removal of the substance or its receptor should reduce spontaneous sleep; and (7) the substance should be part of a biochemical cascade involved in sleep regulation. The following substances meet only one or two of the above criteria. Brief summaries are provided here for completeness with the caveat that none of these substances should be considered as playing a substantive role in physiological sleep regulation until additional investigations are conducted.

Interleukin-2

IL-2 injected into the third ventricle of rats is reported to induce EEG synchronization and behavioral sleep within 5–10 min of administration (95). These effects last from 25 to 140 min depending on the dose, and are also apparent when IL-2 is microinjected into the locus coeruleus (114). Microinjection of IL-2 into the dorsal hippocampus, caudate nucleus, substantia nigra, or ventromedial hypothalamus, however, increases locomotor activity (114). Human recombinant IL-2 injected ICV (62–250 ng) or IV (1000–2000 ng) into rabbits does not alter sleep, although the preparation was active in a thymocyte proliferation assay (115). The failure of human recombinant IL-2 to alter sleep in the rabbit may be due to species specificity as it is not known if human recombinant IL-2 binds to the rabbit IL-2 receptor. Rabbit IL-2 is not commercially available, but rat IL-2 is. Rat IL-2 (25–50 Units) from the same source as that used in the study of DeSarro et al. (95) was injected ICV into rats prior to dark onset. Each of these doses increased SWS during postinjection hours 1–6 relative to values obtained after vehicle (115). An attempt to heat-inactivate this IL-2 preparation was not successful because heating the preparation resulted in a thick gelatinous substance that could not be injected. Therefore, it has not been possible to perform a critical control to determine whether somnogenic effects of IL-2 in the rat are inherent in the protein or due to contamination by somnogenic bacterial products during production. However, IL-2 receptors are found in brain (116), plasma IL-2 levels in humans are higher during sleep than during wakefulness (52,117), and plasma IL-2 levels are higher after sleep deprivation than before (53). Furthermore, IL-1 induces IL-2 synthesis (17), suggesting that some of the somnogenic actions of IL-1 may be mediated by IL-2. Collectively these data suggest that a role for IL-2 in sleep regulation is possible, but several critical experiments remain to be done.

Interleukin-6

Infection, injury, or trauma induce systemic reactions, collectively termed the acute phase response. The full spectrum of the acute phase response is mediated by the interactions of at least four groups of cytokines (IL-1, TNF, IFN, and IL-6) and includes changes in hepatic synthesis of plasma proteins, fever, and enhanced sleep. With the exception of sleep, IL-6 induces the full spectrum of acute phase responses both in vivo and in vitro, whereas IL-1 elicits the full acute phase response in vivo only. IL-1 induces IL-6 (118), IL-6 induces fever (25), and IL-6 is active in thymocyte proliferation assays (119), the classical bioassay for IL-1 activity. Observations such as these suggest that IL-1 actions are mediated, in part, through IL-6, and prompted a study to determine whether IL-6 was somnogenic (25). Rabbits injected ICV with 20–200 ng of human recombinant IL-6 developed fevers in a dose-related manner. Under these conditions, neither the amount of SWS (120) nor EEG slow-wave activity during SWS sleep (121) was consistently altered, even though the magnitude of the IL-6–induced fevers were comparable to those induced by somnogenic doses of IL-1. However, serum or plasma concentrations of IL-6 are correlated with the sleep-wake cycle in humans (62,122), and daytime plasma IL-6 concentrations are elevated in individuals suffering from disorders of excessive daytime sleepiness (123) (see later). These latter data must be interpreted as correlative in nature because there are many factors that could account for increases in IL-6 concentrations. For example, central administration of IL-1 induces increases in circulating IL-6 (124,125), suggesting that increases in brain IL-1 could result in increased systemic IL-6. Until additional information is available concerning the effects on sleep of species-specific IL-6 or the reduction of endogenous IL-6 concentrations or actions, conclusions as to a role for IL-6 in sleep regulation must be viewed with caution.

Interleukin-10/Interleukin-4

IL-10 was originally described as a product of murine type 2 helper T cells that suppressed cytokine production by type 1 helper T cells (126) and was termed "cytokine synthesis inhibitory factor." IL-10 inhibits the synthesis by stimulated monocytes/macrophages of IL-1α, -β, and TNF-α at both the mRNA and protein levels (127). IL-10 administered ICV into rats prior to light onset reduces SWS (128). IL-4 is also an anti-inflammatory cytokine that shares many biological activities with IL-10 (e.g., Refs. 129–132). ICV administration of IL-4 into rabbits reduces SWS and at higher doses also reduces REM sleep (133). The actions of IL-10 and

IL-4 on sleep may be indirect via inhibiting the synthesis of IL-1 and/or TNF. Although IL-10 mRNA is found in brain (134) and microglia produce IL-10 in vitro (135), there is little or no information concerning the presence of receptors for these substances or their actions within the CNS. It is possible that IL-10 and/or IL-4 act directly on sleep mechanisms; EEG slow wave activity during SWS is reduced by IL-10 during time periods when SWS is reduced (M. R. Opp, unpublished data), and IL-10 alters γ-aminobutyric acid–and serotonin-induced calcium channel activity in identified invertebrate neurons (T. K. Hughes, Jr., personal communication). However, determination of the extent to which these cytokines contribute to sleep regulation awaits further investigation.

Fibroblast Growth Factor

Basic and acidic FGF modulate cell proliferation, differentiation, motility, and angiogenesis. Although present in many organs, aFGF is found in large amounts only in the brain (136). FGFs share limited amino acid homology, three-dimensional topology, and biological activities with IL-1. At least four FGF receptors exhibit distinct distribution patterns; three of these receptors are expressed in brain (136). aFGF increases SWS in rats (137) and rabbits (138), whereas bFGF does not. Determination of a potential role for FGF in sleep regulation awaits additional study.

Nerve Growth Factor

NGF enhances the growth and survival of certain sympathetic and sensory neurons. NGF binds to receptors expressed on sensory and sympathetic neurons, nonneuronal cells derived from the neural crest, and on mast cells, B lymphocytes, and monocytes (136). Microinjection of NGF into the nucleus pontis oralis of the pontine reticular formation of cats during the light period of the light-dark cycle rapidly induces a REM sleep–like state that is polygraphically identical to spontaneous REM sleep (139). The amount of time spent in REM sleep during the first postinjection hour increases in a dose-related manner, while SWS and waking are reduced. In contrast, ICV administration of NGF into rabbits during the light period increases both SWS and REMS (140). The increases in REM sleep following ICV administration of NGF are dose-related. Another approach to determine the extent to which NGF might be involved in sleep regulation has been to use the plant toxin saporin coupled to the monoclonal antibody 192 IgG. The monoclonal antibody 192 IgG recognizes the p75 NGF receptor and is specifically internalized in cholinergic basal forebrain neurons containing NGF receptors. Upon internalization, the 192 IgG–saporin complex kills cholinergic basal forebrain neurons without affecting other neuronal types. Such immunolesions of NGF receptor–positive cholinergic neurons in the basal forebrain of rats alters sleep in circadian-dependent fashion; during the light period both SWS and REM sleep are decreased, whereas during the dark period SWS and REMS are increased (141). Data from these immunolesion studies complement those of Yamuy et al. (139) and Takahashi et al. (142); NGF microinjected into the pontine reticular formation or injected into the cerebral ventricular system during the light period increases REM sleep, whereas REM sleep is decreased during the light period in rats in which the cholinergic NGF receptor–positive neurons have been destroyed. Although the mechanisms by which NGF alters sleep are not known, it appears that this growth factor may play a role in REM sleep initiation or maintenance.

Granulocyte-Macrophage Colony-Stimulating Factor

Colony-stimulating factors are cytokines that stimulate pluripotent stem cells to produce hematopoietic cells; they are named according to the type of cells that form colonies on soft agar. GM-CSF acts on bipotential stem cells to produce mononuclear phagocytes and granulocytes. One study (143) reports that SWS increases in a dose-related manner in rats injected ICV with GM-CSF at dark onset. As the dose of GM-CSF is increased, REM sleep is also enhanced. Rats in which GM-CSF was infused for a 10-h period exhibited even greater increases in SWS and REM sleep. The mechanisms for such actions are not clear, and additional studies are required.

III. A Potential Role for Cytokines as Mediators of Excessive Daytime Sleepiness

The major physiological consequences of obstructive sleep apnea include excessive daytime sleepiness (144) and effects on the cardiovascular system (145). The fragmentation of nighttime sleep, which results in individuals feeling unrefreshed upon awakening, has often been thought to contribute to excessive daytime sleepiness. However, the observation that most patients with obstructive sleep apnea do not feel refreshed after short daytime naps (146) suggests that perhaps other factors are involved. We have reviewed data indicating that several cytokines are involved in regulating/modulating sleep. There is increasing evidence that somnogenic cytokines such as IL-1 and TNF exhibit circadian rhythmicity. As such, cytokine concentrations/profiles that deviate from the normal circadian pattern may alter the normal expression of sleep-wake behavior. For the remainder of this chapter, we speculate that increased concentrations of somnogenic cytokines during the daytime, when they are normally low, may mediate or contribute to the excessive daytime sleepiness from which obstructive sleep apnea patients complain.

Although there are few studies that address this hypothesis, those that have been reported suggest there may be an association between circulating cytokines and excessive daytime sleepiness in at least one subset of obstructive sleep apnea patients (see later). However, determination of cytokine profiles from human subjects is generally done from blood, and as such indicates cytokine concentrations in the periphery rather than in the brain. It is not at all clear that cytokine concentrations in the periphery directly reflect or are indicative of cytokine concentrations in the brain. The question of whether information concerning mechanisms regulating a brain behavior such as sleep may be derived from measures obtained from the periphery is an important one. What is clear, however, is that the CNS responds to peripheral events, and there are multiple mechanisms by which peripheral cytokines may signal the brain (147) with subsequent effects on sleep. As such, although changes in peripheral cytokine concentrations may not reflect directly changes in cytokines within brain, circulating cytokines may well be expected to influence or modulate brain activity.

To the best of our knowledge, there are only two published accounts of cytokine profiles in patients with obstructive sleep apnea. Entzian et al. (148) studied 10 hospitalized patients requiring therapy for obstructive sleep apnea. These individuals were obese with a mean respiratory disturbance index of 48.3 ± 12.8 apneas + hypopneas per hour of sleep. Blood samples were collected every 4 h during the day (0800–2000 h) and at 2-h intervals during nighttime sleep. Whole blood cultures stimulated with lipopolysaccharide were used to determine cytokine release. Supernatants from the cultures were assayed for IL-1β, IL-6, TNF-α, and IFN-γ, as well as cortisol and melatonin. The production of each of these substances exhibited clear circadian rhythmicity. There were no statistical differences between normal control subjects and sleep apnea patients for concentrations/profiles of IL-1, IL-6, IFN-γ, cortisol, or melatonin. The circadian rhythm of TNF, however, was dramatically altered in sleep apnea patients; the peak concentrations that occurred during the night in normal control subjects was not present in sleep apnea patients. Rather, sleep apnea patients exhibited increased TNF concentrations in the afternoon, the time period during which concentrations in normal control subjects are at a minimum. It is also interesting to note that in spite of a lack of statistical differences due to inherent interindividual variability, absolute IL-1 concentrations in the sleep apnea patients were more than twice those obtained from normal controls, and IFN-γ concentrations were more than three times those of normal controls. Perhaps the most important finding in this study, however, is the observation that the *alterations in cytokine profiles detected in sleep apnea patients were not normalized by nasal continuous positive airway pressure (CPAP) ventilation therapy.* This is a critical finding because in these patients *sleep fragmentation, arousal frequency, and oxygen tension desaturation were normalized by CPAP therapy.* These observations suggest that the excessive daytime sleepiness of which most obstructive sleep apnea patients complain has a biological basis that cannot be explained solely in terms of nighttime sleep fragmentation.

Recently, Vgontzas et al. (123) published a study in which cytokine profiles were obtained from patient populations of individuals with disorders of excessive daytime sleepiness (123). Three populations were studied; those with obstructive sleep apnea (n = 12), narcoleptics (n = 11), and idiopathic hypersomniacs (n = 8). Single blood samples were drawn in the morning (0600–0700 h) after the completion of the nighttime sleep laboratory recordings. Plasma concentrations of IL-1β, TNF-α, and IL-6 were determined by ELISA. Relative to control subjects, plasma IL-1 concentrations did not differ between the three groups, TNF was elevated in sleep apnea patients and narcoleptics, and IL-6 was elevated only in sleep apnea patients. Correlational analyses indicated that TNF and IL-6 correlated positively with measures of excessive daytime sleepiness; TNF was positively correlated with the degree of nocturnal sleep disturbance and the degree of hypoxia, but not with body mass index, whereas IL-6 concentrations were correlated with degree of nocturnal sleep disturbance, degree of hypoxia, and body mass index. Although the results obtained in these two studies are correlational and do not allow conclusions to be made as to causality, they do provide evidence suggesting that cytokines are elevated in individuals with sleep apnea and provide support for the hypothesis that the excessive daytime sleepiness of which sleep apnea patients complain may be mediated in part by somnogenic cytokines.

However, as stated previously, the reason for elevated cytokine concentrations in patients with sleep apnea was not addressed in either of these studies. If alterations in cytokine concentrations/profiles contribute to excessive daytime sleepiness, what is the biological basis for these changes? Although there are likely to be many factors involved, sleep apnea–associated hypertension may contribute to alterations in cytokine concentrations/profiles. While not all sleep apnea patients are hypertensive and not all individuals with hypertension exhibit altered cytokine profiles (see later), the prevalence of hypertension is much greater in patients with sleep apnea than in the general populace, and there is evidence that cytokine concentrations/profiles are altered during hypertension. For the remainder of this chapter we speculate that immune dysfunction associated with hypertension may be one of several causal factors resulting in altered cytokine profiles reported to occur in sleep apnea patients.

The relationship between sleep apnea and hypertension has been recently reviewed (149–152) and is the subject of other chapters in this volume. For the purpose of this discussion, it is not important whether obstructive sleep apnea results in hypertension during daytime waking (151,152) or daytime hypertension is merely associated with obstructive sleep apnea, because both disorders are found in individuals with similar demographics (149,150). What is important is that the prevalence of hypertension is much higher in apnea patients than in the general population (151). There is evidence of immune dysfunction, including altered cytokine profiles, during hypertension. Although a comprehensive review of the literature implicating immune dysfunction in the etiology of hypertension is beyond the scope of this chapter, many facets of humoral and cellular immunity are altered during hypertension, even though the precise role of immune dysfunction in the etiology of hypertension is not clear (153–157).

The possibility of immune dysfunction leading to hypertension was first addressed by Ebringer and Doyle (158), who described a patient population with essential hypertension in which serum immunoglobulin levels were elevated. Alterations in immunoglobulins are common in subjects with dysfunctional immune systems. Many subsequent studies indicate alterations in immunoglobulin levels during hypertension (reviewed in Ref. 156); significantly elevated serum immunoglobulin levels are found in approximately 20–40% of patients with essential hypertension (155). Furthermore, autoantibodies to nuclear structures and smooth muscle are found more often and in greater concentrations in patients with essential hypertension. In addition to changes in humoral immune components, there are alterations in cellular immunity during hypertension. For example, patients with essential hypertension exhibit delayed hypersensitivity to vascular antigens that is mediated by sensitized

T lymphocytes (reviewed in Refs. 155,156). Further evidence for immune dysfunction as a contributor to hypertension is obtained from animal models such as the spontaneously hypertensive rat (SHR) (reviewed in Ref. 155). SHRs exhibit alterations in T lymphocytes, and serum from SHRs contains antibodies directed against native thymus tissue. Furthermore, T and B cells fail to interact properly for the production of antibodies. These animals develop a measurable hypertension with systolic pressures that often exceed 225 mmHg. When SHRs are chronically administered the immunosuppressant cyclophosphamide, there is a significant attenuation of the hypertension (155). Results of the aforementioned studies, and many others not cited, provide convincing evidence that there is increased prevalence of cellular and humoral immune dysfunction in individuals with hypertension. There are also studies indicating that cytokines are increased in patients with pulmonary hypertension (e.g., Refs. 159,160) and in animal models of pulmonary hypertension (e.g., 161). The associated pathology of pulmonary hypertension (alveolar edema, endothelial injury, right ventricular hypertrophy, etc.) may directly result in the release of cytokines (reviewed in Ref. 160) and may not accurately reflect characteristics of essential hypertension.

There are a few reports in which cytokine concentrations were determined from patients with essential hypertension. Dalekos et al. (162) studied 114 patients with mild to moderate essential hypertension. Inclusion criteria mandated that no antihypertensive drugs had been taken during the preceding 3 months, and normotensive controls were studied in parallel. Blood samples were drawn at 0800 h, and serum IL-1 concentrations that exceeded the mean concentrations found in normotensive controls by three standard deviations were considered elevated. Such elevated serum IL-1 concentrations were detected in 68 of the hypertensive patients (~60%). This initial study was repeated and extended to include groups of patients with essential hypertension, familial hypercholesterolemia, and normotensive controls (163). Elevated serum IL-1 concentrations (values greater than three standard deviations of the mean concentrations obtained from normotensive controls) were detected in 16 of the 38 patients (~57%) with essential hypertension. Furthermore, absolute serum concentrations of IL-1 were significantly higher in patients with essential hypertension than in those with familial hypercholesterolemia. Although we are unaware of additional studies of cytokines and essential hypertension per se, these data support the hypothesis that hypertension-induced elevation in somnogenic cytokines may be one mechanism responsible for excessive daytime sleepiness in at least one subset of obstructive sleep apnea patients.

IV. Conclusions

There is extensive evidence that some cytokines, notably IL-1, TNF, and IFN, possess inherent somnogenic properties and are likely to be involved in sleep regulation; much of this evidence has been reviewed in this chapter. We suggest the possibility that the excessive daytime sleepiness of which most obstructive sleep apnea patients complain may be due, in part, to increases at inappropriate times in the concentrations of somnogenic cytokines, i.e., during daytime wakefulness. This suggestion is based in part on observations that individuals with sleep apnea are more likely to also suffer from hypertension; hypertension is associated with both cellular and humoral immune dysfunction. Although additional preclinical and clinical studies are needed to characterize more fully the extent and precise nature of cytokine alterations during sleep apnea, reports such as those of Entzian et al. (148) and Vgontzas et al. (123) suggest the tantalizing possibility that somnogenic cytokines may be mediators of excessive daytime sleepiness under these conditions.

Acknowledgments

The author was supported, in part, by National Institutes of Health grants MH-52275, MH-54976, and MH-6873 while writing this chapter.

References

1. Krueger JM, Karnovsky ML. Sleep as a neuroimmune phenomenon: a brief historical perspective. Advan Neuroimmunol 1995; 5:5–12.
2. Rothwell NJ, Dantzer RD. Interleukin-1 in the Brain. Oxford: Pergamon Press, 1992.
3. Ransohoff RM, Benveniste EN. Cytokines and the CNS. Boca Raton, FL: CRC Press, 1996.
4. Dinarello CA, Ikejima T, Warner SJC, Orencole SF, Lonnemann G, Cannon JG, et al. Interleukin 1 induces interleukin 1 I. Induction of circulating interleukin 1 in rabbits in vivo and in human mononuclear cells in vitro. J Immunol 1987; 139:1902–1910.
5. Dinarello CA. Biologic basis for interleukin-1 in disease. Blood 1996; 87:2095–2147.
6. Kapás L, Obál F, Jr., Krueger JM. Humoral regulation of sleep. Int Rev Neurobiol 1993; 35:131–160.
7. Obál F, Jr., Payne L, Opp MR, Kapás L, Alföldi P, Krueger JM. Hypothalamic releasing hormones in sleep regulation. In: Smirne S, Franceschi M, Ferini-Strambi L, Zucconi M, eds. Sleep, Hormones and Immunological System. Milano: Masson, 1991: 91–98.
8. Opp MR, Obál F, Krueger JM. Interleukin-1 alters rat sleep: temporal and dose-related effects. Am J Physiol 1991; 260:R52–R58.
9. Krueger JM, Dinarello CA, Chedid L. Promotion of slow-wave sleep (SWS) by a purified interleukin-1 (IL-1) preparation. Fed Proc 1983; 42:356.
10. Krueger JM, Walter J, Dinarello CA, Wolff SM, Chedid L. Sleep-promoting effects of endogenous pyrogen (interleukin-1). Am J Physiol 1984; 246:R994–R999.
11. Tobler I, Borbély AA, Schwyzer M, Fontana A. Interleukin-1 derived from astrocytes enhances slow wave activity in sleep EEG of the rat. Eur J Pharmacol 1984; 104:191–192.
12. Krueger JM, Toth LA, Obál F, Jr., Opp MR, Kimura-Takeuchi M, Kapás L. Infections, cytokines and sleep. In: Smirne S, Franceschi M, Ferini-Strambi L, Zucconi M, eds. Sleep, Hormones and Immunological System. Milano: Masson, 1991:59–70.

13. Krueger JM, Toth LA, Floyd R, Fang J, Kapás L, Bredow S, et al. Sleep, microbes and cytokines. Neuroimmunomodulation 1994; 1(2):100–109.
14. Krueger JM, Toth LA. Cytokines as regulators of sleep. Ann NY Acad Sci 1994; 739: 299–310.
15. Krueger JM, Majde JA. Cytokines and sleep. Int Arch Allergy Immunol 1995; 106: 97–100.
16. Opp MR, Kapás L, Toth LA. Cytokine involvement in the regulation of sleep. P S E B M 1992; 201:16–27.
17. Dinarello CA. Biology of interleukin-1. FASEB J 1988; 2:108–115.
18. Dinarello CA. Interleukin-1 and interleukin-1 antagonism. Blood 1991; 77:1627–1652.
19. Obál F, Jr., Opp MR, Cady AB, Postlethwaite AE, Poppleton H, Seyer JM, et al. Interleukin 1α and an interleukin 1β fragment are somnogenic. Am J Physiol 1990; 259:R439–R446.
20. Krueger JM, Pappenheimer JR, Karnovsky ML. The composition of sleep-promoting factor isolated from human urine. J Biol Chem 1982; 257:1664–1669.
21. Fontana A, Kristensen F, Dubs R, Gemsa D, Weber E. Production of prostaglandin E and an interleukin-1 like factor by cultured astrocytes and C_6 glioma cells. J Immunol 1982; 129:2413–2419.
22. Walter J, Davenne D, Shoham S, Dinarello CA, Krueger JM. Brain temperature changes coupled to sleep states persist during interleukin 1-enhanced sleep. Am J Physiol 1986; 250:R96–R103.
23. Shoham S, Davenne D, Cady AB, Dinarello CA, Krueger JM. Recombinant tumor necrosis factor and interleukin 1 enhance slow-wave sleep. Am J Physiol 1987; 253: R142–R149.
24. Opp MR, Obál F, Jr., Krueger JM. Effects of α-MSH on sleep, behavior, and brain temperature: interactions with IL-1. Am J Physiol 1988; 255:R914–R922.
25. Opp MR, Obál F, Jr., Krueger JM. Corticotropin-releasing factor attenuates interleukin-1 induced sleep and fever in rabbits. Am J Physiol 1989; 257:R528–R535.
26. Walter JS, Meyers P, Krueger JM. Microinjection of interleukin-1 into brain: separation of sleep and fever responses. Physiol Behav 1989; 45:169–176.
27. Opp MR, Krueger JM. Interleukin 1-receptor antagonist blocks interleukin 1-induced sleep and fever. Am J Physiol 1991; 260:R453–R457.
28. Imeri L, Opp MR, Krueger JM. An IL-1 receptor and an IL-1 receptor antagonist attenuate muramyl dipeptide- and IL-1-induced sleep and fever. Am J Physiol 1993; 265:R907–R913.
29. Kapás L, Payne L, Obál F, Jr., Opp MR, Johannsen L, Krueger JM. Sleep in diabetic rats: effects of interleukin 1. Am J Physiol 1991; 260:R995–R999.
30. Opp MR, Obál F, Jr., Payne L, Krueger JM. Responsiveness of rats to interleukin-1: effects of monosodium glutamate treatment of neonates. Physiol Behav 1990; 48:451–457.
31. Obal F, Jr., Fang J, Payne LC, Krueger JM. Growth-hormone-releasing hormone mediates the sleep-promoting activity of interleukin-1 in rats. Neuroendocrinology 1995; 61:559–565.
32. Lancel M, Mathias S, Faulhaber J, Schiffelholz T. Effect of interleukin-1β on EEG power density during sleep depends on circadian phase. Am J Physiol 1996; 270: R830–R837.

33. Gemma C, Imeri L, De Simoni MG, Mancia M. Interleukin-1 induces changes in sleep, brain temperature, and serotonergic metabolism. Am J Physiol 1997; 272:R601–R606.
34. Hansen MK, Krueger JM. Subdiaphragmatic vagotomy blocks the sleep- and fever-promoting effects of interleukin-1β. Am J Physiol 1997; 273:R1246–R1253.
35. Opp MR, Toth LA, Tolley EA. EEG delta power and auditory arousal in rested and sleep-deprived rabbits. Am J Physiol 1997; 41(2):R648–R655.
36. Fang J, Wang Y, Krueger JM. The TNF 55-KD receptor and the IL1 type I receptor are involved in physiological sleep regulation (abstr). Sleep Res. 1997; 26:73.
37. Susic V, Totic S. ''Recovery'' function of sleep: effects of purified human interleukin-1 on sleep and febrile response of cats. Metab Brain Dis 1989; 4(1):73–80.
38. Friedman EM, Boinski S, Coe CL. Interleukin-1 induces sleep-like behavior and alters call structure in juvenile rhesus macaques. Am J Primatol 1995; 35:143–153.
39. Friedman EM, Reyes TM, Coe CL. Context-dependent behavioral effects of interleukin-1 in the rhesus monkey (*Macaca mulatta*). Psychoneuroendocrinology 1996; 21(5): 455–468.
40. Lumpkin MD. The regulation of ACTH secretion by IL-1. Science 1987; 238:452–238.
41. Turnbull AV, Vaughan J, Rivier JE, Vale WW, Rivier C. Urocortin is not a significant regulator of intermittent electrofootshock-induced adrenocorticotropin secretion in the intact male rat. Endocrinology 1999; 140:71–78.
42. Opp MR, Postlethwaite AE, Seyer JM, Krueger JM. Interleukin 1 receptor antagonist blocks somnogenic and pyrogenic responses to an interleukin 1 fragment. Proc Natl Acad Sci USA 1992; 89:3726–3730.
43. Takahashi S, Kapás L, Fang J, Seyer JM, Wang Y, Krueger JM. An interleukin-1 receptor fragment inhibits spontaneous sleep and muramyl dipeptide-induced sleep in rabbits. Am J Physiol 1996; 271:R101–R108.
44. Imeri L, De Simoni MG. Immunological alterations in neurotransmission. In: Lydic R, Baghdoyan HA, eds. Handbook of Behavioral State Control: Cellular and Molecular Mechanisms. Boca Raton, FL: CRC Press, 1999:659–674.
45. Payne LC, Obál F, Jr., Krueger JM. Hypothalamic releasing hormones mediating the effects of interleukin-1 on sleep. J Cell Biochem 1993; 53:309–313.
46. Opp MR, Krueger JM. Anti-interleukin-1β reduces sleep and sleep rebound after sleep deprivation in rats. Am J Physiol 1994; 266:R688–R695.
47. Opp MR, Krueger JM. Interleukin-1 is involved in responses to sleep deprivation in the rabbit. Brain Res 1994; 639:57–65.
48. Takahashi S, Fang J, Kapás L, Wang Y, Krueger JM. Inhibition of brain interleukin-1 attenuates sleep rebound after sleep deprivation in rabbits. Am J Physiol 1997; 273: R677–R682.
49. Borbély AA, Tobler I, Hanagasioglu M. Effect of sleep deprivation on sleep and EEG power spectra in the rat. Behav Brain Res 1984; 14:171–182.
50. Tobler I, Franken P, Scherschlicht R. Sleep and EEG spectra in the rabbit under baseline conditions and following sleep deprivation. Physiol Behav 1990; 48:121–129.
51. Tobler I, Scherschlicht R. Sleep and EEG slow-wave activity in the domestic cat: effect of sleep deprivation. Behav Brain Res 1990; 37:109–118.
52. Moldofsky H, Luc FA, Eisen J, Keystone E, Gorczynski RM. The relationship of interleukin-1 and immune functions to sleep in humans. Psychosom Med 1986; 48(5): 309–318.

53. Moldofsky H, Lue FA, Davidson JR, Gorczynski R. Effects of sleep deprivation on human immune functions. FASEB J 1989; 3:1972–1977.
54. Mackiewicz M, Sollars PJ, Ogilvie MD, Pack AI. Modulation of IL-1β gene expression in the rat CNS during sleep deprivation. NeuroReport 1996; 7:529–533.
55. Ban E, Marquette C, Sarrieau A, Fitzpatrick F, Fillion G, Milon G et al. Regulation of interleukin-1 receptor expression in mouse brain and pituitary by lipopolysaccharide and glucocorticoids. Neuroendocrinology 1993; 58:581–587.
56. Cunningham ET, Jr., DeSouza EB. Interleukin 1 receptors in the brain and endocrine tissues. Immunol Today 1993; 14(4):171–176.
57. Takao T, Tracey DE, Mitchell WM, De Souza EB. Interleukin-1 receptors in mouse brain: characterization and neuronal localization. Endocrinology 1990; 127(6):3070–3078.
58. Breder CD, Dinarello CA, Saper CB. Interleukin-1 immunoreactive innervation of the human hypothalamus. Science 1988; 240:321–324.
59. Van Dam A-M, Brouns M, Louisse S, Berkenbosch F. Appearance of interleukin-1 in macrophages and in ramified microglia in the brain of endotoxin-treated rats: a pathway for the induction of non-specific symptoms of sickness? Brain Res 1992; 588: 291–296.
60. Schöbitz B, De Kloet ER, Holsboer F. Gene expression and function of interleukin 1, interleukin 6 and tumor necrosis factor in the brain. Prog Neurobiol 1994; 44:397–432.
61. Taishi P, Bredow S, Guha-Thakurta N, Obál F, Jr., Krueger JM. Diurnal variations of interleukin-1β mRNA and β-actin mRNA in rat brain. J Neuroimmunol 1997; 75: 69–74.
62. Gudewill S, Pollmächer T, Vedder H, Schreiber W, Fassbender K, Holsboer F. Nocturnal plasma levels of cytokines in healthy men. Eur Arch Psychiat Clin Neurosci 1992; 242:53–56.
63. Lue FA, Bail M, Gorczynski R, Moldofsky H. Sleep and interleukin-1-like activity in cat cerebrospinal fluid (abstr). Sleep Res 1987; 16:51.
64. Hohagen F, Timmer J, Weyerbrock A, Fritsch-Montero R, Ganter U, Krieger S et al. Cytokine production during sleep and wakefulness and its relationship to cortisol in healthy humans. Neuropsychobiology 1993; 28:9–16.
65. Kapás L, Krueger JM. Tumor necrosis factor-beta induces sleep, fever, and anorexia. Am J Physiol 1992; 263(3 pt 2):R703–R707.
66. Vilcek J, Lee TH. Tumor necrosis factor. J Biol Chem 1991; 266:7313–7316.
67. Breder CD, Tsujimoto M, Terano Y, Scott DW, Saper CB. Distribution and characterization of tumor necrosis factor-α-like immuno-reactivity in the murine central nervous system. J Comp Neurol 1993; 337:543–567.
68. Hunt JS, Chen H-L, Hu X-L, Chen T-Y, Morrison DC. Tumor necrosis factor-α gene expression in the tissues of normal mice. Cytokine 1992; 4:340–346.
69. Puccioni-Sohler M, Rieckmann P, Kitze B, Lange P, Albrecht M, Flegenhauer K. A soluble form of tumor necrosis factor receptor in cerebrospinal fluid and serum of HTLV-1-associated myelopathy and other neurological diseases. Neurology 1995; 242:239–242.
70. Hohmann H-P, Brockhaus M, Bauerle PA, Remy R, Kolbeck R, van Loon APGM. Expression of the type A and B tumor necrosis factor (TNF) receptor is independently regulated, and both receptors mediate activation of the transcription factor NF-κB. J Biol Chem 1990; 265:22409–22417.

71. Schall TJ, Lewis M, Koller KJ, Lee A, Rice GC, Wong GHW, et al. Molecular cloning and expression of a receptor for human tumor necrosis factor. Cell 1990; 61:361–370.
72. Schutze S, Machleidt T, Krönke M. The role of diacylglycerol and ceramide in tumor necrosis factor and interleukin-1 signal transduction. J Leukocyte Biol 1994; 56:533–541.
73. Dinarello CA, Cannon JG, Wolff SM, Bernheim HA, Beutler B, Cerami A, et al. Tumor necrosis factor (cachectin) is an endogenous pyrogen and induces production of interleukin 1. J Exp Med 1986; 163:1433–1450.
74. Philip R, Epstein LB. Tumor necrosis factor as immunomodulator and mediator of monocyte cytotoxicity induced by itself, gamma-interferon and interleukin-1. Nature 1986; 323:86–89.
75. Takahashi S, Kapás L, Fang J, Seyer JM, Krueger JM. Somnogenic relationships between interleukin-1 and tumor necrosis factor (abstr). Sleep Res 1996; 25:31.
76. Darko DF, Miller JC, Gallen C, White J, Koziol J, Brown SJ, et al. Sleep electroencephalogram delta-frequency amplitude, night plasma levels of tumor necrosis factor α, and human immunodeficiency virus infection. Proc Natl Acad Sci USA 1995; 92: 12080–12084.
77. Bredow S, Taishi P, Guha-Thakurta N, Obál F, Jr., Krueger JM. Diurnal variations of tumor necrosis factor-α mRNA and α-tubulin mRNA in rat brain. Neuroimmunomodulation 1997; 4:84–90.
78. Floyd RA, Krueger JM. Diurnal variation of TNFα in the rat brain. NeuroReport 1997; 8:915–918.
79. Fang J, Wang Y, Krueger JM. Mice lacking the TNF 55 kDa receptor fail to sleep more after TNFα treatment. J Neurosci 1997; 17:5949–5955.
80. DE Sarro GB, Nistico G. Comparative behavioural, pyrogenic and electrocortical effects of tumor necrosis factor-alpha and interleukin 1 beta in rat. Pharmacol Res 1992; 26 (suppl 2):66–67.
81. Takahashi S, Kapás L, Fang J, Krueger JM. An anti-tumor necrosis factor antibody suppresses sleep in rats and rabbits. Brain Res 1995; 690:241–244.
82. Takahashi LK, Kim H. Relative contributions of pituitary-adrenal hormones to the ontogeny of behavioral inhibition in the rat. Physiol Behav 1995; 57:711–716.
83. Takahashi S, Kapás L, Seyer JM, Wang Y, Krueger JM. Inhibition of tumor necrosis factor attenuates physiological sleep in rabbits. NeuroReport 1996; 7:642–646.
84. Obál F, Jr. Thermoregulation and sleep. Exp Brain Res 1984; (suppl 8):157–172.
85. Obál F, Jr., Rubicsek G, Alföldi P, Sáry G, Obál F. Changes in the brain and core body temperatures in relation to the various arousal states in rats in the light and dark periods of the day. Pflügers Arch 1985; 404:73–79.
86. Parmeggiani PL, Rabini C. Sleep and environmental temperature. Arch Ital Biol 1970; 108:369–387.
87. Parmeggiani PL. Interaction between sleep and thermoregulation. Waking Sleeping 1977; 1:123–132.
88. Krueger JM, Takahashi S. Thermoregulation and sleep: closely linked but separable. In: Blatteis CM, ed. Thermoregulation: Proceedings of the 10th International Symposium on the Pharmacology of Thermoregulation. New York: New York Academy of Sciences, 1997:281–286.
89. Obál FJr, Alföldi P, Rubicsek G. Promotion of sleep by heat in young rats. Pflügers Arch 1995; 430:729–738.

90. Takahashi S, Krueger JM. Inhibition of tumor necrosis factor prevents warming-induced sleep responses in rabbits. Am J Physiol 1997; 272:R1325–R1329.
91. Kapás L, Hong L, Cady AB, Opp MR, Postlethwaite AE, Seyer JM, et al. Somnogenic, pyrogenic, and anorectic activities of tumor necrosis factor-α and TNF-α fragments. Am J Physiol 1992; 263:R708–R715.
92. Palmblad J, Pertrini B, Wasserman J, Kerstedt TA. Lymphocyte and granulocyte reactions during sleep deprivation. Psychosom Med 1976; 41:273–278.
93. Birmanns B, Sapier D, Abramsky O. α-Interferon modifies cortical EEG activity: dose-dependence and antagonism by naloxone. J Neurol Sci 1990; 100:22–26.
94. Dafny N. Interferon modifies EEG and EEG-like activity recorded from sensory, motor, and limbic system structures in freely behaving rats. Neurotoxicology 1983; 4: 235–240.
95. De Sarro GB, Masuda Y, Ascioti C, Audino MG, Nistico G. Behavioral and ECoG spectrum changes induced by intracerebral infusion of interferons and interleukin 2 in rats are antagonized by naloxone. Neuropharmacology 1990; 29(2):167–179.
96. Kimura M, Majde JA, Toth LA, Opp MR, Krueger JM. Somnogenic effects of rabbit and recombinant human interferons in rabbits. Am J Physiol 1994; 267:R53–R61.
97. Krueger JM, Dinarello CA, Shoham S, Davenne D, Walter J, Kubillus S. Interferon alpha-2 enhances slow-wave sleep in rabbits. Int J Immunopharmacol 1987; 9(1):23–30.
98. Reite M, Laudenslager M, Jones J, Crnic L, Kaemingk K. Interferon decreases REM latency. Biol Psychiatry 1987; 22:104–107.
99. Smedley H, Katrak M, Sikora K, Wheeler T. Neurological effects of recombinant human interferon. Br J Med 1983; 286:262–264.
100. Janicki PK. Binding of human alpha-interferon in the brain tissue membranes of rat. Res Comm Chem Patholo Pharmacol 1992; 75:117–120.
101. De Maeyer-Guignard E, De Maeyer JC. Interferons and Other Regulatory Cytokines. New York: John Wiley & Sons, 1988.
102. Krueger JM, Majde JA. Sleep as a host defense: its regulation by microbial products and cytokines. Clin Immunol Immunopathol 1990; 57:188–199.
103. Toth LA. Sleep, sleep deprivation and infectious disease: studies in animals. Advan Neuroimmunol 1995; 5(1):79–92.
104. Toth LA. Microbial modulation of sleep. In: Lydic R, Baghdoyan HA, eds. Handbook of Behavioral State Control: Cellular and Molecular Mechanisms. Boca Raton, FL: CRC Press, 1999:641–657.
105. Toth LA, Rehg JE, Webster RG. Strain differences in sleep and other pathophysiological sequelae of influenza virus infection in naive and immunized mice. J Neuroimmunol 1995; 58:89–99.
106. Fang J, Sanborn CK, Renegar KB, Majde JA, Krueger JM. Influenza viral infections enhance sleep in mice. P S E B M 1995; 210:242–252.
107. Toth LA. Strain differences in the somnogenic effects of interferon inducers in mice. J Interferon Cytokine Res 1996; 16:1065–1072.
108. Kimura-Takeuchi M, Majde JA, Toth LA, Krueger JM. The role of double-stranded RNA in induction of the acute phase response in an abortive influenza virus infection model. J Infect Dis 1992; 166:1266–1275.
109. Buchwald D, Sullivan JL, Komaroff AL. Frequency of ‘‘chronic active epstein-barr virus infection’’ in a general medical practice. JAMA 1987; 257:2303–2307.

110. Nelson KE, Greenberg MA, Mufson MA, Moses VK. The sudden infant death syndrome and epidemic viral disease. Am J Epidemiol 1975; 101(5):423–430.
111. Krueger JM, Obál F, Opp MR, Toth L, Johannsen L, Cady AB. Somnogenic cytokines and models concerning their effects on sleep. Yale J Biol Med 1990; 63:157–172.
112. Krueger JM, Fang J. Cytokines and sleep regulation. In: Lydic R, Baghdoyan HA, eds. Handbook of Behavioral State Control: Cellular and Molecular Mechanisms. Boca Raton, FL: CRC Press, 1999:609–622.
113. Borbély AA. ''Sleep substances'': criteria and physiological basis. In: Inoué S, Krueger JM, eds. Endogenous Sleep Factors. The Hague: SPB Academic Publishing, 1990:31–38.
114. Nisticó G, de Sarro G. Locus ceruleus: site of soporific effects of interleukin-2 in rats. Prog Neuroendocrinimmunol 1990; 3(1):43–48.
115. Opp MR, Krueger JM. Somnogenic actions of interleukin-2: real or artifact. Sleep Res 1994; 23:26.
116. Petitto JM, Huang Z. Molecular cloning of a partial cDNA of the interleukin-2 receptor-beta in normal mouse brain: in situ localization in the hippocampus and expression by neuroblastoma cells. Brain Res 1994; 650:140–145.
117. Uthgenannt D, Schoolmann D, Peitrowsky R, Fehm H-L, Born J. Effects of sleep on production of cytokines in humans. Psychosom Med 1995; 57:97–104.
118. Helle M, Brakenhoff J, De Groot E, Aarden L. Interleukin 6 is involved in interleukin 1-induced activities. Eur J Immunol 1988; 18:957–959.
119. Lotz M, Jirik F, Kabouridis P, Tsoukas C, Kirano T, Kishimoto T, et al. B cell stimulating factor 2/interleukin 6 is a costimulant for human thymocytes and T lymphocytes. J Exp Med 1988; 167:1253–1258.
120. Opp MR, Obál F, Jr., Cady AB, Johannsen L, Krueger JM. Interleukin-6 is pyrogenic but not somnogenic. Physiol Behav 1989; 45:1069–1072.
121. Opp MR, Krueger JM. IL-6: a pyrogenic cytokine that is not somnogenic. In: Dinarello CA, Kluger MJ, Powanda MC, Oppenheim JJ, eds. The Physiological and Pathological Effects of Cytokines. New York: John Wiley & Sons, Inc., 1990:319–324.
122. Bauer J, Hohagen F, Ebert T, Timmer J, Ganter U, Krieger S, et al. Interleukin-6 serum levels in healthy persons correspond to the sleep-wake cycle. Clin Invest 1994; 72: 315.
123. Vgontzas AN, Bixler EO, Papanicolaou DA, Kales A, Stratakis CA, Vela-Bueno A, et al. Rapid eye movement sleep correlates with the overall activities of the hypothalamic-pituitary-adrenal axis and sympathetic system in healthy humans. J Clin Endocrinol Metab 1997; 82:3278–3280.
124. De Simoni MG, Sironi M, De Luigi A, Manfridi A, Mantovani A, Ghezzi P. Intracerebroventricular injection of interleukin 1 induces high circulating levels of interleukin 6. J Exp Med 1990; 171:1773–1778.
125. De Simoni MG, De Luigi A, Gemma L, Sironi M, Manfridi A, Ghezzi P. Modulation of systemic interleukin-6 induction by central interleukin-1. Am J Physiol 1993; 265: R739–R742.
126. Fiorentino DF, Bond MW, Mosmann TR. Two types of mouse T helper cell IV. Th2 clones secrete a factor that inhibits cytokine production by Th1 clones. J Exp Med 1989; 170:2081–2095.
127. Fiorentino DF, Zlotnik A, Mosmann TR, Howard M, O'Garra A. IL-10 inhibits cytokine production by activated macrophages. J Immunol 1991; 147(11):3815–3822.

128. Opp MR, Smith EM, Hughes TK, Jr. IL-10 (cytokine synthesis inhibitory factor) acts in the central nervous system of rats to reduce sleep. J Neuroimmunol 1995; 60:165–168.
129. Cenci E, Romani L, Mencacci A, Spaccapelo R, Schiaffella E, Puccetti P, et al. Interleukin-4 and interleukin-10 inhibit nitric oxide-dependent macrophage killing of Candida albicans. Eur J Immunol 1993; 23(5):1034–1038.
130. Essner R, Rhoades K, McBride WH, Morton DL, Economou JS. IL-4 down-regulates IL-1 and TNF gene expression in human monocytes. J Immunol 1989; 142(11):3857–3861.
131. Fenton MJ, Buras JA, Donnelly RP. IL-4 reciprocally regulates IL-1 and IL-1 receptor antagonist expression in human monocytes. J Immunol 1992; 149(4):1283–1288.
132. Powrie F, Coffman RL. Inhibition of cell-mediated immunity by IL-4 and IL-10. Res Immunol 1993; 144(8):639–643.
133. Kushikata T, Fang J, Wang Y, Krueger JM. Interleukin-4 inhibits spontaneous sleep in rabbits. Am J Physiol 1998; 275:R1185–R1191.
134. Rady PL, Smith EM, Cadet P, Opp MR, Tyring SK, Hughes TK, Jr. Presence of interleukin-10 transcripts in human pituitary and hypothalamus. Cell Mol Neurobiol 1995; 15(2):289–296.
135. Sheng WS, Hu S, Kravitz FH, Peterson PK, Chao CC. Tumor necrosis factor alpha upregulates human microglial cell production of interleukin-10 in vitro. Clin Diagnostic Lab Immunol 1995; 2:604–608.
136. Callard R, Gearing A. The Cytokine FactsBook. San Diego: Academic Press, 1994.
137. Hilaire ZD, Nicolaidis S. Enhancement of slow-wave sleep parallel to the satiating effect of acidic fibroblast growth factor in rats. Brain Res Bull 1992; 29:525–528.
138. Knefati M, Somogyi C, Kapás L, Bourcier T, Krueger JM. Acidic fibroblast growth factor (FGF), but not basic FGF, induces sleep and fever in rabbits. Am J Physiol 1995; 269:R87–R91.
139. Yamuy J, Morales FR, Chase MH. Induction of rapid eye movement sleep by the microinjection of nerve growth factor into the pontine reticular formation of the cat. Neuroscience 1995; 66:9–13.
140. Takahashi N, Krueger J. Nerve growth factor enhances sleep in rabbits. Neurosci Lett 1999; 264(1–3):149–152.
141. Kapás L, Obal F, Jr., Book AA, Schweitzer JB, Wiley RG, Krueger JM. The effects of immunolesions of nerve growth factor-receptive neurons by 192 IgG-saporin on sleep. Brain Res 1996; 712:53–59.
142. Takahashi S, Gala S, Kapás L, Krueger JM. Nerve growth factor enhances sleep in rabbits. Soc Neurosci Abstr 1996; 22:147.
143. Kimura M, McCann SM, Marks GA, Shaffery JP, Kodama T, hang S-Q et al. A novel somnogenic cytokine: Granulocyte-macrophage colony stimulating factor (GM-CSF). Soc Neurosci Abstr 1997; 23:792.
144. Dement WC, Carskadon MA, Richardson G. Excessive daytime sleepiness in the sleep apnea syndrome. In: Dement WC, Guilleminault CG, eds. Sleep Apnea Syndromes. New York: Alan R. Liss, 1978.
145. Shepard JW. Cardiorespiratory changes in obstructive sleep apnea. In: Kryger MH, Roth T, Dement WC, eds. Principles and Practice of Sleep Medicine. Philadelphia: W.B. Saunders Company, 1989:537–551.
146. Kryger MH. Management of obstructive sleep apnea: overview. In: Kryger MH, Roth

T, Dement WC, eds. Principles and Practice of Sleep Medicine. Philadelphia: W.B. Saunders Company, 1989:584–590.
147. Dantzer R. How do cytokines say hello to the brain? Neural versus humoral mediation. Eur Cytokine Net 1994; 5(3):271–273.
148. Entzian P, Linnemann K, Schlaak M, Zabel P. Obstructive sleep apnea syndrome and circadian rhythms of hormones and cytokines. Am J Respirat Crit Care Med 1996; 153:1080–1086.
149. Kryger MH. Controversies in sleep medicine: hypertension [editorial]. Sleep 1997; 20: 789.
150. Stradling J, Davies RJO. Sleep apnea and hypertension—What a mess! Sleep 1997; 20:789–793.
151. Silverberg DS, Oksenberg A. Essential hypertension and abnormal upper airway resistance during sleep. Sleep 1997; 20:794–806.
152. Guilleminault C, Robinson A. Sleep-disordered breathing and hypertension: past lessons, future directions. Sleep 1997; 20:806–811.
153. Norman RA, Jr., Dzielak DJ, Bost KL, Khraibi AA, Galloway PG. Immune system dysfunction contributes to the aetiology of spontaneous hypertension. J Hypertension 1985; 3:261–268.
154. Dzielak DJ. Immune mechanisms in experimental and essential hypertension. Am J Physiol 1991; 260:R459–R467.
155. Dzielak DJ. The immune system and hypertension. Hypertension 1992; 19(suppl 1): 136–144.
156. Fu MLX. Do immune system changes have a role in hypertension? J Hypertension 1995; 13:1259–1265.
157. Lefkos N, Boura P, Boudonas G, Zacharioudaki E, Efthimiadis A, Tsougas M, et al. Immunopathogenic mechanisms in hypertension. Am J Hypertension 1995; 8:1141–1145.
158. Ebringer A, Doyle AE. Raised serum IgG levels in hypertension. Br Med J 1970; 2: 146–148.
159. Okawa-Takatsuji M, Aotsuka S, Uwatoko S, Sumiya M, Yokohari R. Enhanced synthesis of cytokines by peripheral blood monocytes cultured in the presence of autoantibodies against U1-ribonucleoprotein and/or negatively charged molecules: implication in the pathogenesis of pulmonary hypertension in mixed connective tissue disease (MCTD). Clin Exp Immunol 1994; 98:427–433.
160. Gibbons GH. Autocrine-paracrine factors and vascular remodeling in hypertension. Curr Opin Nephrol Hypertension 1993; 2:291–298.
161. Miyata M, Sakuma F, Yoshimura A, Ishikawa H, Nishimaki T, Kasukawa R. Pulmonary hypertension in rats. Int Arch Allergy Immunol 1995; 108:281–286.
162. Dalekos GN, Elisaf MS, Papagalanis N, Tzallas C, Siamopoulos KC. Elevated interleukin-1β in the circulation of patients with essential hypertension before any drug therapy: a pilot study. Eur J Clin Invest 1996; 26:936–939.
163. Dalekos GN, Elisaf M, Bairaktari E, Tsolas O, Siamopoulos KC. Increased serum levels of interleukin-1β in the systemic circulation of patients with essential hypertension: additional risk factor for atherogenesis in hypertensive patients? J Lab Clin Med 1997; 129:300–308.

12

Mechanisms of Hypertension in Obstructive Sleep Apnea

VIREND K. SOMERS

The University of Iowa
Iowa City, Iowa

EUGENE C. FLETCHER

University of Louisville
Louisville, Kentucky

I. Introduction

Approximately 50 million adult Americans have hypertension (1). Obstructive sleep apnea (OSA) afflicts an estimated 15 million American adults (2). There is thus considerable likelihood that both hypertension and sleep apnea will coexist incidentally. However, there is increasing evidence that hypertension and sleep apnea occur as comorbidities to an extent beyond that which would be expected simply from the high prevalence of both these disorders. Recognition of the possible association between sleep apnea and hypertension is evident in the newly released Sixth Report of the Joint National Committee on Prevention, Detection, Evaluation and Treatment of High Blood Pressure (3). Sleep apnea is included as a consideration in those patients with hypertension resistant to conventional therapy.

Attempts to examine the nature of the relationship between blood pressure and sleep apnea are faced with a number of confounding variables, including obesity, antihypertensive therapy, and the difficulty in including adequately matched control subjects. Natural history investigations are limited by ethical concerns regarding randomization of patients with sleep apnea to nontreatment strategies. Thus, of necessity, the majority of the data arise from cross-sectional studies that seek to exclude statistically the influences of potential confounding variables and from studies that follow the effects of treatment of sleep apnea on blood pressure measurements. Studies in humans directed at gaining mechanistic insight into any causal association between sleep apnea and hypertension are limited similarly by factors such as obesity and ongoing sleep apnea therapy. For example, it is important that any control group of seemingly normal obese subjects be evaluated for occult obstructive sleep apnea, since there is a high prevalence of significant sleep apnea even in asymptomatic obese subjects (4). For these reasons, animal models of sleep apnea provide a valuable adjunct to studies of mechanisms linking sleep apnea to increased blood pressure.

This chapter examines the relationship between hypertension and sleep apnea. Potential mechanisms that could explain a causal relationship between these disease states will be explored, drawing from data obtained in studies in both humans and animal models.

II. Evidence Linking Sleep Apnea to Hypertension

The evidence linking OSA to chronic systemic hypertension has been mainly ''guilt by association.'' First, acute elevation of systemic blood pressure (BP) during apnea is a well-described phenomenon. When the apnea is eliminated either by tracheostomy or application of nasal continuous positive airway pressure (CPAP), the acute BP elevation is eliminated. Second, whereas mean systemic BP usually decreases by about 20% during sleep in normal humans, during sleep it remains the same as awake or increases in patients with repetitive nocturnal apnea or in heavy snoring (5–9). This nocturnal rise in sleeping BP or loss of the nocturnal ''dip'' in such individuals is reversed when the snoring and apnea are eliminated (10). Third, there is a high association between the presence of OSA and sustained systemic hypertension. Systemic hypertension occurs in 50% or more of patients with sleep apnea syndrome (11–13). Sustained daytime hypertension has been reversed by effective treatment of apnea, including both tracheostomy (14–16) or nasal CPAP (17–20). Conversely, several studies have shown an approximate 30% incidence of clinically significant sleep apnea in patients with systemic hypertension under treatment (21–24). Fourth, animal studies described below have begun to reproduce chronic BP changes suspected to be caused by OSA.

The finding of OSA in patients with previously diagnosed systemic hypertension is particularly relevant to this discussion since it implies (but remains unproven) that the apnea preceded and caused, or aggravated, the hypertension. The first study to report such a finding examined 16 hypertensive subjects in whom the clinical history suggested sleep apnea and found 11 subjects who had more than 10 apneas per hour (21). Unfortunately, there were no age- or weight-matched controls reported, and the subjects remained on antihypertensive medications during the study. Kales subsequently performed polysomnography on 50 hypertensive and 50 nonhypertensive persons matched for age but not for weight (22). Fifteen, or 30%, of the hypertensive subjects were diagnosed as frank sleep apnea with a mean apnea index of 22.4 events per hour. Fletcher et al. examined the prevalence of sleep apnea in 46 men with essential hypertension and 34 age- and weight-similar normotensive men (23). Three controls and 14 hypertensive men (30%) had sleep apnea defined as greater than 10 apneas per hour of sleep. Williams et al. studied 23 hypertensive subjects and 8 age/weight-matched normotensive controls and found that 35% of the hypertensive subjects had sleep apnea (24). Thus, these data suggest that patients with known hypertension have a greater-than-anticipated prevalence of sleep apnea.

On the other hand, some studies examining hypertensive populations have not demonstrated a higher prevalence of apnea subjects. Hirshkowitz et al. found no difference in apnea index between 38 untreated hypertensive and 53 normotensive males (25). Warley et al. recorded overnight arterial oxygen saturation at home (EEG and respiration not monitored) in 30 men with untreated essential hypertension and compared the data to 30 normotensive age-, height-, and weight-matched controls (26). There were no differences between groups regarding median or lowest saturation or frequency of saturation dips, which were considered to be an estimate of apnea severity.

The resolution of systemic hypertension in treated apnea patients provides circumstantial evidence that apnea caused or contributed to their hypertension. This finding is less clear in patients taken from populations with systemic hypertension who are discovered to have sleep apnea and whose apnea is then treated. In one example, treatment of sleep apnea in eight hypertensive males resulted in a lowering of group mean systolic and diastolic blood pressure from 149/95 to 139/90 mmHg (25). Yet four subjects continued to have a diastolic blood pressure greater than 90 mmHg if taken off of antihypertensive therapy. Other studies have shown improvement of BP in hypertensive patients treated with nasal CPAP. Jennum et al. found that BP dropped substantially in five hypertensive subjects treated for 6 nights (off medication) with nasal CPAP (17). Mayer et al. treated 12 men with sleep apnea and systemic hypertension for 6 months with nasal CPAP and found that mean systolic BP fell from 147 to 126 mmHg while diastolic BP fell from 82 to 69 mmHg ($p < 0.05$) (18). Such findings are not uniform, however. Guilleminault and Suzuki found that in 10 men with sleep apnea treated for 4 weeks (off medication) with effective levels of nasal CPAP, BP did not improve (19). Four individuals did significantly reduce their mean systolic and diastolic blood pressure by 21 and 11 mmHg, respectively. Wilcox et al. examined systemic blood pressure in 19 subjects treated with nasal CPAP for 8 weeks (off medication) and found a reduction in BP in both normotensive and hypertensive subjects (20).

The association between OSA and obesity along with the association between systemic hypertension and obesity make the findings of the above studies difficult to interpret (27–31). Earlier cross-sectional epidemiological data suggest strong associations between central obesity and OSA (30). As a cause of OSA, it is possible that obesity is accompanied by increases in fatty tissue in the pharynx, thereby increasing airway resistance. Obesity could also cause a decrease in functional residual capacity, which can indirectly decrease airway caliber. Obesity itself has been directly implicated as a cause of elevated BP (1,3), reported long before the association between hypertension and OSA was described. In a recent meta-analysis of 194 patients reported with sleep apnea (>10 events/hour), 8% of the variance in diastolic BP was accounted for by body mass index, 4% by age, and 1.7% by apnea index (27). Some larger epidemiological studies that have attempted to control for the presence of obesity continue to suggest a causal association between sleep apnea and systemic hypertension (28–31). A cross-sectional study monitored 147 asymptomatic, working subjects using 24-h ambulatory BP recordings with subjects divided according to the severity of their sleep apnea (28). The results, abstracted in Table 1, show that there is a graduated increase in blood pressure from nonsnorers to snorers with less than 5 apnea-hypopneas per hour to those with more than 5 apneas/h. Another study in 377 consecutive patients referred for a full polysomnographic sleep study with variable prevalences of sleep apnea, obesity, and hypertension showed that age, body mass index, and degree of sleep apnea were all independent predictors of hypertension (29). The relative risk of hypertension associated with age was 4.3, associated with obesity was 2.7, and associated with a diagnosis of sleep apnea was 2.1. Among 1464 consecutive men referred for sleep studies, the degree of sleep apnea was independently related to morning BP, while both obesity and apnea severity were independent risk factors for increased BP (30).

Prospective studies of middle-aged, working populations that address the issue of the relationship between apnea, hypertension, and obesity are now ongoing (32,33). The first in a series of such studies from the Wisconsin Sleep Cohort Study reported a prevalence of sleep-disordered breathing of 9% for women and 24% for men (32). More recent data found an impressive dose-response relationship between sleep-disordered breathing at baseline and the presence of hypertension 4 years later. This association was independent of known confounding factors (33). The odds ratio for hypertension associated with an apnea-hypopnea index above 15 events/h at baseline was 2.9 (95% C.I. of 1.5–5.6).

Table 1 Apnea-Hypopnea Index (apneas plus hypopneas/hour)

	<5 nonsnorers	<5 snorers	>5 apnea
Participants (*n*)	41	53	53
Body mass index (kg/m^2)	25.7	27.6	31.7
Mean apnea-hypopnea index	0.8	1.4	16.6
Waking blood pressure (mmHg)	122/75	124/76	131/80
Sleeping blood pressure (mmHg)	104/62	106/63	113/66

Source: Adapted from Ref. 24.

III. Evidence Linking Sleep Apnea to Cardiovascular Disease

Cardiovascular events, including myocardial infarction and sudden death, follow a circadian variation (34). The peak incidence of these events occurs between 6 a.m. and 12 noon (34). The mechanism underlying this circadian variation is unknown. It is possible that events occurring during sleep may trigger thrombotic or other vascular processes that progress over several hours and manifest only during the subsequent wakefulness hours that follow arousal from sleep. At this time, however, any role for obstructive sleep apnea in the circadian variation of cardiovascular events remains speculative.

What is known is that sleep apnea may be linked to nocturnal cardiac ischemia and nocturnal angina. In a study of 10 consecutive patients with disabling angina and frequent nocturnal angina, Franklin et al. reported that 9 patients were found to have significant sleep apnea (35). Apnea or hypopnea preceded ST depression by about 90 s, even in the absence of any tachycardia. Nocturnal angina and ST depression were attenuated significantly by treatment with CPAP. While Philip and Guilleminault suggest that the frequency of ST depression in patients with sleep apnea may be low, they emphasize the importance of recognition and treatment when this occurs (36). Further support for the concept of sleep apnea precipitating cardiac ischemia in patients with coronary artery disease comes from the work of Koehler and colleagues (37). These investigators studied 30 patients with sleep apnea and noted nocturnal ischemia in 6 patients, 5 of whom had coronary artery disease. Ischemia occurred primarily during rapid eye movement (REM) sleep. In a cohort of patients referred for vascular surgery, Goldman et al. reported the presence of repetitive nocturnal oxygen desaturation and silent myocardial ischemia (38). While Andreas et al. found no evidence of ST depression in sleep apnea patients without clinically evident coronary artery disease on history and exercise testing (39), Hanly and colleagues, in a study of 23 patients with sleep apnea, noted that 7 patients had ST depression during sleep, which was attenuated by CPAP therapy (40). Only 1 of these 7 patients had myocardial ischemia on exercise testing.

Why should sleep apnea patients without ST depression during exercise develop cardiac ischemia during apneic events? This speaks to the combination of stressors induced by apneic episodes, including hypoxemia, increased blood pressure, sympathetic activation, and vasoconstriction. In addition, animal studies suggest that the combination of airway obstruction and arousal elicits increases in coronary vascular resistance of about 24% (41).

There are also firm data implicating sleep apnea in nocturnal arrhythmias. Peripheral chemoreceptor activation by hypoxia, in the absence of lung inflation, elicits the diving reflex. This reflex consists of sympathetic vasoconstriction of peripheral blood vessels (excluding cerebral and coronary circulations) and vagally mediated bradycardia (42,43). The bradycardic response to sleep apnea is blocked by atropine (44,45). Resumption of breathing induces tachycardia, in part due to the vagolytic effects of lung inflation. A pattern of bradycardia alternating with tachycardia is seen frequently as a cyclic variation of the nocturnal EKG in sleep apneic patients (45). This cyclic pattern is mediated primarily by the autonomic nervous system and is attenuated or absent in patients with autonomic neuropathy or Shy-Drager syndrome or in heart transplant recipients.

Vagal activation during apnea may also manifest lower down in the cardiac conduction system, and patients may present with second degree heart block. In a study of 400 sleep apnea patients, Guilleminault et al. noted that almost 50% had cardiac arrhythmias, consisting of nonsustained ventricular tachycardia, sinus arrest, heart block, and premature ventricular contractions (PVCs) (46). All arrhythmias except the PVCs were absent in those patients receiving tracheostomy therapy. It is not clear why some sleep apneics develop bradyarrhythmias and others do not. Factors such as hypoxic chemosensitivity (47) or baroreflex impairment (43) may be involved.

There is also evidence linking sleep apnea to risk factors for cardiovascular disease as well as to more definite cardiovascular endpoints, such as stroke (48,49) and myocardial infarction (50). The ongoing Sleep Heart Health Study is providing important new information in this regard. While this will not be covered in detail for the purposes of this review, epidemiological findings from the Swedish Obese Subjects Study are also of considerable interest. In those subjects reporting loud snoring and observed breathing pauses (suggesting a high likelihood of sleep apnea), there was an increased incidence of chest pain, myocardial infarction, insulin levels, and blood pressure (51).

IV. Circulatory Responses to Sleep

A. Sleep in Normal Subjects

In understanding the responses to sleep in patients with obstructive sleep apnea, it is important to recognize the circulatory responses to sleep in normal subjects. Sleep is classified as non–rapid eye movement (non-REM) and REM sleep. Non-REM sleep occupies the majority of sleep and is itself divided into stages I, II, III, and IV. Stages I and III of non-REM sleep comprise brief, transitional sleep stages. Most non-REM sleep consists of stages II and IV. REM sleep is recognized by rapid eye movements evident on the electrooculogram and loss of postural muscle tone. A number of studies have examined the hemodynamic and autonomic responses to sleep in normal humans (52–54). Non-REM sleep is associated with a progressive reduction in heart rate, blood pressure, and sympathetic nerve traffic as sleep progresses from stages I through to stage IV. This inhibition of the cardiovascular system is most evident during stage IV sleep when heart rate, blood pressure, and sympathetic activity are lowest. By contrast, during REM sleep there is a marked increase in sympathetic activity (about twice the levels seen during wakefulness). Blood pressure and heart rate exhibit intermittent surges. Increases in heart rate and blood pressure are often associated with REM twitches, which are momentary increases in postural muscle tone during REM sleep (54). On average, blood pressure and heart rate during REM are similar to the levels seen during wakefulness. Arousal stimuli occurring during sleep, such as a knock on the door, elicit K complexes on the electroencephalogram, and trigger brief increases in sympathetic activity and consequent rises in blood pressure (54).

These responses to normal sleep provide further insight into the responses to sleep in patients with obstructive sleep apnea. Arousal and increased muscle tone characterize the end of apneic events in patients with sleep apnea. Thus, the sympathetic responses to both arousal and increased muscle tone, acting together with the sympathetic responses to hypoxemia and carbon dioxide retention, would be expected to contribute to increases in blood pressure, evident especially toward the end of apneic events (55).

B. Sleep in Hypertensive Patients

Studies using ambulatory blood pressure–measuring devices have revealed that blood pressure falls as expected during sleep in the majority of patients with hypertension. However, there is a subgroup of hypertensive patients in whom the nocturnal blood pressure decline is attenuated or absent. While there is some controversy as to the reproducibility of the attenuated blood pressure decline during sleep, there is evidence that those hypertensives in whom blood pressure does not decline appreciably during sleep (nondippers) are especially prone to subsequent development of cardiac and vascular events (56). Since blood pressure during sleep in patients with severe sleep apnea may not fall below the levels recorded during wakefulness (55), it has been postulated that those hypertensives classified as nondippers may in fact have undiagnosed obstructive sleep apnea.

In addressing this question, Pankow and colleagues studied 93 patients referred to the sleep laboratory, using noninvasive 24-h blood pressure monitoring (57). They found that the absence of a nocturnal decline in blood pressure was related to apnea severity (Fig. 1). In a corollary to this study, Portaluppi et al. studied 100 newly referred male patients with hypertension (58). Using 24-h blood pressure monitoring with subsequent continuous blood pressure monitoring using the Finapres system, they observed that 11 of the hypertensive patients fell into the nondipper classification (a nighttime blood pressure fall of <10% of the daytime average). They conducted a polysomnographic study of the nondipper hypertensive patients and found that all the nondippers were heavy snorers with 10 of the 11 nondippers having an apnea/hypopnea index greater than 10.

The role of sleep apnea in the nondipper phenomenon, and the associated increased risk in hypertensive patients, is still not fully clarified. Preliminary evidence is, however, very suggestive that sleep-disordered breathing may contribute substantially to the absence of a nocturnal blood pressure decline in hypertensive patients. Whether the increased cardiovascular morbidity that has been linked to the nondipper blood pressure profile is secondary to the higher nocturnal blood pressures, or secondary to the stressors of sleep apnea, or both, remains to be determined.

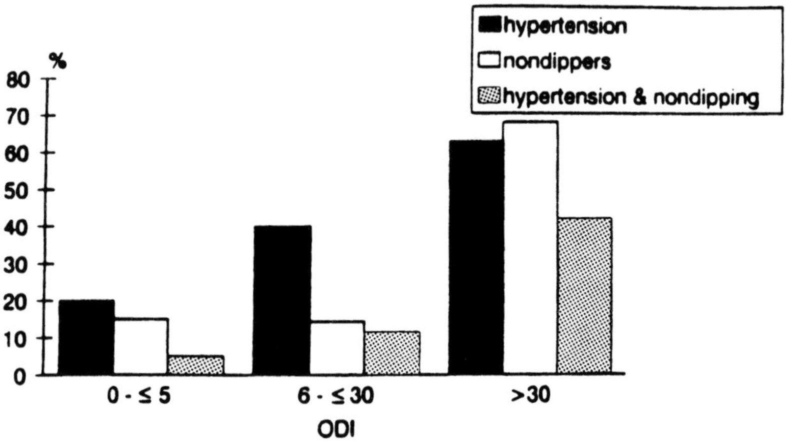

Figure 1 Prevalence (percentage of total number in each group) of hypertension and nondipping in subgroups of 93 patients referred to the sleep laboratory divided according to apnea severity. ODI refers to oxygen desaturation index. Hypertension was defined as a mean daytime blood pressure ≥140/90 mmHg, assessed by noninvasive 24-hour blood pressure measurement. Nondippers were defined as those subjects in whom nighttime blood pressure fell by less than 10% compared to daytime blood pressure. In those patients with severe sleep apnea, the prevalence of both hypertension and the nondipper phenomenon was markedly increased in comparison to patients with mild or minimal sleep apnea. (From Ref. 57.)

V. Generalized Response to Acute Hypoxia and Hypercapnia

Hypoxia with rapid desaturation is the hallmark of acute apnea. Some hypercarbia (usually mild) accompanies this desaturation resulting in variable degrees of asphyxia. Asphyxia is a serious threat to the animal because it jeopardizes organ metabolism and function. Asphyxia stimulates peripheral chemoreceptors resulting in generalized sympathoadrenal-renal discharge to counter the stress of hypoxemia (59,60). Epinephrine is excreted into adrenal venous blood during asphyxia (61). Norepinephrine is produced both by postganglionic neurons of the sympathetic nervous system as well as the adrenal medulla. The peripheral sympathetic nervous system and adrenal medulla act together to preserve homeostasis by increasing cardiac output, modifying blood flow distribution through vasoconstriction and vasodilatation (the latter being dependent upon local reflexes), and altering metabolism to improve oxygen delivery to vital tissues (62–64). The kidney contains both alpha and beta adrenoreceptors, which respond to increased sympathetic activity by increased renin secretion (65). Hypertension in several animal models, including the spontaneously hypertensive rat (SHR), is believed to be related to increased sympathetic nerve activity, perhaps through increased activity of the renin-angiotensin system (60–68).

VI. Acute Circulatory Responses to Obstructive Sleep Apnea

A. Events in the Heart, Coronary Circulation, and Peripheral Vasculature

The effect of asphyxia on the heart and blood vessels has been extensively studied under a variety of settings, including actual and simulated apnea. An excellent explanation of the interaction of chemoreflexes and sympathetic activity in simulated acute apnea in the cat has been recently published by O'Donnell et al. (69). The acute cardiovascular effects of apnea are very similar to those described above for acute hypoxia and include: (1) wide fluctuations in intrathoracic pressure to as low as -90 cmH_2O; (2) gradual fall in blood oxygen and increase in carbon dioxide with stimulation of peripheral chemoreceptors; (3) vagal hypertonia resulting in a fall in heart rate accounted for by hypoxemia, stimulation of baroreceptors, and perhaps apnea; (4) a decrease in left ventricular stroke volume because of decreased left ventricular preload, right ventricular overfilling with septal shift and increased left ventricular afterload; and (5) a surge of sympathetic activity to vascular smooth muscle and perhaps to the adrenal medulla causing vasoconstriction in certain vascular beds (70,71). At termination of the obstructed breathing, release of the bradycardia, normalization of right ventricular preload, and release of left ventricular afterload probably contribute to sudden increases in cardiac output. This, met by constriction of the peripheral vascular bed, results in an acute postapneic increase in blood pressure. These effects appear to be mediated by the sympathetic nervous system, involving the heart, peripheral blood vessels, and probably the kidneys. In humans with severe apnea, urinary catecholamines are elevated and reverse with tracheostomy (72). Both norepinephrine and epinephrine are elevated at night in obstructive sleep apnea, but only epinephrine excretion decreased on a subsequent night with elimination of apneas using nasal CPAP (73). Acute hypoxia simulating apnea has been shown by microneurography to increase postganglionic sympathetic nerve activity as evidenced by an increased muscle sympathetic nerve response (74–76). In humans with borderline hypertension, chemoreflex sensitivity may be increased (77,78). The sympathetic response to chemoreflex activation is especially potentiated in borderline hypertensive humans when apnea and hypoxia are combined (78,79).

Myocardial ischemia is thought to result from a combination of (1) increased left ventricular afterload from the elevated systemic pressure and large negative swings in intrathoracic pressure, (2) sympathoadrenal stimulation, and (3) postapneic tachycardia. All of these may increase myocardial oxygen demand in the face of a diminishing arterial oxygen content due to the episodic hypoxia (80). Furthermore, the α-adrenergic stimulation associated with the sympathetic response could inhibit coronary vasodilatation during apnea (81).

B. Role of Hypoxia and the Chemoreflexes

There is indirect evidence that hypoxia is the main trigger of acute BP elevation during apnea. Shepard found a positive correlation between the level of desaturation and the corresponding elevation of intra-arterial BP in 10 patients with spontaneous apnea (82). Van Den Aardweg and Karemaker examined simulated apneas in normal males with voluntary breathhold under hypoxic conditions (allowing desaturation) and during pretreatment with 100% oxygen (precluding desaturation) (83). Intra-apneic BP rose to abnormal values (>150/95 mmHg) during the hypoxic breathholds but remained stable during hyperoxic apneas, indicating that hypoxia was a necessary component for intra-apneic BP rise. Hedner et al. found a strong correlation between the nadir Sa_{O_2} reached and acute nocturnal BP elevation in 17 apnea subjects studied (84). These authors also found that regardless of resting BP level, OSA patients have an increased pressor response to induced hypoxia, which is not present in nonsnoring, nonapneic controls. Other investigators find a role for arousal and sleep state change in the acute response to apnea. Ringler et al. examined 11 obstructive apnea patients during sleep and found that apneas recorded during oxygen supplementation (eliminating desaturation) were associated with equivalent postapneic mean arterial BP elevations compared to apneas without oxygen supplementation (85). A subsequent study by the same authors had subjects simulate timed obstructive apneas while awake, comparing BP changes during wakefulness to those during sleep apneas of similar duration and negative intrathoracic pressure change (86). Apneas during sleep (accompanied by arousals) produced higher acute BP changes than those produced by apneas while awake (where subjects were already aroused), implying that arousal is an important stimulus to acute elevation of in apnea. Bursts of auditory stimuli during sleep acutely elevate systolic BP up to 20% in normal adults (87).

Chemoreceptors may undergo long-term adaptation in response to hypoxia and hypercarbia and may play a major role in determining baseline BP (88). Abrupt hyperoxia causing deactivation of chemoreceptors will induce a transient fall in arterial BP and sympathetic activity in animals and humans with early hypertension (64,89). Increased ventilatory and sympathetic responsiveness to isocapnic hypoxia has been demonstrated in young subjects with borderline hypertension (77,78). Trzebski and others hypothesize that long-term, repetitive episodic hypoxia during obstructive sleep apnea resets chemoreceptor reflex drive to a higher level, perhaps with elevated sympathetic activity, initiating hypertension (88). Supporting this is the recent finding that hypertensive sleep apnea patients demonstrate an augmented ventilatory response to brief hyperoxic inactivation of chemoreceptors as compared to sleep apnea subjects without hypertension (89). Hypertensive subjects with sleep apnea show an exaggerated BP response to progressive hypoxia not evident in hypertensive subjects without apnea (84). In this study there was also a positive correlation between hypoxic ventilatory response and the pressor response to graded hypoxia. It is thus possible that carotid chemoreceptor output may be reset to a higher level as a result of recurrent episodic asphyxia, causing a chronic increase in sympathetic tone.

In a recent study of otherwise healthy patients with untreated obstructive sleep apnea, a selective potentiation of autonomic, hemodynamic, and ventilatory responses to peripheral chemoreceptor activation by hypoxia was noted (90). Responses to hypercapnia and the cold pressor test were very similar to those seen in closely matched controls in whom sleep apnea was ruled out by polysomnography. Further evidence for an important role of the chemoreflexes is provided by a double-blind controlled study, showing that 100% oxygen, which attenuates tonic peripheral chemoreflex drive, causes significant decreases in heart rate, blood pressure, and sympathetic activity in sleep apnea patients during resting wakefulness (91).

C. Role of the Arterial Baroreflex

Arterial baroreceptors are stretch-activated afferent nerve terminals which lie in the walls of the carotid sinus and aortic arch (92). The baroreceptor afferents are activated by increases in arterial pressure and relay centrally with consequent reductions in sympathetic activity to peripheral blood vessels and to the heart and increased cardiac vagal activity. The resulting vasodilation and bradycardia act to oppose the blood pressure increase. Conversely, baroreflex deactivation, which occurs during reductions in blood pressure, elicits increases in sympathetic activity to peripheral blood vessels and to the heart.

The baroreflexes serve an important role in short-term blood pressure regulation. There is also evidence that baroreflex function is important in long-term maintenance of arterial pressure levels. It is generally accepted that patients with hypertension have impaired baroreflex sensitivity, such that there is an attenuation of sympathetic inhibition and cardiac slowing during increases in blood pressure (93). While it has not been established that the baroreflex impairment contributes to higher blood pressure levels in hypertension, there is evidence that baroreflex impairment may precede the development of hypertension (94).

In considering the baroreflex as a possible mechanism linking sleep apnea and hypertension, it is important to recognize the concept of baroreflex resetting (92). This is a rapidly occurring phenomenon that arises in response to sustained increases or decreases in blood pressure. In brief, when the baroreflexes are exposed to a given pressure level, they seek to maintain blood pressure at that pressure level. Patients with sleep apnea undergo repetitive cyclical oscillations in blood pressure throughout the night. The fluctuations in pressure can be extreme, in the region of 100–150 mmHg. Repetitive exposure of the pressure-sensitive baroreceptor afferents to marked variations in blood pressure over a number of hours of sleep may induce resetting of the baroreflex. Consequently, the baroreflex may function to regulate pressure at a higher level into the following day. In addition, sympathetic activation and catecholamines also act to inhibit baroreflex sensitivity. Patients with sleep apnea have high levels of sympathetic activity as well as higher circulating catecholamine levels. Thus, there is good reason to suppose that patients with sleep apnea have impaired baroreflex sensitivity. Because of baroreflex-mediated restraint on chemoreflex function, impairment of baroreflexes may potentiate chemoreflex function in patients with sleep apnea (95).

Studies investigating baroreflex function in sleep apnea are few and contradictory. This is in large part because of the effects of confounding variables such as age, obesity, and hypertension, each of which is associated with abnormalities in baroreflex function. Ziegler et al. found no difference in baroreflex sensitivity measured at rest in normotensive sleep apneic subjects, in comparison to normal control subjects (96). By contrast, Carlson et al. studied the responses to blood pressure reduction and reported that baroreflex sensitivity was depressed in patients with obstructive sleep apnea (97). However, the patient group in this study had significantly higher blood pressures, were significantly more obese, and were on average 9 years older than the control group. Thus, the difference in baroreflex sensitivity may have been secondary to factors other than obstructive sleep apnea.

Narkiewicz and colleagues compared baroreflex sensitivity in normotensive, otherwise healthy male patients with obstructive sleep apnea to measurements obtained in control subjects closely matched for age and body mass index in whom sleep apnea had been excluded by overnight polysomnography (98). They reported a selective impairment of the sympathetic neural response to baroreceptor deactivation (lowering of blood pressure), but not to baroreceptor activation (raising blood pressure). Thus, the baroreflex abnormality in sleep apnea appears to be limited to the control of sympathetic responses to decreases in blood pressure.

VII. Chronic Circulatory Responses to Obstructive Sleep Apnea

Possible mechanisms for the development of long-term BP elevation in the setting of sleep apnea are: (1) the direct effects of episodic hypoxemia and hypercapnia on chemoreceptors and sympathetic activity; (2) abnormalities in baroreflex function; (3) modification of the cardiovascular system (including fluid balance) in response to marked fluctuations in intrathoracic pressure during obstructed breathing; (4) generalized stress from disruption of sleep; (5) genetic factors; and (6) age. Studies relating these mechanisms to chronic elevated blood pressure are few in number because the evolution of chronic BP elevation in the setting of sleep apnea is very slow and difficult to study. For example, atrial stretch during the repeated Mueller maneuvers of apnea in humans may cause a twofold increase in atrial natriuretic peptide (ANP), which decreases significantly when the apnea is treated with nasal CPAP (99,100). However, increased secretion of ANP with increased urine and sodium excretion (as has been demonstrated in apnea patients) would oppose the development of chronic fluid retention and systemic hypertension (100,101). Plasma renin activity can be extremely difficult to measure accurately in the setting of sleep apnea, but several studies in humans have demonstrated an increase in plasma renin after correction of apnea using nasal CPAP. This would suggest that plasma renin is low during obstructive apnea and not a contributor to elevated BP (102,103). The role of reflex mechanisms such as the chemoreflex and the baroreflex in both acute and chronic responses to sleep apnea have been discussed earlier.

A. Sympathetic Neural Mechanisms

Several animal models of genetic and renal hypertension are believed to have chronically increased sympathetic activity. It is theorized that perhaps an analogous situation in humans exists in response to recurrent obstructive apneas over a period of years. Recurrent activation of the sympathetic nervous system could theoretically lead to a sustained increase in sympathetic activity with either increased vascular tone or some humoral change such as increased catecholamines or renin-angiotensin system activity. Recent studies in humans indeed show that peripheral sympathetic activity may continue after cessation of hypoxia. Morgan et al. administered intermittent asphyxia to five healthy, awake humans over a 20-min period (104). Muscle sympathetic nerve activity climbed throughout the period of asphyxia and remained elevated above control levels for up to 20 min after release of the stimulus. These authors hypothesize that the carotid chemoreceptors are "sensitized" or reset in response to hypoxia. This fits with the theory that long after the nocturnal episodic asphyxia stimulus is terminated, sympathetic activity to the adrenals or peripheral vasculature remains high, promoting diurnal elevation of BP.

Patients with sleep apnea have high levels of sympathetic drive, whether assessed by plasma catecholamines or by direct intraneural recordings using microneurography (Fig. 2). This increased sympathetic activity is apparent even when sleep

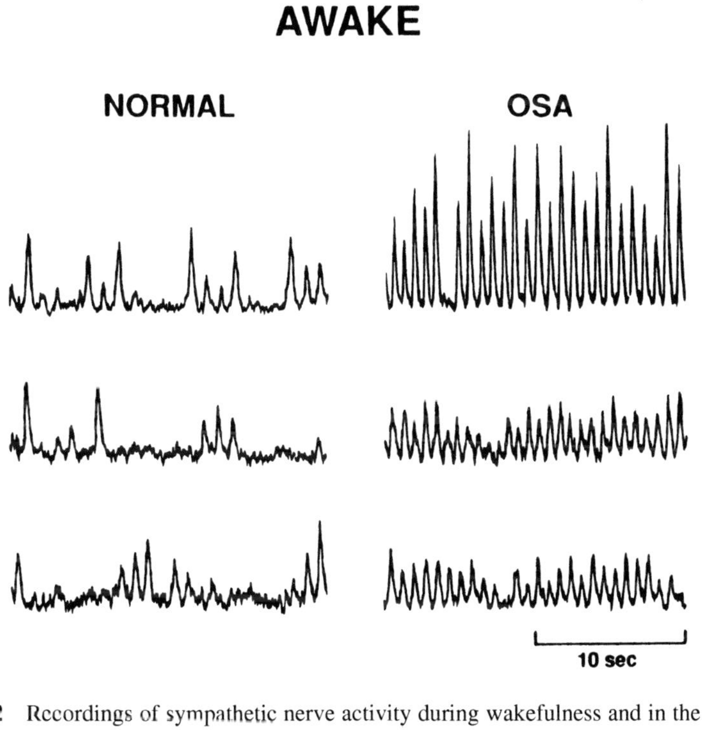

Figure 2 Recordings of sympathetic nerve activity during wakefulness and in the absence of any oxygen desaturation in patients with obstructive sleep apnea (OSA) and age- and gender-matched normal control subjects demonstrating marked elevation of sympathetic burst frequency in patients with sleep apnea. (From Ref. 55.)

apnea patients are awake and breathing normally and in the absence of any oxygen desaturation (55). During sleep, sympathetic activity increases further with consequent increases in nocturnal blood pressure levels (Fig. 3). Acute treatment with CPAP lowers both sympathetic activity and blood pressure during sleep. Hyperoxia lowers blood pressure and sympathetic activity in awake sleep apneic patients, but not in matched control subjects (91). Thus, the sympathetic system is an attractive candidate mechanism to explain higher long-term blood pressure levels in sleep apnea patients. For the reasons stated earlier, definitive proof of this is lacking. In

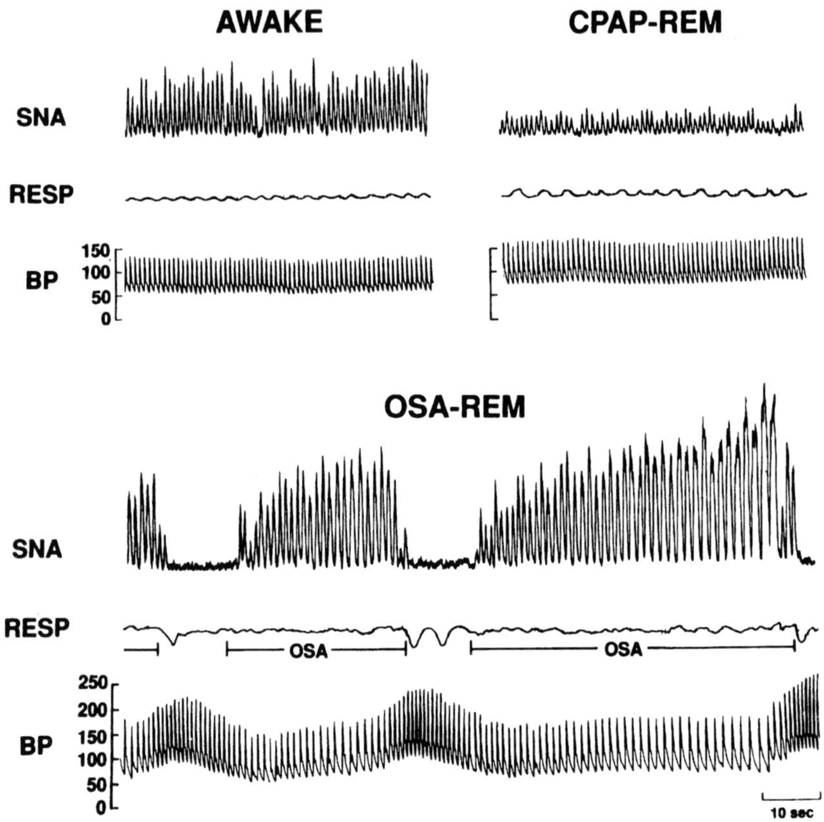

Figure 3 Recordings of sympathetic nerve activity (SNA), respiration (RESP), and intra-arterial blood pressure (BP) in the same subject, when awake (top left), with obstructive sleep apnea during REM sleep (bottom), and with elimination of obstructive sleep apnea by CPAP therapy during REM sleep (top right). SNA is very high during wakefulness, but increases even further secondary to obstructive sleep apnea during REM. BP increases from 130/65 mmHg when awake to 256/110 mmHg at the end of apnea. Elimination of apneas by CPAP results in decreased nerve activity and prevents BP surges during REM sleep. (From Ref. 55.)

an attempt to examine the effects of CPAP therapy on sympathetic activity and blood pressure, Hedner and colleagues found that long-term CPAP was accompanied by reductions in plasma norepinephrine but no reduction in blood pressure (105). Unfortunately, a cohort of untreated sleep apneic patients was not followed.

In a study of normotensive, otherwise healthy patients with sleep apnea, Narkiewicz et al. examined the effects of 1 year of CPAP treatment (106). Measurements of blood pressure, heart rate, and muscle sympathetic nerve activity (MSNA) were obtained at 1 month, 6 months, and 1 year after treatment was started and compared to similar measurements in a cohort of sleep apnea patients who refused treatment. In these normotensive subjects, MSNA decreased after treatment, evident in the measurements obtained at 6 months and 1 year of therapy. However, heart rate and blood pressure were not changed by CPAP. Thus, attenuated sympathetic activation after long-term CPAP therapy is not accompanied by lower blood pressure in normotensive patients. It is possible that blood pressure reduction may be more apparent after treatment of sleep apnea in hypertensive patients.

B. Endothelial Mechanisms

The vascular endothelium and endothelium-related substances may also play a role in increased blood pressure levels in patients with sleep apnea. The studies available are limited and inconclusive. While acetylcholine-induced vasodilation appeared to be impaired in hypertensive sleep apneic patients, a similar impairment was evident in the response to nitroprusside, an endothelium-independent vasodilator (107). The authors of the study suggest that these findings may be a result of incomplete matching of sleep apnea patients and hypertensive controls and/or structural vascular abnormalities. A further important consideration is that the overweight, hypertensive control group did not undergo polysomnographic exclusion of sleep apnea. Thus, the existence and relative importance of endothelium-dependent vasodilator impairment in sleep apnea awaits further clarification.

Endothelin, a potent vasoconstrictor substance released by the endothelium may also be involved. In cell culture, hypoxia results in marked increases in endothelin production (108). Thus, in the intact organism, repetitive hypoxemia from sleep apnea may trigger endothelin production with consequent vasoconstriction and increased blood pressures. Indeed, Phillips et al. have recently demonstrated that plasma endothelin increases strikingly after several hours of untreated obstructive apnea and decreases after several hours of CPAP (109). Changes in endothelin correlated positively with changes in blood pressure. Thus, it is possible that endothelin antagonists may be important in the treatment of resistant hypertension associated with sleep apnea.

C. Abnormalities in Coagulation

A new and potentially exciting area of investigation in the chronic cardiovascular changes of sleep apnea is the change in coagulation that might be induced by chronic episodic hypoxia. Two studies indicate reversible clotting abnormalities that may accompany obstructive sleep apnea. Bokinsky et al. examined spontaneous platelet aggregation and platelet activation in six sleep apnea subjects before and after nasal CPAP (110). Both aggregation and activation were abnormally high on the apnea night and returned to baseline control values after a night of CPAP treatment. In a similar study, Chin et al. examined plasma fibrinogen, hematocrit, and total plasma protein, the latter two parameters used to calculate whole blood viscosity (111). Plasma fibrinogen and whole blood viscosity were elevated following a night of sleep apnea and returned to control levels following the application of nasal CPAP. Cardiovascular events such as stroke, angina, and myocardial infarction may be more common in apnea patients. The implication of these studies is that hypercoagulability is more likely during sleep in patients with episodic hypoxia and cyclic sympathetic nervous system activation. Elimination of this stressful cyclic hypoxia may reduce the risk of vascular occlusion.

VIII. Animal Models of Acute and Chronic Episodic Hypoxia

It may take years before sustained hypertension develops in response to snoring, apnea, and episodic hypoxemia. The development of animal models to simulate the various cardiovascular insults of recurrent apnea may therefore aid in identifying the mechanisms leading to hypertension in apnea patients. The dog (112,113) and rat (114–119) are now being used to study how chronic elevated BP may occur in the setting of repetitive episodic hypoxia and apnea. Brooks et al. have developed a dog model of sleep apnea with repetitive, intermittent occlusion of a tracheostomy using telemetry and real-time EEG sleep staging (113). These authors have shown that intermittent occlusion of the airway daily from 1 to 3 months produces a 15.7 mmHg increase in mean resting awake BP, which reverses after several weeks. Recurrent arousal, although inducing acute BP changes, did not result in sustained elevation of daytime BP.

Small animals can be exposed to rapid swings in ambient oxygen concentration, creating changes in Sa_{O_2} similar to that seen in humans with sleep apnea. In the particular preparation described below, rats are individually housed in cylindrical Plexiglas chambers with snug-fitting lids. Using a timed solenoid valve, 100% nitrogen followed by a compressed air flush can reduce the ambient fractional concentration of oxygen (Fi_{O_2}) to 3–5% for approximately 3–6 s. The cycle is repeated twice per minute during the day for 6–8 hours on consecutive days. Multiple serial arterial blood samples during episodic hypoxia have shown the average nadir level of Sa_{O_2} in this system is 60–80%, well within the range of sleep apnea patients.

Such studies to date in this preparation have demonstrated that recurrent, episodic hypoxia (up to 800 episodes per day) for 35 days can induce increases in mean arterial BP of 10–14 mmHg above baseline in unrestrained rats (114). This increase lasts 1–3 weeks after cessation of episodic hypoxia. It has been demonstrated that such BP elevations are blocked in animals where section of the carotid sinus nerve compromised peripheral chemoreceptor function (115). Furthermore, ablation of the peripheral sympathetic nervous system using intraperitoneal injections of the neurotoxin 6-hydroxy-dopamine also blocks the increase in BP (116). Asphyxia is a stronger stimulus to acute BP elevation compared to hypocapnic hypoxia, but the chronic application of asphyxia to this rat preparation produces no higher daytime elevation of BP than chronic hypocapnic hypoxia (117). It is possible that genetic factors may be involved in the BP response to chronic episodic hypoxia, which could explain why all patients with sleep apnea do not develop systemic hypertension (118).

Finally, recent studies in this model show that bilateral renal artery denervation (ablation of renal sympathetics) eliminates the chronic diurnal BP response, as does bilateral adrenal medullectomy (119). This study suggests that recurrent acute sympathetic nervous system activity works through the kidney to bring about diurnal elevation of BP. The fact that adrenal medullectomy with intact renal nerves also blocked the diurnal BP increase suggests that circulating epinephrine may also be important in regulating BP in the setting of episodic hypoxic stress. There are several possible ways that combined action of adrenal epinephrine and renal artery sympathetics may act together to increase BP chronically. One is that epinephrine enhances presynaptic norepinephrine release and facilitates neurogenic vasoconstriction (120,121). Another is that the renin-angiotensin system may participate in the diurnal BP increase and may be stimulated both by renal artery sympathetics and circulating epinephrine. The most recent study in this rat model shows that the renin-angiotensin system is activated by chronic episodic hypoxia and that the angiotensin-II receptor blocker Losartan prevents the chronic BP response to episodic hypoxia (122).

IX. Summary

Patients with obstructive sleep apnea have high resting awake levels of sympathetic activity. Apneic events increase sympathetic activity and blood pressure further during sleep. Whether repetitive, longstanding sleep apnea is responsible for chronic daytime elevation of blood pressure is not known, although circumstantial evidence is very supportive of this possibility. Definitive evidence linking sleep apnea to the initiation or worsening of hypertension is limited. A plethora of studies of blood pressure, reflex regulation, and vasomotor function in sleep apnea have produced conflicting results. This is in large part due to the absence of carefully controlled studies, where confounding factors such as repeated measurements, blood pressure levels, body mass index, other coexisting disease states, age, and gender have been excluded. Given the high prevalence of undiagnosed sleep apnea in obese individuals, it is also important to exclude OSA in seemingly normal control subjects.

Nevertheless, carefully controlled studies of untreated, otherwise healthy OSA patients are providing new information on mechanisms mediating cardiovascular abnormalities in sleep apnea per se. Recent epidemiological data from the Sleep Heart Health Study (123) and the Wisconsin Sleep Cohort Study (33) are contributing more robust evidence linking sleep apnea to cardiovascular disease generally, and hypertension in particular. Animal models of sleep apnea support the concept that repetitive apnea and oxygen desaturation may be implicated in the genesis of higher blood pressure levels and that elimination of apnea results in blood pressure lowering.

Acknowledgments

The authors would like to acknowledge the assistance of Linda Bang and Kathleen Schroeder, BS. VKS is an Established Investigator of the American Heart Association and is also supported by Grants M01-RR00585, HL 61560, and HL 65176.

References

1. Burt VL, Whelton P, Roccella EJ, et al. Prevalence of hypertension in the US adult population: results from the third National Health and Nutrition Examination Survey, 1988–1991. Hypertension 1995; 25:305–313.
2. National Commission on Sleep Disorders Research. Wake up America: a national sleep alert. Washington, DC: Government Printing Office, 1993.
3. Joint National Committee on Prevention, Detection, Evaluation and Treatment of High Blood Pressure and the National High Blood Pressure Education Program Coordinating Committee. The sixth report of the joint national committee on prevention, detection, evaluation and treatment of high blood pressure. Arch Intern Med 1997; 157:2413–2446.
4. Vgontzas AN, Tan TL, Bixler EO, Martin LF, Shubert D, Kales A. Sleep apnea and sleep disruption in obese patients. Arch Intern Med 1994; 154:1705–1711.
5. Khatri I, Freis E. Hemodynamic changes during sleep. J Appl Physiol 1967; 22:867–873.
6. Littler WA, Honour AJ, Carter RD, Sleight P. Sleep and blood pressure. Br Med J 1975; 3:346.
7. Littler WA. Sleep and blood pressure: further observations. Am Heart J 1979; 97:35–37.
8. Lugaresi E, Coccagna G, Garneti P, Mantovani M, Cirignotta F. Snoring. Electroenceph Clin Neurophysiol 1975; 39:59–64.
9. Lugaresi E, Coccagna G, Cirignotta G, et al. Breathing during sleep in man in normal and pathological conditions. Adv Exp Med Biol 1978; 99:35–45.
10. Mateika JH, Mateika S, Slutsky AS, Hoffstein V. The effect of snoring on mean arterial blood pressure during non-REM sleep. Am Rev Respir Dis 1992; 145:141–146.
11. Guilleminault C, Tilkian A, Dement WC. The sleep apnea syndromes. Ann Rev Med 1976; 27:465–484.
12. Tilkian AG, Guilleminault C, Schroeder JS, Lehrman KL, Simmons FB, Dement WC. Hemodynamics in sleep-induced apnea: studies during wakefulness and sleep. Ann Intern Med 1976; 85:714–719.
13. Kales A, Cadieux RJ, Bixler EO, Soldatos CR, Vela-Bueno A, Misoul CA, Locke TW. Severe obstructive sleep apnea: I. Onset, clinical course, and characteristics. J Chron Dis 1985; 38:419–425.

14. Coccagna C, Mantovani M, Brignani F, et al. Tracheostomy in hypersomnia with periodic breathing. Bull Physiopath Resp 1972; 8:1217–1227.
15. Guilleminault C, Eldridge FL, Simmons FB, Dement WC. Sleep apnea syndrome: can it induce hemodynamic changes? West J Med 1975; 123:7–16.
16. Burack B, Pollack C, Borowiecki B, Weitzman E. The hypersomnia-sleep apnea syndrome: a reversible cardiovascular hazard. Circulation 1977; 56:177.
17. Jennum P, Wildschiodtz G, Christensen NJ, Schwartz T. Blood pressure, catecholamines, and pancreatic polypeptide in obstructive sleep apnea with and without nasal continuous positive airway pressure (nCPAP) treatment. Am J Hyper 1989; 2:847–852.
18. Mayer J, Becker H, Brandenburg U, Penzel T, Peter JH, von Wichert P. Blood pressure and sleep apnea: results of long-term nasal continuous positive airway pressure therapy. Cardiology 1991; 79:84–92.
19. Guilleminault C, Suzuki M. Sleep-related hemodynamics and hypertension with partial or complete upper airway obstruction during sleep. Sleep 1992; 15:S20–S24.
20. Wilcox I, Grunstein RR, Hedner JA, Doyle J, Collins FL, Fletcher PJ, Delly DT, Sullivan CE. Effect of nasal continuous positive airway pressure during sleep on 24-hour blood pressure in obstructive sleep apnea. Sleep 1993; 16:539–544.
21. Lavie P, Ben-Yosef R, Rubin AE. Prevalence of sleep apnea syndrome among patients with essential hypertension. Am J Cardiol 1985; 55:1019–1022.
22. Kales A, Cadieux RJ, Shaw LC, Vela-Bueno A, Bixler EO, Schneck DW, Locke TW, Soldatos CR. Sleep apnoea in a hypertensive population. Lancet 1984; ii:1005–1008.
23. Fletcher EC, DeBehnke RD, Lovoi MS, Gorin AB. Undiagnosed sleep apnea in patients with essential hypertension. Ann Intern Med 1985; 103:190–195.
24. Williams AJ, Houston D, Finberg S, Lam C, Kinney JL, Santiago S. Sleep apnoea syndromes and essential hypertension. Am J Cardiol 1985; 55:1019–1022.
25. Hirshkowitz M, Karacan I, Gurakar A, Williams RL. Hypertension, erectile dysfunction, and occult sleep apnea. Sleep 1989; 12:223–232.
26. Warley ARH, Mitchell AH, Stradling JR. Prevalence of nocturnal hypoxaemia in men with and without hypertension. Q J Med 1988; 68:637–644.
27. Jeong D, Dimsdale JE. Sleep apnea and essential hypertension: a critical review of the epidemiological evidence for co-morbidity. Clin Exp Hyper Theory Pract 1989; A11:1301–1323.
28. Hla KM, Young TB, Bidwell T, Palta M, Skatrud JB, Dempsey, J. Sleep apnea and hypertension; a population based study. Ann Intern Med 1994; 120:382–388.
29. Carlson JT, Hedner JA, Ejnell H, Peterson LE. High prevalence of hypertension in sleep apnea patients independent of obesity. Am J Respir Crit Care Med 1994; 150:72–77.
30. Grunstein R, Wilcox I, Yang TS, Gould Y, Hedner J. Snoring and sleep apnoea in men: association with central obesity and hypertension. Int J Obesity 1993; 17:533–540.
31. Kiselk J, Clark M, Pera V, Rosenberg C, Redline S. The association between hypertension and sleep apnea in obese patients. Chest 1993; 104:775–780.
32. Young T, Palta M, Dempsey J, Skatrud J, Weber S, Badr S. The occurrence of sleep-disordered breathing among middle-aged adults. N Engl J Med 1993; 328:1230–1235.
33. Peppard PE, Young T, Palta M, Skatrud J. Prospective study of the association between sleep-disordered breathing and hypertension. N Engl J Med 2000; 342:1378–1384.

34. Muller JE, Stone PH, Tun ZG, et al. Circadian variation in the frequency of onset of acute myocardial infarction. N Engl J Med 1985; 313:1315–1322.
35. Franklin KA, Nilsson JB, Sahlin C, Naslund U. Sleep apnoea and nocturnal angina. Lancet 1995; 345:1085–1087.
36. Philip P, Guilleminault. Letter to the editor: ST segment abnormality, angina during sleep and obstructive sleep apnea. Sleep 1993; 16:558–559.
37. Koehler U, Dubler H, Glaremin T, Junkermann H, Lubbers C, Ploch T, Peter JH, Pomykaj T, von Wichert P. Nocturnal myocardial ischemia and cardiac arrhythmia in patients with sleep apnea with and without coronary artery disease. Klin Wochenschr 1991; 69:474–482.
38. Goldman MD, Reeder MK, Muir AD, Young JD, Gitlin DA, Casey KR, Smart D, Fry JM. Repetitive nocturnal arterial oxygen desaturation and silent myocardial ischemia in patients presenting for vascular surgery. J Am Geriatr Soc 1993; 41:703–709.
39. Andreas S, Hajak G, Natt P, Auge D, Ruther E, Kreuzer H. ST strecken Veränderungen und Rhythmusstörungen bei obstruktiver Schlafapnoe. Pneumologie 1991; 45:720–724.
40. Hanly P, Sasson Z, Zuberi N, Lunn K. ST-segment depression during sleep in obstructive sleep apnea. Am J Cardiol 1993; 71:1341–1345.
41. Pinto JMB, Garpestad E, Weiss JW, Bergau DM, Kirby DA. Hemodynamic changes associated with obstructive sleep apnea followed by arousal in a porcine model. J Appl Physiol 1993; 75:1439–1443.
42. de Burgh Daly M, Angell-James JE, Elsner R. Role of carotid-body chemoreceptors and their reflex interactions in bradycardia and cardiac arrest. Lancet 1979; 1:764–767.
43. Somers VK, Dyken ME, Mark AL, Abboud FM. Parasympathetic hyperresponsiveness and bradyarrhythmias during apnoea in hypertension. Clin Auton Res 1992; 2:171–176.
44. Zwillich C, Devlin T, White D, Douglas N, Weil J, Martin R. Bradycardia during sleep apnea. J Clin Invest 1982; 69:1286–1292.
45. Guilleminault C, Connolly S, Winkle R, Melvin K, Tilkian A. Cyclical variation of the heart rate in sleep apnoea syndrome: Mechanisms, and usefulness of 24 h electrocardiography as a screening technique. Lancet 1984; 1:126–131.
46. Guilleminault C, Connolly SJ, Winkle RA. Cardiac arrhythmia and conduction disturbances during sleep in 400 patients with sleep apnea syndrome. Am J Cardiol 1983; 52:490–494.
47. Sato F, Nishimura M, Shinano H, Saito H, Miyamoto K, Kawakami Y. Heart rate during obstructive sleep apnea depends on individual hypoxic chemosensitivity of the carotid body. Circulation 1997; 96:274–281.
48. Dyken ME, Somers VK, Yamada T, Ren ZY, Zimmerman MB. Investigating the relationship between stroke and obstructive sleep apnea. Stroke 1996; 27:401–407.
49. Palomaki H, Partinin M, Juvela S, Kaste M. Snoring as a risk factor for sleep-related brain infarction. Stroke 1989; 10:1311–1315.
50. Hung J, Whitford EG, Persons RW, Hillman RW. Association of sleep apnoea with myocardial infarction in man. Lancet 1990; 336:261–264.
51. Grunstein RR, Stenlof K, Hedner J, Sjostrom L. Impact of obstructive sleep apnea and sleepiness on metabolic and cardiovascular risk factors in the Swedish Obese Subjects (SOS) Study. Int J Obes 1995; 19:410–418.

52. Hornyak MM, Cejnar M, Elam M, Malousck M, Wallin BG. Sympathetic muscle nerve activity during sleep in man. Brain 1991; 114:1281–1295.
53. Okada H, Iwase S, Mano T, Sugiyama Y, Watanabe T. Changes in muscle sympathetic nerve activity in sleep curing sleep in humans. Neurology 1991; 41:1961–1988.
54. Somers VK, Dyken ME, Mark AL, Abboud FM. Sympathetic nerve activity during sleep in normal humans. N Engl J Med 1993; 328:303–307.
55. Somers VK, Dyken ME, Clary MP, Abboud FM. Sympathetic neural mechanisms in obstructive sleep apnea. J Clin Invest 1995; 96:1897–1904.
56. Verdecchia P, Schillaci G, Guerrieri M, Getteechi C, Benemio G, Boldrini F, et al. Circadian blood pressure changes and left ventricular hypertrophy in essential hypertension. Circulation 1990; 81:528–536.
57. Pankow W, Nabe B, Lies A, Becker H, Kohler U, Kohl F-V, Lohmann FW. Influence of sleep apnea on 24-hour blood pressure. Chest 1997; 112:1253–1258.
58. Portaluppi F, Provini F, Cortelli P, Plazzi G, Bertozzi N, Manfredini R, Fersini C, Lugaresi E. Undiagnosed sleep-disordered breathing among male nondippers with essential hypertension. J Hypertens 1997; 15:1227–1233.
59. Korner PI, White SW. Circulatory control in hypoxia by the sympathetic nerves and adrenal medulla. J Physiol 1966; 184:272–290.
60. Johnson TS, Young JB, Landsberg L. Sympathoadrenal response to acute and chronic hypoxia in the rat. J Clin Invest 1983; 71:1263–1272.
61. Cannon WB, Hoskins RG. The effects of asphyxia, hypercapnia, and sensory stimulation on adrenal secretion. Am J Physiol 1911; 29:274–279.
62. Liang CS, Gavras H. Renin-angiotensin system inhibition in conscious dogs during acute hypoxemia. J Clin Invest 1980; 62:961–970.
63. Doherty J, Liang C. Arterial hypoxemia in awake dogs. Role of the sympathetic nervous system in mediating the systemic hemodynamic and regional blood flow responses. J Lab Clin Med 1984; 104:665–677.
64. Fukuda Y, Sato A, Suzuki A, Trzebski A. Autonomic and cardiovascular responses to changing blood oxygen and CO_2 levels in the rat. J Auto Nerv Sys 1989; 28:61–74.
65. Heistad DD, Abboud FM. Circulatory adjustments to hypoxia. Circulation 1980; 61: 463–470.
66. Loeffler JR, Stockigt JR, Ganong WF. Effect of alpha and beta adrenergic blocking agents on the increase in renin secretion produced by stimulation of renal nerves. Neuroendocrinology 1972; 10:129–138.
67. Mulvany JJ, Halpern W. Contractile properties of small arterial resistance vessels in spontaneously hypertensive and normotensive rats. Circ Res 1977; 41:19–26.
68. Norman Jr, RA, Dzielak DJ. Role of renal nerves in onset and maintenance of spontaneous hypertension. Am J Physiol 1982; 243:H284–H288.
69. O'Donnell CP, Schwartz AR, Smith PL, Robotham JL, Fitzgerald RS, Shirahata M. Reflex stimulation of renal sympathetic nerve activity ad blood pressure in response to apnea. Am J Respir Crit Care Med 1996; 154:1763–1770.
70. Bonsignore MR, Marrone O, Insalaco G, Bonsignore B. The cardiovascular effects of OSA: analysis of pathogenic mechanisms. Eur Respir J 1994; 7:786–805.
71. Shepard JW, Jr. Hypertension, cardiac arrhythmias, myocardial infarction, and stroke in relation to obstructive sleep apnea. Sleep 1992; 16:S30–S40.
72. Fletcher EC, Miller J, Schaaf JW, Fletcher JG. Urinary catecholamines before and after tracheostomy in OSA and hypertension. Sleep 1987; 10:35–44.

73. Marrone O, Riccobono L, Salvaggio A, Mirabella A, Bonanno A, Bonsignore MR. Catecholamines and blood pressure in obstructive sleep apnea syndrome. Chest 1993; 103:722–727.
74. Blumberg H, Oberle J. Effects of systemic hypoxia and hypercapnia on skin and muscle sympathetic activity in humans (abstr). Pfluger Arch 1985; 403(S):R51.
75. Somers VK, Zavala DC, Mark AL, Abboud FM. Influence of ventilation and hypocapnia on sympathetic nerve responses to hypoxia in normal humans. J Appl Physiol 1989; 67:2095–2100.
76. Somers VK, Zavala DC, Mark AL, Abboud FM. Contrasting effects of hypoxia and hypercapnia on ventilation and sympathetic activity in humans. J Appl Physiol 1989; 67:2101–2108.
77. Trzebski A, Tafil M, Zoltowski M, Przybylski J. Sensitivity of chemoreceptor drive in young men with mild hypertension. Cardiovasc Res 1982; 16:163–172.
78. Somers VK, Mark AL, Abboud FM. Potentiation of sympathetic nerve responses to hypoxia in borderline hypertensive subjects. Hypertension 1988; 11:608–612.
79. Somers VK, Abboud FM. Chemoreflexes—responses, interactions and implications for sleep apnea. Sleep 1993; 16:S30–S34.
80. Chen L, SM Scharf. Systemic and myocardial hemodynamics during periodic obstructive apneas in sedated pigs. J Appl Physiol (in press).
81. Scharf SM, Graver LM, Balaban K. Cardiovascular effects of periodic occlusions of the upper airways in dogs. Am Rev Respir Dis 1992; 146:321–329.
82. Shepard JW Jr. Gas exchange and hemodynamics during sleep. Med Clin North Am 1985; 69:1243–1264.
83. Van Den Aardweg J, Karemaker JM. Repetitive apneas induce periodic hypertension in normal subjects through hypoxia. J Appl Physiol 1992; 72:821–827.
84. Hedner JA, Wilcox I, Laks L, Grunstein RR, Sullivan CE. A specific and potent pressor effect of hypoxia in patients with sleep apnea. Am Rev Respir Dis 1992; 146:1240–1245.
85. Ringler J, Basner RC, Shannon R, Schwartzstein R, Manning H, Weinberger SE, Weiss JW. Hypoxemia alone does not explain blood pressure elevations after obstructive apneas. J Appl Physiol 1990; 69:2143–2148.
86. Garpestad E, Ringler J, Parker JA, Basner RC, Weiss JW. Sleep stage influences the hemodynamic response to obstructive apneas. Am J Respir Crit Care Med 1995; 152: 199–203.
87. Shimizu T, Kogawa S, Tashiro T, et al. Transient elevations of blood pressure in OSA. In: Horne J, ed. Sleep '90. Bochum, Germany: Pontenagel, 1990:182–184.
88. Trzebski A. Arterial chemoreceptor reflex and hypertension. Hypertension 1992; 19: 562–566.
89. Tafil-Klawe M, Thiele AE, Raschcke F, Mayer J, Peter JH, von Wichert W. Peripheral chemoreceptor reflex in obstructive sleep apnea patients: a relationship between ventilatory response to hypoxia and nocturnal bradycardia during apnea events. Pneumonologie 1991; 45:309–312.
90. Narkiewicz K, van de Borne PJH, Pesek CA, Dyken ME, Montano N, Somers VK. Selective potentiation of peripheral chemoreflex sensitivity in obstructive sleep apnea. Circulation 1999; 99:1183–1189.
91. Narkiewicz K, van de Borne PJH, Montano N, Dyken ME, Phillips BG, Somers VK. The contribution of tonic chemoreflex activation to sympathetic activity in blood pressure in patients with obstructive sleep apnea. Circulation 1998; 97:943–945.

92. Chapleau MW, Abboud FM. Mechanisms of adaptation and resetting of the baroreceptor reflex. In: Hainsworth R, Mark AL, eds. Cardiovascular Reflex Control in Health and Disease. London: WB Saunders, 1993:165–193.
93. Mancia G, Ferrari L, Gregorini G, Parati G, Ferrari MC, Pomidossi G, Zanchetti A. Control of blood pressure by carotid sinus baroreceptors in human beings. Am J Cardiol 1979; 44:895–902.
94. Parmer RJ, Cervenka JH, Stone RA. Baroreflex sensitivity and heredity in essential hypertension. Circulation 1992; 85:497–503.
95. Somers VK, Mark AL, Abboud FM. Interaction of baroreceptor and chemoreceptor reflex control of sympathetic nerve activity in normal humans. J Clin Invest 1991; 87: 1953–1957.
96. Ziegler MG, Nelesen RA, Mills PJ, Ancoli-Israel S, Clausen JL, Watkins L, Dimsdale JE. Sleep-disordered breathing: the effect of hypoxia on baroreflexes and pressor sensitivity in sleep apnea and hypertension. Sleep 1995; 18:859–865.
97. Carlson JT, Hedner JA, Sellgren J, Elam M, Wallin BG. Depressed baroreflex sensitivity in patients with obstructive sleep apnea. Am J Respir Crit Care Med 1996; 154: 1490–1496.
98. Narkiewicz K, Pesek, CA, Kato M, Phillips BG, Davison DE, Somers VK. Baroreflex control of sympathetic nerve activity and heart rate in obstructive sleep apnea. Hypertension 1998; 32:1039–1043.
99. Needleman P, Greenwald JE. Atriopeptin: a cardiac hormone intimately involved in fluid, electrolyte and blood pressure homeostasis. N Engl J Med 1986; 314:828–834.
100. Krieger J, Follenius M, Sforza E, Brandenberger G, Peter JD. Effects of treatment with CPAP on ANP and AVP during sleep in sleep apnoea. Clin Sci 1991; 80:443–449.
101. Warley ARH, Stradling JR. Abnormal diurnal variation in salt and water excretion in patients with obstructive sleep apnoea. Clin Sci 1988; 74:183–185.
102. Ehlenz K, Schmidt P, Podzsus T, et al. Plasma levels of atrial natriuretic factor in patients with OSA. Acta Endocrinol 1988; 287(suppl):234–235.
103. Krieger J, Follenius M, Sforza E, Brandenberger G. H_2O and electrolyte metabolism in OSA. In: Home J, ed. Sleep '90. Bochum, Germany: Pontenagel, 1990:429–434.
104. Morgan BJ, Crabtree DC, Palta M, Skatrud J. Combined hypoxia and hypercapnia evokes long-lasting sympathetic activation in humans. J Appl Physiol 1995; 79:205–213.
105. Hedner J, Darpo B, Ejnell H, Carlson J, Caidahl K. Reduction in sympathetic activity after long-term CPAP treatment in sleep apnoea: cardiovascular implications. Eur Respir J 1995; 8:222–229.
106. Narkiewicz K, Kato M, Phillips BG, Pesek CA, Davison DE, Somers VK. Nocturnal continuous positive airway pressure decreases daytime sympathetic traffic in obstructive sleep apnea. Circulation 1999; 100:2332–2335.
107. Carlson JT, Rangemark C, Hedner JA. Attenuated endothelium-dependent vascular relaxation in patients with sleep apnoea. J Hypertension 1996; 14:577–584.
108. Kourembanas S, Marsden PA, McQuillan LP, Faller DV. Hypoxia induces endothelin gene expression and secretion in cultured human endothelium. J Clin Invest 1991; 88: 1054 1057.
109. Phillips BG, Narkiewicz K, Pesek CA, Haynes WG, Dyken ME, Somers VK. Effects of obstructive sleep apnea on endothelin-1 and blood pressure. J Hypertension 1999; 17:61–66.

110. Bokinsky G, Miller M, Ault K, Husband P, Mitchell J. Spontaneous platelet activation and aggregation during obstructive sleep apnea and its response to therapy with nasal CPAP. Chest 1995; 108:625–630.
111. Chin K, Ohi M, Kita H, Noguchi T, Oksuka N, Tsuboi T, Mishima M, Kuno K. Effects of NCPAP therapy on fibrinogen levels in obstructive sleep apnea syndrome. Am J Respir Crit Care Med 1996; 153:1972–1976.
112. O'Donnell CP, Ayuse T, King ED, Schwartz AR, Smith PL, Robotham JL. Airway obstruction during sleep increases blood pressure without arousal. J Appl Physiol 1996; 80:773–781.
113. Brooks D, Horner RL, Kozar LG, Render-Teixeir CL, Phillipson EA. Obstructive sleep apnea as a cause of systemic hypertension. Evidence from a canine model. J Clin Invest 1997; 99:106–109.
114. Fletcher EC, Lesske J, Qian W, Miller CC, Unger T. Repetitive, episodic hypoxia causes diurnal elevation of systemic blood pressure in rats. Hypertension 1992; 19: 555–561.
115. Fletcher EC, Lesske J, Behm R, Miller CC, Unger T. Carotid chemoreceptors, systemic blood pressure, and chronic episodic hypoxia mimicking sleep apnea. J Appl Physiol 1992; 72:1978–1984.
116. Fletcher EC, Lesske J, Culman J, Miller CC, Unger T. Sympathetic denervation blocks blood pressure elevation episodic hypoxia. Hypertension 1992; 20:612–619.
117. Fletcher EC, Bao G, Miller CC. Effect of recurrent episodic hypocapnic, eucapnic, and hypercapnic hypoxia on systemic blood pressure. J Appl Physiol 1995; 78:1516–1521.
118. Fletcher EC, Bao G. The effect of recurrent episodic eucapnic and hypocapnic hypoxia on systemic blood pressure in hypertension prone rats. J Appl Physiol 1996; 81:2088–2094.
119. Bao G, Metreveli N, Li R, Taylor A, Fletcher EC. Blood pressure response to chronic episodic hypoxia: role of the sympathetic nervous system. J Appl Physiol 1997; 83: 95–101.
120. Floras JS, Aylward PE, Victor RG, Mark AL, Abboud FM. Epinephrine facilitates neurogenic vasoconstriction in humans. J Clin Invest 1988; 81:1265–1274.
121. Floras JS, Aylward PE, Mark AL, Abboud FM. Adrenalin facilitates neurogenic vasoconstriction in borderline hypertensive subjects. J Hypertension 1990; 8:443–448.
122. Bao G, Fletcher EC. Renin activity and blood pressure in chronic intermittent hypoxia (abstr). Hypertension 1997; 30(3):509.
123. Nieto FJ, Young TB, Lind BK, Shahar E, Samet JM, Redline S, D'Agnostino RB, Newman AB, Lebowitz MD, Pickering TG. Association of sleep-disordered breathing, sleep apnea, and hypertension in a large community-based study. JAMA 2000; 283: 1829–1836.

13

Cardiac Function in Sleep Apnea

GERALDO LORENZI-FILHO and T. DOUGLAS BRADLEY

University of Toronto
Toronto, Ontario, Canada

I. Introduction

The respiratory and cardiovascular systems must act in concert to transfer oxygen (O_2) and carbon dioxide (CO_2) between the atmosphere and the cells. Accordingly, their control systems must be integrated to ensure that the metabolic needs of the tissues are met under varying conditions in response to demands. Both cyclic changes in breathing and sustained changes in alveolar ventilation exert important effects on the cardiovascular system (1). These effects are particularly prominent in patients with obstructive sleep apnea (OSA), who experience recurrent episodes of asphyxia during sleep associated with cyclic fluctuations in heart rate, blood pressure, cardiac output, and systemic O_2 delivery (2). Therefore, it is not surprising that from the beginning of clinical research in sleep apnea, an association between OSA and cardiovascular disease was recognized. Initially, a high prevalence of nocturnal cardiac arrhythmias, systemic and pulmonary hypertension, and cor pulmonale among patients with OSA was described (3–6). More recently, there is a growing body of evidence implicating OSA in the development or progression of left ventricular (LV) hypertrophy and dysfunction (7,8). For example, a study from our laboratory has demonstrated an association between OSA and certain cases of LV heart failure of otherwise unknown etiology (9). Moreover, the treatment of these patients with continuous positive airway pressure (CPAP) was associated with an improvement in cardiac function measured during the day. These data indicate, first, that elimination of OSA by CPAP was responsible for the improvement in LV function and, second, that OSA was contributing to the development of LV dysfunction in these patients (9).

Cheyne-Stokes respiration in association with central sleep apnea (CSR-CSA) has been a well-recognized complication of severe cardiac failure for over 150 years (10). However, it is only in the last few years that CSR-CSA has attracted more clinical attention since the recognition that it can cause symptoms of a sleep apnea syndrome (11–13). Thus, while sleep apnea can cause cardiovascular disturbances, it is now apparent that cardiac dysfunction can lead to a sleep apnea syndrome. In patients with severe but stable congestive heart failure (CHF), CSR-CSA is common (14–16). More importantly, there is increasing evidence to suggest that CSR-CSA in patients with CHF participates in a vicious cycle that further stresses the failing heart and, in so doing, increases the risk of mortality (17,18). Equally important is the observation that alleviation of CSR-CSA in patients with CHF, through a number of interventions, has been associated with improvements in various aspects of cardiovascular physiology (15,19–21). Nevertheless, CSR-CSA is not yet widely recognized as a clinical problem worthy of diagnosis and specific therapy. This may be because symptoms of paroxysmal nocturnal dyspnea, restless and unrefreshing sleep, daytime somnolence, and fatigue overlap with symptoms of CHF and therefore are not attributed to a sleep-related breathing disorder (16).

In this chapter we will focus and provide our views on the pathophysiological effects of sleep-related breathing disorders on right ventricular (RV) and LV function. The causes and consequences of CSR-CSA in patients with CHF will also be discussed. A concept that will be emphasized throughout is that the multiple burdens associated with sleep apnea disorders not only have acute nocturnal consequences for the cardiovascular system, but also have chronic effects that carry over into the daytime. One good example of this concept is that increases in sympathetic nervous system activity (SNA), resulting from repetitive obstructions or central apneas during sleep, is associated with elevations in SNA during wakefulness as well (22). Treatment of OSA and CSR-CSA in patients with cardiovascular disease will be discussed only briefly, mainly in the context of the evidence it provides for a pathophysiological link between these disorders and right and left ventricular dysfunction.

II. Effects of OSA on the Pulmonary Vessels and Right Ventricle

A. Acute Effects

OSA has profound effects on the pulmonary vasculature manifest by pronounced fluctuations in pulmonary artery pressure (P_{Pa}) with intermittent elevations during sleep that rise above the baseline level during wakefulness (2,23,24). The fluctuations in P_{Pa} parallel the arterial blood pressure (BP) oscillations in that the peak increase occurs at, or just shortly after, the onset of arousal and ventilation. The mechanisms involved in these cyclic elevations in P_{Pa} are summarized in Table 1.

The maximum increase in P_{Pa} generally coincides with the maximum degree of arterial oxyhemoglobin desaturation. Administration of supplemental O_2 markedly attenuates but does not abolish these elevations in P_{Pa} (25). Thus, although hypoxia-induced pulmonary vasoconstriction undoubtedly plays a role in the pathogenesis of these elevations in P_{Pa}, it is probably not the only contributing factor. For example, hypercapnia and acidosis can also induce pulmonary vasoconstriction (26). Accordingly, increasing Pa_{CO_2} during apnea may contribute to elevations in P_{Pa}. This might help to explain why elevations in P_{Pa} are not completely abolished by supplemental O_2.

Recently Laks et al. (27) studied P_{Pa} responses to short exposure to acute hypoxia at two different levels of end-tidal CO_2 in normal subjects and in patients with either moderate or severe OSA. They found similar P_{Pa} increases in response to acute eucapnic and hypercapnic hypoxia in both groups. Normoxic hypercapnia alone was a weak stimulus. There was a marked intersubject and interpatient variability in the pressor response, ranging from 2 to 12 mmHg for a 30% decrease in oxyhemoglobin saturation (Sa_{O_2}) In a subgroup of OSA patients, hypercapnia caused a marked further increase in P_{Pa} in response to hypoxia. In contrast, no such augmentation in P_{Pa} was seen in any of the normal subjects when exposed to hypercapnia. Thus it is unclear to what extent elevations in Pa_{CO_2} cause pulmonary vasoconstriction over and above that due to hypoxia during OSA. It seems that there is interindividual variability in the P_{Pa} response to hypercapnia and that patients with OSA may differ in this response from healthy subjects. However, there are insufficient data to draw firm conclusions on this point.

Table 1 Factors Promoting Acute Increases in Pulmonary Arterial Pressure and Right Ventricular Afterload

Pulmonary vasoconstriction
Hypoxia
Hypercapnia
Exaggerated negative intrathoracic pressure during apnea
Increased transmural pulmonary artery and right ventricle pressure during obstructive apneas
Impairment of left ventricular function and passive rises in pulmonary artery pressure secondary to elevated left-sided cardiac filling pressures
Reduced compliance of the LV due to:
Left ventricular dilation in response to increased BP and exaggerated negative intrathoracic pressure during obstructive apneas
Leftward shift of the interventricular septum during diastole
Hypoxia decreasing LV compliance

When analyzing the P_{Pa} responses during OSA, one should also consider the fact that the pulmonary vasculature is exposed to pleural pressure (Ppl). Exaggerated subatmospheric Ppl during obstructive apneas could increase pulmonary arterial transmural pressure (i.e., the difference between P_{Pa} and Ppl) in the absence of vasoconstriction (28). Marrone et al. (29) demonstrated that transmural systolic P_{Pa} in obstructive apneas, showed rapid changes in synchrony with esophageal pressure swings, and slower changes, related to Sa_{O_2} oscillations. The Sa_{O_2} after each interapneic period returned quickly to the baseline value, no matter to what extent it dropped during each apnea. However, transmural P_{Pa} did not return to the baseline level and progressively increased. This phenomenon was evident only with pronounced dips in Sa_{O_2}. The authors explained their findings on the basis of the time course of the pulmonary vascular response to hypoxia, which lags O_2 desaturation during apneas. Reductions in Sa_{O_2} during sleep apnea generally occur over 10–60 s and revert within a few seconds. Therefore, the increase in P_{Pa} from the beginning to the end of an obstructive apneic cycle may not represent the full response to the level of hypoxia reached during apneas. However, the prolonged elevation in P_{Pa} during the postapneic phase once Sa_{O_2} returns to baseline probably represents the delayed pulmonary vasoconstrictive response to apnea induced hypoxia. Therefore, particularly in patients with severe OSA where recurrent dips in Sa_{O_2} occur, it is possible that the effects of recurrent hypoxia would cause a prolonged increase in P_{Pa} throughout the apneic and ventilatory period during sleep.

Another factor contributing to elevations in P_{Pa} could be transmission of elevated LV filling pressures to the pulmonary vasculature. For example, Buda et al. (30) demonstrated that pulmonary capillary wedge pressure rose during obstructive apneas. This occurred in association with intermittent elevations of systemic blood pressure. They speculated that pulmonary capillary wedge pressure may have risen, via Starling's mechanisms (31,32), secondary to increases in LV afterload resulting from the combined effects of increased systolic BP and generation of markedly subatmospheric Ppl swings during apneas. Exaggerated negative Ppl increases the difference between juxtacardiac and intracardiac pressures, thus increasing systolic LV transmural pressure (LVPtm) (33). The RV will also be exposed to negative Ppl, which increases its afterload over and above that due to elevations in P_{Pa}.

In summary, transient pulmonary hypertension in response to obstructive events during sleep has been well documented. The combination of elevations in P_{Pa} and generation of negative intrathoracic pressure during obstructive apneas leads to intermittent increases in RV afterload. The mechanisms driving these surges in P_{Pa} and RV afterload are part of an integrated response to multiple pathogenic factors acting simultaneously or in rapid succession during obstructive sleep apneas (23).

B. Chronic Effects

Although the above-mentioned mechanisms could account for the intermittent apnea associated elevations in P_{Pa}, they do not readily explain sustained pulmonary hypertension or RV failure (RVF). P_{Pa} characteristically returns to the baseline level on final awakening in patients with OSA (2,24). Such patients usually do not suffer from sustained pulmonary hypertension or RVF, no matter how frequent and severe intermittent nocturnal hypoxia may be (6). While experimental animals may develop RV hypertrophy when exposed to prolonged periods of intermittent severe hypoxia, it has not been shown that this leads to RVF (34).

A number of investigators have demonstrated that sustained pulmonary hypertension and RVF in patients with OSA are almost invariably associated with the presence of both nocturnal and diurnal hypoxia and hypercapnia (6,35,36). For example, in one study, RVF, defined clinically as the presence of an elevated jugular venous pressure, peripheral edema, electrocardiographic evidence of right ventricular hypertrophy, and pulmonary hypertension on a chest radiograph, was found in 12% of patients with OSA (6). Compared with the control group without RVF, those with RVF had similar numbers of apneas and hypopneas during sleep. However, the chief distinguishing feature between the RVF and non-RVF groups was the presence of significantly lower Pa_{O_2} and higher Pa_{CO_2} while awake in the former group (Table 2). Even when the severity of nocturnal apnea-related hypoxia was matched in a subgroup of control subjects, daytime hypoxia and hypercapnia remained the chief distinguishing factors for the presence of RVF. In addition, forced expiratory volume in 1 s (FEV_1) was lower and functional residual capacity and residual volume were higher among the RVF group. Thus, the RVF group had evidence of mild-to-moderate chronic airflow obstruction. However, this in itself would probably not explain awake hypercapnia as the mean FEV_1/forced vital capacity was only 56%. This is a level at which hypercapnia is usually not seen in patients

Table 2 Comparison of Physiological Variables in Obstructive Sleep Apnea Patients with and Without Right Heart Failure

	Without RHF (n = 44)	With RHF (n = 6)	p-value
Age, yr	49 ± 2	49 ± 3	NS
Weight, % ideal	147 ± 7	186 ± 12	<0.05
Apnea and hypopneas, no/h sleep	60 ± 5	57 ± 9	NS
Mean nocturnal Sa_{O_2}, %	90 ± 1	76 ± 3	<0.001
PaO_2, mmHg	75 ± 2	52 ± 4	<0.001
$PaCO_2$, mmHg	36 ± 1	51 ± 2	<0.001
FRC, % pred	98 ± 3	119 ± 11	<0.05
FEV_1, L	3.3 ± 0.1	1.8 ± 0.3	<0.001
FEV_1/FVC, %	76 ± 1	56 ± 5	<0.001
Ventilatory response to CO_2, L/min/mmHg	2.4 ± 0.2	1.2 ± 0.3	<0.01

Data are expressed as mean ± SEM.
RHF, Right heart failure; FRC, functional residual capacity; FEV_1, forced expiratory volume in 1; FVC, forced vital capacity.
Source: Modified from Ref. 6.

with chronic obstructive pulmonary disease (COPD) (37,38). Instead, it appears that CO_2 retention was related to a combination of chronic airflow obstruction, chest wall restriction due to obesity, possibly lower central respiratory drive, and the effects of nocturnal upper airway obstruction (35). Moreover, the severe degree of nocturnal hypoxia observed in the RVF group could be partly attributed to low baseline awake Pa_{O_2} and reduced expiratory reserve volume (6).

The chief conclusion of this study was that the development of RVF in patients with OSA was not due to nocturnal hypoxia alone. Rather, it appeared that hypoxia or hypercapnia while awake was also required so that the pulmonary vasculature was exposed to sustained blood gas derangement. Because these awake blood gas disturbances were associated with mild COPD, these observations gave rise to the notion of an "overlap syndrome" of OSA and COPD. The combination of the two disorders gave rise to cardiopulmonary failure (39). Strong support for these conclusions was subsequently provided by several other investigators (35,36,40,41).

Recent studies have suggested that some OSA patients can have subclinical pulmonary hypertension but not RVF, with no concomitant signs of lung abnormalities or daytime hypoxemia. Laks and associates (42) found a surprisingly high prevalence (42%) of elevated mean P_{Pa} (>20 mmHg) while awake in 100 consecutive patients with OSA. In keeping with previous reports (6,35,40,41) pulmonary hypertension was associated with the presence of abnormal lung function, reduced awake Pa_{O_2} and increased awake Pa_{CO_2}. However, 6 of the 40 patients with pulmonary hypertension had resting arterial Pa_{O_2} of 80 mmHg or higher, suggesting that mild degrees of pulmonary hypertension can be present in the absence of daytime hypoxemia. Sanner et al. (43) studied 92 consecutive patients in whom clinically significant lung disease was excluded. Eighteen (20%) had mild elevations in mean P_{Pa} (range 20–25 mmHg), and of these, 8 (44%) also had increased pulmonary capillary wedge pressure. This suggested that a subclinical degree of LV dysfunction may be common in patients with OSA and, where present, could contribute to a mild degree of pulmonary hypertension. These authors also reported that in a group of 107 patients with OSA, in whom clinically significant lung disease was excluded, 18% had impaired RV ejection fraction (RVEF) and mild RVF (44). RVEF correlated with the apnea-hypopnea index and the extent of nocturnal oxyhemoglobin desaturation, but not with age, body mass index, awake arterial blood gas tensions, sex, lung function, P_{Pa} and LVEF. In addition, 52% of the study subjects with impaired RVEF and 48% of the patients with normal RVEF had daytime pulmonary hypertension at rest or during exercise. Thus, their data do not support the concept that pulmonary hypertension is the cause of reduced RVEF in this subgroup of patients.

Although OSA alone infrequently causes RVF, abolition of OSA by tracheostomy or nasal CPAP can reverse cardiorespiratory complications of OSA even in the presence of obesity and mild-to-moderate COPD (35,45,46). This indicates that while a number of factors contribute to the development of chronic hypercapnia and cor pulmonale in patients with OSA, reversal of OSA alone is sufficient in most cases to improve RV function. Consequently, it seems that there is a threshold level of respiratory disturbance beyond which RV function deteriorates to frank failure. The threshold level of, for instance, OSA that would cause RVF would be lowered in the presence of COPD and vice versa. Thus, the alleviation of one of the major contributing factors to RVF may be sufficient to bring the level of total respiratory disturbance below this threshold level. It remains unclear why reversal of OSA by nocturnal CPAP or tracheostomy leads to reversal of daytime hypercapnia. Relief of upper airway obstruction reduces the mechanical load on the respiratory system, and this may lead to improvement in gas exchange at night. Alteration of the chemical milieu of the brain stem during sleep may be the most important factor. Such an effect probably leads to resetting of the chemoreceptor at night and persistent reduction in the set point for a ventilatory response to CO_2, which persists in the daytime.

Strong support for this mechanism comes from the work of Berthon-Jones and Sullivan (45). They demonstrated that as respiratory failure resolved following institution of nocturnal CPAP therapy in hypercapnic patients with OSA, the threshold Pa_{CO_2} for a ventilatory response during wakefulness shifted to the left. However, the slope of the ventilatory response to CO_2 did not change. The precise mechanism of this phenomenon has not been elucidated. Nevertheless, improved nocturnal and diurnal gas exchange undoubtedly plays a key role in reducing P_{Pa} and reversing cor pulmonale. Relief of highly subatmospheric Ppl and respiratory muscle fatigue or dysfunction may also be of some importance (47). Since cor pulmonale is almost invariably accompanied by respiratory failure, it is likely that the development of respiratory failure precedes the onset of RVF in patients with OSA. Similarly, reversal of respiratory failure is the probable explanation for the reversal of cor pulmonale in these patients (48).

III. Effects of OSA on Left Ventricular Function

A. Acute Effects

There are three key pathophysiological features of OSA that could adversely affect the left ventricle: generation of exaggerated negative Ppl, development of asphyxia during apnea, and arousal from sleep at the termination of apnea. A polysomnographic recording illustrating these features is displayed in Figure 1. Table 3 outlines how these three factors could lead to the development or progression of LV dysfunction or failure.

Exaggerated negative Ppl increases venous return to the right ventricle. The resultant RV distension can lead to a leftward shift of the interventricular septum during diastole, thereby impeding LV filling (49–51). Exaggerated negative Ppl can also reduce the rate of LV relaxation, further increasing the impedance to LV filling and raising LV pressures (30,52). It also leads to increases in LVPtm, an important determinant of LV afterload (33,53). The combined effects of reduced LV preload and increased afterload lead to reduced stroke volume and cardiac output (54). Generation of exaggerated negative Ppl also causes greater reductions in LVEF in pa-

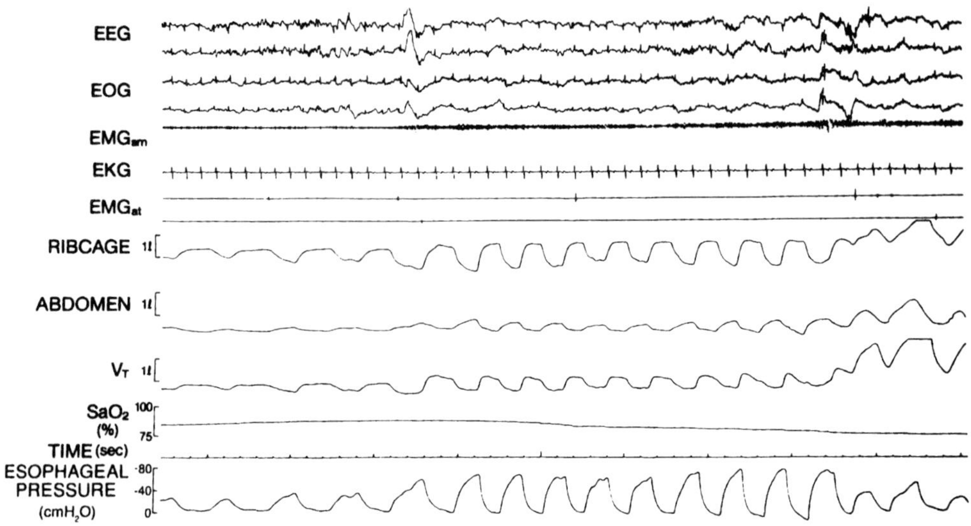

Figure 1 Recording of an obstructive hypopnea in a patient with idiopathic dilated cardiomyopathy during stage 2 sleep. The three key features of obstructive sleep apnea are illustrated. First, paradoxical rib cage motion during hypopnea is accompanied by marked subatmospheric intrathoracic pressure (i.e., esophageal pressure) swings during inspiratory efforts. This negative pressure is generated by the inspiratory muscles, which are being loaded by the upper airway obstruction, and tends to increase left ventricular transmural pressure (i.e., afterload). Second, over the course of the hypopnea, a marked reduction in oxyhemoglobin saturation (Sa_{O_2}) occurs. Third an arousal from sleep (EEG and EMG_{sm} channels) terminates the hypopnea. (From Ref. 9.)

Table 3 Pathophysiological Effects of Obstructive Sleep Apnea on the Left Ventricle

Exaggerated negative intrathoracic pressure during apnea
Increased left ventricular transmural pressure (i.e., afterload)
Increased right ventricular volume with leftward shift of interventricular septum and diastolic filling of the left ventricle
Reduced cardiac output with increased O_2 demand
Apnea-related hypoxia
Reduced myocardial O_2 supply with reduced myocardial contractility, and cardiac ischemia in patients with ischemic heart disease
Increased sympathetic nervous system activity
Increased heart rate and systemic blood pressure promoting hypertrophy
Brady- and ventricular arrhythmias
Arousals
Increased sympathetic nervous system activity
Increased myocardial O_2 demand in the face of reduced O_2 supply

tients with coronary artery disease than in healthy subjects (53,55). This is probably because the diseased myocardium is less capable of compensating for the increased afterload. These hemodynamic disturbances, in combination with apnea-related hypoxia, could predispose to acute cardiac ischemia or pulmonary edema (56,57).

In summary, through one or more of the above mechanisms, generation of exaggerated negative Ppl during Mueller maneuvers or obstructive apneas can induce marked reductions in stroke volume and cardiac output (30,58,59). It probably also contributes to the development of nocturnal ischemia and acute pulmonary edema that have been reported in some patients with OSA (57,60–62). The extent to which each of these factors contributes to reductions in cardiac output probably varies over the course of each apnea and is probably influenced by the presence or absence of coronary artery disease and the underlying contractile state of the myocardium. Accordingly, generation of negative Ppl during OSA probably has more deleterious effects in patients with a diseased than in those with a healthy myocardium (63).

Intermittent hypoxia during obstructive apneas can adversely affect cardiac performance through several mechanisms. Hypoxia causes pulmonary vasoconstriction, increases P_{Pa}, and gives rises to the physiological and clinical consequences described above (2,6,49–51,59,64). Hypoxia can also depress cardiac contractility directly (65) and reduce the rate of relaxation of both ventricles, thus compromising their performance (66). Hypoxia is also a potent stimulator of the sympathetic nervous system (67). This would increase BP and heart rate (HR), which, in turn, would increase metabolic demands of the myocardium in the face of reduced O_2 supply. Acute hypoxia can trigger ischemia in patients with concurrent coronary artery disease (61), which can, in turn, further depress myocardial contractility.

Obstructive apnea is usually terminated by a brief arousal in response to hypoxia, hypercapnia, and ineffectual inspiratory efforts. Arousal from sleep, either alone or in concert with other stimuli discussed below, can provoke increases in SNA, BP, and HR (68,69). Consequent increases in myocardial O_2 demand could be another factor, in addition to reduced supply due to hypoxia, that contributes to cardiac ischemia or arrhythmias. This is liable to be particularly the case in patients with coronary artery disease. In a recent study, the majority of patients referred to a sleep laboratory because of nocturnal angina were found to have OSA (61). Other studies have reported ischemic electrocardiographic changes in patients with OSA even in the absence of coronary artery disease (55).

Activation of the sympathetic nervous system is an important secondary pathophysiological effect of obstructive apneas stemming from the synergistic stimulatory effects of at least five factors: hypoxia, hypercapnia, apnea, reduced cardiac output, and arousal from sleep. At the termination of airway occlusion, BP rises to or above the baseline level just after the peak muscle SNA is reached (22,58,70,71). The principal hemodynamic consequence of this increase in sympathetic nerve traffic is a surge in BP. Muscle SNA and systemic BP tend to peak just after the onset of ventilation, rather than at the termination of apnea (70–72). Regardless of the mechanism, these increases in SNA and systemic BP, along with reductions in intrathoracic pressure, lead to increased LVPtm, not only during, but also after the termination of apneas. They increase LV afterload and render such patients susceptible to the development of myocardial ischemia (55,60,61,73,74) and reduced cardiac output (57,75) tens or hundreds of times each night. In addition, OSA has a number of adverse effects on cardiac rhythm that are related to the severity of hypoxia. These include sinus bradycardia, second-degree heart block, and supraventricular and ventricular ectopy and tachycardia (76–78). Patients with underlying coronary artery disease or CHF are probably especially susceptible to these adverse effects (61).

B. Chronic Effects

There is growing evidence that the acute and repetitive effects of OSA on the cardiovascular system have aftereffects that persist into wakefulness. Daytime muscle SNA and plasma norepinephrine concentrations are higher in such patients than in appropriately matched controls (22,70,79). The mechanisms for this sustained sympathetic activation are unclear but could involve an upward resetting of baseline central sympathetic outflow during the awake state. In addition, repetitive obstructive apneas during sleep have been shown to cause elevation in BP that are sustained into wakefulness (80).

Acute and sustained sympathetic activation has particularly adverse prognostic implications in patients with coexisting heart failure. Survival in CHF is inversely proportional to cardiac noradrenergic drive (81) and to awake plasma norepinephrine concentrations (82). These adverse prognostic relationships are probably a consequence of the detrimental effects of neurally released and circulating catecholamines on cardiovascular homeostasis. Such effects could occur at the level of the myocyte (direct catecholamine toxicity or induction of apoptosis), the myocardial β-receptor complex (number, affinity, or responsiveness to endogenous and exogenous agonists), organ function (altered BP; development of arrhythmias), or functional status of the afflicted patient (83). In addition, because sympathetic activation during sleep arises as a result of apneas and arousals from sleep, not necessarily as a compensatory response to low cardiac output, it may be particularly detrimental to the diseased myocardium. Furthermore, the contractile function of the failing heart is very sensitive to changes in afterload (84). Therefore, recurrent increases in afterload due to OSA are liable to cause more pronounced hemodynamic embarrassment than in subjects with normal cardiac function (53,63). Moreover, recent observations in our laboratory suggest that these adverse hemodynamic effects persist longer into the postapneic period in patients with heart failure than in healthy subjects (63). Over time, these repetitive increases in LV afterload, in association with hypoxia-induced impairment of myocardial contractility, could lead to LV hypertrophy or exacerbation of preexisting heart failure, even in the absence of daytime hypertension (85).

Although the pathogenesis of daytime hypertension in OSA will not be considered in detail herein, hypertension is a common accompaniment of the sleep apnea syndrome. Chronic hypertension has long been recognized as a cardinal factor in the causation of many cases of CHF. For instance, Levy and colleagues (86), using data from a long-term follow-up of a carefully monitored cohort (original Framingham heart study and Framingham offspring study), found that hypertension was the most common risk factor for CHF. During up to 20 years of follow-up, there were 392 new cases of heart failure (out of 5143 subjects); in 91% hypertension antedated the development of CHF. In this study hypertension remained a strong risk factor for CHF even after adjusting for confounding factors such as sex, age, and myocardial infarction. Therefore, any potential causative link between OSA and LV hypertrophy or failure through hypertension would be indirect and subject to a number of confounding variables. Nevertheless, this possible link should not be ignored, given the potential of reversibility of hypertension and LV dysfunction through specific therapy of OSA.

The effects of OSA on the left ventricle of patients who have no overt sign of LV dysfunction have been conflicting. Hedner et al. (85) reported increased LV wall thickness in normotensive patients with OSA compared to normotensive control subjects independent of obesity. On the other hand, Hanly and colleagues (87) found no significant difference in LV dimensions and wall thickness when they compared OSA patients versus snorers with no OSA. The reason for the discrepancy between the results of these two studies is not clear.

More convincing evidence that OSA can have adverse effects on the left ventricle comes from a canine model of OSA. In this model, experimentally induced OSA led to LV systolic dysfunction, as evidenced by a significant reduction in LVEF after 2–3 months (88). In addition, two studies have shown that treatment of OSA was associated with improvements in LV function. Krieger and colleagues (89) studied LV ejection fraction (LVEF) in 29 OSA patients without clinical LV heart failure. Mean LVEF was found to be at the lower limit of normal. After one year of nasal CPAP treatment, LVEF increased by a small but statistically significant amount. However, there was no control group. Malone et al. (9) described a group of eight patients with idiopathic dilated cardiomyopathy and CHF all of whom had severe OSA. Following one month of treatment with nasal CPAP, abolition of OSA was associated with dramatic improvements in LV function. LVEF increased from $37 \pm 4\%$ to $49 \pm 5\%$ ($p < 0.0001$) and was accompanied by improvement in cardiac functional status. Furthermore, secondary withdrawal of CPAP for one week resulted in deterioration of LVEF back to the pre-CPAP treatment level. This study, therefore, provided direct evidence that reversal of OSA in patients with CHF by CPAP could improve LV systolic function and symptoms of CHF. It also provided indirect evidence that OSA could contribute to the development of LV dysfunction in CHF patients without underlying coronary artery disease. Such findings, if found to be reproducible, may well alter the approach to the investigation and treatment of some cases of CHF. They also raise the question as to how many patients with dilated cardiomyopathy of unknown etiology have OSA as a factor contributing to their cardiac disease.

IV. Central Sleep Apnea in Association with Cheyne–Stokes Respiration in Congestive Heart Failure

A. Definition

Cheyne–Stokes respiration is a form of periodic breathing in which apneas and hypopneas alternate with ventilatory periods having a crescendo-decrescendo pattern of V_T. The gradual waxing and waning of ventilation that is almost sinusoidal indicates that CSR is part of a continuum of periodic breathing disorders that arise as a result of oscillations in the chemical stimuli to breathe. The term CSR has been used to describe this abnormal pattern of breathing but not to denote any specific underlying etiology. Cheyne's original description is instructive in this respect and points out the potential complexity and probable multifactorial pathogenesis of CSR (21):

> ''A.B., sixty years of age, of a sanguine temperament, circular chest, and a full habit of body, for years lived a very sedentary life, while he indulged habitually in the luxuries of the table . . . he neglected my directions with regard to diet, nay, his appetite being remarkably keen, he ate more than usual, and took at least a pint of port wine or Madeira daily, as was his habit.'' The patient developed CHF and a cardiac arrhythmia, which was followed by a stroke. He was ''found in bed flushed, speechless and hemiplegic. . . . For several days his breathing was irregular; it would entirely cease for a quarter of a minute, then it would become perceptible, though very low, then by degrees it became heaving and quick, and then it would gradually cease again. This revolution of his breathing occupied about a minute during which there were about thirty acts of respiration.''

Thus, the patient in the original description suffered from both CHF and neurological disease. In addition, the patient also had well-known predisposing factors for the development of OSA, namely obesity and high alcohol intake. Accordingly, it is unclear which was the chief factor responsible for CSR. However, it has long been suggested that the prolonged hyperpnea with the waxing and waning pattern of V_T is a result of a prolonged lung to chemoreceptor circulatory delay and a reduced cardiac output (90). This view has recently been confirmed by the demonstration of an inverse relationship of cardiac output to both circulation time and periodic breathing cycle length in CHF patients with CSR-CSA (91,92). On this basis it is likely that in most patients an element of cardiac dysfunction plays a role in sculpting this abnormal respiratory pattern. In addition, it is not possible to determine whether apneas in the original description were central or obstructive in nature. Most authors have used the term CSR to describe central apneas alternating with prolonged ventilation periods. However, obstructive apneas have also been described in association with a CSR ventilatory pattern (12,93). Therefore, since we will be focusing on central apnea in this section, the term CSR with central sleep apnea (CSR-CSA) will be used throughout.

B. Clinical Features

The first detailed study of CSR-CSA in patients with CHF by Harrison et al. (94) was a classic work in this field. These investigators made several important observations. They recognized that CSR-CSA was most prominent at the onset of sleep (they called this light sleep), that it caused arousals from sleep during the hyperpneic phase, and that during these arousals patients frequently suffered from paroxysmal nocturnal dyspnea. In addition, it was observed that a significant degree of hypoxia could develop as a result of apnea even when oxygenation was relatively normal during wakefulness. Finally, it was suggested that the recurrent exposure to hypoxia and disruption of sleep by arousals and paroxysmal nocturnal dyspnea might be an important contributing factor to the development of fatigue associated with the CHF syndrome. These observations have stood the test of time as evidenced by subsequent confirmatory data (11–13,16,18). It is now recognized that CSR-CSA gives rise to clinical problems largely through its effects during sleep, in agreement with the observations of Harrison et al. (94). These effects are similar to those associated with sleep apnea syndromes and lead to disrupted sleep and its consequences. Hanly and colleagues (95) showed that patients with CHF and CSR-CSA had a sleep latency significantly shorter then CHF patients without this breathing disorder suggesting that they suffered from hypersomnolence. In addition, they demonstrated that patients with CHF and CSR-CSA had more stage 1 and 2 non–rapid eye movement (non-REM) sleep, less rapid eye movement (REM) sleep, and a higher frequency of arousals from sleep than CHF patients without CSR-CSA (95).

C. Mechanisms Leading to Cheyne–Stokes Respiration in Congestive Heart Failure

The mechanisms leading to CSR-CSA in patients with CHF are complex and are a matter of some controversy. In this section we present our views on this subject, which are based largely on experiments and observations in patients with the disorder. Readers wishing to review a more basic, theoretical approach to the pathophysiology of periodic breathing in general are referred to Chapter 3 in this volume. CSR-CSA is a manifestation of instability of the respiratory control system. This control system instability predisposes to wide fluctuations in arterial blood gas tension and ventilation. In addition, CSR-CSA has two distinct phases that are determined by different mechanisms: the hyperpneic phase (91,92) and the central apneic phase. We will first discuss those factors involved in the pathogenesis of central apneas. To accomplish this it will be necessary to briefly review some elements of the normal respiratory control system that maintain homeostasis and then to show how these become disrupted in patients with CHF as summarized in Table 4.

Under normal conditions, ventilation is stable and maintains arterial blood gas tensions within narrow limits through a negative feedback circuit. This negative feedback system consists of a central controller sensitive to fluctuations in Pa_{O_2} and Pa_{CO_2} at the peripheral and central chemoreceptors and a plant (the lungs, chest wall,

Table 4 Stabilizing and Destabilizing Influences on the Respiratory Control System

Stabilizing mechanisms	Destabilizing mechanisms in CHF
Pa_{CO_2} above the apneic threshold	Low Pa_{CO_2} close to apnea threshold due to pulmonary congestion and vagal stimulation
Awake drive to breathe—tends to stabilize breathing (even when Pa_{CO_2} is low)	Sleep onset—removal of awake drive, breathing dependent on chemical drive; instability when $PaCO_2$ is low
Stable sleep without arousals	Arousals from sleep trigger ventilatory overshoot and reductions in Pa_{CO_2} below apnea threshold
Damped ventilatory response to chemical stimuli	Increased ventilatory responsiveness to chemical stimuli (tendency to overshoot)
Upper airway stability with linear response between central drive and ventilation	Variable upper airway resistance with nonlinear relation between central drive and ventilation, tendency to under- and overshoot
Large O_2 and CO_2 reservoir in the lungs	Low FRC determined by pulmonary congestion; FRC even lower when lying down

CHF, congestive heart failure; FRC, functional residual capacity.

and respiratory muscles), which generates ventilation (96). The controlled variables are Pa_{O_2}, Pa_{CO_2}, and pH, which act as negative feedback signals to the central controller. In turn, the central controller maintains blood gas homeostasis by altering its neural output to the respiratory muscles in order to move the chest wall to achieve the appropriate level of ventilation. Pa_{O_2} and Pa_{CO_2} are altered accordingly. Blood gas homeostasis is maintained through certain stabilizing influences inherent in the system. These include respiratory neural control and mechanical factors, as well as central nervous system state. Respiratory neural control factors include maintenance of Pa_{CO_2} well above the threshold for apnea, relatively low gain of the chemoreceptors, a short delay in the transmission of the effects of ventilation on Pa_{O_2} and Pa_{CO_2} to the chemoreceptors (97), and rapid correction of deviations in blood gas tensions toward the desired level. They also include the nonchemical drive to breathe associated with wakefulness that tends to maintain ventilation even when Pa_{CO_2} is driven below the apnea threshold (98). Respiratory mechanical factors include stability and maintenance of upper airway patency allowing the central output to the respiratory muscles to be rapidly translated into airflow in a nonfluctuating manner and a high functional residual capacity acting as a large reservoir of O_2 and CO_2 in the body to damp oscillations in Pa_{O_2} and Pa_{CO_2} during apneas. Stability of central nervous system state prevents abrupt changes in thresholds and gains of the chemoreceptors. As a consequence of these mechanisms, under normal circumstances a nearly optimal balance is struck between stability and speed of response of the control system.

Destabilization of these homeostatic mechanisms predisposes to the development of periodic breathing in general and to CSR-CSA in CHF patients in particular. The key pathophysiological mechanism leading to CSR-CSA is a fluctuation of Pa_{CO_2} above and below the apneic threshold. A number of destabilizing factors could contribute to this fluctuation in Pa_{CO_2}. First, a low Pa_{CO_2} close to the apneic threshold could predispose to the development of central apneas. Under this condition, a relatively small increase in ventilation would drive Pa_{CO_2} below threshold and trigger a central apnea (8,96,99,100). Naughton et al. (100) and Hanly and colleagues (101) have shown that CHF patients with CSR-CSA have lower Pa_{CO_2} both while awake and asleep than those without CSR-CSA. The same is true of patients with idiopathic central sleep apnea (ICSA), a disorder that shares many features of CSR-CSA but which occurs in the absence of cardiac failure (102,103). Second, elevated chemoreceptor responsiveness (gain) could destabilize the respiratory control system by increasing the tendency to hyperventilate, triggering ventilatory overshoot. Among healthy subjects exposed to hypoxia at high altitude, those with the highest chemoreflex responses are the most prone to developing periodic breathing during non-REM sleep (104). Third, shifts in the state of consciousness are likely to destabilize breathing.

As one passes from wakefulness to non-REM sleep, the waking neural drive to breathe is abolished and the behavioral control system is quiescent. Therefore, breathing becomes critically dependent on the metabolic control system (96,105). In addition, during non-REM sleep, the threshold for a ventilatory response to CO_2 is increased, so that a higher Pa_{CO_2} is necessary to stimulate breathing (96,105). If the ambient Pa_{CO_2} during wakefulness is below this new threshold level for sleep, there will be a transient loss of respiratory drive resulting in a central apnea. During the apnea Pa_{CO_2} rises at a rate proportional to metabolic CO_2 production, until it reaches the critical threshold value, and breathing resumes. If sleep becomes firmly established at this point regular breathing follows (103). However, should the central nervous system state shift back momentarily to the awake state, as occurs during arousals from sleep, the increased Pa_{CO_2} level that was present during sleep now represents a state of relative hypercapnia for wakefulness. Consequently, a period of hyperpnea follows, in accordance with the awake ventilatory response to CO_2, resulting in the hyperpneic phase of periodic breathing. As long as the central nervous system state continues to fluctuate between wakefulness and sleep, waxing and waning of the waking neural drive results in alternating periods of hyperpnea and apnea until sleep becomes firmly established. Hence, transitions in sleep-wakefulness state are an ideal setting for the generation of respiratory instability and periodic breathing even in normal humans (96). The magnitude of the fluctuations at sleep onset and the evolution to either a dampening or a perpetuation of periodic breathing over time will depend on several variables. These include the difference between the waking and sleeping Pa_{CO_2} threshold values, the magnitude of the awake ventilatory responses to chemical stimuli, the presence of factors that would augment ventilatory drive during hyperpnea, such as hypoxia, and stability of sleep-wakefulness state (100,102,103,106,108).

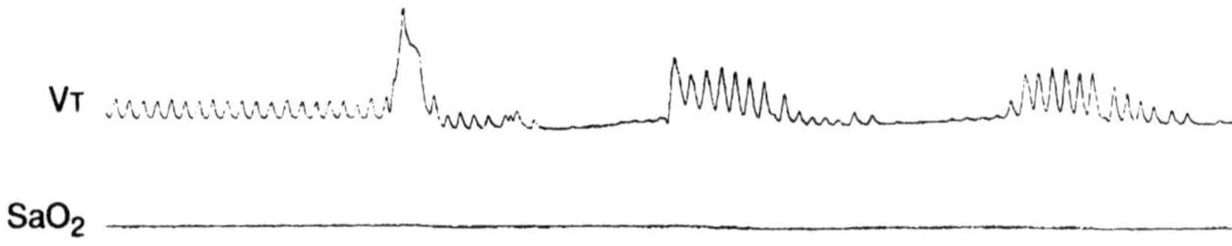

Figure 2 Tidal volume (V_T) and Sa_{O_2} recording from a patient with heart failure and CSR-CSA during stage 2 sleep. This is a typical example of how CSR-CSA is triggered by an abrupt increase in V_T, which occurred in association with an arousal from sleep (not shown) (From Ref. 100.)

In large measure, instability of central nervous system state and respiration are a consequence of arousals from sleep. Xie and colleagues (102) have shown in patients with ICSA that central apneas during stage 2 sleep are triggered and propagated by a relative degree of hyperventilation and hypocapnia. The critical role of arousals in sustaining ventilatory overshoot during periodic breathing was demonstrated by the strong relationship between the grade of arousals and both minute ventilation during hyperpnea and subsequent apnea length. However, arousals did not trigger apneas unless they were associated with increases in ventilation. Therefore, arousal, through promotion of hyperventilation, appears to facilitate rather than to provoke periodic breathing directly. In patients with CSR-CSA, the same principles appear to apply (100).

In patients with CHF, an association between CSR-CSA and low Pa_{CO_2} during both wakefulness and non-REM sleep has been demonstrated in several reports (100,101,109). Naughton et al. (100) found that CHF patients with CSR-CSA had lower Pa_{CO_2} during wakefulness and non-REM sleep than patients without CSR-CSA who had comparable age, LVEF, Pa_{O_2}, and lung-to-chemoreceptor circulatory delay. All episodes of CSR-CSA starting during stage 2 sleep were precipitated by hyperventilation most often, but not always, in association with arousals from sleep (Fig. 2). Furthermore, during episodes of CSR-CSA during stage 2 sleep, Ptc_{CO2} fell on average by 1.5 mmHg, which mirrored a 23% rise in V_I (Fig. 3). In addition, there was a significant inverse correlation between the frequency of apneas and hypopneas and mean Ptc_{CO2} ($r = -0.629$; $p < 0.01$). Accordingly, whereas arousal from sleep acts as a critical defense mechanism to terminate apnea and protect from severe asphyxia in OSA, in CSR-CSA arousal can trigger and propagate central apneas, but without any obvious protective effect.

Further evidence that hyperventilation and hypocapnia are the major factors that trigger central apnea comes from the work of Xie and colleagues (110). They showed that in patients with ICSA, an increase in Pa_{CO_2} of 1–3 mmHg induced either by administration of a CO_2-enriched gas mixture or by addition of dead space virtually eliminated central apneas and hypopneas. We have recently found qualitative and quantitatively similar results in patients with CHF and CSR-CSA (106). Taken together, these data indicate that CSR-CSA has physiological features remarkably

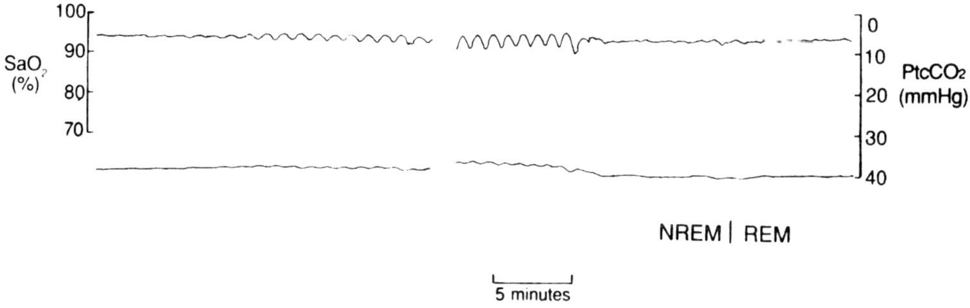

Figure 3 Sa_{O_2} and transcutaneous P_{CO2} (Ptc_{CO2}) during REM and NREM sleep in the same patient as shown in Figure 2 above. The tracing reads from right to left. Periodic dips in Sa_{O_2} indicate the presence of CSR-CSA. Note the absence of CSR-CSA during REM sleep. In NREM sleep CSR-CSA starts abruptly in concert with a reduction in Ptc_{CO2} below 40 mmHg. Ptc_{CO2} oscillates and remains below 40 mmHg throughout CSR-CSA. Later in the night, as Ptc_{CO2} increases back to 40 mmHg, CSR-CSA disappears. In addition, Sa_{O_2} is within normal limits prior to the onset of CSR-CSA and dips only marginally during CSR-CSA, indicating that CSR-CSA typically occurs in the absence of hypoxemia. (From Ref. 100.)

similar to ICSA and that, in both cases, central apneas are critically dependent on a reduction in Pa_{CO_2} below the apneic threshold.

The mechanisms responsible for nocturnal hypocapnia in patients with CSR-CSA have not been fully elucidated. One possible explanation is hypoxia. However, several investigators have shown that both awake $Pa_{O_2}$and mean nocturnal Sa_{O_2} in CHF patients with CSR-CSA are within normal limits and are practically identical to those in CHF patients without CSR-CSA (92,100,101). Experiments in animals and patients with CHF demonstrate that increased LV filling pressures and pulmonary congestion are associated with reduced Pa_{CO_2} (54,107). Recently, Tkacova and colleagues (92) found, in a population of patients with CHF due to nonischemic dilated cardiomyopathy, that despite similar LVEF, LV end-diastolic and systolic volumes were twice as high in patients with CSR-CSA than in those without CSR-CSA. In addition, patients with CSR-CSA had a significantly lower Pa_{CO_2} while awake and lower mean Ptc_{CO2} during stage 2 sleep. Furthermore, the greater the LV end-diastolic volume, the less the rise in Pa_{CO_2} from wakefulness to stage 2 sleep. This relationship suggests that marked LV dilatation in patients with nonischemic dilated cardiomyopathy is associated with a nonchemical drive to breathe that prevents the normal rise in Pa_{CO_2} during the transition from wakefulness to sleep. The most likely explanation for this relationship is that high LV volumes are associated with elevated LV filling pressures. Indeed, Solin and colleagues (111) recently showed that CHF patients with CSR-CSA had significantly higher pulmonary capillary wedge pressures and lower Pa_{CO_2} than patients without CSR-CSA. Lowering of wedge pressure by drugs or CPAP was associated with alleviation of CSR-CSA. Therefore, higher LV volumes and filling pressures are probably associated with greater degrees of pulmonary venous congestion that predispose to hyperventilation and CSR-CSA.

The potential role of hypoxemia in the pathogenesis of CSR-CSA in heart failure is uncertain. In periodic breathing at high altitude, hypoxemia causes hyperventilation and lowers Pa_{CO_2} below the apnea threshold (108). Under these conditions, administration of O_2 removes hypoxic drive, allows Pa_{CO_2} to rise above the apneic threshold abolishing central apneas. The critical dependence of high-altitude periodic breathing on fluctuations in Pa_{CO_2} is further emphasized by the observation that CO_2 inhalation, even in the presence of sustained hypoxia, raises Pa_{CO_2} and abolishes central apneas. However, studies of patients with CHF and CSR-CSA have consistently shown them to be normoxic while awake (100,101,109). Thus hypoxic dips in CSR-CSA are the result, rather than the cause, of central apneas. Nevertheless, the hypoxic dips during apneas could further the tendency to hyperventilate at the termination of central apneas by amplifying the ventilatory response to CO_2 once Pa_{CO_2} rises above the ventilatory threshold (97). Ventilatory overshoot with propagation of CSR-CSA would therefore be facilitated by even mild degrees of apnea-related hypoxia. Dips in Sa_{O_2} would also facilitate arousal from sleep, which in turn contributes to hyperventilation.

A number of studies have investigated the effects of supplemental oxygen in the patients with CHF and CSR-CSA. It must be stressed that most studies were interested in abolishing the dips in Sa_{O_2} rather than understanding how the dips in Sa_{O_2} can contribute to the genesis of CSR-CSA (20,112–114). All studies were consistent in showing a small but significant reduction in the total amount of CSR-CSA. For instance, Hanly et al. (113) showed that low-flow O_2 administered to patients with CHF reduced the duration of CSR-CSA mainly during stage 1 sleep with no significant change during stage 2, slow-wave, or REM sleep. The administration of O_2 was also associated with a more consolidated sleep with a decrease in the number of arousals. Modest reductions in the frequency of central apneas and hypopneas in response to O_2 administration has been confirmed by others (20,113,114). Although not proven, the likely mechanism for this effect is raising Pa_{CO_2} in response to abolition of hypoxic drive. Taken together, these data are consistent with the concept that hypoxia may play a role in aggravating, but is not the major determinant of CSR-CSA in patients with CHF.

Increased ventilatory responsiveness to chemical stimuli is another factor that has been implicated in promoting and or perpetuating CSR-CSA (97,115,116). Augmented gain of the chemoreceptors, which could be primary or, more likely, secondary to pulmonary edema, destabilize the respiratory control system by making it prone to ventilatory overshoot (97,117,118). Wilcox et al. (115) have shown that CHF patients with CSR-CSA have higher central chemoresponsiveness compared to predicted normal values, but did not compare these responses to those in a CHF group without CSR-CSA. In a more recent paper, Javaheri (119) demonstrated increased central ventilatory responsiveness to CO_2 in CHF patients with CSR-CSA than among those without this breathing disorder. In addition, both peripheral and central chemoresponsiveness are increased and are related to a lower than normal

Pa_{CO_2} in patients with ICSA (102). The pathophysiology of this condition is in many respects similar to CSR-CSA (91). Therefore, evidence is mounting that periodic breathing disorders in general, and CSR-CSA in CHF patients in particular, are associated with increased chemoresponsiveness.

Upper airway instability may play a role in the pathogenesis of CSR-CSA. Alex et al. (120) described upper airway occlusion at the onset and at the end of central apneas in patients with CHF. Instability of upper airway resistance could, at least theoretically, promote the development of CSR-CSA. If upper airways resistance increases as ventilation decreases during the decrescendo phase of the hyperpneic portion of CSR-CSA, there will be a tendency to cause an undershoot of ventilation (121). The occasional occluded breath at the onset of central apneas during CSR-CSA (120), as shown in Figure 2, is compatible with this possibility. On the other hand, decreasing resistance as ventilation is increasing during the crescendo phase will facilitate overshoot, rapidly driving Pa_{CO_2} down and setting up conditions for posthyperventilation apneas. In addition, it is possible that upper airway collapse itself can reflexly precipitate central apneas (122). This suggests an important interaction between upper airway and central controller instability in the pathogenesis of some cases of CSR-CSA. Furthermore, patients with ICSA, who share many of the pathophysiological feature of CSR-CSA (102,103,110) have greater upper airway compliance and lung volume–related change in pharyngeal caliber than control subjects (123). These properties are similar to those in patients with OSA (124,125). It has also been recognized that CSR-CSA is more prominent when moving from upright to supine (126). This shift is associated with an increase in venous return to the heart and with narrowing of the upper airway (127). It is noteworthy in this respect that CPAP, which dilates and stabilizes the upper airway (127,128), has been shown to alleviate both ICSA and CSR-CSA (13,15,129). Although CPAP has many other effects that could damp periodic breathing, such as lung inflation and augmentation of cardiac output, stabilization of the upper airway may be an additional factor promoting abolition of central apneas in these conditions. Even though there is no evidence for upper airway occlusion in most cases of CSR-CSA (11), this does not preclude a role for upper airway instability in the pathogenesis of some cases of CSR-CSA. It is possible that the degree to which upper airway instability contributes to the pathogenesis of CSR-CSA will vary from one patient to the next.

CHF patients have a low functional residual capacity, which is further reduced by moving from the upright to the supine position. A large functional residual capacity acts as a large reservoir of O_2 and CO_2 in the body and damps oscillations in Pa_{O_2} and Pa_{CO_2} that would occur during apneas (117,130). Therefore, reductions in functional residual capacity decrease lung O_2 and CO_2 reservoirs and allow greater reductions in Pa_{O_2} and greater increases in Pa_{CO_2} during apneas (117,130). This could contribute to instability of the respiratory control system. However, Naughton et al. (100) have shown that lung volumes in CHF patients with CSR-CSA do not differ from those in patients without CSR-CSA. Thus, the role of reduced lung volume in the pathogenesis of CSR-CSA remains uncertain.

Prolonged circulation time causing time delays in transmitting changes in arterial blood gas tensions within the lungs to the chemoreceptors could theoretically destabilize the respiratory control system. It could do so by changing a negative feedback into a positive feedback system such that ''the right response occurs at the wrong moment'' (117,131). In support of this theory, Guyton et al. (131) induced CSR in sedated dogs by inserting a length of tubing between the heart and brain to prolong the transit time from the lungs to the chemoreceptors. However, CSR was achieved only when the circulatory delay was a few minutes in duration, far exceeding that seen in patients with CHF.

There is now a body of evidence indicating that prolonged circulatory delay is probably not the critical factor predisposing to CSR-CSA. In humans, the circulatory delay for a given chemical stimulus to reach the carotid body from the lungs can be estimated noninvasively. One method that has been used is to determine the time from the end of an apnea until the maximum dip in Sa_{O_2} detected by an oximeter on the ear (which is in close proximity to the carotid body). This lung-to-ear circulation time (LECT) is inversely proportional to the stroke volume and cardiac output in both patients with normal and with abnormal heart function (91,92). Hall et al. (91) compared patients with ICSA, whose cardiac function and LECT are normal, to CHF patients with CSR-CSA. They found that, despite having higher stroke volumes and shorter LECT than the CHF patients with CSR-CSA, those with ICSA had the same low and fluctuating Pa_{CO_2} and high frequency of central apneas during sleep. These data, along with those from other studies (106,110,111), indicate that central apneas in patients with ICSA and CSR-CSA are due to hypocapnia and fluctuations in Pa_{CO_2} below and above the apnea threshold, but are unlikely to be related to the degree of circulatory delay. A number of investigators have also found no significant differences in LECT, LVEF or cardiac output between CHF patients with and without CSR-CSA (17,18,100,111,132).

In the same study it was also observed that the longer periodic breathing cycle length in the CHF patients with CSR-CSA was related to a longer LECT than in the patients with ICSA (Figs. 4 and 5) (91). The relationship between LECT and cycle length was found to be due to the correlation of LECT and hyperpnea length, whereas LECT did not correlate with apnea length (Fig. 6). However, the characteristic ''sculpting'' and prolongation of the hyperpnea in CHF patients was related to their lower cardiac output. Therefore, rather than initiating periodic breathing and central apneas, circulatory delay appears to determine hyperpnea length and, secondarily, cycle length once periodic breathing with central apnea has been established. However, it appears not to affect apnea length, which is influenced by the degree of preceding hyperventilation and hypocapnia (103,133).

In summary, the pathogenesis of CSR-CSA in CHF is complex and is fundamentally related to respiratory control system instability. As discussed above, a constellation of factors contributes to respiratory control system instability in the setting of CHF. Once the summation of these factors reaches a certain threshold level, CSR-CSA ensues. The degree to which each of these factors contributes to the pathogenesis of CSR-CSA probably varies considerably from one individual to the next. Treat-

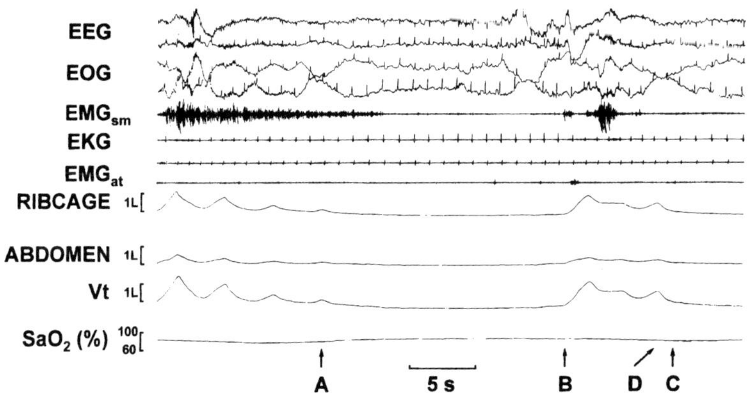

Figure 4 Recording of a central apnea during stage 2 sleep in a patient with idiopathic central sleep apnea. Apnea length (AB) is 18 s, hyperpnea length (BD) is 7 s, total cycle length (AD) is 25 s, and lung to ear circulation time (LECT) from the end of the apnea until the maximum dip in Sa_{O_2} (BC) is 8 s. LECT is short, in keeping with normal cardiac function. Abbreviations as per Figure 1. (From Ref. 91.)

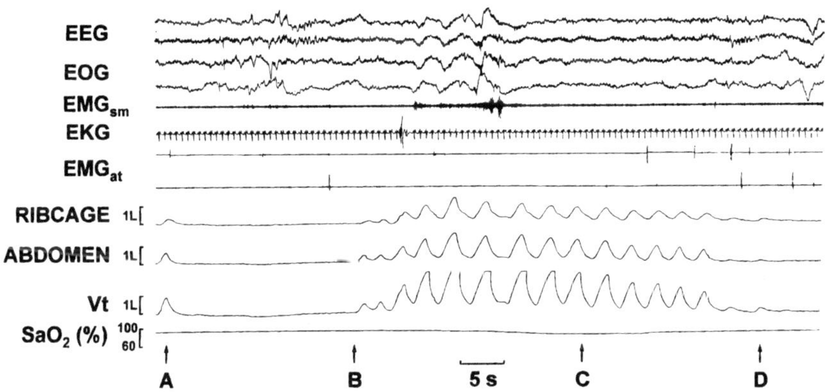

Figure 5 Recording of a central apnea and hyperpnea during stage 2 sleep from a patient with congestive heart failure. It exhibits a crescendo-decrescendo pattern of V_T during hyperpnea that is typical of CSR-CSA. Compared to the patient with idiopathic central sleep apnea (Fig. 4), LECT (BC = 26 s), hyperpnea length (BD = 46 s), and total cycle length (AD = 65 s) are substantially longer, in keeping with lower cardiac output related to heart failure. However, apnea length (AB = 21 s) is similar. Abbreviations as per Figure 1. (From Ref. 91.)

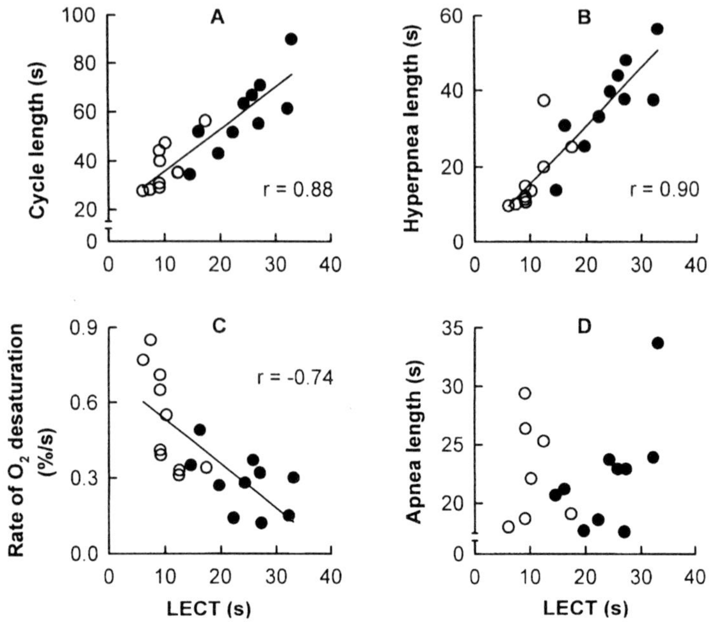

Figure 6 Panels A and B demonstrate the significant direct relationships of periodic breathing cycle length and hyperpnea length to LECT, respectively ($p < 0.001$), in patients with idiopathic central sleep apnea (open circles), whose cardiac function is normal, and heart failure patients with CSR-CSA (closed circles). Panel C shows that the rate of oxyhemoglobin desaturation is inversely related to LECT ($p < 0.001$). However, panel D demonstrates that apnea length is not related to LECT ($p > 0.15$). Abbreviations as per Figure 4. (From Ref. 91.)

ments aimed at relieving this breathing disorder should take the complex interaction of these factors into account.

D. Pathophysiological Consequences of CSR-CSA

Unlike OSA, which probably contributes to the development of CHF, CSR-CSA appears to arise as a result of CHF, as illustrated in Table 5. The question that arises then is: once established, does CSR-CSA constitute an additional burden, analogous to OSA, on the cardiovascular system and contribute to a deterioration of the LV function? Indeed, there is a growing body of evidence suggesting that CSR-CSA is a marker of poor prognosis in patients with CHF. For example, Findley and colleagues (18) reported, in an uncontrolled retrospective study, that patients with CHF who also suffered from CSR-CSA during sleep had a higher mortality rate than patients without CSR-CSA. More recently Hanly et al. (17) prospectively followed a group of 16 patients with stable CHF, 9 of whom had CSR-CSA and 7 of whom

Table 5 Clinical and Pathophysiological Features of CSR-CSA in Patients with Congestive Heart Failure

Prevalence
35–45%
Risk factors
Severe cardiac dysfunction
Low daytime and overnight Pa_{CO_2}
Increased left ventricular volumes
Atrial fibrillation
Pathophysiological consequences of CSR-CSA
Periodic elevations in blood pressure and heart rate during the night
Increased sympathetic nervous system activity (increased overnight urinary and daytime plasma norepinephrine)
Ventricular arrhythmias (?)
Increased mortality risk
Clinical features
Paroxysmal nocturnal dyspnea
Disrupted sleep
Daytime hypersomnolence and fatigue

did not. Despite comparable LVEF, the combined rate of mortality and heart transplantation was significantly higher in the CSR-CSA group. A more recent study by Lanfranchi and colleagues (134) confirmed, in a larger group of patients with CHF, that CSR-CSA is associated with increased mortality in relation to the frequency of respiratory events. These data suggest that CSR-CSA itself may accelerate disease progression in patients with heart failure.

In contrast to obstructive apneas, no inspiratory efforts are made during central apneas (13). On the other hand, a substantial degree of negative Ppl can be generated during hyperpnea. This inspiratory effort is probably one factor provoking arousal from sleep (47,135,136) and paroxysmal nocturnal dyspnea in patients with CHF (7,13,94). BP and HR oscillate in concert with CSR-CSA cycles, very much as they do during OSA (114,137): peaks occur during the hyperpnea and troughs during apnea. The mechanisms mediating these oscillations have not yet been determined. They could be related to the same mechanisms that have been implicated in OSA, including hypoxia and arousals from sleep, both of which can stimulate SNA. However, Franklin and colleagues (114) found that O_2 administration, at a sufficient flow rate to abolish dips in Sa_{O_2}, slightly reduced the frequency of central apneas but did not significantly influence BP or HR oscillations during CSR-CSA. These data indicate that mechanisms other than hypoxic dips are involved in precipitating these surges in BP and HR during CSR-CSA. Regardless of the exact mechanisms, once established, CSR-CSA promotes cyclic increases in BP and HR in concert with the ventilatory cycle (108,129), which may contribute to poor prognosis of CHF patients with CSR-CSA.

As in the case of OSA, CSR-CSA is characterized by sleep fragmentation due to arousals from sleep. Although arousals can occur at the termination of apneas, they frequently occur several breaths into the ventilatory period. This suggests that chemical stimuli are reaching the ventilatory threshold, causing ventilation to resume, before they reach the arousal threshold. When arousals occur after the resumption of breathing, they may not act as a defense mechanism to prevent asphyxia, as is the case in OSA. Indeed, arousals under these conditions may very well be viewed as a pathological phenomenon that promotes CSR-CSA by provoking sleep state instability and hyperventilation. Arousals probably arise from a combination of mild hypoxia and the effort of breathing, particularly when arousals occur after resumption of ventilation. Sleep fragmentation by arousals is probably an important cause of excessive daytime sleepiness and fatigue in patients with CHF and CSR-CSA (13,15,95).

Hypoxia and arousals from sleep are also associated with stimulation of the sympathetic nervous system (22,68,70). Overnight urinary norepinephrine concentrations are markedly higher in CHF patients with CSR-CSA than in those without CSR-CSA and are directly related to the frequency of arousals from sleep and degree of apnea-related hypoxia, but not to LVEF (19). These data strongly suggest, first, that CSR-CSA can trigger sympathetic activation in certain patients with CHF and, second, that the increased SNA in these patients is not simply a compensatory response to low cardiac output, but is directly related to the sleep apnea disorder. It may therefore represent excessive and pathological sympatho-excitation. These changes transcend the sleeping state: in the same study, we observed that daytime plasma norepinephrine concentration was also higher in those with CSR-CSA and was directly related to the frequency of arousals from sleep and the degree of apnea-related hypoxia (19). These higher nocturnal and daytime catecholamine concentrations might aggravate myocardial dysfunction and may be one factor that contributes to the increased risk of death reported in patients with CHF and CSR-CSA (17,18). Thus, CSR-CSA may participate in a vicious pathophysiological cycle involving the cardiovascular, respiratory, and autonomic nervous systems.

Recently, Javaheri and colleagues (109) found that CHF patients with hypocapnia ($Pa_{CO_2} \leq 35$ mmHg) had a higher prevalence of central apneas than those in whom Pa_{CO_2} was > 35 mmHg. In addition, they showed that hypocapnic patients had a higher rate of ventricular tachycardia than the eucapnic patients. The underlying cause of this relationship is unknown. It could be that hypocapnia and alkalosis directly contribute to the frequency of arrhythmias. On the other hand, it could be that CSR-CSA with mild hypoxic dips, arousals from sleep, sympathetic activation, and elevations in BP could trigger ventricular arrhythmias. For instance, Findley and colleagues (138) reported one patient with CHF in whom the timing of ectopic beats was in concert with the CSR-CSA ventilatory cycle and associated dips in Sa_{O_2}. On the other hand, CHF patients with CSR-CSA have larger left ventricles than those without CSR-CSA (90). Since bigger hearts are associated with an increased likelihood of arrhythmias (139), the link between CSR-CSA (and/or low Pa_{CO_2}) with ventricular arrhythmias could be one of association rather than of causality. Nevertheless, since one third of the patients with CHF die of sudden death, presumably related to cardiac arrhythmias (140), this area deserves further investigation.

A detailed discussion of the treatment of CSR-CSA in patients with CHF is beyond the scope of this review. Readers wishing an in-depth discussion of this subject are referred to a recent review article (141). Briefly, since CSR-CSA probably arises from CHF, one of the major aims of therapy is to improve underlying heart failure. Accordingly, the first approach should be to optimize the medical therapy of CHF (142). Failing that, there are a number of other therapeutic options. The most extensively tested treatment over clinically relevant time periods is CPAP. Long-term nightly use of CPAP over 1–3 months has been shown to alleviate CSR-CSA, to increase inspiratory muscle strength and LVEF, and to reduce mitral regurgitation, atrial natriuretic peptide, urinary and plasma norepinephrine levels. It has also been shown to reduce hospital admissions and improve quality of life (13,15,19,143,144). Although supplemental O_2 has been applied to CHF patients with CSR-CSA in a number of studies, most of these were short-term overnight interventions, a time period of little, if any, therapeutic consequence in CHF (112–114). The longest trials were only 2–4 weeks in duration and showed reductions in the severity of CSR-CSA, a decrease in overnight urinary norepinephrine levels, and a modest increase in peak O_2 consumption during graded exercise with nightly use (20,21). However, O_2 has not been shown to improve direct measures of cardiac function or quality of life. Finally, theophylline has been shown to reduce the severity of CSR-CSA over 5 days but has not been shown to improve cardiac function, neurohumoral activity, or quality of life (145). Larger, longer-term randomized trials will be required to determine which, if any, of these interventions are effective for the management of CHF patients with CSR-CSA.

V. Summary

In this chapter we have reviewed evidence for a link between sleep apnea disorders and impairment of RV and LV function. The consensus in the literature is that OSA can contribute to the development of RV dysfunction. There is also evidence that OSA can play a role in the development or aggravation of LV heart failure. However, because of the limited number of studies examining this potential relationship, a consensus on this question has not yet been reached. Because of the obvious clinical importance of this question, more research needs to be directed at the acute and chronic effects of OSA, and of its treatment, on LV function.

There is general agreement that CSR-CSA is a consequence of CHF and that the cause of central apneas is fluctuations in Pa_{CO_2} below the apnea threshold. However, controversy remains as to whether CSR-CSA is simply a consequence of poor cardiac function or whether, once established, it participates in a vicious pathophysiological cycle that leads to progression of heart failure. At the moment there is no consensus as to whether specific therapy of CSR-CSA can lead to improvement in the heart failure syndrome. Nevertheless, there are some promising data on the latter point that provide a strong rationale for the conduct of well-designed controlled clinical trials of therapy for CSR-CSA in patients with CHF.

Acknowledgments

Geraldo Lorenzi-Filho was supported by research fellowships from FAPESP-Brazil, and T. D. Bradley is a Senior Scientist of the Canadian Institutes of Health Research. This work is supported by operating grants MT-11607 and MA-12422 from the Canadian Institutes of Health Research and by the Toronto Rehabilitation Institute.

References

1. Daly MDB. Interactions between respiration and circulation. In: Cherniack NS, Widdicombe JG, eds. Handbook of Physiology, 3rd ed. Bethesda, MD: American Physiological Society, 1986:529–594.
2. Tilkian AG, Guilleminault C, Schroeder JS, Lehrman KL, Simmons FB, Dement WC. Hemodynamics in sleep-induced apnea. Studies during wakefulness and sleep. Ann Intern Med 1976; 85:714–719.
3. Tilkian AG, Guilleminault C, Schroeder JS, Lehrman KL, Simmons FB, Dement WC. Sleep-induced apnea syndrome. Prevalence of cardiac arrhythmias and their reversal after tracheostomy. Am J Med 1977; 63:348–358.
4. Guilleminault C, Tilkian A, Dement WC. The sleep apnea syndromes. Annu Rev Med 1976; 27:465–484.
5. Stradling JR. Sleep apnoea and systemic hypertension. Thorax 1989; 44:984–989.
6. Bradley TD, Rutherford R, Grossman RF, Lue F, Zamel N, Moldofsky H, Phillipson, EA. Role of daytime hypoxemia in the pathogenesis of right heart failure in the obstructive sleep apnea syndrome. Am Rev Respir Dis 1985; 131:835–839.
7. Bradley TD, Floras JS. Pathophysiologic and therapeutic implications of sleep apnea in congestive heart failure. J Card Fail 1996; 2:223–240.
8. Bradley TD. Right and left ventricular functional impairment and sleep apnea. Clin Chest Med 1992; 13:459–479.
9. Malone S, Liu PP, Holloway R, Rutherford R, Xie A, Bradley TD. Obstructive sleep apnoea in patients with dilated cardiomyopathy: effects of continuous positive airway pressure. Lancet 1991; 338:1480–1484.
10. Cheyne J. A case of apoplexy in which the fleshy part of the heart was converted to fat. Dublin Hospital Rep 1818; 2:216–223.
11. Hanly PJ, Millar TW, Steljes DG, Baert R, Frais MA, Kryger MH. Respiration and abnormal sleep in patients with congestive heart failure. Chest 1989; 96:480–488.
12. Dowdell WT, Javaheri S, McGinnis W. Cheyne-Stokes respiration presenting as sleep apnea syndrome. Clinical and polysomnographic features. Am Rev Respir Dis 1990; 141:871–879.

13. Takasaki Y, Orr D, Popkin J, Rutherford R, Liu P, Bradley TD. Effect of nasal continuous positive airway pressure on sleep apnea in congestive heart failure. Am Rev Respir Dis 1989; 140:1578–1584.
14. Javaheri S, Parker TJ, Wexler L, Michaels SE, Stanberry E, Nishyama H, Roselle, GA. Occult sleep-disordered breathing in stable congestive heart failure. Ann Intern Med 1995; 122:487–492.
15. Naughton MT, Liu PP, Bernard DC, Goldstein RS, Bradley TD. Treatment of congestive heart failure and Cheyne-Stokes respiration during sleep by continuous positive airway pressure. Am J Respir Crit Care Med 1995; 151:92–97.
16. Javaheri S, Parker TJ, Liming JD, Corbett WS, Nishiyama H, Wexler L, Roselle, GA. Sleep apnea in 81 ambulatory male patients with stable heart failure. Circulation 1998; 97:2154–2159.
17. Hanly PJ, Zuberi-Khokhar NS. Increased mortality associated with Cheyne-Stokes respiration in patients with congestive heart failure. Am J Respir Crit Care Med 1996; 153:272–276.
18. Findley LJ, Zwillich CW, Ancoli-Israel S, Kripke D, Tisi G, Moser KM. Cheyne-Stokes breathing during sleep in patients with left ventricular heart failure. South Med J 1985; 78:11–15.
19. Naughton MT, Benard DC, Liu PP, Rutherford R, Rankin F, Bradley TD. Effects of nasal CPAP on sympathetic activity in patients with heart failure and central sleep apnea. Am J Respir Crit Care Med 1995; 152:473–479.
20. Andreas S, Clemens C, Sandholzer H, Figulla HR, Kreuzer H. Improvement of exercise capacity with treatment of Cheyne-Stokes respiration in patients with congestive heart failure. J Am Coll Cardiol 1996; 27:1486–1490.
21. Staniforth AD, Kinnear WJM, Starling R, Hetmanski DJ, Cowley AJ. Effect of oxygen on sleep quality, cognitive function and sympathetic activity in patients with chronic heart failure and Cheyne-Stokes respiration. Eur Heart J 1998; 19:922–928.
22. Somers VK, Dyken ME, Clary MP, Abboud FM. Sympathetic neural mechanisms in obstructive sleep apnea. J Clin Invest 1995; 96:1897–1904.
23. Bonsignore MR, Marrone O, Insalaco G, Bonsignore G. The cardiovascular effects of obstructive sleep apnoeas: analysis of pathogenic mechanisms. Eur Respir J 1994; 7: 786–805.
24. Coccagna G, Mantovani M, Brignani F, Parchi C, Lugaresi E. Continuous recording of the pulmonary and systemic arterial pressure during sleep in syndromes of hypersomnia with periodic breathing. Bull Eur Physiopathol Respir 1972; 8:1159–1172.
25. Schroeder JS, Motta J, Guilleminault C. Hemodynamic studies in sleep apnea. In: Guilleminault C, Dement WC, eds. Sleep Anea Syndromes. New York: Alan R. Liss, 1978:177–196.
26. Fishman AP. Chronic cor pulmonale. Am Rev Respir Dis 1976; 114:775–794.
27. Laks L, Bronwyn L, Grunstein RR, Sullivan CE. Pulmonary artery pressure response to hypoxia in sleep apnea. Am J Respir Crit Care Med 1997; 155:193–198.
28. Parish JM, Shepard JW, Jr. Cardiovascular effects of sleep disorders. Chest 1990; 97: 1220–1226.
29. Marrone O, Bonsignore MR, Romano S, Bonsignore G. Slow and fast changes in transmural pulmonary artery pressure in obstructive sleep apnoea. Eur Respir J 1994; 7:2192–2198.
30. Buda AJ, Schroeder JS, Guilleminault C. Abnormalities of pulmonary artery wedge pressures in sleep-induced apnea. Int J Cardiol 1981; 1:67–74.

31. Katz AM. Cardiomyopathy of overload: a major determinant of the progress in congestive heart failure. N Engl J Med 1990; 322:100–110.
32. Sarnof S. Myocardial contractility as described by Starling's law of the heart. Physiol Rev 1955; 35:107–122.
33. Buda AJ, Pinsky MR, Ingels NBJ, Daughters GT, Stinson EB, Alderman EL. Effect of intrathoracic pressure on left ventricular performance. N Engl J Med 1979; 301: 453–459.
34. Nattie EE, Bartler DJ, Johnson K. Pulmonary hypertension and right ventricular hypertrophy caused by intermittent hypoxia and hypercapnia in the rat. Am Rev Respir Dis 1978; 118:653–657.
35. Fletcher EC, Schaaf JW, Miller J, Fletcher JG. Long-term cardiopulmonary sequelae in patients with sleep apnea and chronic lung disease. Am Rev Respir Dis 1987; 135: 525–533.
36. Weitzenblum E, Krieger J, Apprill M, Vallee E, Ehrhart M, Ratomaharo J, Oswald M, Kurtz D. Daytime pulmonary hypertension in patients with obstructive sleep apnea syndrome. Am Rev Respir Dis 1988; 138:345–349.
37. Report of the Medical Research Council Working Party. Long-term domiciliary oxygen therapy in chronic hypoxic cor pulmonale complicating chronic bronchitis and emphysema. Lancet 1981; 1:1364–1368.
38. Bradley TD, Rutherford R, Lue F, Moldofsky H, Grossman RF, Zamel N, Phillipson, EA. Role of diffuse airway obstruction in the hypercapnia of obstructive sleep apnea. Am Rev Respir Dis 1986; 134:920–924.
39. Flenley DC. Sleep in chronic obstructive lung disease. Clin Chest Med 1985; 6:651–661.
40. Chaouat A, Weitzenblum E, Krieger J, Ifoundza T, Oswald M, Kessler R. Association of chronic obstructive pulmonary disease and sleep apnea syndrome. Am J Respir Crit Care Med 1995; 151:82–86.
41. Chaouat A, Weitzenblum E, Krieger J, Oswald M, Kessler R. Pulmonary hemodynamics in the obstructive sleep apnea syndrome. Results in 220 consecutive patients. Chest 1996; 109:380–386.
42. Laks L, Lehrhaft B, Grunstein RR, Sullivan CE. Pulmonary hypertension in obstructive sleep apnoea. Eur Respir J 1995; 8:537–541.
43. Sanner BM, Doberauer C, Konermann M, Sturm A, Zidek W. Pulmonary hypertension in patients with obstructive sleep apnea syndrome. Arch Intern Med 1997; 157:2483–2487.
44. Sanner BM, Konermann M, Sturm A, Muller HJ, Zidek W. Right ventricular dysfunction in patients with obstructive sleep apnoea syndrome. Eur Respir J 1997; 10:2079–2083.
45. Berthon-Jones M, Sullivan CE. Time course of change in ventilatory response to CO_2 with long-term CPAP therapy for obstructive sleep apnea. Am Rev Respir Dis 1987; 135:144–147.
46. Sullivan CE, Berthon-Jones M, Issa FG. Remission of severe obesity-hypoventilation syndrome after short term treatment during sleep with nasal continuous positive airway pressure. Am Rev Respir Dis 1983; 128:177–181.
47. Vincken W, Guilleminault C, Silvestri L, Cosio M, Grassino A. Inspiratory muscle activity as a trigger causing the airways to open in obstructive sleep apnea. Am Rev Respir Dis 1987; 135:372–377.

48. Sullivan CE, Issa FG, Saunders NA. Pathophysiology of sleep apnea. In: Saunders NA, Sullivan CE, eds. Sleep and Breathing. New York: Marcel Dekker, 1984:299–363.
49. Scharf SM, Graver LM, Balaban K. Cardiovascular effects of periodic occlusions of the upper airways in dogs. Am Rev Respir Dis 1992; 146:321–329.
50. Robotham JL, Rabson J, Permutt S, Bromberger-Barnea B. Left ventricular hemodynamics during respiration. J Appl Physiol 1979; 47:1295–1303.
51. Peters J, Fraser C, Stuart RS, Baumgartner W, Robotham JL. Negative intrathoracic pressure decreases independently left ventricular filling and emptying. Am J Physiol 1989; 257:H120–H131.
52. Virolainen J, Ventila M, Turto H, Kupari M. Effect of negative intrathoracic pressure on left ventricular pressure dynamics and relaxation. J Appl Physiol 1995; 79:455–460.
53. Scharf SM, Bianco JA, Tow DE, Brown R. The effects of large negative intrathoracic pressure on left ventricular function in patients with coronary artery disease. Circulation 1981; 63:871–875.
54. Bradley TD, Holloway RM, McLaughlin PR, Ross BL, Walters J, Liu PP. Cardiac output response to continuous positive airway pressure in congestive heart failure. Am Rev Respir Dis 1992; 145:377–382.
55. Hanly P, Sasson Z, Zuberi N, Lunn K. ST-segment depression during sleep in obstructive sleep apnea. Am J Cardiol 1993; 71:1341–1345.
56. Loui WS, Blackshear JL, Fredrickson PA, Kaplan J. Obstructive sleep apnea manifesting as suspected angina: report of three cases. Mayo Clin Proc 1994; 69:244–248.
57. Chaudhary BA, Nadimi M, Chaudhary TK, Speir WA. Pulmonary edema due to obstructive sleep apnea. South Med J 1984; 77:499–501.
58. Morgan BJ, Denahan T, Ebert TJ. Neurocirculatory consequences of negative intrathoracic pressure vs. asphyxia during voluntary apnea. J Appl Physiol 1993; 74:2969–2975.
59. Tolle FA, Judy WV, Yu PL, Markand ON. Reduced stroke volume related to pleural pressure in obstructive sleep apnea. J Appl Physiol 1983; 55:1718–1724.
60. Chan HS, Chiu HF, Tse LK, Woo KS. Obstructive sleep apnea presenting with nocturnal angina, heart failure, and near-miss sudden death. Chest 1991; 99:1023–1025.
61. Franklin KA, Nilsson JB, Sahlin C. Sleep apnoea and nocturnal angina. Lancet 1995; 345:1085–1087.
62. Chaudhary BA, Ferguson DS, Speir WA. Pulmonary edema as a presenting feature of sleep apnea syndrome. Chest 1982; 82:122–124.
63. Bradley TD, Hall MJ, Ando SI, Floras JS. Hemodynamic effects of simulated obstructive apneas in subjects with and without heart failure. Chest 2001; 119:1827–1835.
64. Stoohs R, Guilleminault C. Cardiovascular changes associated with obstructive sleep apnea syndrome. J Appl Physiol 1992; 72:583–589.
65. Kusuoka H, Weisfeldt ML, Zweier JL, Jacobus WE, Marban E. Mechanism of early contractile failure during hypoxia in intact ferret heart: evidence for modulation of maximal Ca^{2+}-activated force by inorganic phosphate. Circ Res 1986; 59:270–282.
66. Cargill RI, Kiely DG, Lipworth BJ. Adverse effects of hypoxaemia on diastolic filling in humans. Clin Sci 1995; 89:165–169.
67. Somers VK, Mark AL, Zavala DC, Abboud FM. Contrasting effects of hypoxia and

hypercapnia on ventilation and sympathetic activity in humans. J Appl Physiol 1989; 67:2101–2106.

68. Hornyak M, Cejnar M, Elam M, Matousek M, Wallin BG. Sympathetic muscle nerve activity during sleep in man. Brain 1991; 114:1281–1295.
69. Morgan BJ, Crabtree DC, Puleo DS, Badr MS, Toiber F, Skatrud JB. Neurocirculatory consequences of abrupt change in sleep state in humans. J Appl Physiol 1996; 80: 1627–1636.
70. Hedner J, Ejnell H, Sellgren J, Hedner T, Wallin G. Is high and fluctuating muscle nerve sympathetic activity in the sleep apnoea syndrome of pathogenetic importance for the development of hypertension? J Hypertens 1988; 6(suppl):S529–S531.
71. Somers VK, Dyken ME, Skinner JL. Autonomic and hemodynamic responses and interactions during the Mueller maneuver in humans. J Appl Physiol 1989; 67:2095–2100.
72. Weiss JW, Remsburg S, Garpestad E, Ringler J, Sparrow D, Parker JA. Hemodynamic consequences of obstructive sleep apnea. Sleep 1996; 19:388–397.
73. Hung J, Whitford EG, Parsons RW, Hillman DR. Association of sleep apnoea with myocardial infarction in men. Lancet 1990; 336:261–264.
74. Galatius-Jensen S, Hansen J, Rasmussen V, Bildsoe J, Therboe M, Rosenberg J. Nocturnal hypoxaemia after myocardial infarction: association with nocturnal myocardial ischaemia and arrhythmias. Br Heart J 1994; 72:23–30.
75. Garpestad E, Parker JA, Katayama H, Lilly J, Yasuda T, Ringler J, Strauss HW, Weiss JW. Decrease in ventricular stroke volume at apnea termination is independent of oxygen desaturation. J Appl Physiol 1994; 77:1602–1608.
76. Shepard JW, Jr. Hypertension, cardiac arrhythmias, myocardial infarction, and stroke in relation to obstructive sleep apnea. Clin Chest Med 1992; 13:437–458.
77. Shepard JW, Jr., Garrison MW, Grither DA, Dolan GF. Relationship of ventricular ectopy to oxyhemoglobin desaturation in patients with obstructive sleep apnea. Chest 1985; 88:335–340.
78. Millar WP. Cardiac arrhythmias and conduction disturbances in the sleep apnea syndrome. Am J Med 1982; 73:317–321.
79. Carlson JT, Hedner J, Elam M, Ejnell H, Sellgran J, Wallin BJ. Augmented resting sympathetic nerve activity in awake patients with obstructive sleep apnea. Chest 1993; 103:1763–1768.
80. Brooks D, Horner RL, Kozar LF, Render-Teixeira CL, Phillipson EA. Obstructive sleep apnea as a cause of systemic hypertension. Evidence from a canine model. J Clin Invest 1997; 99:106–109.
81. Kaye DM, Lambert GM, Lefkovits J, Morris M, Jennings G, Esler MD. Neurochemical evidence of cardiac sympathetic activation and increased central nervous system norepinephrine turnover in severe congestive heart failure. J Am Coll Cardiol 1994; 23: 570–578.
82. Cohn JN, Levine TB, Olivary MT, Garberg V, Lura D, Francis GS, Simon AB, Rector T. Plasma norepinephrine as a guide to prognosis in patients with congestive heart failure. N Engl J Med 1984; 311:819–823.
83. Daly PA, Sole MJ. Myocardial catecholamines and the pathophysiology of heart failure. Circulation 1990; 82:I35–I43.
84. Ross JJ. Afterload mismatch and preload reserve: a conceptual framework for the analysis of ventricular function. Prog Cardiovasc Dis XVIII 1976; 18:254–264.

85. Hedner J, Ejnell H, Caidahl K. Left ventricular hypertrophy independent of hypertension in patients with obstructive sleep apnoea. J Hypertens 1990; 8:941–946.
86. Levy D, Larson MG, Vasan RS, Kannel WB, Ho KKL. The progression from hypertension to congestive heart failure. JAMA 1996; 275:1557–1562.
87. Hanly P, Sasson Z, Zuberi N, Alderson M. Ventricular function in snorers and patients with obstructive sleep apnea. Chest 1992; 102:100–105.
88. Parker JD, Brooks D, Kozar LF, Render-Teixeira CL, Horner RL, Bradley TD, Phillipson EA. Acute and chronic effects of airway obstruction on canine left ventricular performance. Am J Respir Crit Care Med 1999; 160:1888–1896.
89. Krieger J, Grucker D, Sforza E. Left ventricular ejection fraction in obstructive sleep apnea: effects of long-term treatment with nasal continuous positive airway pressure. Chest 1991; 100:917–921.
90. Lange RL, Hecht HH. The mechanism of Cheyne-Stokes respiration. J Clin Invest 1962; 41:42–52.
91. Hall MJ, Xie A, Rutherford R, Ando S, Floras JS, Bradley TD. Cycle length of periodic breathing in patients with and without heart failure. Am J Respir Crit Care Med 1996; 154:376–381.
92. Tkacova R, Hall MJ, Liu PP, Fitzgerald FS, Bradley TD. Left ventricular volume in patients with heart failure and Cheyne-Stokes respiration during sleep. Am J Respir Crit Care Med 1997; 156:1549–1555.
93. Onal E, Lopata M. Periodic breathing and the pathogenesis of occlusive sleep apneas. Am Rev Respir Dis 1982; 126:676–680.
94. Harrison TR, King CE, Calhoun JA, Harrison WG. Cheyne-Stokes respiration as the cause of paroxysmal dyspnea at the onset of sleep. Arch Intern Med 1934; 53:891–910.
95. Hanly P, Zuberi-Khokhar N. Daytime sleepiness in patients with congestive heart failure and Cheyne-Stokes respiration. Chest 1995; 107:952–958.
96. Bradley TD, Phillipson EA. Central sleep apnea. Clin Chest Med 1992; 13:493–505.
97. Khoo MC, Kronauer RE, Strohl KP, Slutsky AS. Factors inducing periodic breathing in humans: a general model. J Appl Physiol 1982; 53:644–659.
98. Skatrud JB, Dempsey JA. Interaction of sleep state and chemical stimuli in sustaining rhythmic ventilation. J Appl Physiol 1983; 55:813–822.
99. Bradley TD, Floras JS. Pathophysiologic and therapeutic implications of sleep apnea in congestive heart failure. J Card Fail 1996; 2:223–240.
100. Naughton M, Benard D, Tam A, Rutherford R, Bradley TD. Role of hyperventilation in the pathogenesis of central sleep apneas in patients with congestive heart failure. Am Rev Respir Dis 1993; 148:330–338.
101. Hanly P, Zuberi N, Gray R. Pathogenesis of Cheyne-Stokes respiration in patients with congestive heart failure. Relationship to arterial PCO_2. Chest 1993; 104:1079–1084.
102. Xie A, Rutherford R, Rankin F, Wong B, Bradley TD. Hypocapnia and increased ventilatory responsiveness in patients with idiopathic central sleep apnea. Am J Respir Crit Care Med 1995; 152:1950–1955.
103. Xie A, Wong B, Phillipson EA, Slutsky AS, Bradley TD. Interaction of hyperventilation and arousal in the pathogenesis of idiopathic central sleep apnea. Am J Respir Crit Care Med 1994; 150:489–495.
104. Lahiri S, Maret K, Sherpa MG. Dependence of high altitude sleep apnea on ventilatory sensitivity to hypoxia. Respir Physiol 1983; 52:281–301.

105. Phillipson EA. Control of breathing during sleep. Am Rev Respir Dis 1978; 118:909–939.
106. Lorenzi-Filho G, Rankin F, Bies I, Merson R, Rosenberg J, Bradley TD. Effects of inhaled CO_2 and O_2 on Cheyne-Stokes respiration in heart failure. Am J Respir Crit Care Med 1998; 157:A776.
107. Churchill ED, Cope O. The rapid shallow breathing resulting from pulmonary congestion and edema. J Exp Med 1929; 49:531–537.
108. Berssenbrugge A, Dempsey J, Iber C, Skatrud J, Wison P. Mechanisms of hypoxia-induced periodic breathing during sleep in humans. J Physiol (Lond) 1983; 343:507–524.
109. Javaheri S, Corbett WS. Association of low $PaCO_2$ with central sleep apnea and ventricular arrhythmias in ambulatory patients with stable heart failure. Ann Intern Med 1998; 128:204–207.
110. Xie A, Rankin F, Rutherford R, Bradley TD. Effects of inhaled CO_2 and added dead space on idiopathic central sleep apnea. J Appl Physiol 1997; 82:918–926.
111. Solin P, Bergin P, Richardson M, Kaye DM, Walters HE, Naughton MT. Influence of pulmonary capillary wedge pressure on central sleep apnea in heart failure. Circulation 1999; 99:1574–1579.
112. Franklin KA, Eriksson P, Sahlin C, Lundgren R. Reversal of central sleep apnea with oxygen. Chest 1997; 111:163–169.
113. Hanly PJ, Millar TW, Steljes DG, Baert R, Frais MA, Kryger MH. The effect of oxygen on respiration and sleep in patients with congestive heart failure. Ann Intern Med 1989; 111:777–782.
114. Franklin KA, Sandstrom E, Johansson G, Balfors EM. Hemodynamics, cerebral circulation, and oxygen saturation in Cheyne-Stokes respiration. J Appl Physiol 1997; 83: 1184–1191.
115. Wilcox I, Grunstein RR, Collins FL, Berthon-Jones M, Kelly DT, Sullivan CE. The role of central chemosensitivity in central apnea of heart failure. Sleep 1993; 16:S37–S38.
116. Ahmed M, Serrette C, Kryger MH, Anthonisen NR. Ventilatory instability in patients with congestive heart failure and nocturnal Cheyne-Stokes breathing. Sleep 1994; 17: 527–534.
117. Cherniack NS, Longobardo GS. Cheyne-Stokes breathing. An instability in physiologic control. N Engl J Med 1973; 288:952–957.
118. Sun SY, Wang W, Zucker IH, Schultz HD. Enhanced peripheral chemoreflex function in conscious rabbits with pacing-induced heart failure. J Appl Physiol 1999; 86:1264–1272.
119. Javaheri S. A mechanism of central sleep apnea in patients with heart failure. N Engl J Med 1999; 341:949–954.
120. Alex CG, Onal E, Lopata M. Upper airway occlusion during sleep in patients with Cheyne-Stokes respiration. Am Rev Respir Dis 1986; 133:42–45.
121. Younes M. The physiologic basis of central apnea and periodic breathing. Curr Pulmonol 1989; 10:265–326.
122. Sullivan CE, Murphy E, Kozar LF. Waking and ventilatory responses to laryngeal stimulation in sleeping dogs. J Appl Physiol 1978; 45:681–689.
123. Bradley TD, Brown IG, Zamel N, Phillipson EA, Hoffstein V. Differences in pharyngeal properties between snorers with predominantly central sleep apnea and those without sleep apnea. Am Rev Respir Dis 1987; 135:387–391.

124. Bradley TD, Brown IG, Grossman RF, Zamel N, Martinez D, Phillipson EA, Hoffstein V. Pharyngeal size in snorers, nonsnorers, and patients with obstructive sleep apnea. N Engl J Med 1986; 315:1327–1331.
125. Brown IG, Bradley TD, Phillipson EA, Zamel N, Hoffstein V. Pharyngeal compliance in snoring subjects with and without obstructive sleep apnea. Am Rev Respir Dis 1985; 132:211–215.
126. Altschule MD, Iglauer A. The effect of position on periodic breathing in chronic cardiac decompensation. N Engl J Med 1958; 259:1064–1066.
127. Brown IG, MacLean PA, Boucher R. Changes in pharyngeal cross-sectional area with posture and applications of continuous positive airway pressure in patients with obstructive sleep apnea. Am Rev Respir Dis 1987; 136:628–632.
128. Sullivan CE, Issa FG, Berthon-Jones M, Eves L. Reversal of obstructive sleep apnea by continuous positive airway pressure applied through the nares. Lancet 1981; 1:862–865.
129. Issa FG, Sullivan CE. Reversal of central sleep apnea using nasal CPAP. Chest 1986; 90:165–171.
130. Longobardo GS, Cherniack NS, Fishman AP. Cheyne-Stokes breathing produced by a model of the human respiratory system. J Appl Physiol 1966; 21:1839–1846.
131. Guyton AC, Crowell JW, Moore JW. Basic oscillating mechanism of Cheyne-Stokes breathing. Am J Physiol 1956; 187:395–398.
132. Hoffman R, Agatston A, Krieger B. Cheyne-Stokes respiration in patients recovering from acute cardiogenic pulmonary edema. Chest 1990; 97:410–412.
133. Datta AK, Shea AA, Horner RL, Guz A. The influence of induced hypocapnia and sleep on the endogenous respiratory rhythm in humans. J Physiol (Lond) 1991; 440: 17–33.
134. Lanfranchi PA, Braghiroli A, Bosimini E, Mazzuero G, Colombo R, Donner CF, Giannuzzi P. 1999. Prognostic value of nocturnal Cheyne-Stokes respiration in chronic heart failure. Circulation 1999; 99:1435–1440.
135. Yasuma F, Kozar LF, Kimoff RJ, Bradley TD, Phillipson EA. Interaction of chemical and mechanical respiratory stimuli in the arousal response to hypoxia in sleeping dogs. Am Rev Respir Dis 1991; 143:1274–1277.
136. Gleeson K, Zwillich CW, White DP. The influence of increasing ventilatory effort on arousal from sleep. Am Rev Respir Dis 1992; 72:985–992.
137. Trinder J, Merson R, Rosenberg J, Fitzgerald F, Kleiman J, Bradley TD. Interactions of ventilation, arousals and blood pressure oscillations during Cheyne-Stokes respiration in patients with heart failure. Am J Respir Crit Care Med 2000; 162:808–813.
138. Findley LJ, Blackburn MR, Goldberger AL, Mandell AJ. Apneas and oscillation of cardiac ectopy in Cheyne-Stokes breathing during sleep. Am Rev Respir Dis 1984; 130:937–939.
139. Francis GS. Development of arrhythmias in the patient with congestive heart failure: pathophysiology, prevalence and prognosis. Am J Cardiol 1986; 57:3B–7B.
140. Goldman S, Johnson G, Cohn JN, Cintron G, Smith R, Francis G. Mechanim of death in heart failure. The vasodilator-heart failure trials. Circulation 1993; 87:VI-24–VI-31.
141. Naughton MT, Bradley TD. Sleep apnea in congestive heart failure. Clin Chest Med 1998; 19:99–113.
142. Dark DS, Pingleton SK, Kerby GR, Crabb JE, Gollub SB, Glatter TR, Dunn MI. Breathing pattern abnormalities and arterial oxygen desaturation during sleep in the

congestive heart failure syndrome. Improvement following medical therapy. Chest 1987; 91:833–836.

143. Granton JT, Naughton MT, Benard DC, Liu PP, Goldstein RS, Bradley TD. CPAP improves inspiratory muscle strength in patients with heart failure and central sleep apnea. Am J Respir Crit Care Med 1996; 153:277–282.
144. Tkacova R, Liu PP, Naughton MT, Bradley TD. Effect of continuous positive airway pressure on mitral regurgitant fraction and atrial natriuretic peptide in patients with heart failure. J Am Coll Cardiol 1997; 30:739–745.
145. Javaheri S, Parker TJ, Wexler L, Liming JD, Lindower P, Roselle GA. Effect of theophylline on sleep-disordered breathing in heart failure. N Engl J Med 1996; 335:562–567.

14

Neuroendocrine Changes in Sleep Apnea

RONALD R. GRUNSTEIN

Royal Prince Alfred Hospital
Sydney, New South Wales, Australia

I. Introduction

Human neuroendocrine and metabolic physiology is often influenced by behavioral states of sleep and wakefulness. Extensive research in this area has flourished due to the development of better assays of endocrine function, paralleling the growth of sleep research stimulated by polysomnography and noninvasive breathing measurement. Data have accumulated on the relative influences of circadian phase or sleep state on hormone secretion, energy expenditure, or end-organ targets of neuroendocrine output. Plasma levels of pituitary and other hormones also spontaneously fluctuate across the 24-h period. These endocrine rhythms have often been labeled either sleep related (when the predominant change in fluctuation is nocturnal) or circadian (when the rhythm appears to be regulated by an internal clock rather than periodic changes in the external environment). The predominant influences are intrinsic circadian rhythmicity and sleep, which interact to varying degrees to produce the characteristic 24-h rhythm of each hormone. Other factors such as meals and exercise may also cause some changes in hormone level (1).

The recognition of breathing disorders in sleep has paralleled the advances in understanding of neuroendocrine biology. However, despite the existence of sleep apnea as a unique mix of sleep fragmentation and hypoxic exposure, little is known about the interrelationships between endocrine and metabolic pathophysiology and sleep apnea. There are a number of areas of common interest. Epidemiological features of sleep apnea include marked male preponderance and an association with obesity and advancing age (2,3). Sleep apnea has also been linked to impaired life quality, sexual dysfunction in adults, poor growth in children, and endocrine conditions such as acromegaly, hypothyroidism, and Cushing's disease. Hormonal treatments such as progesterone have been used therapeutically in sleep apnea, while other treatments such as growth hormone or testosterone may worsen sleep-disordered breathing. Upper body obesity is characteristic in sleep apnea patients, and this type of adiposity is associated with a wide range of metabolic abnormalities, which promote morbidity and mortality (4). One can speculate whether there are links between altered hypothalamic function due to sleep fragmentation and/or hypoxia and positive energy balance in obese patients with sleep apnea.

Sleep apnea may interact with endocrine rhythms via a number of mechanisms. First, repetitive apneas will cause sleep fragmentation and disorganization of sleep stages and cycles. Second, hypoxia may have direct central effects on neurotransmitters (5), which, in turn, will affect hypothalamic-pituitary hormone production. Third, sudden arousal from sleep may produce a central "stress" response leading to hormonal changes (6). Fourth, daytime sleep episodes may interact with daytime hormone rhythms. Finally, all of the above factors may interact and lead to changes in the central control of sleep and endocrine rhythms.

This chapter is aimed at providing a brief neurobiological background to the potential links between endocrine function and sleep apnea, a review of existing data, and some speculation on future avenues of research.

II. Sleep Apnea and Neuroendocrine Changes: Confounding by Other Variables

Assessment of the influence of sleep apnea on endocrine function requires close consideration of confounding factors such as age, obesity, and other associated diseases such as chronic lung disease. Some studies of endocrine function in sleep apnea have ignored this effect. Advancing age has clear effects on many endocrine parameters. However, studies of endocrine function in aging should be interpreted with caution as they may be confounded by age-related diseases (7). Obesity, particularly central adiposity, may influence endocrine function (8). Some of these hormonal changes are reversible with weight reduction, suggesting that a common underlying disorder, for example, in the hypothalamus, may lead to both endocrine dysfunction and obesity. Confounding can be controlled for with multivariate analysis or by treatments that eliminate the disease process, e.g., weight reduction for obesity or CPAP for sleep apnea. However, in analyzing the confounding effect of obesity in sleep apnea, weight reduction may not answer the question as both sleep apnea and obesity could resolve in parallel.

Additional confounding factors include a direct effect of hypoxia on the neuroendocrine axis or even a stress effect of repeated asphyxia in sleep. Hypoxia has long been known to influence certain endocrine parameters, but these studies have been performed in fetal or adult animal models, altitude simulations, or hypocapnic hypoxia in exercise studies (5,9). Most have been performed without measurement of arterial O_2 saturation, and typically the CO_2 level has not been controlled. Studies simulating the type of repetitive hypoxia seen in sleep apnea are unknown. The effects of hypercapnic hypoxic exposure have also not been researched.

The influence of stressors on endocrine function are controversial. The classic "fear and flight" hormones, cortisol and catecholamines, typically rise in response to stress, as do growth hormone and prolactin (10). Testosterone tends to fall following exposure to stressful stimuli (11). Many different endocrine responses to a variety of stressful stimuli have been recorded (6,11,12). There are many disparate views on what constitutes a stressful stimulus as well as significant individual variation in these responses. Most human chronic stress studies have demonstrated gradual adaptation to stimuli. Intermittently chronic stress has rarely been investigated in humans, and virtually all studies occur in the awake patient. In one study we examined the response of patients with sleep apnea who had been on long-term continuous positive airway pressure (CPAP) treatment to sudden withdrawal of this therapy (6). We postulated that sudden reexposure to asphyxia in patients who had lost adaptation to such a stimulus would have produced an increase in catecholamines and adrenocorticotropic hormone (ACTH). However, no such response occurred, suggesting either that the stimulus was not enough to produce an increase in stress hormones or that years of untreated sleep apnea had led to permanent adaptation to the stress.

III. Growth Hormone and Sleep Apnea

A. Growth Hormone Secretion and Sleep

Growth hormone (GH) secretion is closely linked with sleep (13–15) and is therefore of interest when examining the potential neuroendocrine consequences of sleep apnea. GH is a polypeptide released by the anterior pituitary and whose major known function is to stimulate growth (16,17). GH may act directly on tissues, but in most body organs GH acts through an intermediate mediator somatomedin C, now known as IGF-1 (insulin-like growth factor 1), which is synthesized in the liver and other organs in response to GH (18). GH secretion from the pituitary is regulated by two hypothalamic hormones released into the pituitary portal circulation: GHRH (growth hormone–releasing hormone), which stimulates GH output, and somatostatin, which is inhibitory. The control of GH release is mediated through several long and short predominantly negative feedback loops involving GH itself and IGF-1 (17,18).

As GH is secreted in a pulsatile fashion and has a relatively short serum half-life (22 min), a single random GH level provides little information on the 24-h GH production of an individual (18). However, a single IGF-1 level has a high level of correlation with 24-h mean plasma GH and can be used clinically as an index of GH status (18). GHRH has been used pharmacologically as a test of the ability of the pituitary to produce GH in response to stimuli (17). Analogs of somatostatin have been used to inhibit GH production in acromegaly, a state of GH excess (18). These hypothalamic hormones themselves are under the excitatory and inhibitory control of several neurotransmitters including dopamine, serotonin, and norepinephrine (α-adrenergic receptors).

GH secretion is pulsatile and episodic, but, unlike many other hormones, it does not have a dominant independent circadian rhythm. The first studies measuring GH during polygraphically monitored sleep indicated that there was a consistent relationship between GH secretion and slow-wave sleep (SWS) (19,20). Though subsequent investigators have challenged this observation (21,22), recent studies, using more frequent sampling to better characterize GH secretory bursts have found a close association between GH and SWS (13–15). Although the presence of SWS is not obligatory for GH secretion, Van Cauter and coworkers observed that 70% of GH pulses occurring during sleep were associated with SWS (14,15). Another group using 30-s sampling observed maximal GH concentrations within minutes of SWS onset (13). Other work has shown that drugs that enhance SWS such as ritanserin (23) or gammahydroxybuytrate (24) increase GH secretion. GH pulses are closely related to delta wave electroencephalographic activity (25). Experimental arousals during SWS will reduce the magnitude of GHRH-induced GH secretory pulses (15).

Studies of the GH-sleep association are hampered by the lack of an animal model, as GH secretion in sleep is a consistent finding only in humans. Interestingly, only rhesus monkeys with well-developed non–rapid eye movement–rapid eye movement (NREM-REM) sleep cycles had GH secretory peaks in sleep, while animals with fragmented sleep tended to have less secretion at night (26). Humans with fragmented sleep also tend to have less GH secretion. One example of this is aging, when sleep becomes more fragmented, SWS decreases, and GH secretion in sleep diminishes (27). Twenty-four-hour growth hormone production and IGF-1 levels are lower in healthy elderly men compared to younger male subjects. Patients with narcolepsy, although characterized by excessive daytime sleepiness, often have fragmented sleep, and GH secretion occurs irregularly without any relation to sleep cycles (28). Children with psychosocial dwarfism exhibit a decrease in SWS (29).

In obesity, GH production is decreased in both 24-h mean levels and in response to stimuli (8,30). This reduction in GH output is related to increased fat mass rather than weight. Most studies suggest that the reduced GH output in obesity is reversed with weight loss (8,30). IGF-1 levels are also reduced in obesity (31,32).

B. Evidence for Altered GH Secretion in OSA

In a cross-sectional study of 225 men undergoing sleep studies (31), IGF-1 levels (Fig. 1) were reduced in men with sleep apnea, and this was related to the severity

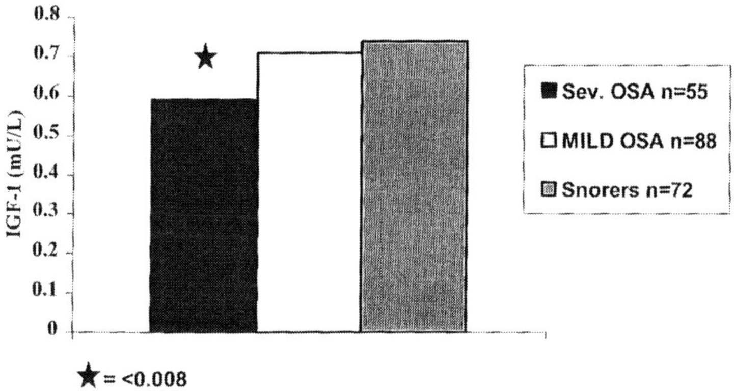

Figure 1 Insulin-like growth factor-1 (IGF-1) levels in patients with severe obstructive sleep apnea (sev. OSA), mild obstructive sleep apnea (mild OSA), and snorers. Severe OSA patients have significantly reduced IGF-1 levels ($p < 0.008$).

of the apnea (both desaturations per hour and minimum oxygen saturation in sleep). The decreased IGF-1 levels were also related to aging and coexisting obesity but also independently to sleep apnea. The role of sleep apnea in these cross-sectional results was confirmed by the reversal of these reduced IGF-1 levels with 3 months of nasal CPAP treatment without any significant accompanying weight change (31) (Fig. 2). As circulating IGF-1 levels are dependent on GH secretion, these data suggested that the lower plasma IGF-1 levels reflected reduced GH secretion.

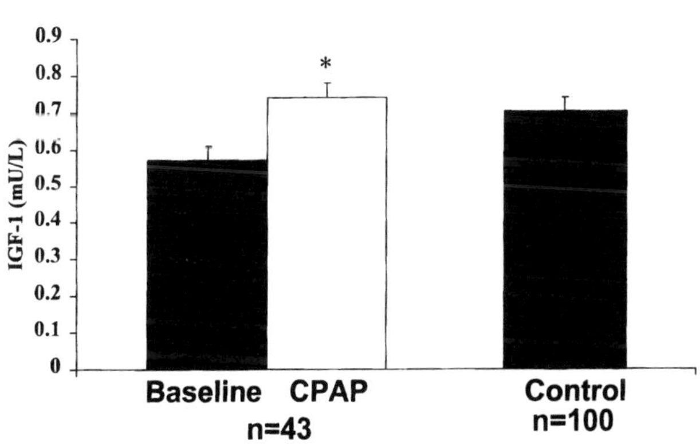

Figure 2 Insulin-like growth factor-1 (IGF-1) levels in 43 men with sleep apnea before (black bar) and after (white bar) 3 months on nasal continuous positive airway pressure (CPAP). These results are contrasted with 100 men of similar age used to establish normative values of IGF-1. $*p < 0.05$.

There are a number of possible reasons why GH secretion may be reduced in sleep apnea. Sleep is fragmented and SWS is markedly reduced or absent in sleep apnea (33), and this may cause a reduction in sleep-entrained GH secretion. Growth hormone concentrations are virtually absent in severe sleep apnea (34–38). However, as discussed previously, reduced GH secretion in sleep apnea may be explained by coexisting central obesity. The best evidence supporting a role for sleep apnea in reducing GH secretion in sleep is provided by studies measuring GH concentrations before and after elimination of sleep apnea without change in confounding variables. Early case studies suggested that both CPAP (36) and tracheostomy (39) led to an increase in GH levels. Other studies measuring GH during sleep pre- and post-CPAP provide further evidence of an increase in sleep-related GH secretion with correction of the sleep-breathing abnormality only (37,38,40,41).

Recently, we compared GH concentrations at baseline, after 1 week of an oral antiandrogen drug, flutamide, for sleep apnea and again after CPAP (38). There was no difference in sleep, breathing, or hormonal variables between the two baseline studies and flutamide. On CPAP treatment, apneic breathing and shifts between sleep stages were markedly reduced, and the average length of SWS epochs were increased. Compared with the baseline studies, there were significant increases in GH concentrations and pulse frequency on CPAP treatment. After CPAP treatment, GH pulses were 11 times more likely to be preceded by an epoch of SWS compared with the baseline (Fig. 3). There was no weight change in the patient explaining these results (38).

These findings suggested that pulsatile GH secretion is facilitated by periods of uninterrupted SWS on CPAP treatment. Fragmentation of SWS by apnea-induced arousals may reduce both the frequency and magnitude of the pulse of GH associated

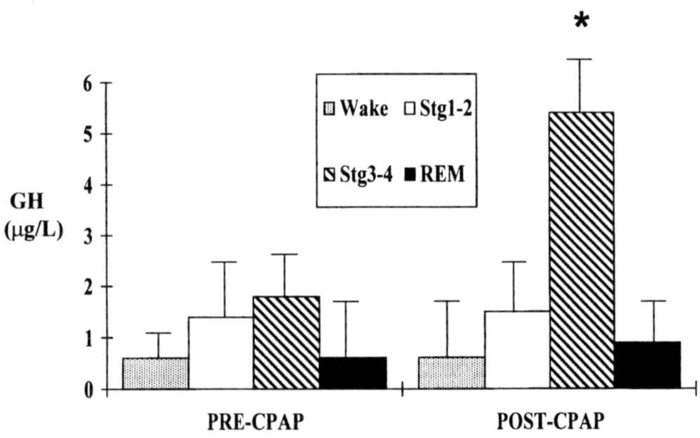

Figure 3 Increased GH concentrations in stage 3–4 sleep compared with other sleep stages in 9 men on nasal CPAP. There is no difference in GH concentrations in different sleep stages during two baseline sleep studies. $*p < 0.05$.

with SWS. Support for this hypothesis is provided by experimental data in healthy volunteers. GH secretion in response to GHRH infusion is enhanced at night particularly in SWS as opposed to REM when the response to GHRH is similar to wakefulness (15). Arousals following GHRH infusion interrupt the normal GH response, which is restored following resumption of sleep (15). As the pulsatile secretion of GH results from the interaction of GHRH and somatostatin at the level of the somatotrope, it is certainly possible that repetitive arousal in sleep apnea may impair the GH response to endogenous bursts of GHRH into the pituitary portal circulation. Interestingly, patients with fibromyalgia are characterized by intrusions of alpha-EEG (awake) activity fragmenting slow-wave sleep, and low GH concentrations have been reported in this condition (42).

The biological significance of reduced GH and IGF-1 levels in sleep apnea is unclear. Severe sleep apnea in the pediatric population is characterized by failure to thrive, short stature, and other growth disturbances that can be corrected by elimination of the upper airway obstruction (39,43). It is possible that impaired GH secretion may play a role in these observations. Detailed studies of GH secretion in otherwise healthy children with sleep apnea are lacking. Waters and coworkers (41) examined GH secretion in sleep in 19 patients with achondroplasia with a mean age of 11 years. Five subjects were restudied after treatment for OSA. In this group of five subjects, improved respiratory distress index and reduced sleep state transitions were not associated with significant changes in GH secretion rate by sleep stage. However, GH secretion peak during the first 2 h of SWS was initially absent, appearing only after treatment of OSA. Other workers have speculated on other mechanisms for poor growth, including increased energy expenditure (44).

Second, a direct effect of intermittent hypoxia on hypothalamic or other central regulation of endocrine rhythms is possible, though we found no independent effect of awake pO_2 or pCO_2 on endocrine function (31). Cornil and coworkers (45) also failed to find an effect of acute and chronic respiratory failure in patients with chronic lung disease on GH secretion. Nevertheless, intermittent severe hypoxemia may well have a different effect centrally than milder sustained hypoxia. Finally, most patients with sleep apnea exhibit daytime sleepiness and decreased activity during the day. Exercise is a stimulus to GH secretion (8). It is possible that reduced exercise and activity in sleep apnea may lead to reduced daytime pulses of GH and decreased IGF-1. With restoration of normal alertness with nasal CPAP, IGF-1 levels could increase. Nevertheless, the precise neurotransmitter changes caused by sleep apnea and their relationship to GH regulation by somatostatin and GHRH secretion remain to be elucidated. The location of the defect in GH secretion is either hypothalamic or pituitary, as tests of pituitary GH reserve, such as the GHRH stimulation test, have not been performed in sleep apnea. However, a hypothalamic origin for reduced secretion is more likely in view of preserved gonadotrophin reserve in sleep apnea (46). Moreover, the potential effects of sleep apnea such as sleep fragmentation are more likely to have effects at the hypothalamic rather than the pituitary level.

C. Possible Implications of Reduced GH Levels in Sleep Apnea

The potential effects of reduced GH concentrations in adults with severe sleep apnea are entirely speculative. The availability of human recombinant GH has permitted detailed clinical studies of the role of GH in adulthood (47,48). These studies, in general, involve the use of recombinant GH in healthy volunteers, healthy elderly, or patients with adult-onset GH deficiency and indicate that the reduced GH concentrations observed in adult sleep apnea have potential clinical sequelae.

These sequelae can be grouped into four main areas: quality of life, body composition, and bone and mineral metabolism. Although sleep fragmentation and related cognitive problems arguably have a dominant role in the impaired quality of life seen in patients with sleep apnea, the reported impaired psychological well-being in growth hormone deficiency (47,48) may also provide a potential mechanism. GH influences central neurotransmitter release (47,48) and thus may affect mood and cognition. GH-deficient adults also have decreased muscle mass and increased body fat, particularly in the central body or visceral regions (47,48). Synthetic GH administration to such patients has positive anabolic effects with increased muscle mass and reduced visceral adipose tissue (47,48). Patients with OSA are typically centrally obese (4), and it is possible that impaired GH secretion in sleep apnea may be involved in maintenance of visceral obesity in these patients. In addition, a number of studies have strongly suggested that GH deficiency is associated with accelerated aging, premature atherosclerosis, and increased cardiovascular mortality (8,47–49). Similar adverse health outcomes occur in sleep apnea, raising the possibility of an etiological role for reduced GH secretion.

In conclusion, sleep apnea is associated with reduced GH concentrations possibly due to less SWS, though an additional effect of intermittent hypoxia cannot be fully excluded. Growth hormone concentrations rise following nasal CPAP treatment. Further research is required to assess the relationship between this rise in GH concentration and health outcomes.

IV. Sleep Apnea and Acromegaly

A. Introduction

Acromegaly is a condition of GH excess in adults characterized by the insidious development of coarsening of facial features, bony proliferation, and soft tissue swelling (18). It is usually secondary to a GH-producing pituitary adenoma, which may be either a micro- or macroadenoma. Rarely, the GH excess commences prior to puberty and closure of the epiphyses, and then the condition is termed gigantism. It occurs with equal frequency in both sexes with a prevalence of 38–60 cases per million. The clinical features may be due to the local effects of an expanding pituitary mass in addition to the effects of excess GH secretion, which include disordered somatic cell growth and insulin resistance (18). The mortality of untreated or partially treated acromegaly is about double the expected rate in healthy subjects matched for age (50). Acromegaly was first described as a clinical entity by Marie in 1886. Ten years later, Roxburgh and Collis (51) described daytime sleepiness and Chappell and Booth (52) observed upper airway obstruction as features of acromegaly but the association between sleep apnea and acromegaly was only described 80 years later (53).

B. Prevalence

Sleep-disordered breathing is extremely common in acromegaly. Earlier studies were hampered by small patient numbers, lack of information on patient selection, as well as limitations in the extent and intensity of monitoring during sleep. Prevalence estimates for sleep apnea in acromegaly in these studies varied from 20 to 40% (54–57). More recent studies have revealed much higher rates of disease. In our studies in Sydney (58), we investigated 63 patients with acromegaly consisting of two groups. Group A (38 patients) were patients referred because of the known diagnosis of acromegaly and a clinical suspicion of sleep apnea. Twenty-five patients (Group B) were referred consecutively from a neuroendocrine clinic at another hospital. Overall, 59 of the 63 patients snored heavily and 50 had more than 5 apneas per hour (Fig. 4). The prevalence of acromegaly has been estimated at between 38 and 60 cases per million (59). As the population base for our sleep disorders center is 5 million people, we estimate there should be 200–300 patients with acromegaly in our referral area. Therefore, our patient group consists of over 20% of that number. Even in our subset of consecutive referrals from another institution where referral was not for sleep apnea symptoms (Group B), 60% of these patients had sleep apnea. Assuming there are 300 patients with acromegaly in our referral base and we found

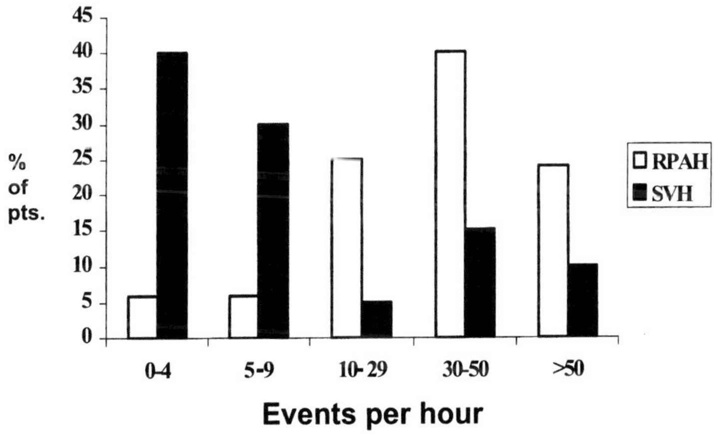

Figure 4 Frequency distribution of sleep-disordered breathing in 53 patients with acromegaly measured by respiratory disturbance index in events/hour. Thirty-three patients were referred to one hospital (RPAH) for clinical suspicion of sleep apnea, 20 consecutive patients with acromegaly from endocrine clinic of another hospital (SVH) with no referral bias.

at least 50 with sleep apnea, then the lowest possible prevalence of sleep apnea in acromegaly is 20% (58). Almost all of our patients were noted to have heavy snoring.

In a Finnish case-control study, Pelttari and coworkers (60) compared the prevalence of sleep apnea in treated acromegaly with a community sample using the static-charged bed respiratory screening device. They found that 10 of their 11 patients had sleep apnea (91%) compared with 29.4% of the general population. In the only other large study of sleep apnea prevalence, Rosenow and coworkers (61) studied 54 patients with treated acromegaly from a larger sample of 100 patients. They excluded patients with previously known sleep apnea. Despite these exclusion criteria, 39% of these remaining 54 patients had sleep apnea. Treatment of acromegaly may also have reduced prevalence as well as the limited monitoring techniques used in the study.

In our acromegaly patient group, sleep apnea was associated with increasing age and tended to be more common in males and females over 50. Obesity does not appear to be a predisposing factor to sleep apnea in acromegaly (58,60). Increases in body mass index in acromegaly may be due to increased muscle mass rather than the increased body fat typically seen in obesity (18).

C. Etiology of Central and Obstructive Sleep Apnea in Acromegaly

Upper airway obstruction due to soft tissue swelling was first reported in 1986 (52). The first reports of the association of sleep apnea with acromegaly suggested that macroglossia was an important etiological factor in producing sleep apnea by narrowing the hypopharynx and collapsing backward in sleep (55). However, endoscopy during apneic periods (62) revealed no posterior movement of the tongue, suggesting that macroglossia was not the primary factor in upper airway obstruction. In this report, primary pharyngeal collapse into the laryngeal vestibule was observed. Attempted treatment with a nasopharyngeal airway past the tongue did not prevent apnea. More recently, Pelttari (60) observed no dynamic narrowing behind the tongue on nasopharyngoscopy.

We have observed a high rate of central apnea in patients with acromegaly (58) (34% of the total group of patients with sleep apnea). Others (54), using full sleep studies, reported that two of their three patients with sleep apnea and acromegaly had predominantly or exclusively central apnea. A waxing and waning central apnea pattern of breathing on static charge sensitive bed studies has also been reported as more common in acromegaly as opposed to typical upper airway obstruction (59).

The high prevalence of central apnea in acromegaly suggests that abnormalities of central respiratory control are involved. This has been supported by our finding that patients with central sleep apnea had significantly lower awake arterial carbon dioxide levels than those with obstructive apnea (58,63), and increased ventilatory responsiveness was observed in the central group (63). Central apnea occurs in association with a wide range of disorders and many potential mechanisms have been described, including disordered central respiratory control (63–66). The precise cause in acromegaly is unclear, but there are possible hypotheses.

Somatostatin immunoreactive nerve cell bodies and terminals have been observed in areas of the medulla involved in respiratory control (67,68). Kalia et al. reported that somatostatin given intracisternally to the rat leads to a rapid inhibition of breathing and apnea (67). Thus, it is possible that defects of central somatostatin pathways will lead to both unrestrained GH secretion (acromegaly) and altered respiratory control (sleep apnea) (63).

Another possible mechanism is that elevated GH or IGF-1 affects central respiratory control, either directly or indirectly, by altering metabolic rate, inducing central apnea. This is supported by the correlation between GH hypersecretion and prevalence of central apnea (58,63). Cardiac failure also induces central apnea (64) and is part of the end stage of acromegaly. In our series we had one patient with left ventricular failure who was greatly disabled by breathlessness. Somatostatin analog treatment was commenced, leading to a rapid improvement in breathlessness and reduction in central apnea without change in left ventricular function. This suggests that heart failure is not the mechanism of central apnea in acromegaly. In fact, cardiac failure was considered a possible explanation in only two of our patients, as none of the other 12 with central apnea had evidence of cardiac disease. Interestingly, apparent central apneas have been observed in beagles exposed to medroxyprogesterone, which in turn causes GH increases and an acromegaly-like condition (69).

Our observations emphasize that whatever the mechanism of central apnea in acromegaly, it is clear that the association between apnea and acromegaly is not simply the result of an airway that is mechanically narrowed by macroglossia and soft tissue swelling. It is unknown whether the increasing clinical use of GH in various patient groups or illicit use of GH in athletes leads to sleep apnea. We observed one case of a child with Turner's syndrome developing sleep apnea after GH (unpublished observation), and others have reported (70) four children developing sleep apnea (two obstructive, two mixed) after GH administration.

D. Disease Activity in Acromegaly and Sleep Apnea

In view of the morbidity and mortality of acromegaly, it is important to define active and inactive (cured) disease. High circulating IGF-1 and GH levels reflect increased GH production and therefore disease activity. Studies describing "cure" following pituitary surgery often use inadequate criteria of disease inactivity (18,71). True cure involves observing a physiological 24-h GH secretion, normal IGF-1 levels, and normal GH responses to glucose. Even in patients with acromegaly and normal IGF-1 and GH profiles, GH secretory patterns are still different from normals (71).

Most studies have observed persisting sleep apnea despite treatment of acromegaly by pituitary surgery. We have found no correlation between disease activity and sleep apnea (58). There were no significant differences in mean GH and IGF-1 levels in patients with and without sleep apnea. There was no relationship between severity of sleep apnea and IGF-1 level. Moreover, four of the five patients who had normal IGF-1 and GH concentrations were found to have sleep apnea. Of the

23 patients with detailed 24-h GH secretory profiles, 16 had sleep apnea (2 predominantly central and 14 predominantly obstructive). In this subgroup with more extensive GH measurements, no significant differences in mean GH and GH pulsatility were found between patients with and without sleep apnea. In contrast, Rosenow has reported lower GH levels in patients with milder sleep apnea (61).

At present it is not known what proportion of patients with both sleep apnea and acromegaly will have complete resolution of their sleep apnea after cure of acromegaly. This will require careful prospective studies accurately monitoring true cure of acromegaly. However, it is clear that sleep apnea does occur in cured acromegaly. The combination of inactive acromegaly and sleep apnea may occur for a number of reasons. Firstly, sleep apnea is a common disorder and may be coincident to acromegaly in patients with other risk factors for sleep apnea. Second, it may take a long time following normalization of growth hormone secretion for effects of acromegaly to resolve, or there may be permanent effects on upper airway function or sleep-breathing regulation.

E. Disease Activity and Central Sleep Apnea

Although we found no relationship between disease activity and sleep apnea, our work has uncovered an important new finding in the link between acromegaly and sleep-disordered breathing (63). As mentioned above, many of our patients had central sleep apnea, and we found that these patients had a much higher IGF-1 and fasting GH levels compared to patients with obstructive apnea (Fig. 5).

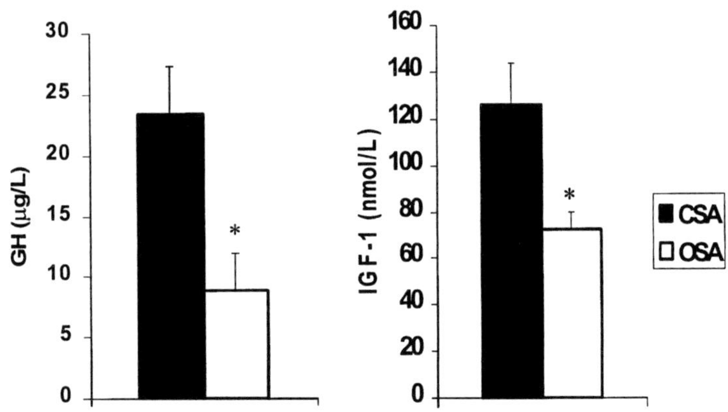

Figure 5 Random growth hormone (GH) and insulin-like growth factor-1 (IGF-1) levels in patients with central (n = 14, black bars, CSA) and obstructive (n = 29, white bars, OSA) sleep apnea. CSA patients have higher levels of GH ($p < 0.001$) and IGF-1 ($p < 0.01$) these than those with OSA. *$p < 0.05$.

F. Somatostatin Analogue (Octreotide) in Sleep Apnea in Acromegaly

Somatostatin, although the main inhibitor of GH secretion, is not effective in acromegaly because of its short serum half-life (18). The newly available long-acting somatostatin analog (SMS 201-995 or octreotide) inhibits GH secretion and is of proven value in the treatment of acromegaly. One report of its effect on sleep apnea in a patient with acromegaly (72) observed a 50% reduction in apnea frequency after 6 days of use. However, there was also a theoretical concern that octreotide could worsen sleep apnea due to the inhibitory effect of somatostatin on respiration (67,68). We investigated the 6-month, stepwise incremental use of octreotide in 19 patients with active acromegaly (73). A 50% decrease occurred in the respiratory disturbance index, and a 40% decrease occurred in total apnea time. Patients reported marked reduction of daytime somnolence and increased feeling of well-being in keeping with the improvement in sleep apnea. A parallel decrease was noted in mean levels of GH and IGF-1. However, no correlation was noted between the decrease in the total amount of sleep time spent in apnea and the decrease in growth hormone levels. The residual respiratory disturbance index after 6 months of treatment was similar in patients who improved, regardless of whether or not biochemical remission (IGF-1 < 35 nmol/L) occurred (73) (Fig. 6).

It is clear that there is no direct relationship between the degree of GH hypersecretion and reduction in apnea. This is not surprising in view of the multifactorial

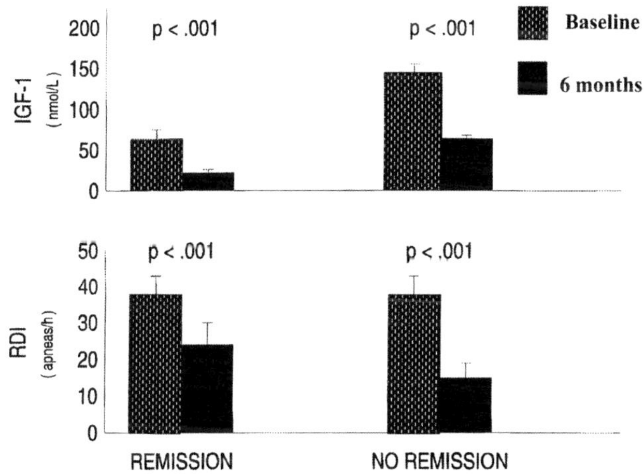

Figure 6 Respiratory disturbance index (RDI) and insulin-like growth factor-1 (IGF-1) in 19 patients with sleep apnea and acromegaly treated with octreotide. Patients are divided into biochemical remission (IGF-1 < 35 nmol/L) and no remission groups. The residual respiratory disturbance index after 6 months of treatment was similar in patients who improved, regardless of whether or not biochemical remission occurred.

etiology of sleep apnea. Acromegaly may induce permanent changes in upper airway structure or control, and this may not simply be changed by GH reduction. It is important to follow up patients with acromegaly in case ongoing therapy with CPAP is needed. Treatment with CPAP in this group in often difficult. Large noses and facial changes make CPAP mask fit a problem. Oily skin secondary to hyperhydrosis (18) may also lead to rapid turnover in mask cushions.

G. Morbidity, Mortality of Acromegaly, and Sleep Apnea

The adverse health risks of both acromegaly and sleep apnea are well established. Both disorders are associated with an increased risk of hypertension (18,74,75). In acromegaly the blood pressure level is sometimes reduced by successful transsphenoidal surgery. One postulated mechanism for hypertension in acromegaly is sodium and water retention secondary to GH overproduction (18).

We have found strong links between hypertension and sleep apnea in our patients with acromegaly, suggesting that sleep apnea may be another important mechanism causing hypertension (58). Over 50% of our patients with both acromegaly and sleep apnea had hypertension. All patients who did not have sleep apnea were normotensive. Patients who were hypertensive had significantly higher respiratory disturbance indices and greater degree of sleep hypoxemia than those who were normotensive. Mean 24-h GH, IGF-1, and degree of obesity were not significantly different in those with hypertension compared to those without hypertension. Using multiple regression, both respiratory disturbance index and age were found to be independent predictors of hypertension (58).

Somnolence has long been recognized as part of the clinical spectrum of acromegaly. Although sleep apnea is the most likely cause, a direct effect of increased GH in promoting sleep and sleepiness has been suggested (74). Alternatively, sleepiness in the absence of sleep apnea may be due to effects of radiotherapy (75). Wright et al. (50) reviewed the causes of death in patients with acromegaly at four London hospitals and found an excess of deaths due to cardiovascular and respiratory causes. They commented, "the excess of deaths due to respiratory disease was an unexpected finding for which there was no obvious explanation." This finding was inexplicable, as there is no apparent excess of chronic lung disease in acromegaly. Lung function is usually normal or supernormal. With our new understanding of the high prevalence of sleep apnea in acromegaly, it is likely that this is the mechanism of deaths at that time attributed to respiratory disease. Another potential link is sleep apnea and upper airway obstruction complicating anesthesia in these patients (76). One recent Swedish report of deaths in acromegaly found 5 postoperative deaths out of 62 total consecutive deaths in patients with acromegaly (59).

V. Sex Hormones and Sleep Apnea

A. The Hypothalamic-Pituitary-Gonadal Axis

Human sexual and reproductive function involves a complex interaction between neural and endocrine events. In humans, pituitary-gonadal function is regulated by the feedback effects of gonadal steroid hormones (progesterones, estrogens, and androgens) and by the hypothalamus (77). The hypothalamus releases luteinizing hormone–releasing hormone (LHRH) under the influence of central neurotransmitters and the feedback of pituitary and gonadal hormones. In response to LHRH, the pituitary releases luteinizing hormone (LH) and follicle-stimulating hormone (FSH). These peptides, in turn, influence the gonads to secrete testosterone (testes) and estrogen and progesterone (ovaries). This very simplistic outline deliberately ignores the role of organs such as the adrenals in sex hormone regulation.

In patients with hypogonadism due to gonadal damage, LH and FSH levels are elevated with decreased gonadal hormone levels. In central lesions, LH and FSH levels do not increase despite reduced gonadal hormone levels. An example of this is the castrated male. LH and FSH levels are high with testosterone levels greatly reduced. In a man with a large pituitary tumor destroying gonadotropin-producing cells, LH and FSH levels are low, as is the testosterone level. Hypothalamic and pituitary lesions can be differentiated by measuring the pituitary response to administered LHRH.

Higher estrogen, decreased total testosterone, and sex hormone–binding globulin (SHBG) levels occur in obesity. The concentration of free testosterone is normal. In massively obese men (>250% above ideal body weight) there can be a decrease in the free testosterone level in spite of the decrease in the sex hormone–binding globulin (78).

Sleep also influences sex hormone levels. LH and testosterone secretion is augmented by sleep (79,80). Testosterone levels fall with prolonged physical stress and sleep deprivation in military exercises (81).

B. Androgens and Sleep Apnea

Low testosterone levels have been reported in men with sleep apnea (82). In our cross-sectional study of 225 men, lower plasma free and total testosterone and SHBG levels were observed in men with sleep apnea. Hormone levels were related to the severity of the sleep apnea (31). No abnormality in prolactin levels were found. The degree of suppression of hormone level by sleep apnea was independent of age, degree of obesity, and presence of awake hypoxemia and hypercapnia. Testosterone levels increase with treatment of sleep apnea using nasal CPAP or even successful uvulopalatopharyngoplasty (31,82).

These androgen abnormalities in sleep apnea (decreased SHBG and free and total testosterone) are qualitatively, as well as quantitatively, distinct from those reported in aging (increased SHBG, decreased free and total testosterone) and obesity (decreased SHBG and total testosterone, normal free testosterone). Importantly, despite the fall in plasma free and total testosterone levels, there was no increase in basal plasma gonadotropin (LH, FSH) levels. These findings, together with the retention of pituitary sensitivity to exogenous gonadotropin-releasing hormone (GNRH) in sleep apnea (46), strongly point to a hypothalamic abnormality as the cause of the fall in testosterone levels. This explanation would be similar to the postulated level of the dysfunction of the GH-IGF-1 axis in sleep apnea. The lack of change in plasma LH levels does not imply that LH secretion is entirely normal in men with sleep apnea, since LH is secreted in an intermittent fashion (79). It is certainly possible that pulsatile LH secretion is abnormal in sleep apnea, but no published data are available.

The potential causes of this hypothalamic abnormality are essentially similar to those involved in reduced GH secretion. Testosterone levels are significantly reduced by sleep deprivation and fragmentation (83). Therefore, sleep fragmentation in sleep apnea may lead to disruption of sleep entrained rhythms in LH and testosterone. Hypoxemia in sleep apnea may be involved because, unlike GH, there are several reports of low sex steroid levels in chronic airflow limitation in studies with small patient numbers (84). In other, larger studies (31), the apparent effects of awake hypoxemia and impaired lung function were entirely accounted for by sleep hypoxemia. It is possible that the sexual dysfunction reported in sleep apnea may be mediated by the sex hormone changes seen in sleep-disordered breathing. The low testosterone levels may also interact with low IGF-1 levels and impair anabolism. Androgens may exacerbate sleep apnea (see below), and it is possible that the fall in androgen levels may be part of an adaptive homeostatic mechanism to reduce sleep-disordered breathing.

Few data are available on sex hormone levels in women with sleep apnea. Mohamed et al. (85) found higher androgen levels in four women with sleep apnea compared with controls, but no information was provided on weight matching. Obese women have higher androgen levels than nonobese (78). Schwartz et al. (86) examined hormone levels in six obese women with sleep apnea and compared them to obese and nonobese controls. Sleep apnea patients had higher free testosterone, SHBG, and dihydroepiandrostenedione sulfate (DHAS) levels. These studies need to be confirmed in larger patient groups but suggest that a link might exist between higher androgen levels (i.e., a more male hormonal profile) and sleep apnea in women.

C. Effect of Sex Hormone Therapy on Sleep Apnea

Testosterone

Several case reports in the early 1980s described development of sleep apnea following testosterone therapy (87–89). Others (90) reported the development of sleep apnea in a 54-year-old woman with renal failure following androgen administration. The sleep apnea resolved on withdrawal of the medication and recurred when the drug was reintroduced. They also observed an increase in supraglottic resistance following androgen administration. These cases certainly suggested that testosterone may be important in the regulation of breathing during sleep and the pathogenesis of sleep apnea. Testosterone also was reported to exacerbate sleep apnea in a 13-year-old male associated with an increase in upper airway collapsibility during sleep (91).

Two studies have systematically examined the sleep-breathing effects of exogenous testosterone on hypogonadal patients. Matsumoto et al. (92) studied five patients and observed development of sleep apnea in one patient and worsening of preexisting sleep apnea in another. There was no effect in the other three patients. Schneider and coworkers (93) investigated 11 hypogonadal men before and after testosterone replacement. There was a significant increase in apneas in the group as a whole, but clinically significant increases occurred in only three patients. The two studies show that testosterone-induced or exacerbated sleep apnea is not a consistent finding in hypogonadal patients. The clinical message from these studies is that patients commencing on androgen replacement should be questioned closely for sleep apnea symptomatology and monitored during the course of their therapy to check if such symptoms develop. The possibility of increasing use of testosterone therapy in eugonadal men will likely bring testosterone-induced apnea into clinical practice.

Progesterone and Estrogen

The low prevalence of sleep apnea in premenopausal women compared to women after the menopause and the increase in sleep-disordered breathing among postmenopausal women has led to studies examining the therapeutic role of progestational hormones in sleep apnea (94,95). Progesterone levels fall after menopause, and progestins have been shown to stimulate ventilation during the luteal phase of the menstrual cycle, in pregnancy, in normal male subjects, and in conditions of alveolar hypoventilation (95).

In general, the therapeutic results for progestins have been disappointing. Recent reports, including a double-blind study at high doses (94), have revealed no improvement in indices of sleep apnea severity. Block et al. (96) were unable to demonstrate a protective effect of progesterone upon postmenopausal females with sleep apnea syndrome. The apparent "protection" of premenopausal status against sleep apnea has provoked some interest in hormone replacement as a therapy for sleep apnea in women. Pickett and coworkers (97) used combined therapy with both progesterones and an estrogen in women who had a surgical menopause. They demonstrated improvement, but the pretreatment apnea severity was very mild. Estrogen alone or in combination with progesterone on sleep-disordered breathing had no effect on sleep apnea in 15 postmenopausal women with moderate obstructive sleep apnea despite a doubling of serum estrogen (98). It is still possible that longer-term or higher-dose treatment may provide more positive results.

Antiandrogens

If testosterone has an apnea-promoting effect, one might postulate that androgen antagonists may improve sleep apnea. The nonsteroidal androgen antagonist flutamide was used for one week in seven males with sleep apnea. Despite endocrine evidence of androgen antagonism, short-term flutamide did not alter sleep-disordered breathing or awake ventilatory drive (99).

VI. Hypothyroidism and Sleep Apnea

A. Introduction and Prevalence

Apneic breathing in myxedema was noted by Massumi and Winnacker (100), and the presence of sleep apnea later confirmed by others (101,107). Though myxedema coma is now rare, in retrospect, many cases were probably due to severe sleepiness and obtundation secondary to severe sleep apnea, coupled with the hypercapnic respiratory failure of sleep apnea.

Several recent studies have questioned the strength of the association between sleep apnea and hypothyroidism. Lin (108) studied 20 hypothyroid patients. All reported snoring, but only two patients had moderate to severe OSA and three had mild OSA. Pelttari and coworkers (109) compared 26 patients with hypothyroidism with 188 euthyroid controls. Fifty percent of the hypothyroid patients and 29.3% of the control subjects had at least some episodes of partial or complete upper airway obstruction. Severe obstruction with episodes of repetitive apnea was present in 7.7% of the patients and in 1.5% of the controls. However, this association was largely explained by coexisting obesity and male gender. It has also been reported that routine thyroid function testing in sleep apnea is not cost effective (110) except in certain high-risk groups such as elderly women. The author is aware of two further large sleep cohort studies currently completed with conflicting conclusions on the strength of the association between sleep apnea and hypothyroidism. It is likely that the prevalence of the association in sleep apnea cohorts is too low and further case-control studies in larger cohorts of sleep apnea patients are needed. In contrast, there are no data from large prospectively collected studies on hypothyroid patients. It has been asserted that the prevalence of sleep apnea in this group is high (106).

B. Response to Thyroid Hormone Replacement

The effect of adequate thyroid hormone replacement on sleep apnea in hypothyroidism has been variable. Orr et al. (103) described three obese patients with myxedema and sleep apnea and reported cure of sleep apnea when they became euthyroid. Other case reports (104–107) describe similar cures. Rajagopal et al. (106) noted a significant reduction in apnea index for both obese and nonobese patients. Mean apnea index fell from 99.5 to <20 in the six obese patients without weight change, and in all patients there was an associated decrease in apnea duration. The three nonobese patients reduced their apnea indices to <5 after achieving euthyroid status.

In contrast, when we reviewed our experience of 10 patients between 1981 and 1985 (107), only two patients had a complete resolution of their sleep apnea when they became euthyroid. Five patients had moderate improvement in their sleep apnea, though they continued to require nasal CPAP, while three patients had worsening in their apnea frequency.

The failure of sleep apnea to resolve after thyroxine treatment supports the view of a chance, rather than causal, association. An alternative explanation may be that hypothyroidism induces long-term changes in upper airway mechanics (111) or breathing control, which do not resolve immediately after a euthyroid state is achieved. However, in one sleep apnea case-control study, past hypothyroidism did not appear to be a risk factor for sleep apnea (111).

C. Risks of Rapid Thyroid Hormone Replacement and Sleep Apnea

Nasal CPAP is an excellent form of therapy in patients with sleep apnea triggered by hypothyroidism for several reasons. Some of these patients will have resolution of sleep apnea when euthyroid and so will only need treatment for the few months required to bring them back to normal thyroid status; clearly, invasive therapies such as tracheostomy would be less appropriate. The second more compelling reason for its use is to prevent cardiovascular complications in the initial stages of replacement therapy. It is well recognized that rapid restoration of the euthyroid state in hypothyroid patients may entail significant cardiovascular morbidity and mortality (107). This is particularly so in the elderly or those with preexisting cardiovascular disease. Certainly there is increased risk in commencing treatment in those patients with coexisting sleep apnea. We observed one male patient with extremely long apneas lasting over 2 min, yet oxyhemoglobin desaturation only fell to 64% (107). Undoubtedly his low metabolic rate and oxygen consumption (reduced to 50% of normal) contributed to his ability to maintain such saturation despite long apneas. After commencing thyroxine treatment there may be a more rapid increase in basal metabolic rate and oxygen consumption than in the clearance of abnormal myxedematous mucoprotein from the upper airway and normalization of depressed ventilatory responses. Long apneas may then be associated with a lower oxyhemoglobin saturation as the oxygen consumption rate is increased, therefore posing a major risk of dangerous hypoxemia for a patient with compromised coronary blood supply.

Sleep apnea may be an important factor in worsening coronary artery disease or sudden death in some patients early in their course of treatment for hypothyroidism. In our patient series, two female patients had cardiac complications after commencing thyroxine prior to a sleep study and the use of nasal CPAP therapy. One had a myocardial infarction with residual nocturnal angina after her thyroxine dosage was increased. Her nocturnal angina resolved after nasal CPAP was commenced. Another had nocturnal ventricular arrhythmias and unstable angina noted after thyroxine was commenced. Both complications resolved with CPAP therapy. We are also aware of an elderly obtunded patient with myxedema and witnessed long apneas who died in her sleep 24 hours after commencing a minimal dose of 25 μg of thyroxine. No sleep study had been performed and no CPAP treatment commenced. Abouganem et al. (112) reported extreme bradycardia and hypotension complicating sleep apnea in a patient with myxedema successfully managed with nasal CPAP prior to commencing thyroxine. Orr (103) described a myxedematous patient with OSA and cardiac arrhythmias who had a tracheostomy performed resolving both the OSA and arrhythmias.

D. Mechanisms

Several mechanisms have been suggested to explain the association between sleep apnea and hypothyroidism. Upper airway patency may be impaired by physical narrowing, impaired function of upper airway muscles, and reduced central drive to upper airway muscles. In hypothyroidism, mucoproteins can be deposited in the tongue and pharyngeal tissues (103,104), narrowing the airway. Airway narrowing is exacerbated by an increase in muscle volume, including the genioglossus (107). In addition, upper airway muscle function may be impaired by hypothyroid myopathy. Myopathy is a well-recognized feature of hypothyroidism and is present in approximately one third of patients. We found evidence of hypothyroid myopathy in three patients with evidence of impaired supraglottic resistance suggesting upper airway muscle weakness (107). These patients displayed a marked increase in supraglottic resistance when awake in the supine compared to the erect posture; this difference was no longer present after effective thyroid replacement. Impaired ventilatory drive has been frequently observed in earlier studies of hypothyroidism, but typically in association with obesity.

Recent studies of ventilatory drive in hypothyroidism have revealed conflicting results in both initial and posttreatment results (113). None of the studies with larger patient numbers provided simultaneous measurements of sleep-disordered breathing and ventilatory control (113). In view of the effect of sleep apnea on respiratory control (114,115), this may explain some of the difficulties in data interpretation. The presence of both central and obstructive apneas as well as failure of some patients to respond at all to thyroid hormone suggests that a combination of mechanisms operate in hypothyroid patients leading to sleep apnea. Upper airway patency will be affected in most patients, and in some, abnormalities of central drive to upper airway muscles will exist. Patients with obesity and hypothyroidism are probably at added risk of developing sleep apnea and, when compared to normal weight patients, do not improve as readily following thyroid hormone replacement as normal weight patients.

VII. Other Hormones and Sleep Apnea

In a preliminary report, Rapaport et al. (116) found that nocturnal ACTH levels in patients with sleep apnea fell on the first night of CPAP treatment compared to a night with untreated sleep apnea. They interpreted these findings as demonstrating the ‘‘stress’’ effect of sleep apnea. In contrast, no effect on plasma cortisol, ACTH, or catecholamines was observed with CPAP withdrawal in long-term users (6). Morning cortisol levels appear unaffected by sleep apnea (31). Patients with corticosteroid excess secondary to Cushing’s disease are characterized by truncal obesity, hypertension, and depression. In the only published data, about one-third of patients appear to have sleep apnea (117).

VIII. Neuroendocrine Changes, Obesity, and Sleep Apnea: Potential Interactions

A. Central Obesity and Sleep Apnea

The health risks of obesity are well known (118). However, while there are clear deleterious effects of morbid obesity, recent work has demonstrated that obesity is a heterogeneous disorder. Body fat distribution, i.e., predominantly upper body obesity, is often a more crucial determinant of morbidity and mortality than total adiposity (118,119). In terms of measurement, this means that morbidity and mortality are more closely related to waist-hip ratio (an elevated ratio is a measure of upper body obesity) than body mass index (BMI) This concept has clarified many of the confusing contradictory research in the health risks of obesity. Upper body obese individuals have increased risk of cardiovascular and cerebrovascular disease, diabetes, hypertension, hyperlipidemia, hyperuricemia, and insulin resistance relative to lower body obese individuals (119). The clustering of diseases associated with upper body obesity is really a rediscovery of the concept of ''android'' obesity (excess fat in the upper body) versus ''gynoid'' obesity (excess fat in the gluteofemoral region). This concept was first described by Vague (120), who suggested that cardiovascular disease, gout, and diabetes were more prevalent in android obesity. He stated that ''the region situated between the first three cervical vertebrae and particularly over the atlas, is the only site where, at equal weights, fat is normally more abundant in the male than in the female.''

Obesity is the most common metabolic abnormality in sleep apnea. In sleep apnea, the predominant pattern of obesity is central (121). There is a plethora of data linking central obesity to poor health outcomes (118–123). Clearly the health risks of obesity and sleep apnea are similar and data analysis is complicated by mutual confounding variables (121). Attempts at separating out the two disorders have suggested that both are additive in the pathogenesis of obesity-related morbidity.

B. Does Sleep Apnea Promote Central Obesity?

Obesity is a powerful epidemiological predictor of sleep apnea (2–4), and weight reduction may lead to marked improvement in sleep apnea severity (124). However, there are certainly fewer data addressing the reverse possibility—that sleep apnea may promote the development of obesity (125). Unfortunately, no long-term longitudinal studies of sleep apnea development exist. Over 50% of the first 100 patients commenced on home CPAP had a measured weight loss of greater than 5 kg at the time of long-term follow-up (126). In addition, we have frequently observed dramatic weight loss following commencement of nasal CPAP in patients who have previously been resistant to active weight loss programs. It is tempting to think that chronic intermittent hypoxia and sleep fragmentation over years in sleep apnea can lead to changes in central control of energy regulation, appetite control, feeding, and metabolism which would promote weight gain and thus worsen sleep apnea further. Moreover, if this is the case, could this vicious cycle be broken by successful CPAP therapy? Or are there clear interindividual differences in underlying hypothalamic function leading to divergent responses in energy balance in patients with sleep apnea?

During sleep, energy expenditure (EE) typically fails, relative to the awake basal state (127). In severe sleep apnea, sleep EE appears to increase during apneic sleep and falls with CPAP therapy (128). This would seem to be paradoxical—such EE changes would favor weight loss prior to CPAP and weight gain after CPAP. However, the 24-h EE may be different in untreated sleep apnea with reduced spontaneous physical activity (fidgeting, routine physical activities) due to fatigue and sleepiness producing a net decrease in EE, despite increased EE in sleep due to respiratory effort and sleep fragmentation. Other intriguing data suggest that patients with sleep apnea may have altered serotoninergic sensitivity in the hypothalamus. Hudgel and coworkers observed that the cortisol response to L-5-HTP, a serotonin precursor, was elevated relative to control nonapneic subjects and was not readily explained by changes in weight (129). Subsequent data have shown that treatment with nasal CPAP reverses the elevated cortisol response to serotoninergic stimulation (130). These investigators have speculated that the exaggerated cortisol responses in sleep apnea indicate supersensitivity of postsynaptic serotoninergic receptors in the hypothalamus caused by a serotoninergic ''deficient'' state induced by sleep apnea. Certainly short periods of sleep deprivation in humans and animals produce evidence of increased serotonin turnover (131)—whether chronic sleep

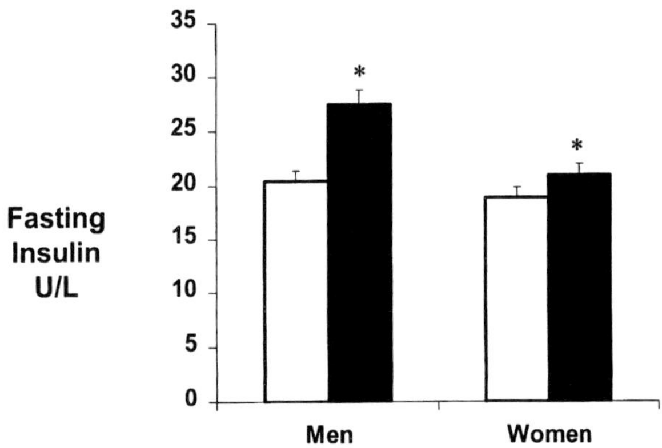

Figure 7 Fasting insulin levels are higher in severely obese men ($p < 0.008$) and women ($p < 0.01$) with a high likelihood of sleep apnea (black bars, $n = 338$ men and 155 women) versus those with low likelihood sleep apnea (white bars, $n = 216$ men and 481 women). $^*p < 0.05$. (Adapted from Ref. 112.)

fragmentation and hypoxemia in sleep apnea produces serotonin depletion in the hypothalamus and other regions is entirely speculative.

Interestingly, there are parallel findings of a serotonin-deficient state in central obesity (123). Bjorntorp (123) has described a cluster of disorders associated with central obesity including abnormalities of the hypothalamic–pituitary–end-organ axes (low growth hormone and testosterone, high cortisol), a ''defeat'' reaction to stress with psycho-social disability and carbohydrate craving promoted by a low serotoninergic state. Specific serotoninergic agonists have been used as treatments in central obesity. The observed low testosterone and GH in sleep apnea also occurs in central obesity. In central obesity, recombinant GH appears to reduce central body fat (48). Restoration of GH secretion during sleep with nasal CPAP in sleep apnea may have similar effects. A recent report suggests that nasal CPAP will reduce visceral fat deposits without change in BMI in patients with sleep apnea (132).

Another area of common ground is insulin sensitivity. Central obesity is associated with hyperinsulinemia and insulin resistance (123). Certainly some data also point to increased insulin levels in sleep apnea independent of weight and central obesity (133) (Fig. 7). Nasal CPAP also improves insulin sensitivity in NIDDM (134). However, in community cohorts, any relationship between sleep apnea and insulin resistance appears to be mediated by obesity (135). Other areas of speculative interest include products of fat mass, which include the hypothalamic weight regulator leptin and certain cytokines such as tumor necrosis factor-α (TNF-α) (136). TNF-α is involved in promoting sleep (137) and also, via separate actions, insulin resistance (136). Recent data indicate that the circadian rhythm of TNF-α, measured by a bioassay, is altered in sleep apnea compared with controls (138). The rhythm

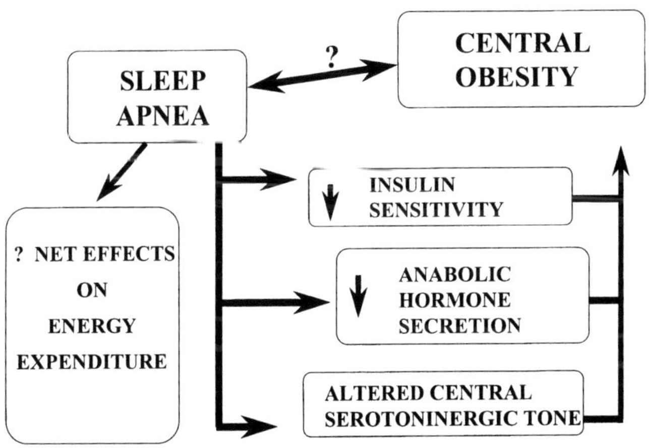

Figure 8 Putative metabolic and hormonal factors interacting in sleep apnea potentially leading to weight gain. See text for details.

is not normalized by nasal CPAP. TNF-α levels, measured by direct assay, are elevated in sleep apnea and related to severity of disease. It is possible that TNF-α may be involved in exacerbating somnolence, low activity levels, and even promoting insulin resistance in sleep apnea.

Leptin has only recently been discovered; it promotes motor activity, energy expenditure, and weight loss (139). One brief report suggests that a plasma leptin (one sample only) is increased in sleep apnea and reduced with nasal CPAP (140). Leptin levels are high in obesity due to increased production and leptin ''resistance'' at the hypothalamic level (139). Moreover, leptin production appears to be pulsatile with nocturnal components (141). Could control of sleep apnea with nasal CPAP improve leptin sensitivity (suggested by lower leptin levels) and promote weight loss by this mechanism? At this stage of knowledge, there is no direct evidence of a coherent unifying mechanism or series of mechanisms to suggest that sleep apnea will promote weight gain. Inactivity, sleepiness, low levels of anabolic hormones, altered central serotoninergic ''tone,'' TNF-α, and other cytokines may all promote central fat accumulation (Fig. 8). Future research into the links between central obesity, neuroendocrine function, and sleep apnea may provide not only insights into the pathophysiology of sleep-breathing disorders, but also clues to novel pharmacological therapies.

References

1. Van Cauter E, Refetoff S. Multifactorial control of the 24 hour secretory profiles of pituitary hormones. J Endocrinol Invest 1985; 8:381–391.
2. Young T, Palta M, Dempsey J, Skatrud J, Weber S, Badr S. Occurrence of sleep disordered breathing among middle-aged adults. N Engl J Med 1993; 328:1230–1235.
3. Bearpark H, Elliott L, Grunstein R, Cullen S, Schneider H, Althaus W, Sullivan C. Snoring and sleep apnea: a population study in Australian men. Am J Respir Crit Care Med 1995; 151:1459–1465.
4. Grunstein RR, Wilcox I, Yang TS, Gould Y, Hedner JA. Snoring and sleep apnoea in men: association with central obesity and hypertension. Int J Obesity 1993; 17:533–540.
5. Pastuszko A, Wilson DF, Erecinska. M. Neurotransmitter metabolism in rat brain synaptosomes: effect of anoxia and pH. J Neurochem 1982; 38:1657–1667.
6. Grunstein RR, Stewart DA, Lloyd H, Akinci M, Cheng N, Sullivan CE. Acute withdrawal of nasal CPAP in obstructive sleep apnea does not cause a rise in stress hormones. Sleep 1996; 19:774–782.
7. Handelsman DJ, Staraj S. Testicular size: the effects of aging, malnutrition, and illness. J Androl 1985; 6:144–151.
8. Veldhuis JD, Iranmanesh A. Physiological regulation of the human growth hormone (GH)–insulin-like growth factor type I (IGF-I) axis: predominant impact of age, obesity, gonadal function, and sleep. Sleep 1996; 19:S221–S224.
9. Sutton JR. Effect of acute hypoxia on the hormonal response to exercise. J Appl Physiol 1977; 42:587–592.
10. Kanaley JA, Weltman JY, Veldhuis JD, Rogol AD, Hartman ML, Weltman A. Human

growth hormone response to repeated bouts of aerobic exercise. J Appl Physiol 1997; 83:1756–1761.

11. Gonzalez-Santos MR, Gaja-Rodriguez OV, Alonso-Uriarte R, Sojo-Aranda I, Cortes-Gallegos V. Sleep deprivation and adaptive hormonal responses of healthy men. Arch Androl 1989; 22:203–207.
12. Chrousos GP. Ultradian, circadian, and stress-related hypothalamic-pituitary-adrenal axis activity—a dynamic digital-to-analog modulation. Endocrinology 1998; 139: 437–440.
13. Holl RW, Hartman ML, Veldhuis JD, Taylor WM, Thorner MO. Thirty-second sampling of plasma growth hormone in man: correlation with sleep stages. J Clin Endo Metab 1991; 72:854–861.
14. Van Cauter E, Kerkofs M, Caufriez A, van Onderbergen A, Thorner MO, Copinschi G. A qualitative estimation of growth hormone secretion in normal man: reproducibility and relation to sleep and time of day. J Clin Endo Metab 1992; 74:1441–1450.
15. Van Cauter E, Caufriez A, Kerkofs M, van Onderbergen A, Thorner MO, Copinschi G. Sleep, awakenings, and insulin-like growth factor 1 modulate the growth hormone (GH) secretory response to GH-releasing hormone. J Clin Endocrinol Metab 1992; 74:1451–1459.
16. Veldhuis JD, Iranmanesh A, Weltman A. Elements in the pathophysiology of diminished growth hormone (GH) secretion in aging humans. Endocrine 1997; 7:41–48.
17. Merriam GR, Buchner DM, Prinz PN, Schwartz RS, Vitiello MV. Potential applications of GH secretagogues in the evaluation and treatment of the age-related decline in growth hormone secretion. Endocrine 1997; 7:49–52.
18. Melmed S. Acromegaly. N Engl J Med 1990; 322:966–977.
19. Takahashi Y, Kipnis DM, Daughaday WH. Growth hormone secretion in sleep. J Clin Invest 1968; 47:2079–2090.
20. Sassin JF, Parker DC, Mace JW, Gotlin RW, Johnson LC, Rossman LG. Human growth hormone release: relation to slow-wave sleep and sleep-waking cycles. Science 1969; 165:513–515.
21. Steiger A, Herth T, Holsber F. Sleep electroencephalography and the secretion of cortisol and growth hormone in normal controls. Acta Endocrinol (Copenh) 1987; 116:36–43.
22. Jarett DB, Greenhouse JB, Miewald JM, Fedorka IB, Kupfer DJ. A reexamination of the relationship between growth hormone secretion and slow wave sleep using delta wave analysis. Biol Psych 1990; 27:497–509.
23. Gronfier C, Luthringer R, Follenius M, Schaltenbrand N, Macher JP, Muzet A, Brandenberger G. A quantitative evaluation of the relationships between growth hormone secretion and delta wave electroencephalographic activity during normal sleep and after enrichment in delta waves. Sleep 1996; 19:817–824.
24. Van Cauter E, Plat L, Scharf MB, Lepoult R, Cespedes S, Hermite-Baleriaux M, Copinschi G. Simultaneous stimulation of slow-wave and growth hormone secretion by gamma-hydroxbutyrate in normal young men. J Clin Invest 1997; 100:745–753.
25. Steiger A, Holsboer F. Neuropeptides and human sleep. Sleep 1997; 20:1038–1052.
26. Quabbe HJ, Gregor M, Bumke-Vogt C, Eckhof A, Witt I. Twenty-four-hour pattern of growth hormone secretion in the rhesus monkey: studies including alterations of the sleep/wake and sleep stage cycles. Endocrinology 1981; 109:513–522.
27. Vermeulen A. Nyctohemeral growth hormone profiles in young and aged men: correlation with somatomedin C levels. J Clin Endocrinol Metab 1987; 64:884–888.

28. Higuchi T, Takahashi Y, Takahashi K, Niimi Y, Miyasita A. Twenty-four-hour secretory patterns of growth hormone, prolactin, and cortisol in narcolepsy. J Clin Endocrinol Metab 1979; 49:197–204.
29. Taylor BJ, Brook CGD. Sleep EEG in growth disorders. Arch Dis Childhood 1986; 61:754–760.
30. Iranmanesh A, Veldhuis JD. Clinical pathophysiology of the somatotropic (GH) axis in adults. Endo Metab Clin North Am 1992; 21:783–817.
31. Grunstein RR, Handelsman DJ, Lawrence S, Blackwell C, Caterson ID, Sullivan CE. Neuroendocrine dysfunction in sleep apnea: reversal by nasal continuous positive airway pressure. J Clin Endo Metab 1989; 68:352–358.
32. Rasmussen MH, Frystyk J, Andersen T, Breum L, Christiansen JS, Hilsted J. The impact of obesity, fat distribution, and energy restriction on insulin-like growth factor-1 (IGF-1), IGF-binding protein-3, insulin, and growth hormone. Metabolism 1994; 43: 315–319.
33. Issa FG, Sullivan CE. The immediate effects of nasal continuous positive airway pressure treatment on sleep pattern in patients with obstructive sleep apnea syndrome. Electroencephalogr Clin Neurophysiol 1986; 136:755–761.
34. Miles LE, Austin S, Guilleminault C. Secretion of glucose, growth hormone and cortisol during sleep in patients with obstructive sleep apnea. In: Guilleminault C, Dement WC, eds. Sleep Apnea Syndromes. New York: Liss, 1978:323–332.
35. Clark RW, Schmidt HS, Malarkey WB. Disordered growth hormone and prolactin secretion in primary disorders of sleep. Neurology 1979; 23:855–857.
36. Grunstein R, McNamara SG, Caterson I, Turtle JR, Sullivan CE. Nocturnal growth hormone secretion in sleep apnoea: changes with CPAP therapy. Aust NZ J Med 1986 (suppl 3); 16:629.
37. Saini J, Krieger J, Brandenberger G, Wittersheim G, Simon C, Follenius M. Continuous positive airway pressure treatment. Effects on growth hormone, insulin and glucose profiles in obstructive sleep apnea patients. Horm Metab Res 1993; 25:375–381.
38. Grunstein RR. Metabolic aspects of sleep apnea. Sleep 1996; 19:S218–S220.
39. Goldstein SJ, Wu RHK, Thorpy MJ, Shprintzen RJ, Marion RE, Saenger P. Reversibility of deficient sleep entrained growth hormone secretion in a boy with achondroplasia and obstructive sleep apnea. Acta Endocrinol (Copenh) 1987; 16:95–97.
40. Cooper BG, White JES, Ashworth L, Alberti KGMM, Gibson GJ. Hormonal and metabolic profiles in subjects with obstructive sleep apnea syndrome and the acute effects of nasal continuous positive airway pressure treatment. Sleep 1995; 18:172–179.
41. Waters KA, Kirjavainen T, Jimenez M, Cowell CT, Sillence DO, Sullivan CE. Overnight growth hormone secretion in achondroplasia: deconvolution analysis, correlation with sleep state, and changes after treatment of obstructive sleep apnea. Pediatr Res 1996; 39:547–553.
42. Bennett RM, Clark SR, Campbell SM, Burckhardt CS. Low levels of somatomedin C in patients with the fibromyalgia syndrome. Arthritis Rheum 1992; 35:1113–1116.
43. Stradling JR, Thomas G, Williams P, Warley AH, Freeland A. Effect of adenotonsillectomy on nocturnal hypoxemia, sleep disturbance and symptoms in snoring children. Lancet 1990; 335:249–253.
44. Marcus CL, Carroll JL, Koerner CB, Hamer A, Lutz J, Loughlin GM. Determinants of growth in children with OSA syndrome. J Pediatrics 1994; 125:556–562.
45. Cornil A, Glinoer D, Leclerq R, Copinschi G. Adrenocortical and somatotrophic secre-

tions in acute and chronic respiratory insufficiency. Am Rev Respir Dis 1975; 112: 77–81.

46. Stewart DA, Grunstein RR, Sullivan CE, Handelsman DJ. Neuroendocrine changes in sleep apnea are not related to a pituitary defect. Sleep Res 1989; 18:308.
47. Bengtsson BA, Edin S, Lann L, et al. Treatment of adults with growth hormone (GH) deficiency with recombinant human GH. J Clin Endo Metab 1993; 76:309–317.
48. Johannsson G, Marin P, Lonn L, Ottosson M, Stenlof K, Bjorntorp P, Sjostrom L, Bengtsson BA. Growth hormone treatment of abdominally obese men reduces abdominal fat mass, improves glucose and lipoprotein metabolism, and reduces diastolic blood pressure. J Clin Endocrinol Metab 1997; 82:727–734.
49. Carroll PV, Christ ER, Bengtsson BA, Carlsson L, Christiansen JS, Clemmons D, Hintz R, Ho K, Laron Z, Sizonenko P, Sonksen PH, Tanaka T, Thorne M. Growth hormone deficiency in adulthood and the effects of growth hormone replacement: a review. Growth Hormone Research Society Scientific Committee. J Clin Endocrinol Metab 1998; 83:382–395.
50. Wright AD, Hill DM, Lowy C, Fraser TR. Mortality in acromegaly. Q J Med 1970; 39:1–16.
51. Roxburgh F, Collis AJ. Notes on a case of acromegaly. Br Med J 1896; ii:63–65.
52. Chappell WF, Booth JA. A case of acromegaly with laryngeal symptoms and pharyngeal symptoms. J Laryng Otol 1896; 10:142–150.
53. Laroche C, Festal G, Poenaru S, Caquet R, Lemaigre D, Auperin A. Une observation de respiration periodique chez une acromegalie. Ann Med Intern 1976; 127:381–385.
54. Perks WH, Horrocks PM, Cooper RA, et al. Sleep apnea in acromegaly. Br Med J 1980; 280:894.
55. Mezon BJ, West P, MaClean JP, Kryger M. Sleep apnea in acromegaly. Am J Med 1980; 69:615–618.
56. Hart TB, Radow SK, Blackard WG, Tucker HSG, Cooper KR. Sleep apnea in active acromegaly. Arch Intern Med 1985; 145:865–866.
57. Pekkarinen T, Partinen M, Pelkonen R, Iivanainen M. Sleep apnea and daytime sleepiness in acromegaly: relationship to endocrinological factors. Clin Endocrinol 1987; 27:649–654.
58. Grunstein RR, Ho KY, Sullivan CE. Acromegaly and sleep apnea. Ann Intern Med 1991; 115:527–532.
59. Bengtsson B-A, Edenm S, Ernst I, Oden A, Sjogren B. Epidemiology and long term survival in acromegaly. Acta Med Scand 1988; 223:327–335.
60. Pelttari L. Polo O, Rauhala E, Vuoriluoto J, Aitasalo K, Hyyppa MT, Kronholm E, Irjala K, Viikari Nocturnal breathing abnormalities in acromegaly after adenomectomy. J Clin Endocrinol (Oxf) 1995; 43:175–182.
61. Rosenow F, Reuter S, Deuss U, Szelies B, Hilgers RD, Winkelmann W, Heiss WD. Sleep apnoea in treated acromegaly: relative frequency and predisposing factors. Clin Endocrinol (Oxf) 1996; 45:563–569.
62. Cadieux RJ, Kales A, Santen RJ, Bixler EO, Gordon R. Endoscopic findings in sleep apnea associated with acromegaly. J Clin Endocrinol Metab 1982; 55:18–22.
63. Grunstein RR, Ho KY, Berthon-Jones M, Stewart D, Sullivan CE. Central sleep apnea is associated with increased ventilatory response to carbon dioxide and hypersecretion of growth hormone in patients with acromegaly. Am J Respir Crit Care Med 1994; 150:496–502.

64. Naughton MT, Bradley TD. Sleep apnea in congestive heart failure. Clin Chest Med 1998; 19:99–113.
65. Neubauer JA. Mechanisms of apnea. Curr Opin Pulm Med 1995; 1:491–497.
66. White, D. Central sleep apnea. In: Kryger MH, Roth T, Dement WC. Principles and Practice of Sleep Medicine. Philadelphia: WB Saunders, 1989; 513–524.
67. Kalia M, Fuxe K, Agnati LF, Hokfelt T, Harfstrand A. Somatostatin produces apnea and is localised in medullary respiratory nuclei: a possible role in apneic syndromes. Brain Res 1984; 296:339–344.
68. Chen ZB, Hedner T, Hedner J. Local application of somatostatin in the rat ventrolateral brain medulla induces apnea. J Appl Physiol 1990; 69:2233–2238.
69. Concannon P, Altszuler N, Hampshire J, Butler WR, Hansel W. Growth hormone, prolactin, and cortisol in dogs developing mammary nodules and an acromegaly-like appearance during treatment with medroxyprogesterone acetate. Endocrinology 1980; 106:1173–1177.
70. Gerard JM, Garibaldi L, Myers SE, Aceto T Jr, Kotagal S, Gibbons VP, Stith J, Weber C. Sleep apnea in patients receiving growth hormone. Clin Pediatr Phila 1997; 36: 321–326.
71. Frohman LA. Acromegaly: what constitutes optimal therapy? J Clin Endocrinol Metab 1996; 81:443–445.
72. Chanson P, Timsit J, Benoit O, et al. Rapid improvement in sleep apnea of acromegaly after short term treatment with somatostatin analogue SMS 201-995. Lancet 1986; 1: 1270–1271.
73. Grunstein RR, Ho KK, Sullivan CE. Effect of octreotide, a somatostatin analog, on sleep apnea in patients with acromegaly. Ann Intern Med 1994; 121:478–483.
74. Minniti G, Moroni C, Jaffrain-Rea ML, Bondanini F, Gulino A, Cassone R, Tamburrano G. Prevalence of hypertension in acromegalic patients: clinical measurement versus 24-hour ambulatory blood pressure monitoring. Clin Endocrinol (Oxf) 1998; 48: 149–152.
75. Silverberg DS, Oksenberg A. Essential and secondary hypertension and sleep-disordered breathing: a unifying hypothesis. J Hum Hypertens 1996; 10:353–363.
76. Southwick JP, Katz J. Unusual airway difficulty in the acromegalic patient-indications for tracheostomy. Anesthesiology 1979; 51:72–73.
77. Veldhuis JD, Evans WS, Johnson ML, Willis MR, Rogol AD. Physiological properties of the luteinizing hormone pulse signal: impact of intensive and extended venous sampling paradigms on its characterization in healthy men and women. J Clin Endocrinol Metab 1986; 62:881–891.
78. Glass AR. Endocrine aspects of obesity. Med Clin North Am 1989; 73:139–160.
79. Pincus SM, Mulligan T, Iranmanesh A, Gheorghiu S, Godschalk M, Veldhuis JD. Older males secrete luteinizing hormone and testosterone more irregularly, and jointly more asynchronously, than younger males. Proc Natl Acad Sci USA 1996; 93:14100–14105.
80. Pietrowsky R, Meyrer R, Kern W, Born J, Fehm HL. Effects of diurnal sleep on secretion of cortisol, luteinizing hormone, and growth hormone in man. J Clin Endocrinol Metab 1994; 78:683–687.
81. Elman I, Breier A. Effects of acute metabolic stress on plasma progesterone and testosterone in male subjects: relationship to pituitary-adrenocortical axis activation. Life Sci 1997; 61:1705–1712.

82. Santamaria JD, Prior JC, Fleetham JA. Reversible reproductive dysfunction in men with obstructive sleep apnea. Clin Endocrinol 1988; 28:461–470.
83. Akerstedt T, Palmblad J, de la Torre B, Marana R, Gillberg M. Adrenocortical and gonadal steroids during sleep deprivation. Sleep 1980; 3:23–30.
84. Semple PD, Beastall GH, Brown TM, Stirling KW, Mills RJ, Watson WS. Sex hormone suppression and sexual impotence in hypoxic pulmonary fibrosis. Thorax 1984; 39:46–51.
85. Mohamed G, Lopata M, Kukreja J, Schraufnagel D. Androgen levels in women with sleep apnea syndrome. Am Rev Respir Dis 1983; 127:A237.
86. Schwartz SM, Fry JM, Eskin BA, Wallace T. Hormonal status in premenopausal women with obstructive sleep apnea. Sleep Res 1989; 18:243.
87. Sandblom RE, Matsumoto AM, Schoene RB, et al. Obstructive sleep apnea induced by testosterone administration. N Engl J Med 1983; 308:506–510.
88. Strumpf IJ, Reynolds SF, Vash P, Tashkin DP. A possible relationship between testosterone, central control of ventilation, and the Pickwickian syndrome. Am Rev Respir Dis 1978; 117:A183.
89. Harman E, Wynne JW, Block AJ. The effect of weight loss on sleep disordered breathing and oxygen desaturation in morbidly obese men. Chest 1982; 82:291–293.
90. Johnson MW, Anch AM, Remmers JE. Induction of the obstructive sleep apnea syndrome in a woman by exogenous androgen administration. Am Rev Respir Dis 1984; 129:1023–1025.
91. Cistulli PA, Grunstein RR, Sullivan CE. Effect of testosterone administration on upper airway collapsibility during sleep. Am J Respir Crit Care Med 1994; 149:530–532.
92. Matsumoto AM, Sandblom RE, Schoene RB, Lee KA, Giblin EC, Pierson DJ, Bremner WJ. Testosterone replacement in hypogonadal males: effects on obstructive sleep apnea, respiratory drives and sleep. Clin Endocrinol (Oxf) 1985; 22:713–717.
93. Schneider BK, Pickett CK, Zwillich CW, Weil JV, McDermott MT, Santen RJ, Varano LA, White DP. Influence of testosterone on breathing during sleep. J Appl Physiol 1986; 61:618–624.
94. Robinson RW, Zwillich CW. The effects of drugs on breathing during sleep. Clin Chest Med 1985; 6:603–614.
95. Cook WR, Benich JJ, Wooten SA. Indices of severity of obstructive sleep apnea syndrome do not change during medroxyprogesterone acetate therapy. Chest 1989; 96: 262–266.
96. Block AJ, Wynne JW, Boysen PG, Lindsey S, Martin C, Cantor B. Menopause, medroxyprogesterone and breathing during sleep. Am J Med 1980; 70:506–510.
97. Pickett CK, Regensteiner JG, Woodard WD, Hagerman DG, Weil JV, Moore LG. Progestigin and estrogen reduce sleep-disordered breathing in post-menopausal women. J Appl Physiol 1989; 66:1656–1661.
98. Cistulli PA, Barnes DJ, Grunstein RR, Sullivan CE. Effect of short-term hormone replacement in the treatment of obstructive sleep apnoea in postmenopausal women. Thorax 1994; 49:699–702.
99. Stewart DA, Grunstein RR, Berthon-Jones M, Handelsman DJ, Sullivan CE. Androgen blockade does not affect sleep-disordered breathing or chemosensitivity in men with obstructive sleep apnea. Am Rev Respir Dis 1992; 146:1389–1393.
100. Massumi RA, Winnaker JL. Severe depression of the respiratory center in myxedema. Am J Med 1964; 36:876–882.

101. Duron B, Quinchard J, Fullana N. Nouvelles recherches sur le mechanisme des apnecs du syndrome de pickwick. Bull Physiopathol Respir 1972; 8:1277–1288.
102. Yamamoto T, Hirose N, Miyoshi K. Polygraphic study of periodic breathing and hypersomnolence in a patient with severe hypothyroidism. Eur Neurol 1977;15:188–193.
103. Orr WC, Males JL, Imes NK. Myxedema and obstructive sleep apnea. Am J Med 1981; 70:1061–1066.
104. Skatrud J, Iber C, Ewart R, Thomas G, Rasmussen H, Schultze B. Disordered breathing during sleep in hypothyroidism. Am Rev Respir Dis 1981; 124:325–329.
105. Millman RP, Bevilacqua J, Peterson DD, Pack AI. Central sleep apnea in hypothyroidism. Am Rev Respir Dis 1983; 127:504–507.
106. Rajagopal KR, Abbrecht PH, Derderian SS, Pickett C, Hofeldt F, Tellis CJ, Zwillich CW. Obstructive sleep apnea in hypothyroidism. Ann Intern Med 1984; 101:471–474.
107. Grunstein RR, Sullivan CE. Hypothyroidism and sleep apnea. Mechanisms and management. Am J Med 1988; 85:775–779.
108. Lin CC, Tsan KW, Chen PJ. The relationship between sleep apnea syndrome and hypothyroidism. Chest 1992; 102:1663–1667.
109. Pelttari L, Rauhala E, Polo O, Hyyppa MT, Kronholm E, Viikari J, Kantola I. Upper airway obstruction in hypothyroidism. J Intern Med 1994; 236:177–181.
110. Winkelman JW, Goldman H, Piscatelli N, Lukas SE, Dorsey CM, Cunningham S. Are thyroid function tests necessary in patients with suspected sleep apnea? Sleep 1996; 19:790–793.
111. Petrof BJ, Kelly AM, Rubinstein NA, Pack AI. Effect of hypothyroidism on myosin heavy chain expression in rat pharyngeal dilator muscles. J Appl Physiol 1992; 73: 179–187.
112. Abouganem D, Taylor AL, Donna E, Baum GL. Extreme bradycardia during sleep apnea caused by myxedema. Arch Intern Med 1987; 147:1497–1499.
113. Ladenson PW, Goldenheim PG, Ridgeway EC. Prediction and reversal of blunted ventilatory responsiveness in patients with hypothyroidism. Am J Med 1988; 84:877–891.
114. Grunstein RR, Sullivan CE. Neural control of respiration during sleep. In: M Thorpy, ed. Handbook of Sleep Disorders. New York: Marcel Dekker, 1990. 77–102.
115. Kimoff RJ, Brooks D, Horner RL, Kozar LF, Render-Teixeira CL, Champagne V, Mayer P, Phillipson EA. Ventilatory and arousal responses to hypoxia and hypercapnia in a canine model of obstructive sleep apnea. Am J Respir Crit Care Med 1997; 156: 886–894.
116. Rapaport D, Rothenberg SA, Hollander CS, Goldring RM. Obstructive sleep apnea (OSA) alters ultradian rhythm of ACTH secretion. Am Rev Respir Dis 1989; 139: A80.
117. Shipley JE, Schteingart DE, Tandon R, Starkman MN. Sleep architecture and sleep apnea in patients with Cushing's disease. Sleep 1992; 15:514–518.
118. Kissebah AH, Freedman DS, Peiris AN. Health risks of obesity. Med Clin North Am 1989; 73:111–138.
119. Bjorntorp P. Obesity. Lancet 1997; 350:423–426.
120. Vague J. The degree of masculine differentiation of obesities. A factor determining predisposition to diabetes, atherosclerosis, gout, and uric calculous disease. Am J Clin Nutr 1956; 4:20–34.
121. Grunstein RR, Stenlof K, Hedner J, Sjostrom L. Impact of self reported sleep apnea symptoms on psycho-social performance in the Swedish Obese Subjects (SOS) Study. Sleep 1995; 18:635–643.

122. Vanhala MJ, Pitkajarvi TK, Kumpusalo EA, Takala JK. Obesity type and clustering of insulin resistance-associated cardiovascular risk factors in middle-aged men and women. Int J Obes Relat Metab Disord 1998; 22:369–374.
123. Bjorntorp P. Neuroendocrine abnormalities in human obesity. Metabolism 1995; 44(2 suppl 2):38–41.
124. Strobel RJ, Rosen RC. Obesity and weight loss in obstructive sleep apnea: a critical review. Sleep 1996; 19:104–115.
125. Grunstein RR. Endocrine and metabolic disturbances in obstructive sleep apnea. In: NA Saunders, CE Sullivan, eds. Sleep and Breathing. 2d ed. New York: Marcel Dekker 1993:449–481.
126. Grunstein RR, Dodd MJ, Costas L, Sullivan CE. Home nasal CPAP for sleep apnea—acceptance of home therapy and its usefulness. Aust NZ J Med 1986; 16:635
127. Bonnet MH, Berry RB, Arand DL. Metabolism during normal, fragmented and recovery sleep. J Appl Physiol 1991; 71:1112–1118.
128. Stenlof K, Grunstein RR, Hedner J, Sjostrom L. Energy expenditure in obstructive sleep apnea: effects of treatment with continuous positive airway pressure. Am J Physiol 1996; 271:E1036–E1043.
129. Hudgel DW, Gordon EA, Meltzer HY. Abnormal serotonergic stimulation of cortisol production in obstructive sleep apnea. Am J Respir Crit Care Med 1995; 152:186–192.
130. Hudgel DW, Gordon EA. Serotonin-induced cortisol release in CPAP-treated obstructive sleep apnea patients. Chest 1997; 111:632–638.
131. Heiser P, Dickhaus B, Opper C, Schreiber W, Clement HW, Hasse C, Hennig J, Krieg JC, Wesemann W. Platelet serotonin and interleukin-1 beta after sleep deprivation and recovery sleep in humans. J Neural Transm 1997; 104:1049–1058.
132. Chin K, Nakamura T, Narai N, Shimziu K, Kita Y, Oku M, Mishima M, Ohi M. Changes in intraabdominal visceral fat in patients with obstructive sleep apnea syndrome following long term nasal CPAP therapy. Am J Respir Crit Care Med 157:A58, 1998.
133. Grunstein RR, Stenlof K, Hedner J, Sjostrom L. Impact of obstructive sleep apnea and sleepiness on metabolic and cardiovascular risk factors in the Swedish Obese Subjects (SOS) Study. Int J Obesity 1995; 151:410–418.
134. Brooks B, Cistulli PA, Borkman M, McGee S, Ross G, Grunstein RR, Sullivan CE, Yue D. Effect of nasal continuous positive airway pressure treatment on insulin sensitivity in patients with Type II diabetes and obstructive sleep apnea. J Clin Endocrinol Metab 1994; 79:1681–1685.
135. Stoohs RA, Facchini F, Guilleminault C. Insulin resistance and sleep-disordered breathing in healthy humans. Am J Respir Crit Care Med 1996; 154:170–174.
136. Katsuki A, Sumida Y, Murashima S, Murata K, Takarada Y, Ito K, Fujii M, Tsuchihashi K, Goto H, Nakatani K, Yano Y. Serum levels of tumor necrosis factor-alpha are increased in obese patients with noninsulin-dependent diabetes mellitus. J Clin Endocrinol Metab 1998; 83:859–862.
137. Vgontzas AN, Papanicolaou DA, Bixler EO, Kales A, Tyson K, Chrousos GP. Elevation of plasma cytokines in disorders of excessive daytime sleepiness: role of sleep disturbance and obesity. J Clin Endocrinol Metab 1997; 82:1313–1316.
138. Entzian P, Linnemann K, Schlaak M, Zabel P. Obstructive sleep apnea syndrome and circadian rhythms of hormones and cytokines. Am J Respir Crit Care Med 1996; 153: 1080–1086.

139. Tataranni PA. From physiology to neuroendocrinology: a reappraisal of risk factors of body weight gain in humans. Diabetes Metab 1998; 24:108–115.
140. Saarelainen S, Lahtela J, Kallonen E. Effect of nasal CPAP treatment on insulin sensitivity and plasma leptin. J Sleep Res 1997; 6:146–147.
141. Licinio J, Mantzoros C, Negrao AB, Cizza G, Wong ML, Bongiorno PB, Chrousos GP, Karp B, Allen C, Flier JS, Gold PW. Human leptin levels are pulsatile and inversely related to pituitary-adrenal function. Nat Med 1997; 3:575–579.

15

Cardiovascular Consequences of Obstructive Sleep Apnea

Insights from Animal Models

DINA BROOKS and ELIOT A. PHILLIPSON

University of Toronto
Toronto, Ontario, Canada

I. Introduction

Epidemiological studies have identified obstructive sleep apnea (OSA) as a risk factor for hypertension, myocardial infarction, stroke, and sudden death (1–3), but the physiological mechanisms underlying these associations have not been defined. Progress in studying the long-term complications of OSA has been hampered by the fact that by the time patients with OSA come to clinical attention, the disorder and its possible long-term sequelae have usually been present for several years. In addition, patients with OSA often present with confounding conditions, such as obesity, that predispose them to cardiovascular diseases. Furthermore, elucidation of the possible underlying mechanisms that link OSA with the development of cardiovascular disease requires that several physiological measurements (some of which are invasive) be made over extended periods of time, a requirement that is generally not feasible in patients with the disorder.

Given the limitations in studying the mechanisms and consequences of OSA in patients with the disorder, both natural and induced animal models of OSA have become an important focus of investigation. For example, spontaneous sleep-disordered breathing, which has been described in brachycephalic canine breeds such as the English bulldog, provides several important investigative advantages (4,5). In particular, this model can be used to examine the primary causes of apnea and the neural mechanisms controlling the upper airway dilator muscles during sleep (6). However, the apneas in the bulldog are limited predominantly to rapid eye movement (REM) sleep, whereas in human OSA, apneas occur in both non-REM and REM sleep. Furthermore, the English bulldogs generally have sleep-disordered breathing by the time they are acquired, precluding studies in the "predisease" state that would distinguish the primary defects and secondary consequences of the disorder (7). Thus, several investigators have induced OSA in animal models, including newborn lambs and adult pigs and dogs, for short (up to 48 h) and long time periods (up to 3 months) (8–12). These induced models can be used to investigate the cardiovascular consequences of apneas and to examine the mechanisms underlying these consequences. Episodic hypoxia has also been induced experimentally (in the rat) to investigate the cardiovascular effects of this stimulus alone, without upper airway occlusion (13).

In this chapter we will review the evidence derived from induced animal models that implicate OSA in the pathogenesis of cardiovascular disease. The immediate effects of apnea on the cardiovascular system and the long-term effects of OSA on blood pressure (BP) and cardiac function will be the focus of the review.

II. Description of Models of OSA

A. Short-Term Induced Models

Lamb Model

The first induced model of repeated upper airway occlusion in conscious animals was described by Fewell and colleagues (8). Lambs 8–14 days of age were instrumented for recording of the electroencephalogram (EEG), electrooculogram, nuchal and diaphragmatic electromyogram (EMG), BP, and arterial oxygen saturation. The lambs breathed through a fenestrated tracheostomy tube placed in the trachea. A balloon-tipped catheter was inserted into the tracheostomy tube so that airflow could be obstructed by inflation of the balloon. The animals were monitored with a closed-circuit video system, and occlusions were initiated by the investigators whenever the animals fell asleep. With arousal from sleep, the obstruction was released by deflation of the balloon. The model was induced in five lambs for a period of 17–30 h and resulted in a longer time to arousal from active sleep in response to airway occlusion and a greater decrease in arterial oxygen saturation at the point of arousal. Although the model mimicked human OSA in some respects, it required continuous human intervention, as well as physical attachments between the animals and the recording apparatus, thereby precluding its long-term application.

Porcine Model

A similar model of repeated upper airway occlusion during sleep has been described in pigs (9). Ten pigs were instrumented for recording of the EEG, electrooculogram and nuchal EMG, and for measurement of cardiovascular variables (coronary blood flow, arterial BP, and heart rate). A modified tracheostomy tube was placed in the trachea to allow obstruction of the upper airway during sleep. The pigs were housed in fiberglass open-topped boxes during the experiments and were monitored by the investigators from an adjacent room. Changes were measured in arterial BP, heart rate (HR), and coronary blood flow during wakefulness, non-REM sleep, and REM sleep, and in response to airway occlusion. This model was also limited in terms of long-term applicability.

Rat Model

One aspect of OSA, intermittent hypoxia, has been studied extensively by Fletcher and colleagues (13), who produced repetitive hypoxia in the rat that simulated the recurrent hypoxia of sleep apnea. The rats were subjected to a hypoxic environment (3–5% nadir ambient oxygen concentration) every 30 s, 7 h per day for up to 35 days. Daytime blood pressure was measured periodically. However, the rats in this model were not subjected to airway occlusion and its associated changes in intrathoracic pressure. Furthermore, the hypoxic events were not synchronized to sleep state and may not have been associated with the arousal responses that are typical of OSA.

Canine Models

Three different canine models of induced upper airway occlusion have been described, the first being a short-term model (12 h) in conscious dogs (11), the second a short-term model in anesthetized dogs (10), and the third a long-term model (3 months) in conscious dogs (7,12). In the first model, dogs were instrumented for recordings of the EEG, electrooculogram, and nuchal EMG, and for measurement of BP. The leads were exteriorized and attached to the recording apparatus in an adjacent room. The animals were monitored by closed-circuit television for 12 h. Upper airway obstruction was induced by the investigators through the inflation of a balloon in the endotracheal tube whenever sleep was exhibited, and with arousal from sleep, the airway obstruction was released. This model in the dog is similar to those described above in the lamb and pig (8,9). These short-term models involve the recording of electrophysiological variables through exteriorized leads and the induction of airway occlusion through a custom-designed tracheostomy whenever sleep is detected. Thus, these models provide insight into the immediate and short-term consequences of recurrent upper airway occlusion during sleep.

The second model of induced OSA involved anesthetized dogs that were instrumented for the measurement of cardiac output, heart rate, arterial BP, left ventricular end-diastolic and end-systolic transmural pressure, coronary blood flow, and myocardial contractility (10). With the animals breathing 100% oxygen, airway occlusion was produced by clamping the endotracheal tube at end-expiration for 60 s, then unclamping the tube for the next 60 s. The changes in cardiovascular variables were measured over 7 consecutive cycles of airway occlusion. Although the use of anesthesia simplified the measurement of cardiovascular variables, anesthesia can independently affect cardiovascular function (14–16), thereby complicating the interpretation of data. Furthermore, the time over which measurements can be made in anesthetized animals is limited. Therefore, the anesthetized preparation is not suitable for long-term studies of the consequences of OSA.

Finally, Kimoff and colleagues (7) and later Brooks et al. (12) described a novel long-term canine model of OSA. The dogs were tracheostomized, and a special custom-designed valve was connected to the endotracheal tube through which the dog breathed. Sleep state was monitored on-line by a computer that used telemetered signals from implanted EEG and nuchal EMG electrodes to make a judgment about sleep-wake state. The valve was controlled by radiofrequency signals and was programmed to close when the dog fell asleep and to open when the animal aroused. Kimoff et al. (7) first applied this model of OSA to two dogs for a 5-day period. A slightly modified version was later applied in four dogs for up to 4 months (12). The model simulated closely human OSA by producing repeated episodes of airway occlusion and arousal from sleep. A second computer received and stored cardiovascular variables from the dog (17). Because the model used biotelemetry and computer technology, there were no physical attachments between the dog and the monitoring apparatus, allowing the dog to move about freely. In addition, the system functioned without human intervention, except for routine monitoring and maintenance.

III. Immediate Hemodynamic Effects of OSA

Airway occlusion in OSA results in five physiological events that are associated with hemodynamic consequences: (1) progressive hypoxia, the magnitude of which (at least in humans) is dependent on apnea duration, lung volume, and baseline oxygen saturation (18,19); (2) progressive hypercapnea that is relatively less severe than the hypoxia, due to the buffering ability of the body for carbon dioxide (20); (3) negative intrathoracic pressure generated by the futile inspiratory efforts against the closed airway; (4) arousal from sleep, which results in restoration of upper airway patency and resumption of airflow; and (5) increases in sympathetic nervous system activity.

A. Effects of Apnea on BP

In patients with OSA, arterial BP may increase by 15–50 mmHg in response to apnea, with the peak rise coinciding with arousal from sleep and the resumption of ventilation (21–24). Following arousal, BP typically remains elevated for 10–15 s before returning slowly to control levels (23). This pattern of BP change in humans is also observed in dogs during obstructive apneas (11,25).

Studies in patients and in animal models have attempted to elucidate the relevant contribution of the different stimuli, particularly hypoxia and arousal from sleep, on the BP response to obstructive apneas. Ringler and colleagues (24) concluded that hypoxemia alone does not account for the increases in BP associated with obstructive apneas in humans. In contrast, Iwase et al. (26) demonstrated that administration of supplemental oxygen before an apnea prevents the postapneic increase in BP in anesthetized dogs, thus implicating an important role for hypoxia. Furthermore, O'Donnell and coworkers (27) demonstrated in conscious dogs that the acute increase in BP associated with an apnea was only partially attributable to arousal, since termination of apneas prior to arousal still resulted in a significant BP surge (Fig. 1). However, Brooks et al. (25) found a weak correlation in conscious dogs between the changes in BP and the fall in Sa_{O_2} during apneas in non-REM sleep, but a somewhat stronger correlation in REM sleep. These apparent discrepancies may relate to the finding of O'Donnell and coworkers (11), who demonstrated a significant correlation between the change in mean arterial BP and the degree of hypoxia only for obstructions in which Sa_{O_2} fell below 80%. In the study by Brooks et al. (25), only airway occlusions in REM sleep resulted in Sa_{O_2} levels below 80%. Thus, in the absence of severe hypoxia, other stimuli associated with airway occlusion, particularly arousal from sleep, appear to play a more important role in causing the acute increases in BP, whereas in the presence of severe hypoxia, the contribution of other stimuli becomes proportionately less.

Long-term changes in the acute responses to obstructive apneas during sleep were also examined in the canine model by Brooks et al. (25). OSA of 3–4 months duration resulted in progressive lengthening of the time to arousal in response to acute airway occlusion and in greater desaturation, peak inspiratory pressures, and surges in blood pressure during the occlusions. Long-term sleep fragmentation, without airway obstruction, also resulted in similar alterations in the acute responses to airway occlusion. These findings suggest that changes in the responses to acute airway occlusion during the course of long-term OSA can be attributed predominantly to the associated sleep fragmentation, rather than to other stimuli.

B. Effects of Apnea on Cardiac Function

The effects of a decrease in intrathoracic pressure induced by the Mueller maneuver (i.e., voluntary inspiration against a closed glottis) or by upper airway obstruction are complex (28). The resulting decrease in right atrial pressure initially enhances venous return to the right heart and increases right ventricular volume (29,30). As a result, the intraventricular septum may shift to the left, leading to decreased left ventricular compliance and stroke volume (29,31–35). However, the rise in venous return to the right heart is limited by collapse of the great veins at the entrance to the thoracic cavity (36–38). Right ventricular afterload may also increase as a result of hypoxic pulmonary vasoconstriction. The lower intrathoracic pressure during occluded inspiratory efforts also increases the transmural pressure gradient across the right and left ventricles and thereby increases their afterload (28,30,39,40). The increase in afterload and the decrease in compliance of the left ventricle may lead to

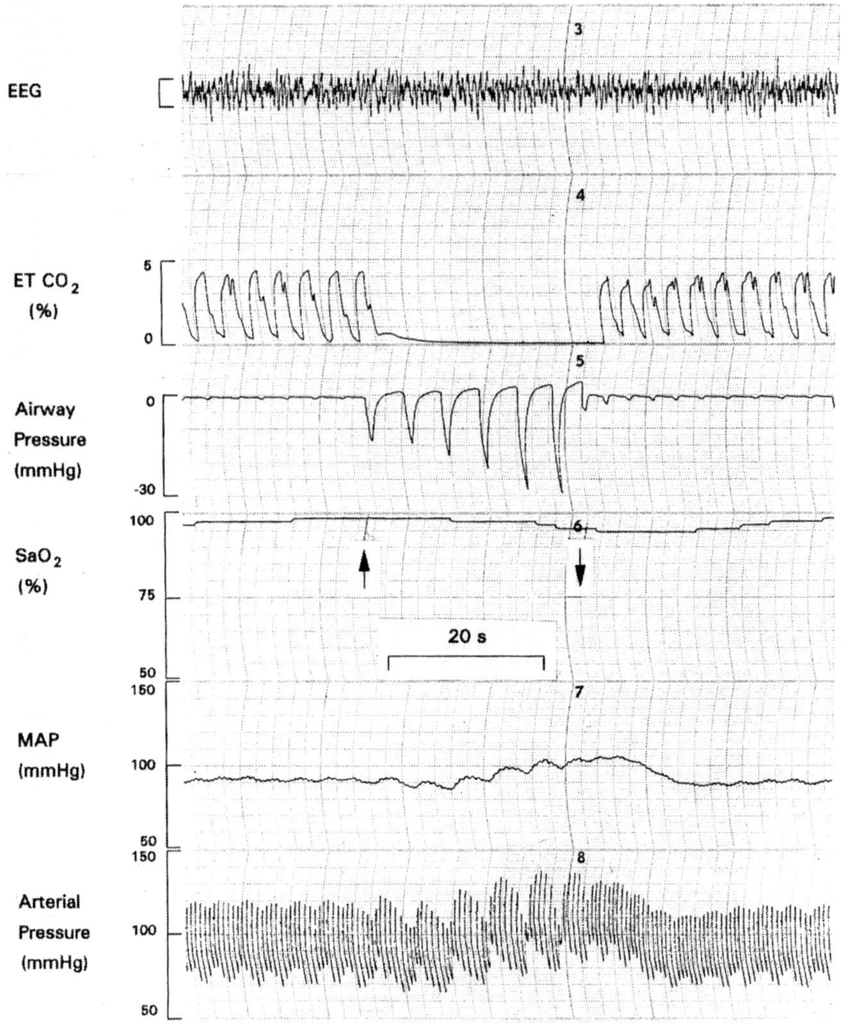

Figure 1 Demonstration of the use of an animal model to investigate mechanisms involved in the acute increases in blood pressure associated with obstructive sleep apneas. Tracings (from the top down) show the EEG, end-tidal CO_2 concentration, airway pressure, arterial O_2 saturation, mean arterial BP, and arterial blood pressure in a sleeping dog. Upper airway was occluded (up arrow) and released (down arrow) during non-REM sleep, without inducing arousal from sleep. Note the increase in BP associated with the obstructive apnea, despite the absence of arousal. (From Ref. 27.)

an increase in left ventricular end-diastolic pressure and left atrial pressure (20), as indicated by an increase in pulmonary capillary wedge pressure during apneas (41). These hemodynamic changes result in an increase in intrathoracic blood volume, and in heart size, as demonstrated by direct fluoroscopic examination (42).

Recent evidence from a long-term canine model of OSA confirms that during obstructive sleep apneas, left ventricular transmural pressure increases (Fig. 2). At the same time, there is also a progressive increase in left ventricular end-systolic volume during the occluded inspiratory effort. The combination of increased left ventricular systolic transmural pressure and end-systolic volume represents an increase in left ventricular wall tension and stress (43) and almost certainly results in an increase in myocardial metabolism and O_2 requirements. Indeed, acute studies in anesthetized dogs and pigs have demonstrated that inspiratory resistive loading or periodic upper airway occlusion induce increases in myocardial O_2 demand, resulting in coronary vasodilation and increased coronary blood flow under normal conditions (9,10,44). As a result, in the presence of experimental coronary artery stenosis, periodic airway occlusion induces evidence of outright myocardial ischemia and of systolic and diastolic dysfunction (10). Taken together, these studies could account for the reported clinical and epidemiological association between OSA and myocardial ischemia (1). The increase in left ventricular end-systolic volume during OSA observed in the canine model is also associated with a decrease in stroke volume (45,46) and may contribute to the reported association between OSA and cerebral infarction (1,42,47–49).

IV. Long-Term Hemodynamic Effects of OSA

A. Effects of OSA on Nighttime BP

Given that periods of upper airway obstruction result in acute transient increases in arterial BP, it is not surprising that long-term OSA in the dog results in nighttime hypertension that resolves following cessation of OSA (12). Long-term recurrent arousals from sleep in response to acoustic stimulation (without airway occlusion) resulted in the *same* degree of nighttime hypertension. Whether arousals produced by acoustic stimuli are physiologically equivalent in all respects to those produced by OSA is not clear. Nevertheless, since the arousal and apnea indices in the two protocols were matched, the findings suggest that the long-term nocturnal BP increases associated with OSA are largely the result of recurrent arousal from sleep.

B. Effects of OSA on Daytime BP

The long-term application of an induced model of OSA in the dog has provided the first definitive evidence of a direct link between OSA and systemic hypertension. Specifically, OSA of 1–3 months duration resulted in progressive increases in daytime mean arterial BP (Fig. 3) to a maximum of 16 mmHg. Following cessation of OSA, daytime hypertension resolved slowly over a period of 1–3 weeks. In contrast,

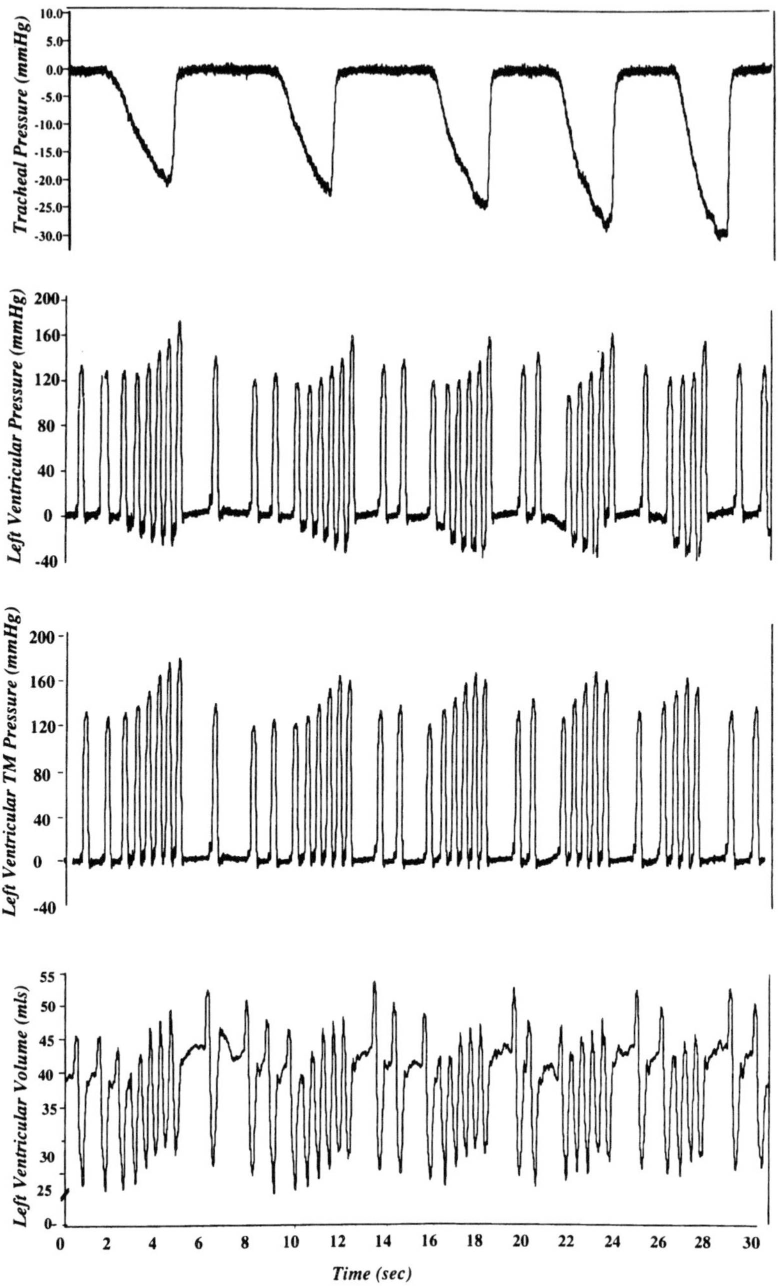

Figure 2 Demonstration of the use of an animal model to investigate the impact of obstructive sleep apnea on left ventricular (LV) function. Tracings (from the top down) show tracheal pressure, LV pressure, LV transmural pressure, and LV volume in a sleeping dog during long-term (3 months) OSA. Note that during the occluded inspiratory efforts (indicated by the negative tracheal pressure swings) there was an increase in both LV transmural pressure and end-systolic volume. (From Ref. 46.)

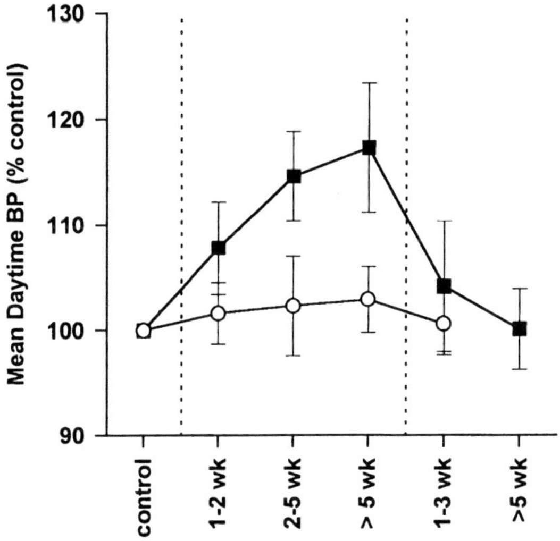

Figure 3 Demonstration of the use of a long-term animal model of OSA to establish an etiological link between OSA and daytime hypertension and to investigate the mechanisms involved. Data points (solid squares) represent mean (±SEM) of mean arterial BP in four dogs, measured during quiet wakefulness during a control phase (to the left of the first dashed line), during several weeks of OSA (between the two dashed lines), and following cessation of OSA (to the right of the second dashed line). Note that OSA was associated over several weeks with a progressive increase in BP that resolved following cessation of OSA. In contrast, when the same dogs were subjected in a separate protocol to sleep fragmentation by acoustic stimuli without airway occlusion (open circles), there was no increase in daytime BP. (From Ref. 12.)

sleep fragmentation without airway obstruction did not produce a significant increase in daytime BP (Fig. 3).

Several stimuli associated with OSA may contribute to the development of daytime hypertension, including the repetitive episodes of hypoxia and hypercapnea, disruption of sleep architecture, and fluctuations in intrathoracic pressure during the occluded respiratory efforts. However, the results of the study by Brooks et al. (12) indicate that disruption of sleep architecture by recurrent arousals is not the critical underlying stimulus, suggesting that hypoxia and/or fluctuations in intrathoracic pressure may be of greater importance. Support for the role of hypoxia can be derived from the observation that rats subjected to chronic (35 days) intermittent hypoxia patterned after the hypoxia of sleep apnea develop sustained elevations of BP (13). This increase in BP involved the activation of the carotid chemoreceptors, in that carotid body denervation prevented the increase in BP (50). The increase in BP was mediated through increased sympathetic activity and could be prevented by pharmacological sympathectomy (51).

C. Effects of OSA on Cardiac Function

In recent years, the notion has begun to emerge that OSA may have a long-term impact on left ventricular function. For example, patients with OSA have been reported to have a thicker than normal left ventricular wall even in the absence of systemic hypertension (52). In patients with cardiomyopathy and OSA, improvements in left ventricular ejection fraction have been demonstrated following abolition of the OSA with nasal continuous positive airway pressure during sleep (53–55). These clinical findings suggest that OSA may have adverse effects on left ventricular function. This notion is also supported by evidence from animal models. For example, in the rat model of episodic hypoxia (that mimics the recurrent hypoxia of OSA), exposure for 35 days resulted in an increase in left ventricular/body weight ratio and left ventricular size (13). Repeated exposure to negative intrathoracic pressure may also contribute to left ventricular impairment by increasing left ventricular afterload and may stimulate left ventricular hypertrophy (40). The systemic hypertension and frequent surges in nighttime BP associated with OSA could also contribute to left ventricular dysfunction (56). Direct evidence implicating OSA in left ventricular dysfunction was derived from the long-term canine model of OSA, in which there was a reduction in left ventricular ejection fraction and increase in left ventricular end-systolic volume after several weeks of OSA, even during the waking, daytime hours when the dogs were not being subjected to airway occlusion (46). Whether these changes were related to chronic episodic left ventricular loading by the obstructive apneas or to the development of sustained daytime hypertension, or to a combination of these factors, has not yet been determined.

V. Conclusions

Induced animal models of OSA are subject to several limitations, the most obvious being that such models cannot be used to investigate the mechanisms that initiate upper airway occlusion during sleep. In addition, in those models in which the induced airway occlusion is at the level of the trachea, the lack of input from receptors in the oropharynx (as occurs in human OSA) could theoretically alter the responses to the occlusion.

Despite these limitations, induced animal models of OSA have allowed investigations of mechanisms involved in OSA that would not be feasible in patients and have thereby provided considerable insight into the acute and chronic cardiovascular effects of recurrent upper airway occlusion during sleep. For example, as outlined in this chapter, such models have established a direct etiological link between OSA and sustained daytime hypertension, thus confirming the relationship first identified by epidemiological and clinical studies. In addition, the animal models of OSA have allowed investigation of the mechanisms underlying such relationships. In this sense, the continued use of animal models will further considerably our understanding of the clinical consequences of OSA and will ultimately impact on the management of patients with this disorder.

References

1. Koskenvuo M, Kaprio J, Telakivi T, Partinen M, Heikkila K, Sarna S. Snoring as a risk factor for ischemic heart disease and stroke in men. Br Med J 1987; 294:16–19.
2. He J, Kryger MH, Zorick FJ, Conway W, Roth T. Mortality and apnea index in obstructive sleep apnea. Experience in 385 male patients. Chest 1988; 94:9–14.
3. Hla KM, Young TB, Bidwell T, Palta M, Skatrud JB, Dempsey J. Sleep apnea and hypertension. A population-based study. Ann Intern Med 1994; 120:382–388.
4. Amis TC, Kurpenshoek C. Patterns of breathing in brachycephalic dogs. Am J Vet Res 1986; 47:2200–2204.
5. Hendricks JC, Kovalski RJ, Kline LR. Phasic respiratory muscle patterns and sleep-disordered breathing during rapid-eye movement sleep in the English bulldog. Am Rev Respir Dis 1991; 144:1112–1120.
6. Pack A. Invited editorial. Canine model of obstructive sleep apnea. J Appl Physiol 1994; 76:1409–1410.
7. Kimoff RJ, Makino H, Horner RL, Kozar LF, Lue F, Slutsky AS, Phillipson EA. Canine model of obstructive sleep apnea: model description and preliminary application. J Appl Physiol 1994; 76:1810–1817.
8. Fewell JE, Williams BJ, Szabo JS, Taylor BJ. Influence of repeated upper airway obstruction on the arousal and cardiopulmonary response to upper airway obstruction in lambs. Pediatr Res 1988; 23:191–195.
9. Pinto JMB, Garpestad E, Weiss JW, Bergau DM, Kirby DA. Hemodynamic changes associated with obstructive sleep apnea followed by arousal in a porcine model. J Appl Physiol 1993; 75:1439–1443.
10. Scharf SM, Graver LM, Balaban K. Cardiovascular effects of periodic occlusions of the upper airway in dogs. Am Rev Respir Dis 1992; 146:321–329.
11. O'Donnell CP, King ED, Schwartz AR, Robotham JL, Smith PL. Relationship between blood pressure and airway obstruction during sleep in the dog. J Appl Physiol 1994; 77:1819–1828.
12. Brooks D, Horner RL, Kozar LF, Render-Teixeira CL, Phillipson EA. Obstructive sleep apnea as a cause of systemic hypertension. Evidence from a canine model. J Clin Invest 1997; 99:106–109.
13. Fletcher EC, Lesske J, Qian W, Miller III CC, Unger T. Repetitive, episodic hypoxia causes diurnal elevation of blood pressure in rats. Hypertension 1992; 19:555–561.
14. Chelly JE, Rogers K, Hysing ES, Taylor A, Hartley C, Merin RG. Cardiovascular effects of an interaction between calcium blocking drugs and anesthetics in chronically instrumented dogs. I. Verapamil and halothane. Anesthesiology 1986; 64:560–567.
15. Chiueh CC, Kopin IJ. Hyperresponsivity of spontaneously hypertensive rat to indirect measurement of blood pressure. Am J Physiol 1978; 234:H690–H695.
16. Seyde WC, McGowan L, Lund N, Duling B, Longnecker DE. Effects of anesthetics on regional hemodynamics in normovolemic and hemorrhaged rats. Am J Physiol 1985; 249:H164–H173.
17. Brooks D, Horner RL, Kozar LF, Waddell TK, Render CL, Phillipson EA. Validation of a telemetry system for long-term measurement of blood pressure. J Appl Physiol 1996; 81:1012–1018.
18. Bradley TD, Martinez D, Rutherford R, Lue F, Grossman RF, Moldofsky H, Zamel N,

Phillipson EA. Physiological determinants of nocturnal arterial oxygenation in patients with obstructive sleep apnea. J Appl Physiol 1985; 59:1364–1368.
19. Shepard JW Jr. Gas exchange and hemodynamics during sleep. Med Clin North Am 1985; 69:1243–1264.
20. Parish JM, Shepard JW. Cardiovascular effects of sleep disorders. Chest 1990; 97: 1220–1226.
21. Tilkian AG, Guilleminault C, Schroeder JS, Lehrman KL, Simmons FB, Dement WC. Hemodynamics in sleep-induced apnea: studies during wakefulness and sleep. Ann Intern Med 1976; 85:714–719.
22. Motta H, Guilleminault G, Schroeder JS, Dement WC. Tracheostomy and hemodynamic changes in sleep-induced apnea. Ann Intern Med 1978; 89:454–458.
23. Shepard JW Jr. Hemodynamics in obstructive sleep apnea. In: Fletcher EC, ed. Abnormalities of Respiration During Sleep: Diagnosis, Pathophysiology and Treatment. Orlando: Grune and Stratton, 1986:39–61.
24. Ringler J, Basner RC, Shannon R, Schwartzstein R, Manning H, Weinberger SE, Weis JW. Hypoxemia alone does not explain blood pressure elevations after obstructive apneas. J Appl Physiol 1990; 69:2143–2148.
25. Brooks D, Horner RL, Kimoff RJ, Kozar LF, Render-Teixeira CL, Phillipson EA. Effect of obstructive sleep apnea versus sleep fragmentation on responses to airway occlusion. Am J Respir Crit Care Med 1997; 155:1609–1617.
26. Iwase N, Kikuchi Y, Hida W, Miki H, Taguchi O, Satoh M, Otake S, Takishima T. Effects of repetitive airway obstruction on O_2 saturation and systemic and pulmonary arterial pressure in anesthetized dogs. Am Rev Respir Dis 1992; 146:1402–1410.
27. O'Donnell CP, Ayuse T, King ED, Schwartz AR, Smith PL, Robotham JL. Airway obstruction during sleep increases blood pressure without arousal. J Appl Physiol 1996; 80:773–781.
28. Scharf SM. Cardiovascular effects of airways obstruction. Lung 1991; 169:1–23.
29. Scharf S, Brown R, Tow DE, Parisi AE. Cardiac effects of increased lung volume and decreased pleural pressure in man. J Appl Physiol 1979; 47:257–262.
30. Buda AJ, Pinsky MR, Ingel NB Jr, Daughters GT, Stinson EB, Alderman EL. Effect of intrathoracic pressure on left ventricular performance. N Engl J Med 1979; 301:453–459.
31. Taylor RR, Corell JW, Sonnenblick EH, Ross J. Dependence of ventricular distensibility on filling of the opposite ventricle. Am J Physiol 1967; 213:711–718.
32. Shiomi T, Guilleminault C, Stoohs R, Schnittger I. Leftward shift of the interventricular septum and pulsus paradoxus in obstructive sleep apnea syndrome. Chest 1991; 100: 894–902.
33. Tolle FA, Judy WV, Yu PL, Markand ON. Reduced stroke volume related to pleural pressure in obstructive sleep apnea. J Appl Physiol 1983; 55:1718–1724.
34. Brinker JA, Weiss JL, Lappe DL, Rabson JL, Summer WR, Permutt S, Weisfeldt ML. Leftward septal displacement during right ventricular loading in man. Circulation 1980; 61:626–633.
35. Guzman PA, Maughan WL, Yin FC, Eaton LW, Brinker JA, Weisfeldt ML, Weiss JL. Tansseptal pressure gradient with leftward septal displacement during the Mueller manoeuvre in man. Br Heart J 1981: 46:657–662.
36. Natori H, Tamaki S, Kira S. Ultrasonographic evaluation of ventilatory effect on inferior vena cava configuration. Am Rev Respir Dis 1979; 120:421–427.

37. Condos WRJ, Latham RD, Hoadley SD, Pasipoularides A. Hemodynamics of the Mueller maneuver in man: right and left heart micromanometry and Doppler echocardiography. Circulation 1987; 76:1020–1028.
38. Guyton AC, Adkins LH. Quantitative aspects of the collapse factor in relation to venous return. Am J Physiol 1954; 177:523–527.
39. Marrone O, Bellia V, Ferrara G, Milone F, Romano L, Salvaggio A, Stallone A, Bonsignore G. Transmural pressure measurements. Importance in the assessment of pulmonary hypertension in obstructive sleep apneas. Chest 1989; 95:338–342.
40. Bradley TD, Floras JS. Pathophysiologic and therapeutic implications of sleep apnea in congestive heart failure. J Card Fail 1996; 2:223–240.
41. Buda AJ, Schroeder JS, Guilleminault C. Abnormalities of pulmonary artery wedge pressures in sleep-induced apnea. Intl J Cardiol 1981; 1:67–74.
42. Lugaresi E, Cirignotta F, Coccagna G, Montagna P. Clinical significance of snoring. In: Saunders NA, Sullivan CE, eds. Sleep and Breathing. New York: Marcel Dekker, 1984:283–298.
43. Grossman W, Jones D. McLaurin LP. Wall stress and patterns of hypertrophy in the human left ventricle. J Clin Invest 1975; 56:56–64.
44. Peters J, Ihle P. Coronary and systemic vascular response to inspiratory resistive breathing. J Appl Physiol 1992; 72:905–913.
45. Schneider H, Schaub CD, Andreoni KA, Schwartz AR, Smith PL, Robotham JL, O'Donnell CP. Systemic and pulmonary hemodynamic responses to normal and obstructed breathing during sleep. J Appl Physiol 1997; 83:1671–1680.
46. Parker JD, Brooks D, Kozar LF, Render-Teixeira CL, Horner RL, Bradley TD, Phillipson EA. Acute and chronic effects of airway obstruction on canine left ventricular performance. Am J Respir Crit Care Med 1999: 160:1888–1896.
47. Partinen M, Palomaki H. Snoring and cerebral infarction. Lancet 1985; 2:1325–1326.
48. Palomaki H, Partinen M, Juvela S, Kaste M. Snoring as a risk factor of sleep-related brain infarction. Stroke 1989; 20:1311–1315.
49. Shepard JW Jr. Hypertension, cardiac arrhythmias, myocardial infarction, and stroke in relation to obstructive sleep apnea. Clin Chest Med 1992; 13:437–458.
50. Fletcher EC, Lesske J, Behm R, Miller CC III, Straus H, Unger T. Carotid chemoreceptors, systemic blood pressure, and chronic episodic hypoxia mimicking sleep apnea. J Appl Physiol 1992; 72:1978–1984.
51. Fletcher EC, Lesske J, Culman J, Miller CC III, Unger T. Sympathetic denervation blocks blood pressure elevation in episodic hypoxia. Hypertension 1992; 20:612–619.
52. Hedner J, Ejnell H, Caidahl K. Left ventricular hypertrophy independent of hypertension in patients with obstructive sleep apnea. J Hypertension 1990; 8:941–946.
53. Malone S, Liu PP, Holloway RM, Rutherford R, Xie A, Bradley TD. Obstructive sleep apnoea in patients with dilated cardiomyopathy: effects of continuous positive airway pressure. Lancet 1991; 338:1480–1484.
54. Krieger J, Grucker D, Sforza E, Chambron J, Kurtz D. Left ventricular ejection fraction in obstructive sleep apnea. Effects of long-term treatment with nasal continuous positive airway pressure. Chest 1991; 100:917–921.
55. Tal A, Lieberman A, Margulis G, Sofes S. Ventricular dysfunction in children with obstructive sleep apnea. Ped Pulmonol 1988; 4:139–143.
56. Bradley TD. Right and left ventricular functional impairment in sleep apnea. Clin Chest Med 1992; 13:459–479.

16

Simplified Diagnostic Tests for Obstructive Sleep Apnea and Its Variants

JOHN R. STRADLING

Churchill Hospital
Oxford, England

ROBERT J. O. DAVIES

University of Oxford
Churchill Hospital
Oxford, England

I. Evolution of Sleep Studies in Obstructive Sleep Apnea

Our understanding of the pathophysiology of obstructive sleep apnea (OSA) is constantly evolving, and therefore it is not surprising that the approach to diagnostic tests should also be evolving. In the early days of OSA, patients presented with hypersomnolence and were investigated in neurophysiology sleep laboratories, usually run by experienced neurologists or psychiatrists. These laboratories had a long history of sleep investigation, centered on the EEG and its varying patterns during sleep. Routine sleep studies in the 1960s consisted of EEG, EMG, and EOG monitoring in order to stage sleep, with particular interest in rapid eye movement (REM) sleep and its latency. Indeed in some laboratories a reduction in REM latency was part of the diagnosis of endogenous depression, and many sleep studies were carried out in the investigation of this disorder (1). It is not surprising therefore that when the first comprehensive reports of OSA began to appear they came from neurophysiology units with great expertise in sleep staging and polysomnography (PSG) (2–4). Emphasis was placed on neurophysiological monitoring, demonstrating poor sleep and the predominance of apneas during REM sleep. Simple signal transducers, such as oro-nasal thermistors and ribcage/abdominal mercury strain gauges, were added to polysomnography to document the irregular breathing that was usually dramatically abnormal. Since the obstructive apneas were so obvious, these were the first abnormalities to be defined, counted, and then referred to as the apnea index (the number of apneas per hour of sleep). At the time it seemed obvious that these were the primary abnormality that caused the patient's presenting symptom of hypersomnolence. However, there was no way to prove that all the patient's symptoms were due only to the apneas, although none of a group of 20 normal subjects (aged 40–60 years) had >4 apneas per hour (5). In the absence of anything better, or significant dissent, the standard way to investigate these patients became full polysomnography with EEG, EMG, EOG, oro-nasal airflow, ribcage, abdominal monitoring, with Sa_{O_2} added later following the wider availability of reliable pulse oximeters. No analysis was ever made as to whether this approach accurately defined the disease in a quantitative way that could produce useful thresholds for predicting likely therapeutic responses and benefits, or indeed adverse consequences. However, this approach identified thousands of patients who were helped initially by tracheotomy and subsequently, since 1981, nasal continuous positive airway pressure (CPAP) (6). This technique became established in the literature in a way that was perhaps not justified by its origins, based as they were on face validity, rather than a full understanding of the condition. It became the gold standard of investigation against which to assess other techniques, which would fall by the wayside if they could not mimic an apnea index derived from polysomnography. Full polysomnography was defended on a variety of grounds, including the importance of proving sleep and demonstrating REM periods, but, as pointed out by Guilleminault and Partinen in 1990 (7), reimbursement arrangements related to this expensive investigation may have played their part in its persistence.

Paradoxically, changing financial pressures have now become one of the main reasons for reviewing the value of full polysomnography, which remains expensive even when partially automated. Health economics and a better understanding of the pathophysiology of OSA have led us to reexamine whether simpler and less expensive approaches to its diagnosis may be just as good as polysomnography, and hopefully even better.

II. Which Physiological Variables May Provide Useful Information During a Sleep Study?

Our current general understanding of symptomatic OSA is that it is one end of a spectrum of upper airway narrowing during sleep, largely due to the withdrawal of compensatory pharyngeal dilator mechanisms accompanying the loss of the awake stimulus (8,9). With sleep onset, even in normal individuals, there are usually increases in upper airway resistance (10) and sometimes the appearance of inspiratory flow limitation (11). Greater increases in upper airway resistance lead to more inspiratory flow limitation, then snoring appears at some specific point, followed by hypoventilation (when compensatory mechanisms are inadequate), and finally complete occlusion causes apneas. In response to this continuous spectrum of upper airway narrowing are the body's compensatory actions. One of these will be increased inspiratory effort to maintain adequate ventilation, but there are also reflexes that may increase upper airway tone and limit the narrowing (12–14). To reverse this narrowing requires more activation of the pharyngeal dilator muscles. This will usually occur with a return of sleep state toward, or into, wakefulness and the attendant general increase in activation of all postural muscles that accompanies this arousal. The dominant arousal stimulus is likely to be the increased inspiratory effort (15,16) (Fig. 1), although hypoxia and hypercapnia are also arousal stimuli in their own right (17–19). It is generally believed that it is the sleep fragmentation that causes most of the daytime symptoms of OSA, although increased inspiratory effort may contribute directly (20). The hypoxemia present in some patients may produce additional cognitive defects (21). It is not clear what particular aspect of apneas and sleep fragmentation are critical to the development of daytime symptoms. For example, does the resulting sleepiness depend more on apnea length, their number, the length of undisturbed interarousal intervals, or the degree of return to full arousal with each event (22)? Thus, it is likely that measurement of upper airway narrowing, increased inspiratory effort, and some aspect of sleep fragmentation are important in trying to establish if a patient's hypersomnolence is likely to result from sleep fragmentation due to sleep apnea or one of its variants.

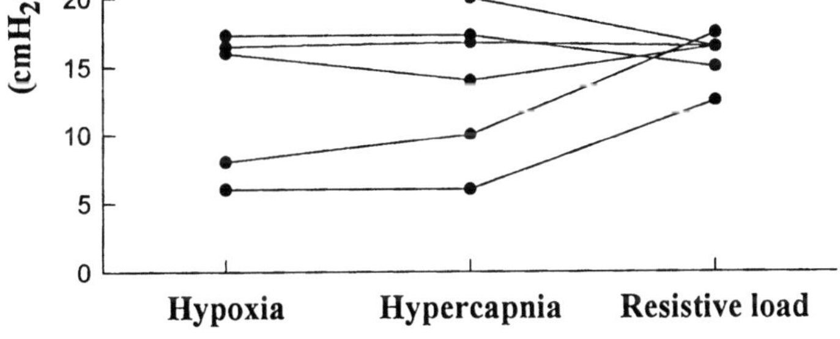

Figure 1 Normal sleeping subjects were challenged with progressive hypoxia, progressive hypercapnia, and an added inspiratory resistive load. Esophageal pressure was monitored and the inspiratory effort reached on the breath prior to arousal measured. Note the interindividual variation in inspiratory effort at arousal, which is largely independent of the actual stimulus. This suggests that the degree of inspiratory effort is the common arousing stimulus across the three experimental conditions. (From Ref. 15.)

Other consequences of OSA include the profound autonomic and cardiovascular changes with each apnea that can lead to systolic blood pressure falls of >50 mmHg with each frustrated inspiratory effort (pulsus paradoxus) and rises of >80 mmHg with each arousal (23) (Fig. 2). Some authors believe that these profound cardiovascular changes may cause adverse complications and suggest that treatment should be recommended for OSA, even in the absence of any daytime symptoms (24), particularly if there is underlying coronary heart disease (25). Such disagreements are important sources of confusion when discussing the place of simplified diagnostic tests in OSA.

Most evidence for an adverse effect of OSA on diurnal blood pressure comes from epidemiology studies (26–30) where the level of OSA apparently provoking hypertension is usually somewhat below that seen in sleep clinics and usually in otherwise asymptomatic individuals who are unlikely to want nasal CPAP therapy. For the purposes of this discussion we are assuming that the majority of sleep clinics dealing with sleep apnea patients offer treatment in an attempt to relieve day-to-day symptoms and rarely try to reduce the chances of some future cardiovascular event, such as a myocardial infarction or stroke. There is no convincing evidence that treatment would do this, and it is unlikely that an individual without significant hypersomnolence will comply closely for many years with an intrusive treatment such as nasal CPAP. The presence of less severe initial symptoms has been shown

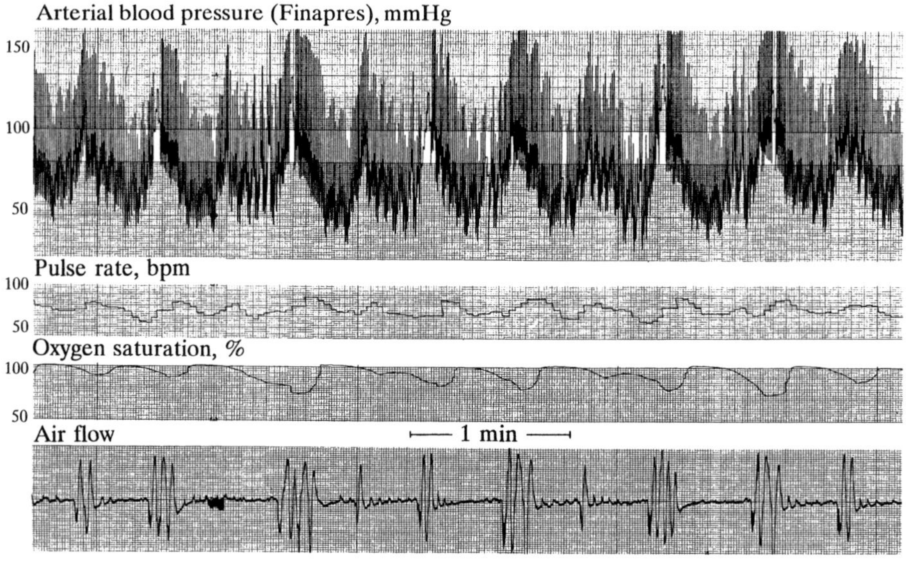

Figure 2 Monitoring of beat-to-beat blood pressure (Finapres), pulse rate, oxygen saturation, and oro-nasal airflow over 8 minutes in a sleeping patient with OSA. Note the large rises in BP at the end of each apnea and the increasing respiratory swings during the obstructive apneas.

by some groups to reduce compliance with CPAP (31–33). Should a much simpler and less unpleasant treatment appear, then risk reduction data and "numbers needed to treat" analyses will be required to justify its use for the prevention of cardiovascular events. This is exactly the same approach that we use currently to assess intervention to reduce cardiovascular risk in asymptomatic subjects such as cholesterol-lowering drugs (34) and anticoagulants in atrial fibrillation (35).

A final reason for assessing the degree of OSA, usually in an otherwise asymptomatic individual, is when pharyngeal surgery is contemplated for the social inconvenience of snoring. Due to the poor success rate of pharyngeal surgery in curing OSA and snoring (36,37), and its potential adverse consequences in those who may subsequently require nasal CPAP (38), it is regarded as unwise to operate on individuals with significant OSA. In this context, "significant" needs, of course, to be defined. There is probably no particular cut-off point, but the more severe the OSA, the less advisable the surgical option. Again, this approach is poorly supported by evidence, and the way sleep studies are used to influence surgical decisions varies from center to center. However, simplified diagnostic tests cannot be validated in this situation unless we specify meaningful outcomes, for example, does a particular test identify those who do well with pharyngeal surgery (long-term relief of obstruction and noise, with no adverse side effects), as opposed to those who do not?

III. Limitations of Current Sleep Study Variables

Apneas were the first pathological events to be recognized (2), followed by obstructive hypopneas (39), with or without attendant hypoxemia. The addition of hypopneas allowed the recognition of severely sleep fragmented individuals who sometimes had few complete apneas.

A. Hypopneas and Upper Airway Resistance Syndrome Apneas

Following this widening of the criteria for a pathological event came the more recent recognition that upper airway narrowing with inspiratory flow limitation, without apparent hypopnea or hypoxemia, could also lead to sleep fragmentation (40). Although there was usually a history of snoring in such individuals, during a sleep study there could be periods where upper airway narrowing without snoring led to a compensatory increase in inspiratory effort and recurrent arousal from sleep (upper airway resistance syndrome). This fitted nicely with the observation that in most patients with sleep apnea it was probably the increase in inspiratory effort that was the dominant arousal stimulus (15), rather than hypoxemia or hypercapnia (Fig. 1). The final proof that these nonapneic events were truly similar to conventional apneas and hypopneas was provided by a similar beneficial response to a trial of nasal CPAP therapy (40). These nonapneic events leading to arousal had not previously been spotted on polysomnography recordings analyzed conventionally for apnea/hypopnea index (AHI) and sleep stages. The importance attached to these events by some has led to the recommendation that routine esophageal pressure monitoring is essential to document the increases in inspiratory effort that result from upper airway narrowing and hence lead to arousal (20,41).

B. Correlation Between Sleep-Related Events and Daytime Function

The correlation between events measured on a conventional sleep study and daytime symptoms has usually been very poor (42). This has greatly limited our ability to use the sleep study to answer the simple clinical question, "Can this individual's symptoms be explained by sleep fragmentation?" In sleep clinic populations, those with OSA are not that much sleepier than those who turn out to have just snoring (43–45). This poor correlation could have several explanations. As mentioned before, we do not know which events are responsible for symptoms or how best to measure them. Our ability to measure the symptoms themselves, either objectively or subjectively, is also not very good, with limited agreements between similar objective tests multiple sleep latency test (MSLT), multiple wakefulness test (MWT) (46,47) and between the objective and subjective tests (Epworth Sleepiness Scale, ESS) (48,49). Finally there is considerable night-to-night variation of sleep study respiratory indices, particularly in the mild-to-moderate part of the spectrum, with a significant proportion of patients crossing arbitrary thresholds between two separate studies (50–52). Despite all these reasons for a poor correlation between symptoms and sleep study indices, many centers still use fixed thresholds (such as 15 apneas per hour) to make clinical decisions (e.g., whether to offer nasal CPAP therapy).

The correlation between various indices of daytime impairment and measures of "sleep apnea" activity has been looked at by several laboratories. Cheshire et al. (42) looked at the relationship between a variety of measures of daytime impairment and a variety of indices of fragmented sleep (Table 1). None of the EEG definitions of sleep fragmentation (3 or 1.5 s return of alpha or theta rhythm) correlated with objective sleepiness measured with the MSLT in a group of 29 patients with >15 apneas or hypopneas per hour of sleep. There were correlations between performance tests and respiratory indices of sleep apnea severity, but less so with most of the EEG markers of arousal, except for a 1.5 s definition, which also required EMG activation for more than 1.5 s. This would suggest that putting extra effort into counting EEG microarousals, over and above simple respiratory measurements, is unlikely to produce clinically useful increases in our ability to diagnose those individuals with sleep apnea who are likely to respond to treatment. Rees et al. (53) showed that not all apneas end in visible EEG arousal, but always ended in autonomic evidence of arousal (e.g., blood pressure rises). Earlier work had already shown blood pressure (BP) rises to be very sensitive markers of arousing stimuli (54). Martin et al. (55) were able to show that "subcortical" or "autonomic" arousals induced in normal subjects were capable of producing objective increases in daytime sleepiness and mood changes. Thus, although subcortical arousals may be important in contributing to daytime symptoms, there has been little evidence that these, or recognizable but brief EEG arousals, are any better at predicting sleepiness than the simpler respiratory indices of sleep apnea.

Table 1 Correlations Between Sleepiness (MSLT), Various Daytime Measures of Cognitive Function, and Various Nighttime Measures of Sleep Apnea Severity in 29 Patients with OSA[a]

	MSLT	Simple reaction time test	Trail making test	IQ decrement	Block design
AHI	NS	0.58	NS	0.45	0.57
>4% Sa_{O_2} desaturation index	NS	0.42	NS	0.47	0.33
Lowest Sa_{O_2}	NS	NS	0.56	0.40	NS
Arousal index, 1.5-s EMG rise with EEG speeding	NS	NS	NS	NS	0.41
Arousal index, 1.5-s EEG speeding with *any* EMG rise	NS	0.61	NS	0.44	0.47

[a] >15 apneas or hypopneas per hour of sleep. NS = not significant.
Source: Ref. 42.

C. Use of Outcomes to Measure the Relevance of Sleep-Related Events

Our own unit has also explored predictors of both initial daytime sleepiness and the improvement in sleepiness seen following a month of CPAP therapy (56,57), the purpose of the latter being to identify that portion of the sleepiness specifically due to problems with upper airway narrowing during sleep. Forty-one patients referred to the sleep laboratory, ranging from normal to severe sleep apnea, had baseline measures of sleepiness. All received CPAP (whether clinically indicated or not, median compliance 5 h/night) and measures of sleepiness repeated at one month. The sleep study derivatives included respiratory variables (AHI, Sa_{O_2} dip rate), EEG variables, autonomic variables [beat-to-beat blood pressure measured indirectly using pulse transit time (58) and heart rate rises], and body movements from a video image processing system. Interestingly, all these sleep study measures of sleep fragmentation correlated significantly both with baseline sleepiness and its improvement with nasal CPAP, measured subjectively [ESS (59)] and objectively [behavioral MWT (60)]. However, the best correlates of nasal CPAP responsive sleepiness were the measure of body movement from the video image processing system and >4% Sa_{O_2} dips per hour (Table 2). The EEG markers and autonomic markers appeared to be somewhat less satisfactory (although not significantly so). This suggests that it may be the bigger arousals leading to body movement that are most responsible for daytime symptoms of sleepiness and that chasing ever-more-sensitive markers of arousals will bring no useful clinical benefit in this situation.

In epidemiological surveys looking at sleep apnea, the correlation between sleep study measures of apnea and daytime symptoms has been poor or nonexistent

Table 2 Correlations of Both Baseline Sleepiness (subjective, ESS: objective, MWT) and Change in Sleepiness Following 1 Month of CPAP Therapy with Various Initial Measures of OSA Severity in 41 Patients Presenting to the Sleep Clinic with a History of Snoring and Given CPAP Regardless of Sleep Study Severity[a]

	Baseline (pre-CPAP)		Improvements in test on CPAP	
	ESS	MWT	ΔESS	ΔMWT
ASDA arousal index	0.50 ($p = 0.001$)	−0.51 ($p = 0.0007$)	−0.38 ($p = 0.02$)	0.43 ($p = 0.006$)
1.5-s arousal index	0.49 ($p = 0.001$)	−0.49 ($p = 0.0007$)	−0.38 ($p = 0.02$)	0.43 ($p = 0.006$)
Neural net EEG analysis of arousals	0.46 ($p = 0.02$)	−0.51 ($p = 0.0007$)	−0.50 ($p = 0.001$)	0.54 ($p = 0.0003$)
Movement index (from video)	0.40 ($p = 0.01$)	−0.53 ($p = 0.0004$)	−0.63 ($p < 0.0001$)	0.60 ($p < 0.0001$)
Autonomic arousal index	0.52 ($p = 0.0005$)	−0.49 ($p = 0.001$)	−0.42 ($p = 0.006$)	0.44 ($p = 0.004$)
AHI	0.41 ($p = 0.008$)	−0.41 ($p = 0.007$)	−0.53 ($p = 0.0004$)	0.52 ($p = 0.0005$)
>4% Sa_{O_2} desaturation index	0.39 ($p = 0.013$)	−0.41 ($p = 0.006$)	−0.67 ($p < 0.0001$)	0.58 ($p < 0.0001$)

[a] On the whole, measures of CNS arousal best predict baseline sleepiness, but measures of respiratory events best predict improvement with CPAP.
Source: Ref. 56.

(61–63). This suggests very strongly that all apneas and hypopneas are not the same in their ability to cause symptoms and that some cofactor needs to be present to generate daytime symptoms, perhaps the degree of arousal required to break them (19,22,64).

As argued in the preceding section, a new approach to sleep studies seems to be indicated. It is clear that polysomnography cannot, and should not, be regarded as a gold standard as it has never been properly validated as a tool to measure the actual pathological process resulting from reduced upper airway tone with sleep onset. In addition, it has not been validated as a tool to answer some of the usual clinical questions about patients with possible sleep apnea:

1. Can this patient's symptoms be explained by sleep apnea or related condition?
2. Is nasal CPAP likely to be beneficial?
3. What are the chances that pharyngeal surgery will be safe and beneficial?

If polysomnography is inadequate in this way, what are the alternatives in terms of both alternative physiological variables to measure and their clinical value?

From a respiratory clinician's point of view, a beneficial symptomatic response to CPAP is perhaps the outcome of interest, and future diagnostic approaches could perhaps be assessed according to their ability to predict a favorable subjective response to this therapy, e.g., using the ESS. Unfortunately, placebo responses will contaminate a subjective response and require accounting for. Alternatively, the gold standard might be an objective response to CPAP, e.g., using improvements in the MWT, although again placebo responses might still be present. However, in a recent sham placebo-controlled trial of CPAP, no placebo response was found for the MWT, although there was one for the ESS and measures of self-assessed health status (SF-36) (65). In addition, it is not clear what improvements in MWT should be regarded as a clinically useful positive response. Our attempts to find the most relevant marker of sleep fragmentation on a sleep study, described earlier, explored both subjective and objective nasal CPAP responsiveness as the reference standard (56).

The best diagnostic approach to assessing the likely efficacy of CPAP in reversing symptoms might not be the same as that required to predict future adverse cardiovascular events (should they exist), particularly, for example, if sleep fragmentation is the cause of sleepiness while hypoxemia the cause of hypertension. Similarly, trying to predict beneficial outcome following pharyngeal surgery from a sleep study might depend more on whether hypopneas predominated rather than apneas. Thus, in reality, we do not have one clear gold standard against which to evaluate new limited diagnostic tests. Virtually none of the published studies looking at simplified diagnostic techniques have used this outcomes approach; most have relied on a conventional comparison with polysomnography.

The next section explores some of the techniques currently available to monitor OSA and its variants that could be used outside the laboratory and reviews what evidence there is that they provide a useful contribution to the clinician's decision making. Unfortunately, this evidence is usually derived only from their ability to mimic conventional polysomnography, either in a correlation analysis with AHI or in a specificity/sensitivity analysis to predict an AHI above or below certain arbitrary thresholds.

IV. Measurement of Upper Airway Narrowing and Increased Inspiratory Effort

A. Upper Airway Narrowing

The primary pathology in OSA and its variants (sleep-induced upper airway narrowing) can be measured or inferred, directly or indirectly, by measuring several different signals. For example, continuous measures of upper airway resistance using a face mask with a pneumotachograph and esophageal balloon would be one of the most direct gold standard approaches available. An alternative would be the forced oscillation technique via a face mask (66). At the other end of the spectrum, the least direct approaches would be snoring and oximetry. Clearly the nearer one can get to the primary pathology the better, but sometimes this may be at the expense of invasiveness and therefore inappropriate in a limited sleep study.

Table 3 lists the signals that could be used to measure upper airway narrowing and increased inspiratory effort. The forced oscillation technique involves oscillating a known volume of air in and out of the nose and mouth via a face mask at about 5 Hz. The pressure in the mask is measured, and the pressure swings at 5 Hz will be proportional to the degree of upper airway resistance (66). The requirement for a face mask and a good seal will reduce its usefulness in limited studies. In addition, the data obtained will be in a format unfamiliar to those accustomed to AHI values, for example, a histogram of numbers of breaths at various degrees of upper airway resistance, or the median and centile values of the resistance for all breaths across the night.

Airflow limitation is a concept well understood by physiologists interested in airway narrowing. Expiratory airflow limitation during a forced maneuver is seen on flow volume loops from patients with a large airway obstruction, such as a tracheal tumor. In this situation the airflow rises but is locked at a reduced value by the fixed narrowing of the airway and the onset of turbulent flow. Thus, despite increasing expiratory effort no increase in airflow is achieved, and this is what is meant by flow limitation (67), a property of Starling resistors. Sometimes the airway narrowing is not rigid and may vary in size depending on the phase of respiration, hence flow limitation may only be present in expiration, inspiration, or only part of either. This is what appears to happen in the pharynx during inspiration. If the pharyngeal airway is not held open sufficiently, then inspiratory airflow will rise to a limited and reduced maximum and stay reduced until the end of inspiration. Sometimes a higher flow will be obtained briefly before the pharyngeal walls are sucked in by the subatmospheric pressures generated by the inspiration. This gives rise to the characteristic flow-limited inspiratory pattern rather than the normal smooth sinusoidal shape (Fig. 3). It should be appreciated that this ''characteristic'' pattern of a transient peak followed by flow limitation will not always be present if the pharynx is already narrowed at inspiratory onset and if the degree of narrowing changes during the course of the inspiration for some reason [e.g., recruitment of defense reflexes (12,13)]. It has been quite difficult to automate the analysis of inspi-

Table 3 Markers of Increased Upper Airway Narrowing and Increased Inspiratory Effort

Upper airway narrowing	Increased inspiratory effort
Face mask and esophageal pressure	Esophageal pressure
Forced oscillation technique	Ribcage/abdominal paradox
Inspiratory airflow limitation	Supraclavicular/sternal notch depression
Snoring	Inspiratory blood pressure swings
Apneas/hypopneas	Fast component of electrostatic bed signals

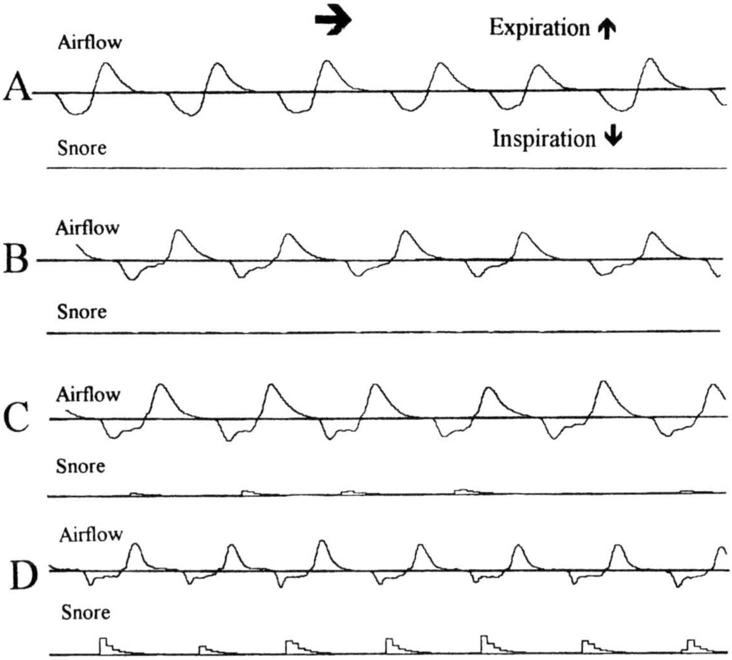

Figure 3 Nasal "airflow" tracings using nasal cannulae connected to a pressure transducer (inspiration downward). Four separate tracings from one individual; A, unobstructed, noiseless inspiration; B, moderate inspiratory flow limitation with no noise; C, moderate inspiratory flow limitation with quiet snoring; D, marked inspiratory flow limitation with louder snoring.

ratory flow limitation, probably for these reasons. The Sydney group has explored its use quite extensively and incorporated successfully a measurement of airflow limitation, derived from the shape of the inspiratory flow curve, as the feedback signal in an automatic CPAP machine (68,69). Airflow limitation is most accurately measured using a face mask and pneumotachograph, although measuring pressure just inside the nares produces a very similar shaped signal (70–72). If a sampling tube (often a nasal cannula designed for O_2 administration) of sufficient diameter is used, so that a small degree of resistance to airflow in the nares is produced, then the system behaves somewhat like a pneumotachograph. If a square root transformation of the signal is generated, then the similarity to a pneumotachograph signal is even better (70). Thermistors cannot be used for this purpose as their time constants are too long to reproduce the flow limitation patterns with sufficient precision (73,74). Good correlations exist between measures of airflow limitation and actual upper airflow narrowing (Fig. 4) (71,72). At present the ability of this signal and its all-night analysis to represent the full spectrum of upper airway narrowing seen

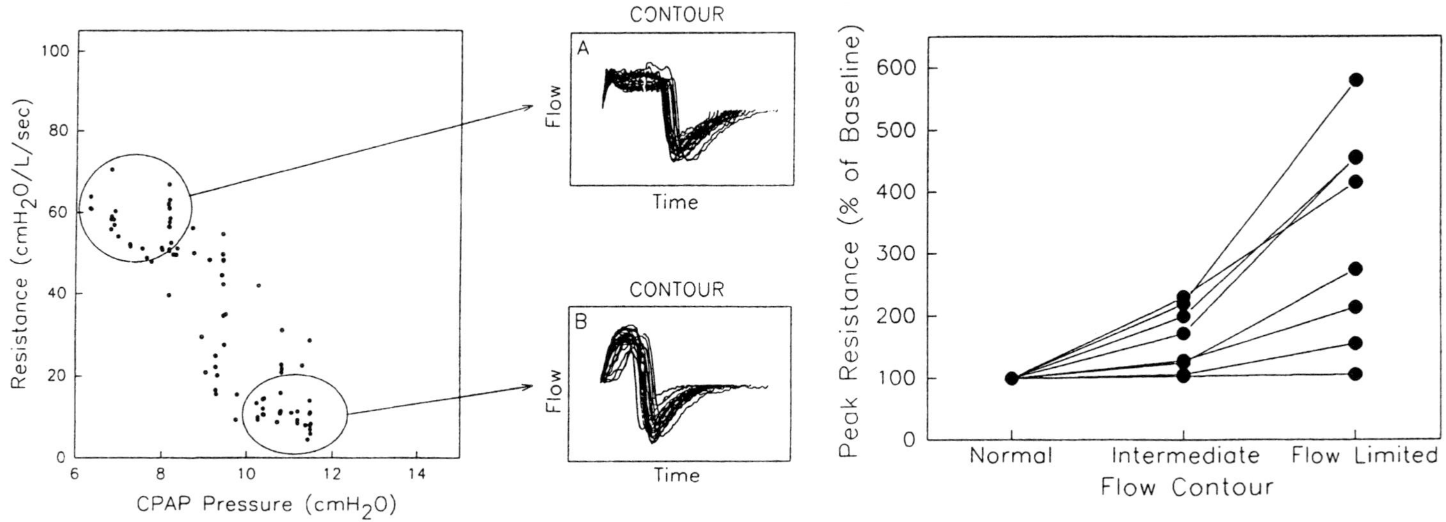

Figure 4 Measurements of upper airway resistance (from esophageal pressure and flow through a nose mask) while CPAP pressure was varied in one patient with OSA. Note that at low CPAP pressures (left end of left graph) the inspiratory resistance is high and the flow contour severely flow limited. At higher pressures the inspiratory flow contour is nicely rounded and not flow limited. The righthand graph relates upper airway resistance with hand scoring of inspiratory flow contours in eight subjects. (From Ref. 71.)

across normal subjects, snorers, and OSA has not been verified. However, it appears that even normal subjects get some degree of airflow limitation on some breaths (11), so that sensitivity is unlikely to be a problem, but specificity may be.

At some point, as the pharynx narrows, audible vibrations will occur. Snoring can come from different pharyngeal locations, and presumably its occurrence will depend on factors other than simply the pharyngeal dimensions and resistance. Thus, the point at which snoring begins will not mean the same degree of narrowing or flow limitation across all individuals (75), the most extreme example of this being the reduction or abolition of low-frequency snoring by pharyngeal surgery, sometimes in the absence of any effect on pharyngeal obstruction and apneas. In addition, Guilleminault's group has shown, particularly in women, that airflow limitation to the point of awakening can occur with no snoring (76,77). Thus, the measurement of snoring is only a qualitative marker of the presence of upper airway narrowing with potentially limited specificity and sensitivity. However, due to its ease of measurement from either pharyngeal, nasal, forehead, chest, or room microphones, it is an ideal signal to incorporate into a limited monitoring system. For example, the MESAM system from Germany (snoring, body position, heart rate, and oximetry) incorporates a pharyngeal microphone but limits the snoring resolution to three levels (Fig. 5). In an assessment of this device in patients referred to a sleep lab, its performance against a conventional AHI of 10/h depended mainly on the oxygen desaturation index, with a poor specificity and better sensitivity for the "snoring

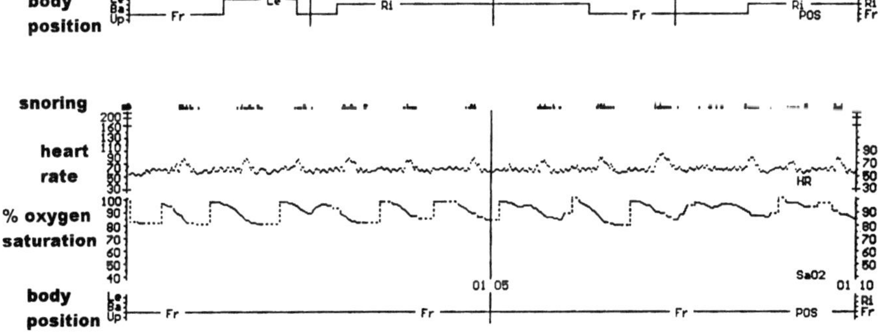

Figure 5 Two tracings from a MESAM portable recorder in a subject with OSA; top tracing is 2 h, bottom tracing is 10 min. Each tracing, top down, consists of snoring (three levels), heart rate, oximetry, and posture. In the bottom tracing, note the clear evidence of interapneic snoring, desaturations, and arousal-related rises in pulse rate.

index'' (27% and 96%, respectively) versus 97% and 92% for the desaturation index (78). Remmers' group (79) used a combination of oximetry and snoring (suprasternal skin microphone) for a portable sleep apnea monitor. The snoring signal was analyzed for intersnore intervals between 10 and 120 s (presumed apneas) accompanied by falls in Sa_{O_2} of >3%. The respiratory disturbance index (RDI) calculated in this way in a group of patients referred to the sleep lab–produced sensitivity and specificity values ranging between 84 and 90% and 95 and 98%, respectively, depending on the exact polysomnographic definition of OSA. The algorithms used in this device were honed to simulate conventional AHI (employing Sa_{O_2} dip criteria), and thus its ability to recreate AHI is not surprising. A second larger study (80), using the device at home as well as the lab, found a far better correlation between simultaneous lab polysomnography AHI and their RDI than between a home and lab RDI. This highlights the problem of night-to-night variation in this kind of work. The cause of systematic bias between home and lab studies was a tendency for patients to sleep longer on their backs when in the laboratory. This group's most recent publication has demonstrated that ≥4% Sa_{O_2} dips/h from the oximeter signal, carefully analyzed, has a correlation on its own with AHI of 0.97, and the inclusion of snoring added nothing to its performance. Others have not found such good correlations with AHI (81), likely due to the use of different oximeters and different analysis algorithms (see later).

Other home monitors have used the same signals as PSG, particularly nasal flow, to generate an RDI. Most of the discrepancies between home and laboratory studies in an early paper using the Edentrace device were probably due to night-to-night variation (82). This paper also used falls in Sa_{O_2} to help classify respiratory events, and thus significant technical differences between home and laboratory studies would not have been expected.

B. Increased Inspiratory Effort

Attempts to estimate the rise in inspiratory effort in response to pharyngeal narrowing have centered on pleural pressure measurements, direct and indirect. Esophageal pressure has been measured conventionally with an esophageal balloon, or a pressure tipped catheter, passed via the nose. Most laboratories have not adopted this as a routine, although a few have (20,41). Only one group (83) has moved this measurement out of the lab using a solid-state transducer on a fine catheter passed via the nose. They showed that conventional apneas and hypopneas could be recognized, but a more sophisticated analysis looking at nonapneic/hypopneic increases in pleural pressure was not done.

During a loaded inspiration with marked subatmospheric pressures, there will tend to be dysynchronous movements of the ribcage (RC) and abdomen (AB) due to a difference in the ''strength'' of the two compartments. Usually there is paradoxical inward drawing of the ribcage (either partially or complete) as the diaphragm descends and the abdomen moves out (Fig. 6). Measurement of this paradox has been

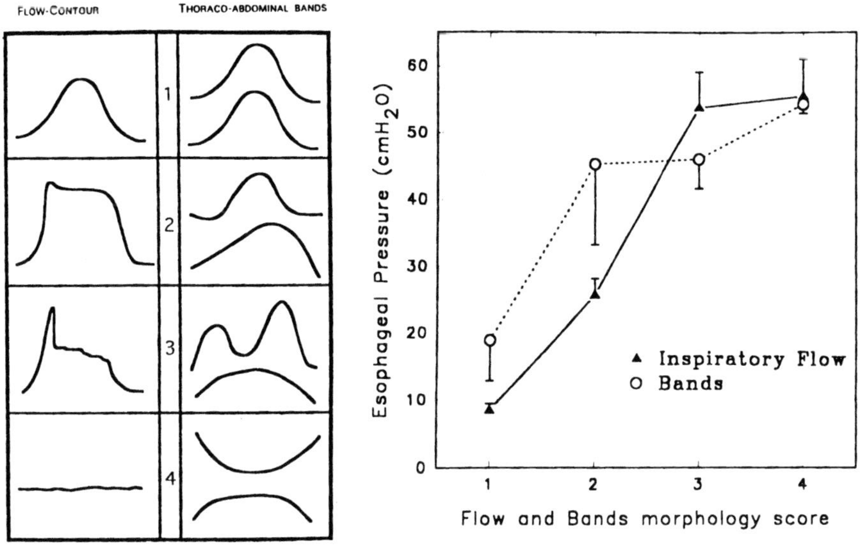

Figure 6 Comparison of two noninvasive measures of upper airway narrowing and increased inspiratory effort. The lefthand diagram shows the development of paradoxical movement of the ribcage/abdominal bands (righthand panels) as inspiratory flow limitation develops (lefthand panels), through to complete apnea. The visual scorings of these two phenomena (1–4) are then tolerated with the size of the inspiratory esophageal pressure swings. (From Ref. 72.)

shown to correlate with upper airway narrowing and increased inspiratory effort (72). It is conveniently displayed as the phase angle of an RC/AB plot and is available in a commercial system (Densa Ltd., Flint, UK). There is no published formal comparison with other diagnostic techniques. This device has been used in a published study looking at its value during a CPAP titration night (84) where it produced identical outcomes to conventional PSG in terms of the pressures prescribed (yet another outcome measure).

A simple system using an electrostatic mattress to measure body movements has also been able to identify a marker of obstructed breathing (85). This relies on detecting the fast components of respiratory movements (''spikes'') that are usually only present during periods of upper airway loading. This is a promising approach, but it has not yet been shown reliably to identify those individuals with upper airway obstruction likely to respond to treatment.

Another, more indirect, approach to monitoring pleural pressure has been the use of suprasternal or supraclavicular (86) skin indrawing. These areas of skin are quite close to the pleural surface and, if the fatty layer is not too great, will be drawn in during inspiration. Various devices have been used, but, like the ribcage/abdomen paradox, they have not gained wide acceptance, partly, we suspect, because these kinds of measurements do not produce an index of upper airway narrowing directly comparable to the AHI, as discussed earlier.

The final approach to be discussed in this section is the use of inspiratory blood pressure falls (pulsus paradoxus). Because the heart and thoracic aorta are in the chest, any intrathoracic pressures to which they are subjected will be added to, or subtracted from, the arterial pressure measured outside the thoracic cavity. In a way one can view the arterial tree as a fluid-filled manometer line into the chest. This reflection of pleural pressure by the arterial tree has been recognized for a long time and has been used in the assessment of asthma severity (87). Recently its use in estimating inspiratory effort during upper airway obstruction has been described (88,89). Noninvasive and qualitative measurements of beat-to-beat blood pressure have only been possible since the invention of the Finapres (90) and a portable device to measure beat-by-beat pulse wave velocity (or pulse transit time) (91). The Finapres device (Ohmeda 2300, Englewood, CO; Portapres/Finometer, TNO, Amsterdam, The Netherlands) uses a photoplethysmographic volume clamp technique that makes the pressure in a cuff around the finger match the arterial pressure in the digital arteries. The tracings so produced are remarkably similar to peripheral

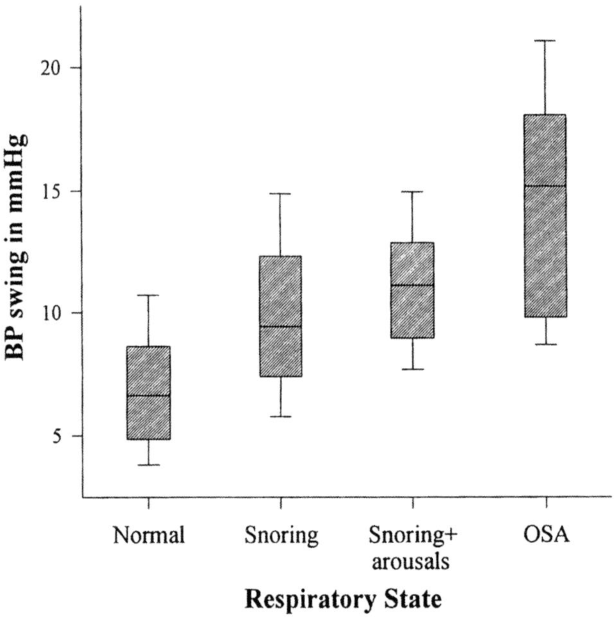

Figure 7 Measurement of the inspiratory swings in systolic BP, using the Finapres, during multiple periods of breathing during sleep classified into four levels of upper airway obstruction. Note that as the degree of upper airway obstruction increases, so does the size of the inspiratory systolic BP swings, reflecting the increasing inspiratory effort. (From Ref. 89.)

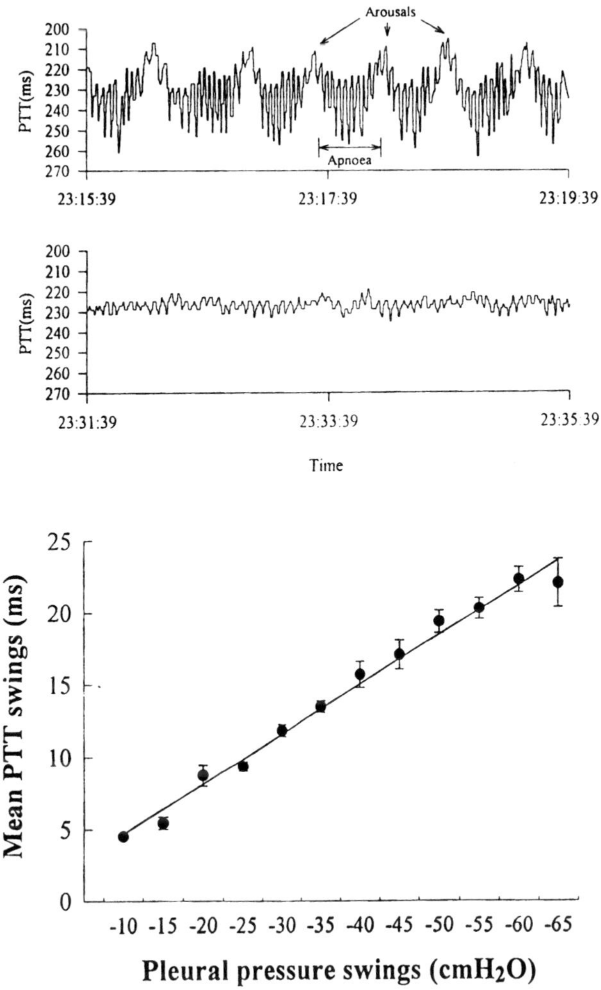

Figure 8 Use of pulse transit time as a surrogate of beat-to-beat blood pressure changes. The top two tracings are from a patient with OSA, off and on nasal CPAP. The tracings are inverted so that rises in BP (falls in PTT) are upwards. Note the rise in BP with each arousal and large inspiratory falls with each frustrated inspiratory effort (compare with Fig. 2). On CPAP (second trace) the arousal-related rises in BP disappear and the size of the inspiratory swings are greatly diminished. The bottom tracing shows the correlation between inspiratory swings in esophageal pressure (during a CPAP titration study, when the airway pressure was deliberately raised and lowered to produce a range of inspiratory efforts) and inspiratory swings in PTT. Data from one subject, esophageal pressure swings grouped in 5 cmH_2O bins. (From Ref. 96.)

intra-arterial line tracings, and the respiratory swings are easily seen and measured (Fig. 2). The sizes of the swings are very similar to, and correlate well with, the sizes of the pleural pressure swings (88). Davies et al. used the Finapres device to measure inspiratory BP swings during different periods where the breathing was normal, snoring, snoring with arousals, and frank OSA (89,92). There was a progressive increase across these groups as one would predict, and it appeared promising as a noninvasive measure of inspiratory effort (Fig. 7). Although there is a semi-portable version of the Finapres device, it is still not very practical for home sleep studies (93). An alternative device for measuring beat-to-beat blood pressure relies on measurement of pulse wave velocity (or pulse transit time; Parametric Recorders, London, UK; Sunrise Medical, Somerset, Pennsylvania; Stowood Scientific Instruments, Oxford, UK) (94,95). Changes in the time taken for the pulse shock wave to travel from the opening aortic valve to the periphery depend mainly on blood pressure. The approximate time taken for the pulse wave to travel from the aortic valve to the index finger is about 200 ms. As blood pressure rises, the wall tenses and the pulse shock wave travels faster. For convenience, the start time is identified from the R wave of the ECG, thus adding the left ventricular isometric contraction time to the overall measurement. The arrival time is conveniently measured with the use of a finger oximeter probe, using the transmittance signal from either of the two available infrared frequencies. The change in R wave to finger transit time for every 1 mmHg change in BP is approximately 1 ms (96). Rather serendipitously, during falls in intrathoracic pressure the left ventricular contraction time is also prolonged, which contributes to the overall lengthening of R wave to finger pulse transit time (PTT) (97). The limitation of this technique is that a value is only available with each heart beat and it therefore undersamples a waveform with the frequency of breathing. This is circumvented by measuring each inspiratory change in PTT breath-by-breath but averaging over several breaths. Used in this way it clearly measures changes in inspiratory effort in patients with OSA (96,98) (Fig. 8) and differentiates between normal subjects, snorers, and those with OSA. The Grenoble group has also found that the use of PTT tracings could differentiate obstructive from central apneas nearly as well as esophageal pressure tracings (99,100). More recently they have established its use in recognizing partially obstructed breaths that can lead to arousal (101,102).

V. Measurement of Sleep Fragmentation

Although the EEG has been viewed as the closest we can get to the signal implying symptomatic sleep disturbance noninvasively, this may not be true. A number of different methods can be used to identify sleep disturbance (see Table 4). Recent data have suggested that arousing events that only have autonomic consequences (rise in heart rate and BP) may produce daytime sleepiness even if they do not propagate from the brain stem up into the frontal cortex (103). Frontal EEG elec-

Table 4 Markers of Sleep Disturbance

EEG	Autonomic	Others
Microarousals	Heart rate rises	Body movements
Conventional arousals	BP rises	Sudden reductions in RC/AB paradox
Sleep state changes	Skin vasoconstriction	Sudden reductions in airflow limitation
Amount of stage 1 and 2 vs. 3 and 4		

trodes (F_3, A_2) will pick up more microarousals than temporal ones (C_3, A_2) (104), but autonomic markers will pick up even more (54,58). Thus, once again we have no gold standard measurement of sleep fragmentation that best predicts daytime symptoms.

A. EEG Measures of Sleep Fragmentation

Conventional derivatives of all night EEG monitoring that were felt to reflect quality of sleep in OSA were the amount of stage 1 and 2 sleep state changes and the number of epochs (20 or 30 s) after sleep onset that were subsequently scored awake or movement time (105). This approach fails to reflect accurately the sort of sleep fragmentation seen in OSA, and most laboratories that still use EEG have moved onto microarousal scoring. Many laboratories have their own definition, but the definition advanced by the American Sleep Disorders Association is no more arbitrary than any other (106). They defined a microarousal as an EEG frequency increase of ≥3 s, including theta, alpha, and/or frequencies greater than 16 Hz, but not spindles. In practice, many laboratories score any discernible rise in EEG frequency (hopefully excluding spindles) of 3 s or more. This definition only requires a rise in EMG amplitude when in REM sleep, whereas other well-recognized microarousal definitions required EMG rises during non-REM sleep as well (42). Rather surprisingly, even the most sensitive arousal definitions do not seem to predict daytime sleepiness in a group of sleep clinic patients better than respiratory variables (42). In addition, interlab agreement on the scoring of these microarousals is not particularly good (107).

However, it is possible to measure EEG with ambulatory recorders, initially done with small tape recorders (Oxford Medilog) and more recently with solid-state digital recorders. Add to this some form of automatic analysis and this approach does become an attractive option for home monitoring. Computerized EEG analysis was never very successful in mimicking the manually based epoch scoring techniques, particularly in abnormal sleep, but it shows greater promise in characterizing the fluctuating sleep depth seen in sleep and breathing disorders (Fig. 9) (22, 108–111).

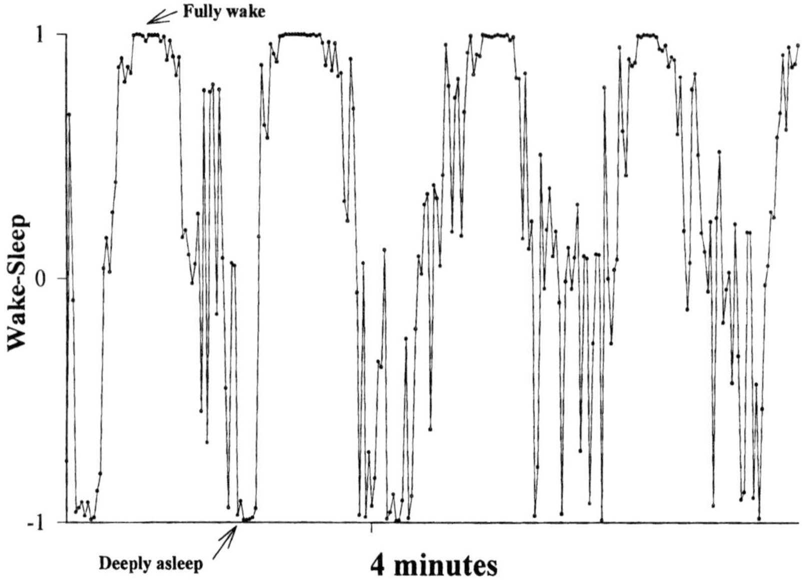

Figure 9 Second-by-second tracings of EEG sleep depth in a patient with OSA measured by the neural network technique described by Pardey et al. (109). +1 on the axis is where the previously trained neural network classifies the EEG as ''maximally awake,'' and −1 is where the classification is ''maximally asleep'' (corresponding to maximal slow wave activity). Note the enormous swings; the ''deepest'' periods occurring prior to abrupt arousal are often bursts of K complexes with identical characteristics, of course, to slow waves when using an analysis window of 1 s.

B. Autonomic Measures of Sleep Fragmentation

The process of arousal, either spontaneous or in response to an outside stimulus, begins in the brain stem, travels upward via two pathways (112–114), and then radiates through the whole cortex. Habituation of EEG responses to external noises by sleeping humans, but with preservation of an autonomic response (115), shows us that this propagation upward of an ''arousal'' is in some way controlled and not inevitable. For example, the exhausted mother of a new baby will wake to its cry but sleep through the morning alarm call. The extent to which the arousals at the end of a respiratory event generate daytime sleepiness may depend on whether the increased upper airway resistance can be cleared without ''having to wake up the whole cortex'' (64). Thus, autonomic markers of arousal may be too sensitive and document all potentially arousing events, rather than just those that cause daytime symptoms.

The early portable sleep recorder, the MESAM, documented heart rate variability (Fig. 5) but did not formally incorporate this into its automatic analysis. Our work on autonomic responses to arousal during sleep showed that transient heart

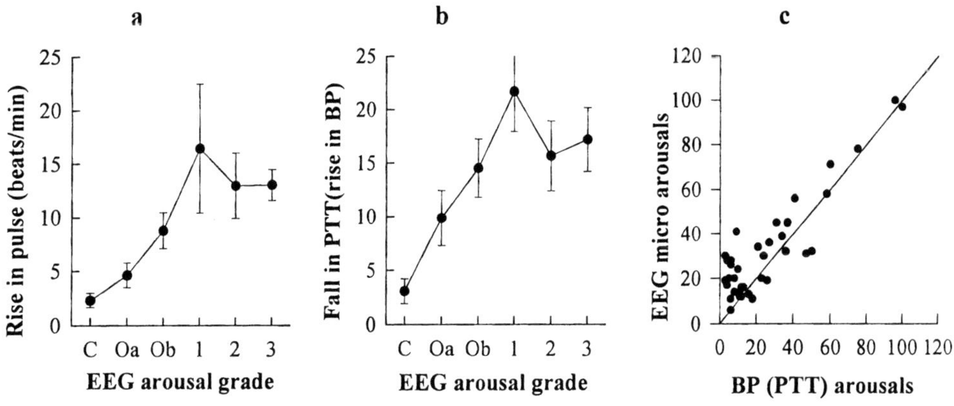

Figure 10 Graphs (a) and (b) show the relationship between graded EEG arousals and two autonomic consequences (heart rate rise and BP rise, measured by pulse transit time analysis) in normal subjects exposed to auditory tones during non-REM sleep. Arousal grading: C, control period (no auditory stimulus); Oa, no discernible change in EEG or EMG in response to stimulus; Ob, "deepening" of EEG with the appearance of greater slow wave activity or K complexes only; 1, increase in high frequency EEG or EMG (or both) for less than 3 s; 2, increase in high frequency EEG or EMG (or both) for between 3 and 10 s; 3, increase in high frequency EEG or EMG (or both) for more than 10 s. (From Ref. 58.) The righthand graph (c) compares the number of arousals per hour defined by BP rises (using PTT) with the number of arousals defined by EEG [ASDA criteria (106)] in 40 patients monitored in the sleep laboratory for possible OSA. (From Ref. 116.)

rate (HR) rises could certainly occur in response to external noises in the absence of discernible EEG changes (58) (Fig. 10). In addition, a significant correlation between "heart rate" arousals (rises in BPM of >10) and other indices of sleep apnea severity (e.g., AHI) in a group of 41 sleep clinic patients has been demonstrated (r = 0.38) (116).

The availability of noninvasive beat-to-beat blood pressure monitors has allowed the recognition that BP rises may be even more sensitive than heart rate at detecting arousals (58) (Fig. 10) and correlated even better than HR with the AHI in 41 sleep clinic patients (r = 0.56 vs. 0.38 for HR, although this difference did not reach statistical significance) (116). Once again, autonomic markers of arousal have not been shown to be clinically superior to conventional markers of sleep apnea severity in their ability to predict daytime symptoms or response to treatment (Table 2) (56,57). However, the preliminary data suggest that they are likely to be as good and, when measured using pulse transit time (an indirect measure of BP), are considerably easier to monitor at home (requiring only EEG electrodes and an oximeter probe) and subsequently analyze than conventional polysomnographic channels (56,57,116).

Movements during the sleep period are usually indicative of arousal. Early work showed that body movements were much more common during stages 1 and 2 of sleep than during stages 3 and 4 (117). A study comparing EEG microarousals with body movements visible on video recordings concluded that in sleep clinic patients there was usually detectable movement if the arousal was more than 2 s in length (118). It is possible to log movement of any part of the body from video recordings using automatic video processing systems (Fig. 11) (119,120). As described in an earlier section, Bennett et al. (56,57) have shown that body movements measured in this way are more predictive of daytime sleepiness and its improvement on nasal CPAP than either EEG, respiratory, or autonomic markers of sleep fragmentation (Table 2). Other approaches monitoring body movements during sleep have used wrist worn actigraphs (121–123), and it is clear that useful information can be obtained. These have been shown to differentiate sleep from wake and allow the

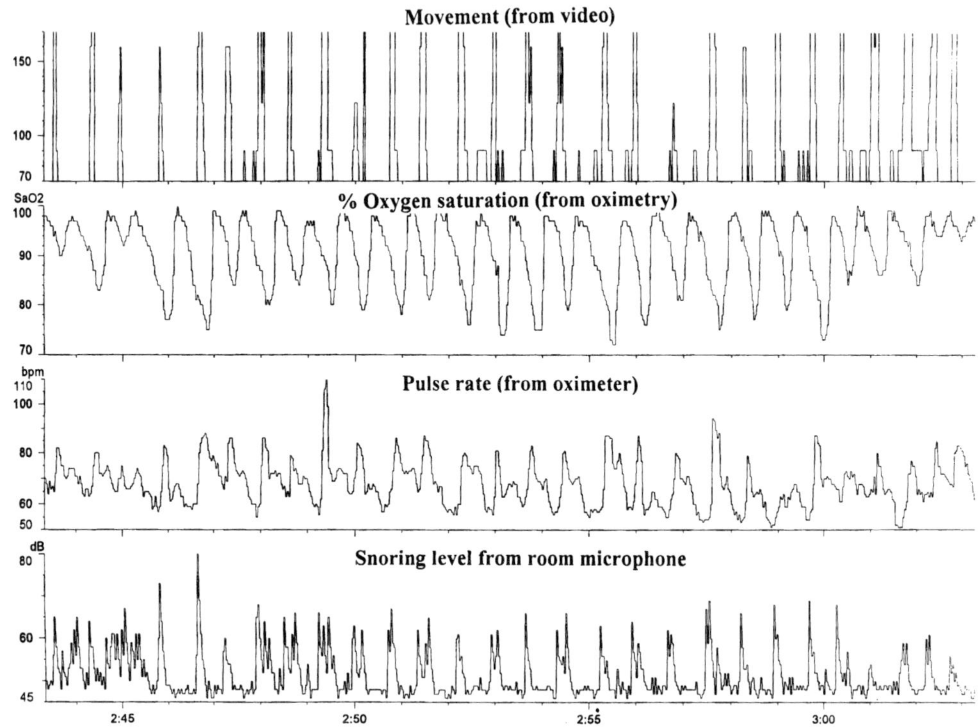

Figure 11 Twenty-minute tracing of a patient with sleep apnea using only oximetry and video recordings (Visi-Lab, Stowood Scientific Instruments, Oxford, UK). The top tracing is body movement (derived from digitally processing the video signal), the second tracing is oximetry, the third is heart rate, and the fourth is snoring. Movement and heart rate tracings provide information on sleep disturbance, oximetry, and snoring on respiratory abnormalities.

construction of a sleep/wake hypnogram (124,125), but it is not yet clear whether they pick up the relevant microarousals of sleep apnea (123), which sometimes produce head movement without arm movement. A head-mounted actigraphy system may be better in this respect (126). Body movements can also be automatically logged by the electrostatic bed system mentioned earlier.

If sleep disturbance is being provoked by upper airway narrowing and increased inspiratory effort, then following an arousal, with reopening of the upper airway, abnormalities of these signals should suddenly reverse. For example, inspiratory flow limitation usually disappears on awakening, as does RC/AB paradox. The rapid disappearance of flow limitation (104) and RC/AB paradox (127) have been proposed as markers of arousal from obstructive respiratory events, and in preliminary study, sudden changes in RC/AB paradox do correlate with EEG arousals (123).

VI. Non-EEG Sleep Study Systems

The term ''limited sleep study'' has come to mean almost any sleep study not employing EEG. Douglas et al. showed that the addition of EEG did not help in the diagnosis of sleep clinic patients when most of these patients were being investigated for possible OSA (81). However, this study was done at a time when AHI was still regarded as the main abnormality, and the importance of microarousals had not been fully appreciated. Although it is clearly possible to design non-EEG systems that produce results that mimic AHI, the extra diagnostic ability that may be lost by not taking account of microarousals has not been established. It is also argued that not recording EEG in a sleep study denies the reporter other essential information, for example, the absence of a real sleep time by which to divide the number of respiratory events. However, even if the time in bed is 10% or so greater than sleep time, the error in an RDI so introduced is less than the night-to-night variation (50–52) and only a problem if arbitrary thresholds are used for therapeutic decisions. It is also argued that it is essential to document REM sleep since OSA can be worse then. Douglas and colleagues showed that REM sleep did not occur in only 9% of laboratory polysomnographic studies (81). Of these, 4.5% had OSA diagnosed anyway, with repeat studies on the other 4.5% did not change the diagnosis. Finally, it is argued that the absence of an EEG tracing prevents the diagnosis of other conditions. The two other main diagnoses made in sleep laboratories are narcolepsy and periodic limb movement disorder. Early-onset REM sleep is characteristic of narcolepsy, but it occurs in normal subjects and patients with other sleep fragmentation syndromes (128–132), particularly REM sleep–dominant ones such as the nocturnal hypoventilation syndromes (e.g., scoliosis, postpolio syndrome). Narcolepsy is best diagnosed from history, HLA typing, and MSLTs that show two or more REM sleep onset periods in the absence of a sleep disruption or deprivation syndrome. Thus, it is unlikely that the presence or absence of early onset REM on a sleep study would be the critical investigation that made or excluded the diagnosis of narcolepsy.

Several limited sleep study systems do monitor leg movements, and thus EEG is not necessary for this diagnosis. Even in systems that do not measure leg movements, if there are multiple and regular unexplained microarousals (about every 30 or 40 s), this would lead one to perform a more extensive study including leg movements. Evidence of such sleep fragmentation could come from any one of the techniques described earlier.

One of the earliest limited sleep study systems to gain acceptance was the MESAM monitor (Madaus, Freiburg, Germany). The MESAM-4 device monitors snoring (three levels only), oxygen saturation (oximetry), heart rate, and posture (Fig. 5) (133). Several centers have evaluated this monitor in sleep clinic populations, all against polysomnography as the gold standard (134–141). Although there are automatic analyses available for heart rate, snoring, and oxygen desaturations, most studies have found that the majority of the signal lies in the oximeter channel with little extra predictive value from heart rate or snoring analysis (134). Hand scoring of all channels, however, was usually better than automatic scoring, although a more sophisticated automatic Sa_{O_2} dip analysis gave r values against AHI (>0.9) at least as good as the r values of two nights of AHI measurements against each other (135). Using cut-off AHI values of >10 or more produced sensitivity and specificity values of over 80%, the exact figures of course depending on whether the cut-off point on the oxygen desaturation index was set for high specificity or high sensitivity. These studies on patients referred to a sleep clinic (high prior probability) showed that a monitoring device relying heavily on the oximetry channel for its usefulness can provide acceptable sensitivity and specificity figures. It is not known if those subjects missed by less than 100% sensitivity or ''overdiagnosed'' by less than 100% specificity are clinically disadvantaged as a consequence.

Because of the reasonable agreement between laboratory AHI and MESAM 4 in patients, this device has been used outside the laboratory in populations with a low prior probability of having OSA, truck drivers (142), and random samples (143). It is unlikely that the sensitivity/specificity figures found in sleep clinic patients with high prior probabilities of having OSA will be the same in such populations with low prior probabilities. Unfortunately we have no evidence on which to assess their diagnostic performance based on outcomes relevant to these populations. AHI as an indicator of disease in randomly selected populations has been called into question (64), particularly given the lack of significant relationship between AHI and symptoms of sleepiness in a large Wisconsin cohort study (62,64) or in a similar Australian study (63).

The dependence of the MESAM on its oximetry channel for most of its diagnostic ability suggests that oximetry-alone studies may have a role to play. Many authors have looked at this with varying success. There are very different algorithms for counting respiratory events, particularly the calculation of any baseline prior to registering a dip as well as the size of the dip itself. Furthermore, there are subtle characteristics of Sa_{O_2} dipping that aid a visual analysis, which are missed by computer algorithms, hence manual review and scoring are recommended by some. For example, Douglas et al. (81) found a poor correlation between counted Sa_{O_2} dips and AHI, but visual inspection of the tracings produced a much better sensitivity. Others have found much better correlations between Sa_{O_2} dip rate and AHI than these authors, the difference probably being due to the nature of the oximeter and the method of analysis (135,144–153) (Fig. 12).

The two potential limitations of oximetry alone are due to the presence of upper airway obstructive events that can lead to arousal without detectable hypoxia and respiratory oscillations producing transient hypoxia without arousal, a particular problem when the resting Sa_{O_2} is already low. This low baseline Sa_{O_2} means that quite minor oscillations in ventilation, leading to small changes in Pa_{O_2}, produce large changes in Sa_{O_2} due to the increasing steepness of the hemoglobin dissociation curve (154). The particular oximeter used, its speed of response, the sampling frequency, and the experience of the interpreter will all influence its value. However, clearly abnormal tracings and clearly normal tracings in all studies seem reliably to pick out the ends of the spectrum of snoring and sleep apnea, particularly when combined with clinical data (146,147,150). Remmers and colleagues (79,152,155), originally looking at a multichannel device, have shown that careful analysis of Sa_{O_2} tracings alone can mimic AHI, giving sensitivity/specificity levels in excess of 80%, with no extra diagnostic information coming from the snoring channel. Furthermore, most disagreement between AHI and Sa_{O_2} dip rates occurred at high AHI levels, where misdiagnosis was unlikely.

Another commonly used limited sleep study system validated against PSG is the Edentrace (Nellcor, Hayward, CA) (82,156,157). This device measures oro/nasal

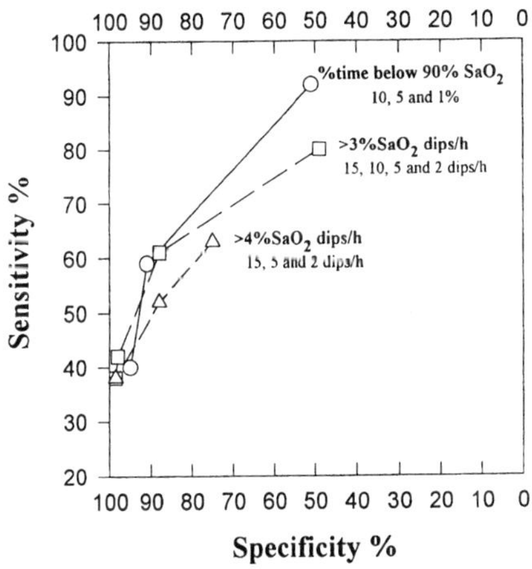

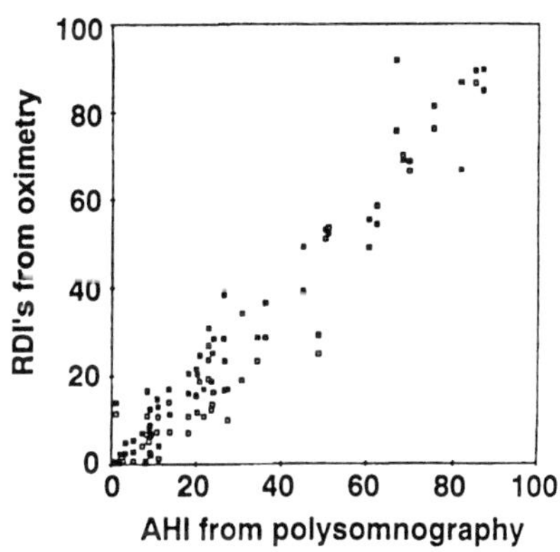

Figure 12 (Left) Three receiver operator characteristics (ROC) curves plotting the sensitivity against specificity of three oximetry derivatives (at various thresholds) regarding their ability to recognize an AHI of ≥15/h. (From Ref. 150.) (Right) Plot of RDIs from oximetry (using either desaturation or resaturation events) against simultaneous AHIs from polysomnography in 53 patients being investigated for possible OSA. (From Ref. 135.)

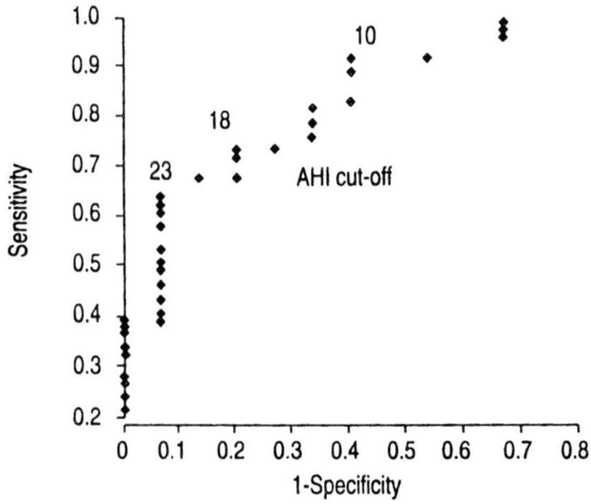

Figure 13 Receiver operator characteristics (ROC) curves for AHI measurements using the Edentrace (Nellcor, Hayward, CA) at home compared to a laboratory polysomnography AHI of >10 per hour. (From Ref. 156.)

airflow by thermistor, chest wall impedance, Sa_{O_2}, heart rate, snoring, and body position. Two of the published studies achieved correlations of over 0.9 between polysomnography and Edentrace AHI values. Parra et al. (156) produced full sensitivity/specificity ROC curves for an AHI > 10 allowing the performance of the Edentrace at any chosen threshold to be read off (Fig. 13). As with the MESAM system, sensitivity/specificity values over 70% are achievable.

The commercial home-monitoring system utilizing the measurement of ribcage/abdominal phase angle is the DENSA (Densa Ltd., Flint, UK). One group (158,159) has published on this device using a variety of derivatives from oro/nasal airflow, ribcage/abdominal movement, oximetry, and body position. This group also found sensitivity and specificity values in excess of 80% when compared to a polysomnography AHI of >10. As is often the case, visual scoring of these tracings

Figure 14 Printouts from an Autoset system (ResMed, Sydney, Australia). On the left are diagnostic tracings using nasal cannulae and oximetry. Signals, top down, are Sa_{O_2}, snoring, estimated relative ventilation, flattening index (estimate of inspiratory flow limitation, 0.15 considered lower limit of normal), cumulative hour-by-hour apnea count, cumulative hour-by-hour respiratory irregularity count, and record of apnea length. Note the periods of snoring, "abnormal" flow limitation, and an abnormal RDI with little hypoxemia. The tracings on the right are from a CPAP titration night using a nasal mask and oximetry. Signals, top down, are Sa_{O_2}, snoring, estimated ventilation, CPAP pressure delivered according to the internal algorithm, flattening index, mask leak, apnea count, and respiratory irregularity count.

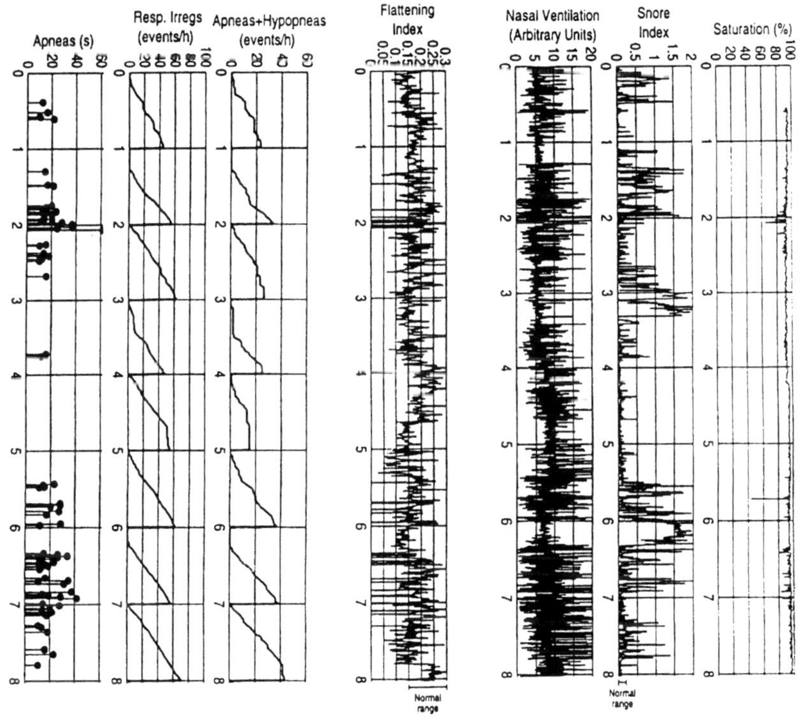

Apneas (s)
Resp. Irregs (events/h)
Apneas+Hypopneas (events/h)
Flattening Index
Nasal Ventilation (Arbitrary Units)
Snore Index
Saturation (%)
Normal range
Normal range

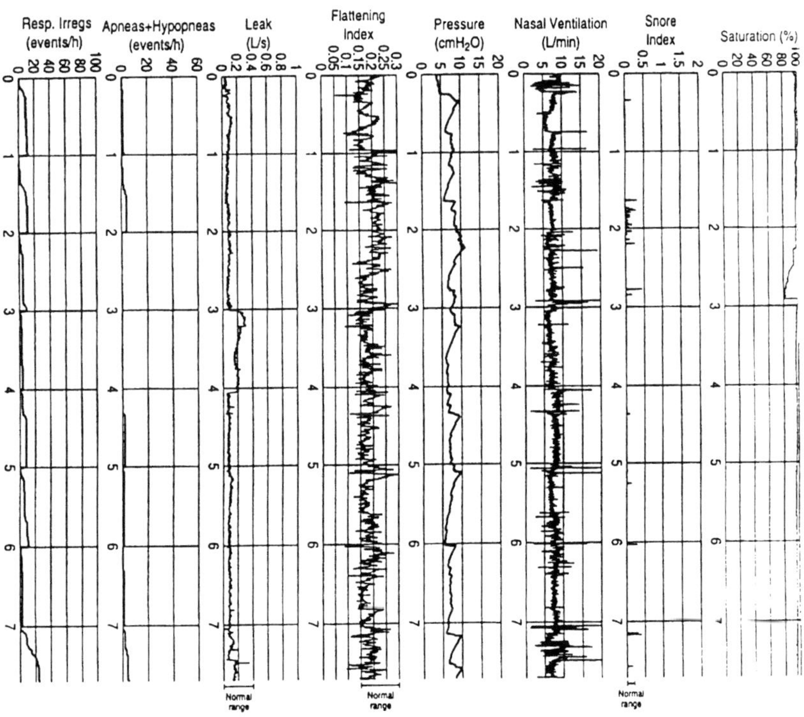

Resp. Irregs (events/h)
Apneas+Hypopneas (events/h)
Leak (L/s)
Flattening Index
Pressure (cmH_2O)
Nasal Ventilation (L/min)
Snore Index
Saturation (%)
Normal range
Normal range
Normal range

was better than any of the automatic ones. These studies come from one of the first groups to recognize that because AHI alone is not the final arbiter of CPAP therapy, the value of a limited study should be assessed, in conjunction with symptoms, as to its ability to predict who will benefit from CPAP.

The work from our unit looking at predictors of CPAP responsive sleepiness was mentioned earlier (56). Movement arousals (from video signals), ''automatic'' arousals, and >4% Sa_{O_2} dip rates were all at least as good as EEG markers of sleep fragmentation at predicting improvement in objective sleepiness following nasal CPAP therapy at one month. Longer-term acceptance of nasal CPAP therapy (at 6 months) was also best predicted from the movement arousals, ''autonomic'' arousals, and >4% Sa_{O_2} dip rates, and less well from the EEG markers of sleep fragmentation (unpublished observations). Our usual sleep-monitoring system (Visi-Lab, Stowood Scientific Systems, Oxford, UK) monitors body movement (video processing), Sa_{O_2} and pulse rate (from oximetry), and snoring from a room microphone (Fig. 11). Thus, when using the pragmatic clinical endpoint of CPAP benefit as the gold standard, it seems that full polysomnography does not have anything to add over and above the simpler respiratory, movement, and autonomic measures of sleep apnea severity.

More recently a device called the Autoset has been introduced. This is a portable monitor that can be used either diagnostically or as an automatic CPAP titration machine. In the diagnostic mode, oximetry is monitored along with airflow by pressure transducer, via nasal cannulae, to provide an AHI, respiratory event index, snoring, as well as an index of inspiratory flow limitation (Fig. 14). Two studies have shown, not surprisingly, that this approach can provide AHI values very similar to those derived from polysomnography (160,161). In addition, the Autoset can be used with a nasal mask in its automatic CPAP titration mode, when again indices of inspiratory flow limitation, apneas, desaturations, and snoring are all available for inspection along with the CPAP pressure found by the algorithm (Fig. 14). Thus much more than an AHI is available, although the intrusion of a nasal CPAP mask is likely to be greater than simple nasal prongs, and no assessment of its ability to identify CPAP responsiveness sleepiness has been published. It seems likely on an intuitive basis that actually measuring the required CPAP pressure overnight will provide a good index of likely CPAP responsiveness, since it is directly related to the primary pathology in OSA, the tendency for the pharynx to collapse (the closing pressure).

VII. Conclusions

It is quite clear that there are many simplified sleep study systems available that can be tuned to mimic AHI values obtained by full polysomnography. However, AHI is not a gold standard that allows one to recognize important clinical endpoints (e.g., CPAP responsiveness, UPPP success). Thus, it is difficult to know whether simplified systems that do not agree with a polysomnography AHI (or give different styles of output) are either better or worse at predicting these clinical endpoints. It is likely that superior and cheaper systems will continue to evolve once studies are performed using clinical endpoints as the reference. In addition, studies dissecting out the real causes of daytime symptoms in OSA and its variants should help speed up the process of selecting the most useful sleep study predictor in those patients who are likely to benefit from nasal CPAP or some other effective treatment. Limited studies on snorers, designed to predict favorable response to pharyngeal surgery, may need very different physiological signals, since that clinical endpoint is so different. It is not possible at present to recommend the ideal limited sleep study system for recognizing significant sleep-induced upper airway obstruction. Technology is evolving quickly, and manufacturers are introducing novel sensors and approaches to analysis. The prospective buyer must be satisfied that such devices measure something related to upper airway obstruction, something related to sleep fragmentation, and that this will identify those individuals likely to benefit from treatment. It is hoped that this chapter will provide the appropriate information to allow clinicians to ask the right questions for themselves about new monitoring devices. In our view it is still the case that the experience of the interpreting physician is more important than the specific technical details of the equipment in use.

References

1. Benca RM, Obermeyer WH, Thisted RA, Gillin JC. Sleep and psychiatric disorders. A meta-analysis. Arch Gen Psych 1992; 49:651–668.
2. Gastaut H, Tassinari CA, Duron B. Etude polygraphique des manifestations episodiques (hypniques et respiratoires), diurnes et nocturnes, du syndrome de Pickwick. Rev Neurol 1965; 112:568–579.
3. Lugaresi E, Coccagna G, Mantovani M, Lebrun R. Some periodic phenomena arising during drowsiness and sleep in man. Electroencephalog Clin Neurophysiol 1972; 32: 701–705.
4. Guilleminault C, Tilkian A, Dement WC. The sleep apnea syndromes. Ann Rev Med 1976; 27:465–484.
5. Guilleminault C, Van den Hoed J, Mitler MM. Sleep apnea syndromes. In: Guilleminault C, Dement WC, eds. Clinical Overview of the Sleep Apnea Syndromes. New York: Alan R Liss, 1978:1–12.
6. Sullivan CE, Issa FG, Berthon-Jones M, Eves L. Reversal of obstructive sleep apnoea by continuous positive airway pressure applied through the nares. Lancet 1981; 1:862–865.
7. Guilleminault C, Partinen M. Obstructive Sleep Apnea Syndrome. New York: Raven Press, 1990.
8. Lugaresi E, Mondini S, Zucconi M, Montagna P, Cirignotta F. Staging of heavy snorers' disease. A proposal. Bull Eur Physiopathol Respir 1983; 19:590–594.
9. Lugaresi E, Cirignotta F, Gerardi R, Montagna P. Snoring and sleep apnea: natural history of heavy snorers disease. In: Guilleminault C, Partinen M, eds. Obstructive Sleep Apnea Syndrome: Clinical Research and Treatment. New York: Raven Press, 1990:25–36.
10. Wiegand L, Zwillich CW, White D. Collapsibility of the human upper airway during normal sleep. J Appl Physiol 1989; 66:1800–1808.

11. Rees K, Wraith PK, Berthon-Jones M, Douglas NJ. Shape of the inspiratory flow time profile versus resistance in normal subjects. Am J Respir Crit Care Med 1998; 157: A651.
12. Horner RL, Innes JA, Murphy K, Guz A. Evidence for reflex upper airway dilator muscle activation by sudden negative airway pressure in man. J Physiol Lond 1991; 436:15–29.
13. Henke KG, Sullivan CE. Effects of high-frequency oscillating pressures on upper airway muscles in humans. J Appl Physiol 1993; 75:856–862.
14. Chadwick GA, Crowley P, Fitzgerald MX, O'Regan RG, McNicholas WT. Obstructive sleep apnea following topical oropharyngeal anesthesia in loud snorers. Am Rev Respir Dis 1991; 143:810–813.
15. Gleeson K, Zwillich CW, White DP. The influence of increasing ventilatory effort on arousal from sleep. Am Rev Respir Dis 1990; 142:295–300.
16. Yasuma F, Kozar LF, Kimoff J, Bradley TD, Phillipson EA. Interaction of chemical and mechanical respiratory stimuli in the arousal response to hypoxia in sleeping dogs. Am Rev Respir Dis 1991; 143:1274–1277.
17. Douglas NJ, White DP, Weil JV, Pickett CK, Zwillich CW. Hypercapnic ventilatory response in sleeping adults. Am Rev Respir Dis 1982; 126:758–762.
18. Douglas NJ, White DP, Weil JV, Pickett CK, Martin RJ, Hudgel DW, et al. Hypoxic ventilatory response decreases during sleep in normal men. Am Rev Respir Dis 1982; 125:286–289.
19. Berry RB, Gleeson K. Respiratory arousal from sleep: mechanisms and significance. Sleep 1997; 20:654–675.
20. Zamagni M, Sforza E, Boudewijns A, Petiau C, Krieger J. Respiratory effort. A factor contributing to sleep propensity in patients with obstructive sleep apnea. Chest 1996; 109:651–658.
21. Naegele B, Thouvard V, Pepin JL, Levy P, Bonnet C, Perret JE, et al. Deficits of cognitive executive functions in patients with sleep apnea syndrome. Sleep 1995; 18: 43–52.
22. Stradling JR, Pitson DJ, Bennett LS, Barbour C, Davies RJO. Variation in the arousal pattern following obstructive events in obstructive sleep apnea. Am J Respir Crit Care Med 1999; 159:130–136.
23. Ali NJ, Davies RJO, Fleetham JA, Stradling JR. The acute effects of continuous positive airway pressure and oxygen administration on blood pressure during obstructive sleep apnea. Chest 1992; 101:1526–1532.
24. Peter JH, Koehler U, Grote L, Podszus T. Manifestations and consequences of obstructive sleep apnoea. Eur Respir J 1995; 8:1572–1583.
25. Schafer H, Koehler U, Ploch T, Peter JH. Sleep-related myocardial ischemia and sleep structure in patients with obstructive sleep apnea and coronary heart disease. Chest 1997; 111:387–393.
26. Lugaresi E, Cirignotta F, Coccagna G, Piana C. Some epidemiological data on snoring in cardiocirculatory disturbances. Sleep 1980; 3:221–224.
27. Hla KM, Young TB, Bidwell T, Palta M, Skatrud JB, Dempsey J. Sleep apnea and hypertension. Ann Intern Med 1994; 120:382–388.
28. Young T, Peppard P, Palta M, Hla KM, Finn L, Morgan B, et al. Population-based study of sleep-disordered breathing as a risk factor for hypertension. Arch Intern Med 1997; 157:1746–1752.
29. Gislason T, Benediktsdottir B, Bjornsson JK, Kjartansson G, Kjeld M, Kristbjarnar-

son H. Snoring, hypertension, and the sleep apnea syndrome. An epidemiologic survey of middle-aged women. Chest 1993; 103:1147–1151.
30. Olson LG, King MT, Hensley MJ, Saunders NA. A community study of snoring and sleep-disordered breathing. Health outcomes. Am J Respir Crit Care Med 1995; 152: 717–720.
31. Kribbs NB, Pack AI, Kline LR, Smith PL, Schwartz AR, Schubert NM, et al. Objective measurement of patterns of nasal CPAP use by patients with obstructive sleep apnea. Am Rev Respir Dis 1993; 147:887–895.
32. Waldhorn RE, Herrick TW, Nguyen MC, O'Donnell AE, Sodero J, Protolicchio SJ. Long-term compliance with nasal continuous positive airway pressure therapy of obstructive sleep apnea. Chest 1990; 97:33–38.
33. Rolfe I, Olson LG, Saunders NA. Long-term acceptance of continuous positive airway pressure in obstructive sleep apnea. Am Rev Respir Dis 1991; 144:1130–1133.
34. de Faire U, Ericsson CG, Grip L, Nilsson J, Svane B, Hamsten A. Retardation of coronary atherosclerosis: the Bezafibrate Coronary Atherosclerosis Intervention Trial (BECAIT) and other angiographic trials. Cardiovasc Drugs Ther 1997; 11(suppl 1): 257–263.
35. Anonymous. Risk factors for stroke and efficacy of antithrombotic therapy in atrial fibrillation. Analysis of pooled data from five randomized controlled trials. Arch Intern Med 1994; 154:1449–1457.
36. Sher AE, Schechtman KB, Piccirillo JF. The efficacy of surgical modifications of the upper airway in adults with obstructive sleep apnea syndrome. Sleep 1996; 19:156–177.
37. Miljeteig H, Mateika S, Haight JS, Cole P, Hoffstein V. Subjective and objective assessment of uvulopalatopharyngoplasty for treatment of snoring and obstructive sleep apnea. Am J Respir Crit Care Med 1994; 150:1286–1290.
38. Mortimore IL, Bradley PA, Murray JA, Douglas NJ. Uvulopalatopharyngoplasty may compromise nasal CPAP therapy in sleep apnea syndrome. Am J Respir Crit Care Med 1996; 154:1759–1762.
39. Gould GA, Whyte KF, Rhind GB, Airlie MA, Catterall JR, Shapiro CM, et al. The sleep hypopnea syndrome. Am Rev Respir Dis 1988; 137:895–898.
40. Guilleminault C, Stoohs R, Duncan S. Snoring (I). Daytime sleepiness in regular heavy snorers. Chest 1991; 99:40–48.
41. Guilleminault C, Stoohs R, Clerk A, Cetel M, Maistros P. A cause of excessive daytime sleepiness. The upper airway resistance syndrome. Chest 1993; 104:781–787.
42. Cheshire K, Engleman H, Deary I, Shapiro C, Douglas NJ. Factors impairing daytime performance in patients with the sleep apnoea/hypopnoea syndrome. Arch Intern Med 1992; 152:538–541.
43. Crocker BD, Olson LG, Saunders NA, Hensley MJ, McKeon JL, Allen KM, et al. Estimation of the probability of disturbed breathing during sleep before a sleep study. Am Rev Respir Dis 1990; 142:14–18.
44. Viner S, Szalai JP, Hoffstein V. Are history and physical examination a good screening test for sleep apnea? Ann Intern Med 1991; 115:356–359.
45. Whyte KF, Allen MB, Jeffrey AA, Gould GA, Douglas NJ. Clinical features of the sleep apnoea/hypopnoea syndrome. Q J Med 1989; 72:659–666.
46. Sangal RB, Thomas L, Mitler MM. Maintenance of wakefulness test and multiple sleep latency test. Measurement of different abilities in patients with sleep disorders. Chest 1992; 101:898–902.

47. Sangal RB, Thomas L, Mitler MM. Disorders of excessive sleepiness. Treatment improves ability to stay awake but does not reduce sleepiness. Chest 1992; 102:699–703.
48. Johns MW. Sleepiness in different situations measured by the Epworth Sleepiness Scale. Sleep 1994; 17:703–710.
49. Olson LG, Cole MF, Ambrogetti A. Correlations among Epworth Sleepiness Scale scores, multiple sleep latency tests and psychological symptoms. J Sleep Res 1998; 7:248–253.
50. Chediak AD, Acevedo Crespo JC, Seiden DJ, Kim HH, Kiel MH. Nightly variability in the indices of sleep-disordered breathing in men being evaluated for impotence with consecutive night polysomnograms. Sleep 1996; 19:589–592.
51. Mosko SS, Dickel MJ, Ashurst J. Night-to-night variability in sleep apnea and sleep-related periodic leg movements in the elderly. Sleep 1988; 11:340–348.
52. Stradling JR, Mitchell J. Reproducibility of home oximetry tracings. J Amb Mon 1989; 2:203–208.
53. Rees K, Spence DPS, Earis JE, Calverley PMA. Arousal responses from apneic events during non rapid-eye-movement sleep. Am J Respir Crit Care Med 1995; 152: 1016–1021.
54. Davies RJO, Belt PJ, Robert SJ, Ali NJ, Stradling JR. Arterial blood pressure responses to graded transient arousal from sleep in normal humans. J Appl Physiol 1993; 74: 1123–1130.
55. Martin SE, Wraith PK, Deary IJ, Douglas NJ. The effect of nonvisible sleep fragmentation on daytime function [see comments]. Am J Respir Crit Care Med 1997; 155: 1596–1601.
56. Bennett LS, Langford BA, Stradling JR, Davies RJO. Sleep fragmentation indices as predictors of daytime sleepiness and nCPAP response in OSA. Am J Respir Crit Care Med 1998; 158:778–786.
57. Bennett LS, Barbour C, Langford B, Stradling JR, Davies RJ. Health status in obstructive sleep apnea: relationship with sleep fragmentation and daytime sleepiness, and effects of continuous positive airway pressure treatment. Am J Respir Crit Care Med 1999; 159:1884–1890.
58. Pitson D, Chhina N, Knijn S, van Herwaaden M, Stradling J. Changes in pulse transit time and pulse rate as markers of arousal from sleep in normal subjects. Clin Sci 1994; 87:269–273.
59. Johns MW. Daytime sleepiness, snoring, and obstructive sleep apnea. The Epworth sleepiness scale. Chest 1993; 103:30–36.
60. Bennett LS, Stradling JR, Davies RJO. A behavioural test to assess daytime sleepiness in obstructive sleep apnoea. J Sleep Res 1997; 6:142–145.
61. Stradling JR, Crosby JH. Predictors and prevalence of obstructive sleep apnoea and snoring in 1001 middle aged men. Thorax 1991; 46:85–90.
62. Young T, Palta M, Dempsey J, Skatrud J, Weber S, Badr S. The occurrence of sleep-disordered breathing among middle-aged adults. N Engl J Med 1993; 328:1230–1235.
63. Olson LG, King MT, Hensley MJ, Saunders NA. A community study of snoring and sleep-disordered breathing. Symptoms. Am J Respir Crit Care Med 1995; 152:707–710.
64. Stradling JR, Davies RJO. Is it necessary to record sleep? Sleep 1996; 19:S251–S254.
65. Jenkinson C, Davies RJO, Mullins R, Stradling JR. Randomised prospective parallel

trial of therapeutic nasal continuous positive airway pressure (NCPAP) against subtherapeutic NCPAP for obstructive sleep apnoea. Lancet 1999; 353:2100–2105.

66. Farre R, Rotger M, Montserrat JM, Navajas D. A system to generate simultaneous forced oscillation and continuous positive airway pressure. Eur Respir J 1997; 10: 1349–1353.
67. Pride NB, Permutt S, Riley RL, Bromberger Barnea B. Determinants of maximal expiratory flow from the lungs. J Appl Physiol 1967; 23:646–662.
68. Berthon Jones M. Feasibility of a self-setting CPAP machine. Sleep 1993; 16:S120–S121.
69. Teschler H, Berthon Jones M, Thompson AB, Henkel A, Henry J, Konietzko N. Automated continuous positive airway pressure titration for obstructive sleep apnea syndrome. Am J Respir Crit Care Med 1996; 154:734–740.
70. Montserrat JM, Farre R, Ballester E, Felez MA, Pasto M, Navajas D. Evaluation of nasal prongs for estimating nasal flow. Am J Respir Crit Care Med 1997; 155:211–215.
71. Condos R, Norman RG, Krishnasamy I, Peduzzi N, Goldring RM, Rapoport DM. Flow limitation as a noninvasive assessment of residual upper-airway resistance during continuous positive airway pressure therapy of obstructive sleep apnea. Am J Respir Crit Care Med 1994; 150:475–480.
72. Montserrat JM, Ballester E, Olivi H, Reolid A, Lloberes P, Morello A, et al. Time-course of stepwise CPAP titration. Behavior of respiratory and neurological variables. Am J Respir Crit Care Med 1995; 152:1854–1859.
73. Ballester E, Badia JR, Hernandez L, Farre R, Navajas D, Montserrat JM. Nasal prongs in the detection of sleep-related disordered breathing in the sleep apnoea/hypopnoea syndrome. Eur Respir J 1998; 11:880–883.
74. Norman RG, Ahmed MM, Walsleben JA, Rapoport DM. Detection of respiratory events during NPSG: nasal cannula/pressure sensor versus thermistor. Sleep 1997; 20:1175–1184.
75. Stoohs R, Skrobal A, Guilleminault C. Does snoring intensity predict flow limitation or respiratory effort during sleep? Respir Physiol 1993; 92:27–38.
76. Guilleminault C, Stoohs R, Clerk A, Simmons J, Labanowski M. Excessive daytime somnolence in women with abnormal respiratory efforts during sleep. Sleep 1993; 16: S137–S138.
77. Guilleminault C, Stoohs R, Philip P, Lababowsky M, Simmons J, Clerk A. Determinants of daytime sleepiness: the role of sleep fragmentation and the role of respiratory effort in women. Sleep Res 1993; 22:204.
78. Stoohs R, Guilleminault C. MESAM 4: an ambulatory device for the detection of patients at risk for obstructive sleep apnea syndrome (OSAS). Chest 1992; 101:1221–1227.
79. Issa FG, Morrison D, Hadjuk E, Iyer A, Feroah T, Remmers JE. Digital monitoring of sleep-disordered breathing using snoring sound and arterial oxygen saturation. Am Rev Respir Dis 1993; 148:1023–1029.
80. Flemons WW, Remmers JE. The diagnosis of sleep apnea: questionnaires and home studies. Sleep 1996; 19:S243–S247.
81. Douglas NJ, Thomas S, Jan MA. Clinical value of polysomnography. Lancet 1992; 339:347–350.
82. Redline S, Tosteson T, Boucher MA, Millman RP. Measurement of sleep-related breathing disturbances in epidemiologic studies. Assessment of the validity and reproducibility of a portable monitoring device. Chest 1991; 100:1281–1286.

83. Tvinnereim M, Mateika S, Cole P, Haight J, Hoffstein V. Diagnosis of obstructive sleep apnea using a portable transducer catheter. Am J Respir Crit Care Med 1995; 152:775–779.
84. Montserrat JM, Alarcon A, Lloberes P, Ballester E, Fornas C, Rodriguez Roisin R. Adequacy of prescribing nasal continuous positive airway pressure therapy for the sleep apnoea/hypopnoea syndrome on the basis of nighttime respiratory recording variables. Thorax 1995; 50:969–971.
85. Kirjavainen T, Polo O, McNamara S, Vaahtoranta K, Sullivan CE. Respiratory challenge induces high frequency spiking on the static charge sensitive bed (SCSB). Eur Respir J 1996; 9:1810–1815.
86. Tobin MJ, Jenouri GA, Watson H, Sackner MA. Noninvasive measurement of pleural pressure by surface inductive plethysmography. J Appl Physiol 1983; 55:267–275.
87. Knowles GK, Clark TJ. Pulsus paradoxus as a valuable sign indicating severity of asthma. Lancet 1973; 2:1356–1359.
88. Lea S, Ali NJ, Goldman M, Loh L, Fleetham J, Stradling JR. Systolic blood pressure swings reflect inspiratory effort during simulated obstructive sleep apnoea. In: Horne J, ed. Sleep 90. Bochum: Pontenagel Press, 1990:178–181.
89. Davies RJO, Vardi-Visy K, Clarke M, Stradling JR. Identification of sleep disruption and sleep disordered breathing from the systolic blood pressure profile. Thorax 1993; 48:1242–1247.
90. Molhoek GP, Wesseling KH, Settels JJM, Van Vollenhoven E, Weeda HWH, De Witn B, et al. Evaluation of the Penaz servo-plethysmo-manometer for the continuous, non-invasive measurement of finger blood pressure. Basic Res Cardiol 1984; 79:598–609.
91. Brock J, Pitson D, Stradling JR. Use of pulse transit time as a measure of changes in inspiratory effort. J Amb Mon 1993; 6:295–302.
92. Davies RJO, Crosby J, Vardi-Visy K, Clarke M, Stradling JR. Non-invasive beat to beat arterial blood pressure during non-REM sleep in obstructive sleep apnoea and snoring. Thorax 1994; 49:335–339.
93. Imholz BP, Langewouters GJ, van Montfrans GA, Parati G, van Goudoever J, Wesseling KH, et al. Feasibility of ambulatory, continuous 24-hour finger arterial pressure recording. Hypertension 1993; 21:65–73.
94. Gribbin B, Steptoe A, Sleight P. Pulse wave velocity as a measure of blood pressure change. Psychophysiology 1976; 13:86–90.
95. Pollak MH, Obrist PA. Aortic-radial pulse transit time and ECG Q-wave to radial pulse wave interval as indices of beat-by-beat blood pressure change. Psychophysiology 1983; 20:21–28.
96. Pitson DJ, Sandell A, van den Hout R, Stradling JR. Use of pulse transit time as a measure of inspiratory effort in patients with obstructive sleep apnoea. Eur Respir J 1995; 8:1669–1674.
97. Pitson DJ, Chhina N, Knijn S, van Herwaaden M, Stradling JR. Mechanism of pulse transit time lengthening during obstructed inspiration. J Amb Mon 1995; 8:101–105.
98. Pitson DJ, Stradling JR. Value of beat-to-beat blood pressure changes, detected by pulse transit time, in the management of the obstructive sleep apnoea/hypopnoea syndrome. Eur Respir J 1998; 12:685–692.
99. Argod J, Pepin JL, Levy P. Differentiating obstructive and central sleep respiratory events through pulse transit time. Am J Respir Crit Care Med 1998; 158:1778–1783.
100. Smith RP, Argod J, Pepin J, Levy PA. Pulse transit time: an appraisal of potential clinical applications. Thorax 1999; 54:452–458.

101. Loiodice C, Selck M, Loire M, Levy P, Pepin JL. [Measurement of respiratory effort (esophageal pressure) and estimation of resistance of the upper airway in polysomnography: indications, limitations and results.] Neurophysiol Clin 1998; 28:507–520.
102. Smith RP, Argod J, Pepin JL, Levy P. Comparison between two measurements of respiratory effort oesophageal pressure (PES) and pulse transit time (PTT) when scoring non-apneic obstructive respiratory events (NAOP). Eur Respir J 1999; 14(suppl 30):406S.
103. Rauscher H, Formanek D, Zwick H. Nasal continuous positive airway pressure for nonapneic snoring? Chest 1995; 107:58–61.
104. O'Malley EB, Farkas DT, Norman RG, Walsleben JA, Rapoport DM. Frontal EEG arousals are associated with autonomic changes. Am J Respir Crit Care Med 1997; 155(part 2):A775.
105. Rechtschaffen A, Kales A. A Manual of Standardised Terminology, Techniques and Scoring System for Sleep Stages of Human Subjects. Washington, DC: National Institutes of Health, 1968.
106. Bonnet M, Carley D, Carskadon M, Easton P, Guilleminault C, Harper R, et al. EEG arousals: scoring rules and examples. A preliminary report from the Sleep Disorders Atlas Task Force of the American Sleep Disorders Association. Sleep 1992; 15(2): 173–184.
107. Drinnan MJ, Murray A, Griffiths CJ, Gibson GJ. Inter-observer variability in recognising arousal in respiratory sleep disorders. Am J Respir Crit Care Med 1998; 158:358–362.
108. Kemp B. A proposal for computer-based sleep/wake analysis. J Sleep Res 1993; 2: 179–185.
109. Pardey J, Roberts S, Tarassenko L, Stradling J. A new approach to the analysis of the human sleep-wakefulness continuum. J Sleep Res 1996; 5:201–210.
110. Davies RJO, Bennett LS, Barbour C, Tarassenko L, Stradling JR. Second by second patterns in cortical electroencephalograph and sub-cortical (systolic blood pressure) arousal during Cheyne-Stokes breathing. Eur Respir J 1999; 14:940–945.
111. Khoo MC, Anholm JD, Ko SW, Downey R, 3rd, Powles AC, Sutton JR, et al. Dynamics of periodic breathing and arousal during sleep at extreme altitude. Respir Physiol 1996; 103:33–43.
112. Steriade M. Arousal: revisiting the reticular activating system. Science 1996; 272:225–226.
113. Hilton SM. The defence-arousal system and its relevance for circulatory and respiratory control. J Exp Biol 1982; 100:159–174.
114. Sforza E, Nicolas A, Lavigne G, Gosselin A, Petit D, Montplaisir J. EEG and cardiac activation during periodic leg movements in sleep: support for a hierarchy of arousal responses. Neurology 1999; 52:786–791.
115. Johnson LC, Lubin A. The orienting reflex during waking and sleeping. Electroencephalogr Clin Neurophysiol 1967; 22:11–21.
116. Pitson DJ, Stradling JR. Autonomic markers of arousal during sleep in patients undergoing investigation for obstructive sleep apnoea, their relationship to EEG arousals, respiratory events and subjective sleepiness. J Sleep Res 1998; 7:53–60.
117. Wilde-Frenz J, Schulz H. Rate and distribution of body movements during sleep in humans. Percept Motor Skills 1983; 56:275–283.
118. Vos PJE, Stradling JR. Assessment of sleep times and movement arousals from video recordings. J Amb Mon 1991; 4:35–42.

119. Stradling JR, Thomas G, Belcher R. Analysis of overnight sleep patterns by automatic detection of movement on video recordings. J Amb Mon 1988; 1:217–222.
120. Morielli A, Ladan S, Ducharme FM, Brouillette RT. Can sleep and wakefulness be distinguished in children by cardiorespiratory and videotape recordings? Chest 1996; 109:680–687.
121. Sadeh A, Alster J, Urbach D, Lavie P. Actigraphically based automatic bedtime sleep/wake scoring: validity and clinical applications. J Amb Mon 1989; 2:209–216.
122. Sadeh A, Hauri PJ, Kripke DF, Lavie P. The role of actigraphy in the evaluation of sleep disorders. Sleep 1995; 18:288–302.
123. Drinnan MJ, Murray A, White JE, Smithson AJ, Gibson GJ, Griffiths CJ. Evaluation of activity-based techniques to identify transient arousal in respiratory sleep disorders. J Sleep Res 1996; 5:173–180.
124. Mullaney DJ, Kripke DF, Messin S. Wrist actigraphic assessment of sleep time. Sleep 1980; 3:83–92.
125. Cole RJ, Kripke DF. Progress in automatic sleep/wake scoring by wrist actigraph. Sleep 1988; 17:331.
126. Mamelak A, Hobson JA. Nightcap: a home-based sleep monitoring system. Sleep 1989; 12:157–166.
127. Atkins NCM, Stone PA, Davies J, Smith E, Woodcock A. The development and resolution of paradox in relation to respiratory events during sleep. Am Rev Respir Dis 1992; 145:A173.
128. Bishop C, Rosenthal L, Helmus T, Roehrs T, Roth T. The frequency of multiple sleep onset REM periods among subjects with no excessive daytime sleepiness. Sleep 1996; 19:727–730.
129. Miyasita A, Fukuda K, Inugami M. Effects of sleep interruption on REM-NREM cycle in nocturnal human sleep. Electroencephalogr Clin Neurophysiol 1989; 73:107–116.
130. Park JD, Radtke RA. Hypersomnolence in myotonic dystrophy: demonstration of sleep onset REM sleep [letter]. J Neurol Neurosurg Psychiatry 1995; 58:512–513.
131. Staner L, Van Veeren C, Linkowski P. Clinical correlates of sleep onset REM periods in major depression. Acta Psychiatr Belg 1994; 94:104–105.
132. Takeuchi T, Miyasita A, Sasaki Y, Inugami M, Fukuda K. Isolated sleep paralysis elicited by sleep interruption. Sleep 1992; 15:217–225.
133. Penzel T, Amend G, Meinzer K, Peter JH, von Wichert P. MESAM: a heart rate and snoring recorder for detection of obstructive sleep apnea. Sleep 1990; 13:175–182.
134. Esnaola S, Duran J, Infante Rivard C, Rubio R, Fernandez A. Diagnostic accuracy of a portable recording device (MESAM IV) in suspected obstructive sleep apnoea. Eur Respir J 1996; 9:2597–2605.
135. Rauscher H, Popp W, Zwick H. Quantification of sleep disordered breathing by computerised analysis of oximetry, heart rate and snoring. Eur Respir J 1991; 4:655–659.
136. Rihs F, Mathis J, Gugger M, Hess CD. [Screening for sleep apnea: clinical use of MESAM IV and Apnoe-Check]. Schweiz Med Wochenschr 1995; 125:995–1002.
137. Koziej M, Cieslicki JK, Gorzelak K, Sliwinski P, Zielinski J. Hand-scoring of MESAM 4 recordings is more accurate than automatic analysis in screening for obstructive sleep apnoea. Eur Respir J 1994; 7:1771–1775.
138. Stoohs R, Guilleminault C. Investigations of an automatic screening device (MESAM) for obstructive sleep apnoea. Eur Respir J 1990; 3:823–829.
139. Roos M, Althaus W, Rhiel C, Penzel T, Peter JH, von Wichert P. [Comparative use

of MESAM IV and polysomnography in sleep-related respiratory disorders.] Pneumologie 1993; 47(suppl 1):112–118.
140. Duran Cantolla J, Esnaola Sukia S, Rubio Aramendi R, Egea Santaolalla C. [Validity of a portable recording system (MESAM IV) for the diagnosis of sleep apnea syndrome.] Arch Bronconeumol 1994; 30:331–338.
141. Hoch B, Amend G, Mosebach U, Penzel T, Peter JH, Schneider H, et al. [Assessment of the MESAM and Biox 3700 early warning methods for the diagnosis of sleep-related respiratory disorders in young men.] Pneumologie 1991; 45(suppl 1):217–222.
142. Stoohs RA, Bingham LA, Itoi A, Guilleminault C, Dement WC. Sleep and sleep-disordered breathing in commercial long-haul truck drivers. Chest 1995; 107:1275–1282.
143. Bearpark H, Elliott L, Grunstein R, Cullen S, Schneider H, Althaus W, et al. Snoring and sleep apnea. A population study in Australian men. Am J Respir Crit Care Med 1995; 151:1459–1465.
144. Farney RJ, Walker LE, Jensen RL, Walker JM. Ear oximetry to detect apnea and differentiate rapid eye movement (REM) and non-REM (NREM) sleep. Screening for the sleep apnea syndrome. Chest 1986; 89:533–539.
145. Pepin JL, Levy P, Lepaulle B, Brambilla C, Guilleminault C. Does oximetry contribute to the detection of apneic events? Mathematical processing of the Sa_{O_2} signal. Chest 1991; 99:1151–1157.
146. Williams AJ, Yu G, Santiago S, Stein M. Screening for sleep apnea using pulse oximetry and a clinical score. Chest 1991; 100:631–635.
147. Rauscher H, Popp W, Zwick H. Model for investigating snorers with suspected sleep apnoea. Thorax 1993; 48:275–279.
148. Series F, Marc I, Cormier Y, La Forge J. Utility of nocturnal home oximetry for case finding in patients with suspected sleep apnea hypopnea syndrome. Ann Intern Med 1993; 119:449–453.
149. Levy P, Pepin JL, Deschaux Blanc C, Paramelle B, Brambilla C. Accuracy of oximetry for detection of respiratory disturbances in sleep apnea syndrome. Chest 1996; 109:395–399.
150. Gyulay S, Olson LG, Hensley MJ, King MT, Allen KM, Saunders NA. A comparison of clinical assessment and home oximetry in the diagnosis of obstructive sleep apnea. Am Rev Respir Dis 1993; 147:50–53.
151. Bennett LS, Davies RJO, Stradling JR. American Journal of Respiratory and Critical Care Medicine 1999; 159:A795.
152. Vazquez JC, Tsai WH, Flemons W, Masuda A, Brant R, Hajduk E, et al. Automated analysis of digital oximetry in the diagnosis of obstructive sleep apnea. Thorax 2000; 55:302–307.
153. Olson LG, Ambrogetti A, Gyulay SG. Prediction of sleep-disordered breathing by unattended overnight oximetry. J Sleep Res 1999; 8:51–55.
154. Stradling JR, Lane DJ. Nocturnal hypoxaemia in chronic obstructive pulmonary disease. Clin Sci 1983; 64:213–222.
155. Eisele JH, Jain SK. Circulatory and respiratory changes during unilateral and bilateral cranial nerve IX and X block in two asthmatics. Clin Sci 1971; 40:117–125.
156. Parra O, Garcia-Esclasans N, Montserrat JM, Garcia Eroles L, Ruiz J, Lopez JA, et al. Should patients with sleep apnoea/hypopnoea syndrome be diagnosed and managed on the basis of home sleep studies? Eur Respir J 1997; 10:1720–1724.
157. Whittle AT, Finch SP, Mortimore IL, Mackay TW, Douglas NJ. Use of home sleep

studies for diagnosis of the sleep apnoea/hypopnoea syndrome. Thorax 1997; 52: 1068–1073.
158. Lloberes P, Montserrat JM, Ascaso A, Parra O, Granados A, Alonso P, et al. Comparison of partially attended night time respiratory recordings and full polysomnography in patients with suspected sleep apnoea/hypopnoea syndrome. Thorax 1996; 51:1043–1047.
159. Carrasco O, Montserrat JM, Lloberes P, Ascasco C, Ballester E, Fornas C, et al. Visual and different automatic scoring profiles of respiratory variables in the diagnosis of sleep apnoea-hypopnoea syndrome. Eur Respir J 1996; 9:125–130.
160. Bradley PA, Mortimore IL, Douglas NJ. Comparison of polysomnography with ResCare Autoset in the diagnosis of the sleep apnoea/hypopnoea syndrome. Thorax 1995; 50:1201–1203.
161. Gugger M, Mathis J, Bassetti C. Accuracy of an intelligent CPAP machine with in-built diagnostic abilities in detecting apnoeas: a comparison with polysomnography. Thorax 1995; 50:1199–1201.

17

New Developments in Positive Pressure Therapy for Sleep Apnea

MARK H. SANDERS

Montefiore University Hospital
University of Pittsburgh School of Medicine
Pittsburgh, Pennsylvania

FREDERIC SÉRIÈS

Laval University
Laval Hospital
Sainte-Foy, Quebec, Canada

I. Introduction

The capability of continuous positive airway pressure (CPAP), delivered through a noninvasive interface to maintain upper airway patency during sleep in patients with obstructive sleep apnea/hypopnea (OSA/H) has been well established (1–11). Sériès et al. have confirmed the hypothesis of Sullivan and coworkers that the primary mechanism of action is through pneumatic splinting of the airway (1,12). As a consequence of stabilizing the upper airway during sleep in OSA/H patients, CPAP therapy is associated with improved daytime alertness and improvement in at least some parameters of cognitive function (13–18). While the effectiveness of nasal CPAP in maintaining upper airway patency during sleep in OSA/H patients is undisputed, suboptimal patient compliance with this therapy is equally undisputed (19–25). Since these two facts became evident, the thrust of technology has been directed towards modifying existing or developing new techniques and modalities that would be equally effective but more readily accepted and consistently utilized by patients. These efforts have resulted in an increasing number of interface options from which patients may choose as well as a modest broadening of available positive pressure modalities.

II. Developments in Interface Technology

A. Nasal Interfaces

In its initial description, CPAP was delivered by a customized nasal mask, which was fabricated from medical grade silicon rubber (1). Subsequent early reports described use of customized nasal interfaces using dental acrylic material (26), commercially available nasal masks developed to deliver nitrous oxide (4), and pediatric size anesthesia masks (6). By the mid-1980s, nasal masks, constructed specifically for application of CPAP via the nasal route, became commercially available, and in North America became the standard of care. In Europe, however, it appears that customized nasal interfaces have remained in relatively more widespread use (27). It is intuitively obvious that both approaches have inherent advantages, and the clinician, as well as the patient, must assess the relative values of a customized fit, availability, ease of replacement, and cost.

The need to accommodate to the wide variability of facial configurations in the population of OSA/H patients has spawned a great diversity of mask design. The clinician and the patient can *almost* always find a mask that provides a reasonably comfortable fit and effectively sealed mask/skin interface. Alternatives to nasal masks, cushioned nasal prongs, have been available for the last decade (28). The limited surface area over which a leak-free seal must be maintained is a conceptual advantage, and indeed, one group of investigators reported in abstract form that approximately one half of their patients preferred the prongs during the in-laboratory CPAP titration (29). These authors noted that an individual's preference for mask or prongs may vary over time. Sanders and coworkers noted that there was no systematic difference in therapeutic pressure requirement across the various interfaces (30). It may therefore be reasonable to provide patients with several types of styles of interface to use.

B. Oro-Nasal Masks

Mouth leaks represent a potentially significant problem during positive pressure application via the nasal route. It is remarkable that such leaks are not an even greater clinical problem than they are in the OSA/H patient population. In this regard, it has been postulated that nasopharyngeal pressurization moves the soft palate against the tongue, thereby precluding airflow into the oropharynx (31–33). Nonetheless, mouth leaks may occur, especially in patients who have undergone uvulopalatopharyngoplasty (34). The adverse consequences of such leaks include reduction of mask pressure below the level required to maintain upper airway patency and/or sleep disruption, as has been demonstrated in patients undergoing nasal noninvasive positive pressure ventilatory assistance for nonapneic ventilatory insufficiency (35,36). Unfortunately, in our clinical experience, chin straps designed to keep the mouth closed are of limited use and often ineffective in preventing leakage. Alternatively, some patients are unable to comfortably breathe exclusively through the nasal route and are therefore unable to utilize nasal interfaces. Under these circumstances, selected patients may use an interface that permits breathing through either the oral or nasal route. Such oro-nasal masks have recently been demonstrated to provide an acceptable alternative to nasal interfaces (37,38). In one series, approximately 10% of OSA/H patients were unable to use a nasal interface. These individuals were, however, able to accept positive pressure therapy using an oro-nasal interface (37).

It is evident that nasal interfaces will not be replaced by universal application of oro-nasal interfaces. In a randomized trial of nasal versus oro-nasal masks, Mortimore et al. (39) reported that most but not all patients preferred the former and that average hours of nightly use was greater with the nasal mask. The important point, however, is for clinicians to provide patients with interface alternatives and that all patients will not express the same preference.

Although they are effective for positive pressure delivery, certain precautions must be taken when using oro-nasal interfaces. An alternative source of air entrainment must be available to the patient if there is loss of electical power or mechanical failure associated with cessation of positive pressure administration. Incorporation of a low-pressure alarm into the positive pressure system should be considered for patients who are unable to readily remove the mask themselves. Similarly, the mask and headgear must also be designed for rapid removal in the event that the patient becomes nauseated and is likely to vomit. With the mouth covered, the clinician and the patient must be cognizant of the risk for aspiration of gastric contents. Patients should be counseled to avoid ingestion of food or beverages for at least several hours before using positive pressure via an oro-nasal interface.

A commercially available mouthpiece has been employed to deliver noninvasive positive pressure ventilatory assistance exclusively via the oral route to patients with chronic ventilatory insufficiency (40–42). When nasal leakage occurred, cotton pledgets were employed to occlude the nares. This technique has not been widely applied to OSA/H patients. Given the knowledge regarding the effectiveness of oro-nasal interfaces, there is no conceptual reason to expect that mouthpiece application of positive pressure would be inadequate in OSA/H patients. Concerns regarding mouthpiece interfaces still exist, however, with respect to interference with speech and potential alteration of dental occlusion (42). Clearly, there are too few data regarding the utility of exclusively oral interfaces in OSA/H patients to permit any conclusions to be made at the present time.

III. Adjuncts to CPAP

A. Pressure Ramping

Some patients may find the sensation associated with CPAP to be sufficiently uncomfortable that it interferes with their ability to fall asleep. In recent years, pressure ramps have been incorporated in CPAP devices to reduce the pressure to which patients are initially exposed after turning on the CPAP device. The clinician may prescribe a rate at which the pressure subsequently increases, thereby manipulating the interval until the predetermined therapeutic level of CPAP is reached. In this manner, the application of lower, albeit less-than-therapeutic pressure provides patients with an opportunity to fall asleep. Although pressure ramps almost certainly facilitate sleep onset in some patients, to our knowledge there are no data indicating how frequently this adjunct is prescribed, nor have there been any peer-reviewed trials to assess the impact of this adjunct on patient acceptance and compliance with CPAP therapy. In our experience, some patients for whom pressure ramping is prescribed either never use it or rapidly discontinue using it after acclimatizing to CPAP.

Pressure ramping is not without its potentially negative aspects. Since the patient may be asleep on less than the therapeutic pressure, it is conceivable that some degree of oxyhemoglobin desaturation may occur. Although conceptually, the duration of such desaturation might be limited to the duration of the ramp (generally $\leq$ 30 min), Pressman and coworkers recently reported a patient who repetitively awoke throughout the night to reset the ramp mechanism and therefore experienced notable desaturation as well as sleep fragmentation (43). Until recently, a clinician would have difficulty detecting such "ramp abuse." However, software now incorporated into CPAP units will track patterns of CPAP usage across specific and sequential 24-h periods, reporting the pressure profiles characterizing the pattern of usage.

B. Humidification

It is well recognized that nasopharyngeal complaints, including nasal congestion, dryness, and rhinorrhea, are common among CPAP users (32). The nature and severity of these complaints vary widely across the patient populations utilizing CPAP, and indeed, all users do not express these complaints. Clinicians have attempted to address these complaints by prescribing oral antihistamines, topical α-adrenergic agents, cholinergic sprays, agents that stabilize mast cells, and topical nasal steroids. The impact of these interventions is variable, at best. Thus, our incomplete understanding of the pathogenesis of these problems has been particularly frustrating. Some insight in this regard has recently been provided by Richards et al. (44), who observed that raising the relative humidity of inspired air delivered via CPAP attenuates the increase in nasal resistance that would otherwise occur during augmentation of nasal airflow during a substantial mouth leak. These investigators hypothesized that exposure to air with low relative humidity evokes inflammatory mediator release, which in turn causes clinical symptoms. This is a plausible scenario, and incorporation of a heated humidifier into the CPAP circuit may be a reasonable approach in symptomatic patients. Massie and coworkers (45) recently reported the results of a randomized cross-over study examining the impact of heated humidification versus no humidification versus a cold passover humidifier on various aspects of CPAP therapy. Daily CPAP use by patients receiving heated humidification was greater with statistical but arguably clinical significance relative to those patients who used a cold passover humifier or no humidification (patients receiving heated humification had an average of 22 min and 35 min more daily usage than those receiving a passover humidifier or no humidification, respectively). Patients receiving heated humidification with CPAP were more refreshed on awakening and reported greater satisfaction with CPAP than the other two groups. However, there was no difference in side effects between the groups with respect to heated versus cold passover humidifiers. Although 76% of the patients chose the heated humidifier over the cold passover humidifier, some patients preferred no humidification at all or requested to have the option to use one or the other at any given time, e.g., using the less cumbersome passover humidifier when traveling. In light of the above information, and in as much as heated humidifiers add measurably to the cost of care, it remains questionable whether heated humidifiers should be used as opposed to selectively prescribed. The clinician should assess the potential benefits of heated humidification on an individual basis since the potential costs of an untreated patient due to CPAP intolerance and/or surgical failure are likely to be substantial.

Increasing the relative humidity of inspired air on CPAP need not mandate use of a humidifier incorporated into the device circuit. Martins de Araujo and colleagues (46) recently demonstrated that while a heated humidifier increased the relative humidity of inspired air in the presence of mouth leaks on nasal CPAP, it did not restore the humidity to the level measured in the absence of mouth leaks. In contrast, use of an oro-nasal interface with CPAP without a humidifier was associated with delivery of the same relative humidity as breathing without CPAP, regardless of whether the mouth was open or closed. The authors concluded that clinicians have the option of using either a humidifier or oral-nasal mask to address problems related to low inspired relative humidity. They cautioned, however, that currently available humidifiers may not fully restore relative humidity and that not all patients accept an oro-nasal interface.

IV. Bi-Level Positive Pressure

In addition to inspiratory collapse, the inherent instability of the upper airway during sleep in OSA/H patients makes it susceptible to collapse even during expiration, despite the absense of negative intrapharyngeal pressure (47–51). It has been demonstrated, however, that the pressure required to maintain upper airway patency during expiration is less than that needed to maintain upper airway patency during inspiration in order to prevent clinically and physiologically significant obstructive apneas and hypopneas (52). By providing bi-level positive pressure, the magnitude of the applied expiratory pressure may be adjusted independently of the inspiratory pressure in contrast to conventional CPAP, which is defined by equal levels of positive pressure during inspiration and expiration. Thus, patients may be successfully treated at lower positive pressure during exhalation than would be possible using CPAP.

There are limited published data addressing the relative benefits of bi-level positive pressure therapy compared with CPAP. In one study assessing the efficacy of combining diagnostic efforts and initiation of positive pressure therapy in a single night (''split-night'' polysomnography), CPAP therapy was precluded by intolerance in 14% of patients in whom development of a bi-level positive pressure prescription was subsequently possible (30). In a recent comparison of long-term patient compliance using CPAP and bi-level positive pressure, the greater dropout rate in the OSA/H group randomized to receive CPAP suggested to the investigators that patient acceptance of bilevel positive pressure may be better (53). However, in these study participants who remained in the study during the one-year follow-up period, there was no difference in compliance between CPAP and bi-level as defined by average number of hours used per day.

Bi-level positive pressure may be useful, however, as a salvage therapy for patients who are intolerant of CPAP. Resta et al. (54) reported that 23% of 130 sleep apnea patients were either unable to tolerate CPAP or were ineffectively treated by this modality. These individuals were successfully treated with bi-level positive pressure. Patients requiring bi-level pressure were more obese, more likely to have obstructive airways disease and to be hypercapnic than patients who were successfully treated with CPAP.

The pressure differential between inspiratory and expiratory positive pressures may augment ventilation. This may be useful in those individuals who have a combination of OSA/H and alveolar hypoventilation and who continue to experience oxyhemoglobin desaturation during sleep despite maintenance of upper airway patency on CPAP (55). Normalization of arterial carbon dioxide tension during wakefuless may occur after a period of nocturnal ventilatory assistance, and ultimately it may be possible to satisfactorily convert patients to conventional CPAP therapy (55).

The clinician might consider using bi-level positive pressure in patients who are intolerant of the sensation of exhaling against the level of expiratory positive pressure that is associated with a therapeutic level of CPAP. A small proportion of individuals complain of chest wall discomfort in conjunction with stretching of chest wall structures during CPAP therapy. This may be related to CPAP-induced elevation of functional residual capacity (56), which may be minimized with reduction of applied expiratory pressure. As discussed above, bi-level positive pressure may be useful in patients with combined OSA/H-hypoventilation syndromes.

V. Central Sleep Apnea

A detailed discussion of the treatment of central sleep apnea is beyond the scope of this chapter. However, although it has been previously reported that CPAP therapy is effective in eliminating central apneas that occur in patients who otherwise have predominancy OSA/H (57), clinical experience indicates that there is a measurable OSA/H patient population who develop "central" apneas on CPAP therapy. Although often of no recognizable clinical consequence, some individuals may exhibit oxyhemoglobin desaturation or arousals as a result of these events. In these patients, the availability of a back-up rate to deliver positive pressure after a clinician-designated apnea interval may be useful. It is important, however, to avoid hyperventilation, which could contribute to further reduction of ventilatory drive and promote central apnea or enhance predisposition to upper airway occlusion during the central apnea events (58–63).

VI. Positive Airway Pressure in the Pediatric Population

Although in the technical sense, positive pressure therapy for OSA/H in children is not a new modality, appreciation of its value for these patients is evolving, and it merits wider clinical consideration in this population.

The exact prevalence of OSA/H in the pediatric and adolescent populations has not been adequately eludicated. A recent paper estimated the prevalence in children from 6 months to 6 years of age to be at least 2.9% (64). Adeno-tonsillar enlargement and craniofacial abnormalities constitute substantial risk factors in this population. In the former circumstance, tonsillectomy and adenoidectomy has been the therapeutic approach of choice. However, this surgery may be associated with notable medical morbidity, particularly in children who have co-existent craniofacial abnormalities, cor pulmonale, morbid obesity, failure to thrive, age <2 years, and severe OSA/H by polysomnography (65) Rosen et al. (65) reported that CPAP or bi-level positive pressure is useful in addressing postoperative complications associated with OSA/H in patients who were ≤ 15 years of age.

Gonsalez et al. (66) and Jarund and Lauritzen (67) have also recently reported the use of CPAP in the care of patients with craniofacial dysostoses. These investigators documented the utility of nasal CPAP in pediatric patients who still exhibited OSA/H after attempts at surgical correction of craniofacial dysostoses. Jarund and Lauritzen recommended that, when possible, craniofacial surgery be deferred until skeletal growth is completed and that nasal CPAP be employed as an interim treatment. Waters et al. (68) published their experience in treating 80 OSA/H patients, ≤ 15 years of age, with nasal CPAP. This therapy successfully ameliorated OSA/H in 90% of children (mean pressure: 7.9 cm H_2O). Ten percent of the children were CPAP failures due to the presence of hypoventilation or development of central apneas. Compliance with positive pressure therapy in the pediatric population appears to be no worse than in the adult population, although less completely studied. In this regard, however, Guilleminault et al. (69) stressed the importance of a supportive family and frequent communication between the patient, family, and physicians. Clinicians who treat children with positive pressure therapy by mask should be aware, however, that there is a risk for developing mid-face hypoplasia related to the orthopedic impact of the mask/headgear (107). It has been suggested that children below the age of 12 are at the greatest risk for this complication and these patients should receive maxillomandibular evaluations at least yearly (107).

VII. Flow-Dependent Positive Airway Pressure

The nasal airway contributes measurably to airflow resistance for which the positive pressure prescription must account in order to deliver a therapeutic level of pressure to the collapsible segment of the airway in OSA/H patients. Nasal resistance varies with airflow, and Farrè and coworkers (70) recently described a variation of bi-level positive airway pressure in which the magnitude of positive pressure varies over the duration of the ventilatory cycle according to an algorithm relating airflow and resistance (71). Thus, flow-dependent positive airway pressure differs from currently available bilevel and CPAP applications that provide constant pressure throughout inspiration but is similar in that a constant, baseline level of expiratory pressure may be applied. It also differs from proportional assist ventilation in which inspiratory pressure varies according to airway resistance and respiratory system elastance (72). At the present time, there have been no published clinical trials of this device. It is not known how this system will function in the presence of mask or mouth leaks or in the environment of varying nasal resistance or varying critical closing pressure of the collapsible segment (P_{crit}). Studies will also be needed to determine if this technique enhances patient acceptance and compliance.

VIII. Automatic CPAP Therapy

A. Potential Advantages and Clinical Relevance

The effective positive pressure levels (P_{eff}) generally corresponds to the level of pressure that abolishes apneas, hypopneas, and snoring with prevention of oxyhemoglobin desaturation and maintenance of good sleep continuity in all sleep stages and in all body positions. Traditionally, P_{eff} is determined during a polysomnographic study during which the attending technician progressively increases the positive pressure level in response to observed obstructive sleep-disordered breathing events and ''respiratory-related arousals.'' P_{eff} level represents the pressure required to normalize sleep and breathing during the first treatment night in a sleep laboratory. However, P_{eff} may vary in different clinical situations such as with changing body, neck, and jaw position (73–75). It also depends on sleep stages, upper airway collapsibility being greater during stages I–II and REM than during slow wave sleep (73). This is illustrated by the significant decrease in P_{eff} during slow-wave sleep compared to other sleep stages (76). For these reasons, it is considered that P_{eff} has not been accurately determined if the patient has not been observed during sleep in the supine position and in REM sleep during the titration study. Furthermore, changes in P_{eff} can also originate from modifications in upper airway characteristics. Changes in upper airway vascular tone have been shown to influence upper airway collapsibility (75). On the other hand, mechanical properties such as upper airway hysteresis may also dramatically influence the pressure-flow relationship. Condos et al. reported that the pressure that abolishes flow limitation is 2–5 cmH_2O higher during ascending compared with the descending levels of positive pressure (77). P_{eff} may also vary during the course of CPAP therapy (78) and dramatically decrease after weight loss (79). All of these elements suggest that positive pressure requirements are dynamic in nature and may change within the course of a single night and from one night to another on a short- and long-term basis. Accordingly, prescribing the single pressure determined to be effective during an in-laboratory trial for home CPAP therapy may conceivably over- or undertreat the OSA/H patient at any given time. Therefore, continuous adaptation of the pressure settings to the patient's need could represent a more physiological approach to CPAP therapy.

B. Theory and Principles

Consideration of the dynamic changes in upper airway function that may occur during sleep has led to development of devices that continuously adjust the magnitude of delivered positive pressure. In general, these devices can be classified into two different categories represented by *auto-titrating* and *automatic* CPAP machines. In this chapter, the auto-titrating CPAP machines are defined as those designed to facilitate determination of a single P_{eff} that would be therapeutic in the home environment. The pressure setting is then adjusted at this P_{eff} level on a conventional, fixed CPAP machine to be used as chronic treatment. Automatic CPAP machines that can be used without a formal titration sleep study represent the other category. These machines could also theoretically be used to determine a single P_{eff} that maintains upper airway patency under ''worst-case'' collapsibility conditions but are practically designed for home CPAP therapy with continuous adjustments of the positive pressure level in response to the patient's physiological demands.

Auto-titrating CPAP, atomatic CPAP, and the different models in each category vary by the type and number of parameters that are analyzed during the night, the signal processing of these parameters, the thresholds that are used to define abnormal breathing events, and the algorithm by which pressure is changed. The airflow can be measured with a pneumotachograph located in the device circuit between the mask and the exhaust port or incorporated within the CPAP machine. The pneumotachograph signal is used to measure total ventilation and to identify apneic and hypopneic events, according to algorithm-based criteria. Similarly, the airflow signal may also be used to identify specific airflow characteristics. Several reports have described usefulness of flow-contour analysis in determining the positive pressure level that minimizes respiratory efforts by eliminating flow-limited breaths (77,80). When the positive pressure level is progressively raised, obstructive apneic and hypopneic events are converted in flow-limited breathing events characterized by a persistent flattening or plateauing of inspiratory flow indicative of elevated inspiratory resistance, and then to normal nonobstructed breaths (Fig. 1). Analyzing the shape of the inspiratory flow contour may therefore be used to determine the CPAP level that prevents flow limitation (81).

Ventilation can also be measured by analyzing the changes in the CPAP compressor speed that are required to maintain a constant pressure level during inspiration and expiration. In currently available CPAP machines, the delivered airflow is closely regulated to maintain the pressure level at the prescribed magnitude throughout the respiratory cycle by increasing and decreasing the compressor speed during the inspiration and expiration using a servo-control mechanism. The corresponding changes in the compressor speed can be used to estimate the difference between the

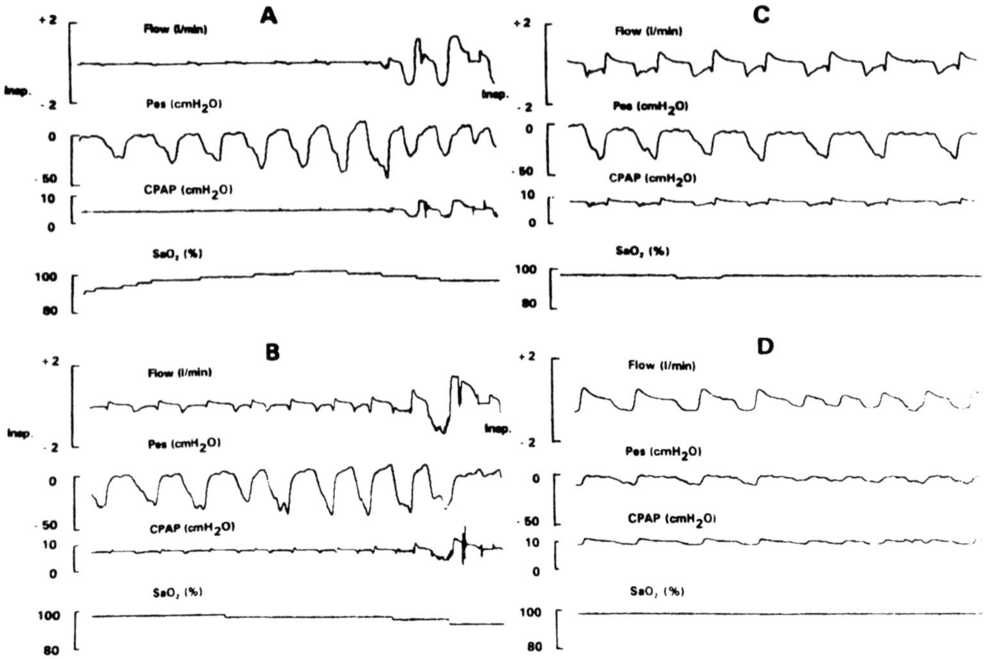

Figure 1 Changes in instantaneous flow, esophageal pressure swings, and arterial oxygen saturation with increasing positive pressure level. The rise in the CPAP level turns a typical obstructive apnea (A), into an obstructive hypopnea (B), then into stable flow limitation with no desaturation (C), and then into normal respiration (D). Ventilatory unstability is observed in A and B only with the presence of apneic and hypopneic events, but an increase in inspiratory efforts with low inspiratory flow values and flow plateauing is observed until the effective pressure has been reached (A, B, C). (From Ref. 80.)

maximum inspiratory and expiratory flow. Stability of the breath-by-breath changes in the speed of the compressor indicates stable breathing. Breathing disorders are associated with a decrease in the inspiratory-expiratory difference in the compressor flow regime, since inspiratory flow demands on the system are diminished resulting in a decreased pressure drop within the system and therefore less need for pressure compensation (76).

Upper airway resistance can be assessed by the forced oscillation technique, which entails introducing small pressure oscillations into the nasal mask with pressure and flow recording to determine oscillatory impedance (78). This provides a continuous recording of respiratory resistance that has been found to decrease in parallel with inspiratory efforts until the effective pressure level has been reached (83). A different approach can be used to discriminate apneas associated with a patient (i.e., ''central'' apnea) or occluded upper airway by measuring the changes in airflow induced by low-amplitude, high-frequency changes in mask pressure (84).

Episodes of snoring may also be analyzed with a high-frequency pressure transducer to identify fluttering in the inspiratory and expiratory pressure signal (84,85).

It is clear that there are notable differences between auto-CPAP machines concerning the number of signals that are analyzed; furthermore, the integration of these variables into the algorithms of pressure change varies dramatically from one apparatus to another. For these reasons, the results of clinical studies obtained with one machine may differ substantially from those of other auto-CPAP machines. Therefore, in auto-CPAP therapy, in contrast to conventional fixed CPAP treatment, the results of validation studies obtained with one apparatus cannot be extrapolated to other machines.

C. Determining the Effective Pressure Level—Auto-Titrating CPAP

As reflected by a review of the literature, it appears that there is an exponentially increasing interest of sleep researchers in auto-titrating CPAP with numerous abstracts and peer-reviewed papers (21 in the last 3 years) employing various designs to study the efficiency of a variety of devices. In this update of the clinical evaluation of these machines, we have limited the present review to published articles. We are aware that important developments are going to occur that may be relevant to some important issues that we presently address.

D. Specific Advantages

Auto-titrating CPAP machines are proposed to be used in the hospital or home environment to provide insight into the single best pressure that maintains a patent airway across the full spectrum of physiological challenges. If this procedure is accurate, it should mminimize the delay for initiating CPAP therapy that is associated with scheduling an in-laboratory titration, improve the availability of sleep laboratories for obligatory sleep studies, and reduce the cost of treatment.

E. Clinical Studies

Two clinical studies have evaluated the accuracy of the Auto-Set® self-titrating machine, and one investigated the AutoAdjust® apparatus. Importantly, in all of these studies the auto-titration procedure was performed in a hospital environment, and the two Auto-Set studies were under the supervision of the attending sleep technician or nurse. Studies evaluating AutoSet compared the acute effects of manual and auto-CPAP titration on sleep and respiratory variables (86). The pressure prescription is derived from the cumulative pressure over time and corresponds to the pressure at or below which 95% of the night is spent after deleting the periods with leaks greater than 0.4 L/S. In both studies, sleep architecture, sleep fragmentation, obstructive breathing frequency, and desaturation improved with the auto-titrating device in the 20 patients studied. Teschler et al. found that the reduction of the apnea + hypopnea index was better achieved during the auto-titrating night than during manual titration and that the P_{eff} to be prescribed according to AutoSet recording was 1.3 ± 0.3 cm H_2O higher than the one determined during the manual procedure (84). Importantly, however, these results may be accounted for by methodological differences between the two titrating procedures: during manual titration there was no recording of flow, and no attempt was made to eliminate snoring and flow limitation, which are the goals of the AutoSet machine. In contrast to the study of Teschler et al., Lloberes and coworkers observed no difference in the P_{eff} measured during auto- or manual titration (86), even though no attempt was made to abolish flow limitation. Interestingly, the arousal and awakening indices were not increased during the auto-CPAP trial, and there was no evidence that the fluctuating positive pressure induced sleep fragmentation. Mask leaks associated with inappropriate increases in mask pressure significantly interfered with pressure regulation in 4 of 20 patients in the study by Teschler et al. (84). This precluded an auto-titration procedure in one subject. In the other patients, excessive mask leaks represented less than 15% of the night. This study may be open to criticism because these periods were deleted from the analysis of cumulative pressure time for P_{eff}. It must be emphasized that no central apneas with an open upper airway were observed in either study. CPAP compliance measured at 3 months in the 20 enrolled patients was similar in patients whose prescribed fixed pressure level was determined by auto-titration compared to conventionally titrated subjects (4.9 ± 0.3 h and 4.7 ± 0.2 h per night respectively, mean ± SEM). Effective pressure measured with the AutoSet machine has been found to remain unchanged during CPAP therapy over 8 months of follow-up (87).

The practical advantages of the auto-titration procedure have been evaluated by Stradling et al. using the AutoAdjust machine (88). One hundred and thirteen patients were randomly allocated to a manual or auto-titration procedure to determine the effective pressure level to be prescribed for use at home with a fixed CPAP machine. Titration nights were done during a conventional sleep study, but no details were provided regarding the need for, or degree of technician intervention during auto-titration. Inappropriate increases in pressure in response to normal nonobstructive hypopneas during REM sleep were prevented by modifying the definition of hypopneic events to reflect a 60% reduction in ventilation for more than 40 s. The investigators determined the prescribed pressure for use at home during a subsequent review of the sleep and respiratory variables. The prescribed value corresponded to the lowest pressure that abolished most of the obstructive events. The efficacy of CPAP therapy was estimated by the willingness of the patients to continue on CPAP therapy for 6 weeks after titration. The manual and auto-titration groups had a similar proportion of patients who wanted to continue on CPAP (64% and 73%, respectively) and who were undecided (23% and 25%, respectively). Persistent hypersomnolence was observed in some patients in whom treatment was designated as successful and more frequently in undecided patients, but it is not known if this could be related to persistent abnormalities during sleep. The percentage of treatment failures (defined as the patient had "given up and unwilling to try CPAP again") was 13% in the conventional titration group and 2% in the automatic titration group ($p <$

0.05). There is no clear explanation for this difference, and the main conclusion was that an automatic determination of the effective pressure does not reduce medium-term CPAP acceptance.

Another approach for determining P_{eff} consists in the continuous acquisition of cardiorespiratory and sleep variables and mask pressure at the positive pressure level automatically changes during the night. This was done by Juhasz et al. (89) with the Vitalog® HMS-5000 system driving a BiPAP machine set in the IPAP mode in 21 OSA/H patients during in-laboratory recordings followed by a conventional CPAP titration night. The algorithm of pressure change consisted in 1 cmH_2O presure rise every 5 min over a 6 cmH_2O interval in a 30-min cycle. At the end of the night, the identification of the effective pressure level was done during a review of the recording to identify the pressure that abolished apneas, hypopneas, snoring, and desaturation. The titration procedure was successful in 72% of patients, but it required technician intervention in the remaining 28% in order to change from a varaible pressure to a fixed pressure mode due to inability to fall asleep, repetitive central apneas, and inappropriate pressure increases in response to nonobstructive breathing disorders. Five patients developed secondary alveolar hypoventilation due to increasing CPAP with the presence of central sleep apnea in two patients. This undesirable machine behavior was particularly evident in patients with congestive heart failure. There was no difference between the effective pressure measured by manual titration and the pressure determined after review of the machine-controlled CPAP changes in the 19 patients who completed the automatic titration night (8.4 $\pm$ 2.3 and 8.1 $\pm$ 2.4 cmH_2O, respectively). It should be noted that this was the only report that specifically notes the inclusion of patients with cardiopulmonary diseases. Other studies either excluded these individuals or did not mention this issue in the study population.

F. Conclusion

The results of the above-mentioned studies suggest that auto-titrating machines may adequately estimate the maximim pressure level required to maintain upper airway patency during sleep in OSA/H patients. However, it is important to note that the above-mentioned studies were completed in an attended situation. While several studies reported technician intervention, others did not comment in this regard, and it cannot be assumed that such intervention did not occur. Since the rationale for use of these devices is to reduce the technician-intense nature of positive pressure titration, to improve availability and patient access to therapy, and to reduce the cost of the titration procedure, it is critical to demonstrate the efficacy of this modality in an unmonitored environment. An important and often overlooked issue is that these CPAP devices, applied in an auto-titration manner, still require human expertise to manually review tracings, identify inappropriate pressure changes, and determine the effective pressure level. This strategy increases the confidence we can have for these machines but obviously means that CPAP titration is still dependent on the expertise of a clinician. Finally, since patients with associated lung and/or cardiovascular diseases may have significant sleep-related breathing disorders which are independent of upper airway dysfunction (expiratory flow limitation, alveolar hypoventilation, periodic breathing, central sleep apneas) that can nonetheless modify ventilation and airflow contour, further studies are required to establish the safety of such procedures in these patients.

The aim of automatic CPAP is to extend the application of the auto-titrating machine to chronic home CPAP therapy. Surprisingly, most of the studies that have been conducted on the presently available machines only investigated machines' behavior during a single night and in the monitored environment of a sleep laboratory. It could be argued that it should be possible to use some of the previously described, auto-titrating machines for home automatic CPAP therapy, but technical requirements such as pneumotachograph requirement may limit its application at home for others.

G. In-Laboratory Clinical Studies

The effectiveness of an automatic CPAP machine driven by the forced oscillation technique signal (Somnosmart, Weinmann, Germany) has been evaluated in 11 men (90). Following the manual titration night, the device was used for two consecutive nights where the upper pressure limit was fixed to 15.5 cmH_2O or individually determined, the minimal pressure being set to 4 cmH_2O. The awake impedence value was used as a reference to quantify sleep-related changes in respiratory impedence. The frequency of obstructive events (apnea, hypopnea, snoring) significantly decreased with the two automatic CPAP setting. The total and respiratory-related arousals also significantly dropped but the former remained quite high during the auto-CPAP nights. No comparison was available with the results of the manual titration night, and no mention was made on the need for technician intervention. The mean CPAP pressure levels delivered during the automatic CPAP nights were significantly less than the manual titration level.

The efficacy of the AutoAdjust apparatus used in the automatic adjustable mode has been compared to fixed CPAP in 12 patients who had a previous conventional in-laboratory CPAP titration study and a minimal 2-week period of home CPAP therapy with a fixed CPAP (91). The machine was used with default settings that allow pressure changes from 3 cmH_2O to 5 cmH_2O above the prescribed pressure level. No mention was made on the need for technician intervention during the night using the automatic CPAP. The percentage of total sleep time spend in slow wave sleep was significantly higher with AutoAdjust than with fixed CPAP (8.5 ± 7.5 and $4.6 \pm 6.05\%$, respectively; $p < 0.05$), inverse results being observed for the time spent in stage II. Since the frequency of respiratory and spontaneous arousals was the same with the two CPAP modes, no clear explanation can be given for this finding. The apnea and hypopnea indices observed during automatic CPAP therapy were below the normal threshold considered in this study (15 events/sleep hour). During the automatic CPAP night, subjects spent $63.1 \pm 34.2\%$ below the pressure prescribed for fixed CPAP use. No information was given concerning the relationship between sleep stage and body position on positive pressure changes. These results seem promising, but as discussed previously, conclusions can be made only after demonstration that this efficacy persists during home CPAP therapy. It is important to note that automatic CPAP benefits would be largely improved if the machine could be used without a previous titration night.

Different results were published by Sharma et al. using the Virtuoso® machine in a similar study design except that they included 20 untreated patients (92). Using the automatic CPAP device, intervention of the technician was required in 5 patients in order to reset the CPAP machine. Total sleep time, sleep architecture, and sleep fragmentation were similarly improved during the two treatment modes. Breathing abnormalities improved with each treatment mode, the difference in apnea + hypopnea index (manual 3.8 ± 3.1; automatic 6.1 ± 5.3) and in the percent total sleep time below various levels of SaO_2 (manuals 0.8 ± 2.4% below 85% SaO_2; automatic 4.2 ± 16.2% below 85% SaO_2) being nonsignificant. CPAP failure to increase the pressure was noted in 5 subjects. The maximal pressure level applied was significantly less during the auto-titration procedure (10.1 ± 3.8 vs. 12.3 ± 3.8 cmH_2O; $p < 0.05$). It was concluded that the investigated prototype should not be used for auto-titration studies without the supervision of a technologist or for long-term home use without previous in-laboratory testing.

Lofaso et al. evaluated the efficacy of an automatic CPAP machine (REM plus®) with an algorithm that was modified to adjust the pressure only in response to snoring (93). In 15 untreated OSA/H patients the apnea + hypopnea index decreased from 51 ± 31/h to 12 ± 21/h. A decrease was observed in 12 patients, while no benefit was found in 3 subjects (1 nonheavy snorer and 2 mouth-breathers). Inspiratory flow limitation persisted once snoring had been abolished, and there was a notable intersubject variability in the degree with which sleep fragmentation improved during automatic CPAP therapy (arousal index 13 ± 20 events/h, mean ± SD). Furthermore, significant desaturation persisted during CPAP therapy with 39 ± 101 min recorded with oxyhemoglobin saturation below 90%.

The results of the two last studies of devices that used an algorithm of pressure changes based on mask pressure vibration suggest that it may not reflect the optimal algorithm for determining the effective pressure level. It is reasonable to state that according to the results of the above-mentioned studies, automatic CPAP may have some improper behavior in some patients, with the possibility of patient intolerance and/or suboptimal treatment. Therefore, determination of P_{eff} may be difficult in patients with unsatisfactory responses to one night of automatic CPAP therapy.

H. In-Home Studies

Besides its utility for determining the single most effective positive pressure level, the previously described AutoSet machine has also been used as an automatic CPAP machine in a 2 week home clinical trial (94). It was found that the mean overnight pressure level was 57 ± 7% (mean ± SEM) of the prescribed fixed pressure level. No information was provided on CPAP compliance or on the impact of CPAP on diurnal sleepiness.

Meurice et al. compared the efficacy of the Morphèe Plus® automatic CPAP machine and conventional CPAP therapy on sleep and breathing characteristics and neuropsychological performance in 16 untreated patients with sleep apnea/hypopnea syndrome (76). A manual CPAP titration procedure was done to determine the effective pressure level (P_{eff}). Patients were then randomly allocated to either automatic CPAP or fixed CPAP for a 3-week period of home CPAP therapy. The positive pressure was allowed to change inside a P_{eff} +2 and −4 cmH_2O range. Similar improvement in sleep and breathing variables was observed during a sleep study performed after 3 weeks of therapy. Automatic pressure changes were not associated with arousals or awakenings. In the automatic CPAP group, the mean overnight pressure level was significantly lower than the previously measured, manually titrated effective pressure level, P_{eff}(8.4 ± 2.8 and 9.1 ± 3.1 cmH_2O, respectively). In this group, 49.3 ± 15% of the time that CPAP was used over 3 weeks of therapy was spent at a pressure below P_{eff}. Subjective and objective daytime sleepiness (Epworth questionnaire, maintenance of wakefulness tests) and psychometric tests (trail-making test) were similarly improved in the two treatment groups. Interestingly, home CPAP compliance, assessed by the number of hours per night during which a positive pressure was applied, significantly differed between the two treatment groups (6.5 ± 1 h in the automatic CPAP group and 5.1 ± 1.1 h in the fixed CPAP group; $p = 0.02$) (Fig. 2). These results demonstrated the efficacy of this machine when used at home in an unattended environment.

The need to determine the reference pressure and therefore to complete a titra-

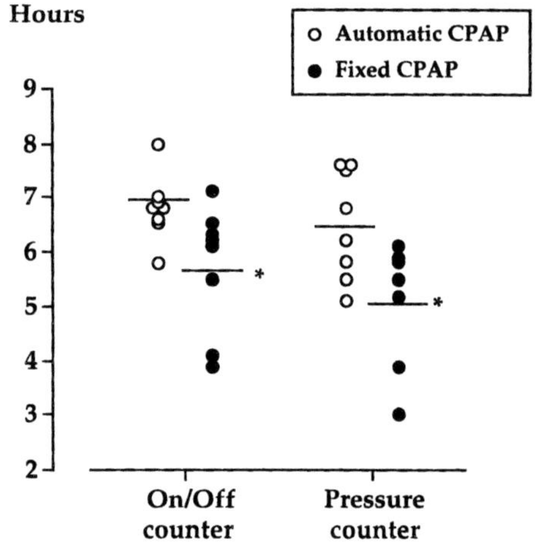

Figure 2 Individual values of CPAP compliance in patients treated with conventional CPAP and with automatic CPAP (Morphée Plus) in a 3-week home trial. The number of hours the machine was turned on and the number of hours a positive pressure was applied is higher in the automatic CPAP group. (From Ref. 76.)

tion sleep study when using the Morphèe Plus may obviously interfere with its usefulness as an automatic CPAP machine. This limitation can be bypassed by estimating P_{eff}, the effective pressure level using a predictive formula that incorporates data addressing body mass index, neck circumference, and the apnea + hypopnea index (95). This strategy was evaluated in 36 newly diagnosed untreated OSA/H patients (apnea + hypopnea index = 43.6 ± 19.8) whose estimated pressure level (see below for pressure determination) was below 15 cmH_2O (96). Following conventional CPAP titration sleep study, patients were randomly assigned to fixed CPAP mode with a pressure level set at the P_{eff}, or automatic CPAP mode using P_{eff} as the reference pressure, or automatic CPAP mode with the P_{ref} set at an estimated effective pressure level. In the automatic CPAP mode, allowed pressure changes were within a range of 3 cmH_2O above and 4 cmH_2O below the reference pressure. The estimated P_{eff} was significantly less than the measured P_{eff} (9.7 ± 2.2 cmH_2O and 11.2 ± 2.0 cmH_2O, respectively; $p = 0.001$). Sleep and breathing characteristics similarly improved across the three groups as assessed by a sleep study performed while the patient was wearing the test CPAP modality (Fig. 3). Borderline abnormal apnea + hypopnea index values persisted in two subjects on the fixed CPAP and two subjects in the automatic CPAP estimated groups. This index remained abnormal (apnea + hypopnea index = 19.3) in one patient in the estimated P_{eff} group whose estimated pressure was substantially underestimated. Sleep fragmentation was significantly reduced with all three CPAP modes. Across

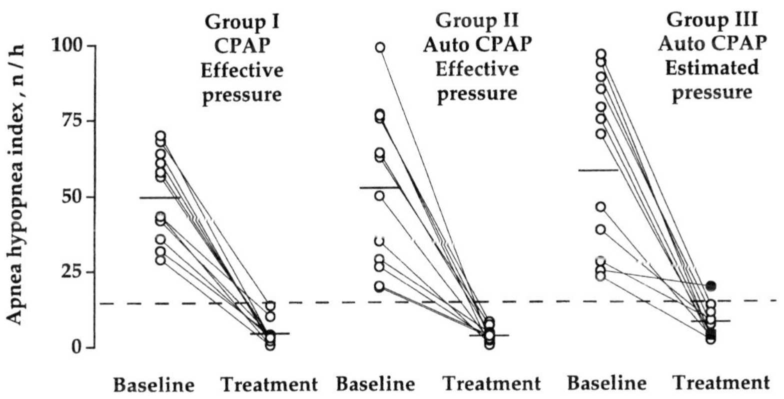

Figure 3 Individual values of the respiratory disturbance index measured at baseline and after 3 weeks of CPAP therapy in patients receiving (1) conventional CPAP, (2) automatic CPAP with a reference pressure measured during a titration sleep study, and (3) automatic CPAP with an estimated value of the reference pressure. The same CPAP apparatus was used in the three groups. The apnea + hypopnea index remained abnormal in one patient of this last group whose estimated pressure was underestimated by more than 4 cmH_2O. The dashed line represent the normal apnea + hypopnea threshold. (From Ref. 97.)

the three treatment groups, a persistent arousal index of >15/h was observed in nine subjects (periodic leg movements in one patient in each group). Subjective and objective diurnal sleepiness improved similarly in the three groups.

The previously described sleep stage dependence of the delivered positive pressure level (76) was also observed in the two automatic CPAP groups with a 1.4 cmH_2O mean difference between stages I–II and III–IV, and 0.8 cmH_2O difference between stages I–II and REM sleep. In the two automatic CPAP groups, the mean CPAP level measured during the home treatment period was significantly less than the effective pressure level (9.5 ± 2.4 cmH_2O and 11.1 ± 2.4 cmH_2O, respectively; $p < 0.0001$). In these two groups, 51.0 ± 7.9% of the CPAP time was recorded at or below the reference pressure.

The effective pressure time index (ratio of the number of hours CPAP is applied and the number of hours the machine is turned on) was significantly higher in the two automatic CPAP groups than in the fixed CPAP group. This difference in effective pressure time index was not related to the use of different interfaces (i.e., nasal mask or nasal prongs interface) since these were similarly distributed in the three treatment modes. Six subjects of the two automatic CPAP groups and three subjects of the constant CPAP group received CPAP treatment for more than 7 h per night at least 5 days per week ($p > 0.05$).

A potentially useful observation was a strong negative correlation between the percentage of CPAP time spent below reference pressure during the treatment period and the difference between effective and estimated pressure. This can be helpful to adjust the pressure settings during Morphée Plus automatic CPAP therapy according to the fact that the adequate reference pressure level can be reliably estimated by the percentage of CPAP time spent below actual reference pressure. The accuracy of this new strategy in automatic CPAP therapy was assessed in a new cohort of 30 untreated sleep apnea patients, 15 of whom were treated with auto-CPAP at home without a titration sleep study, and the other 15 receiving fixed CPAP therapy with the same machine, after a conventional manual CPAP titration (97). A printout of the CPAP trend was obtained after 2 weeks of treatment to measure the percentage of CPAP time spent below P_{ref}. P_{ref} adjustments were made, if necessary, according to the CPAP time $<P_{eff}$, effective and estimated pressure difference relationship. The reference pressure had to be increased in eight patients with an amount of pressure change of 3.0 ± 2.1 cmH_2O (range 1–4 cmH_2O). Interestingly, a significant improvement in treatment use was observed following pressure adjustment (5.9 ± 1.1 to 6.5 ± 0.8 h/night; $p < 0.05$). Similar excellent clinical and polysomnographic responses were observed in the experimental and conventional treatment groups after at least 2 weeks of adequate P_{ref} setting. At the control visit, the effective pressure time index was significantly higher in the automatic CPAP group (93.4 ± 4.0%) than in the conventional CPAP group (88.6 ± 8.1%). Therefore, with a careful follow-up, the Morphée Plus apparatus can be safely used with an estimated value of the P_{ref} using a dedicated algorithm of reference pressure change. Independently of the use of a new algorithm of pressure setting, these results are interesting since they demonstrate the feasibility to initiate automatic CPAP therapy during an unattended home trial.

Another application of this relationship could be to determine the effective pressure level during a home fixed CPAP trial. We prospectively evaluated this procedure in 42 newly diagnosed subjects using the Morphée Plus set with an estimated P_{ref} to perform an initial home titration period, then determining the effective pressure level according to the CPAP time less than, or equal to the reference pressure level, and setting this P_{eff} level on a fixed CPAP machine for several weeks of home CPAP therapy (98). Determination of the appropriate size of nasal mask, patient education regarding the interface, and demonstration of the procedures to operate the machine were made by a home care company. Treatment compliance was high during the home titration phase as assessed by the number of hours the machine was used (6.6 ± 1.5 h/night) and the number of hours a positive pressure was applied (5.9 ± 1.4 h/night) during this study period. At the end of the automatic CPAP trial, the mean calculated pressure setting was 1 ± 1 cmH_2O higher than estimated P_{ref}. At the end of the fixed CPAP period at home, a significant improvement was observed in sleep and breathing characteristics (sleep architecture, sleep fragmentation, apnea + hypopnea index, nocturnal desaturation), with a normalization of the apnea + hypopnea index (<10/h) in all but two subjects. The arousal index with CPAP was 15.9 ± 6.7/h and the frequency of respiratory-related arousals was normal (<15/h) in all but two patients in whom the apnea + hypopnea index remained abnormal. Patients were seen at follow-up after 6.5 ± 2.8 months of CPAP treatment using the pressure setting determined during the auto CPAP trial. Eighty-six percent of them were still on CPAP. The number of hours the machine was turned on from the beginning of fixed CPAP therapy was 6.1 ± 1.7 h per night.

This treatment strategy has the advantage of establishing an effective level CPAP based on data collected over several nights but not requiring any hospital equipment or dedicated room. In contrast, the current practice of in-laboratory fixed CPAP titration permits identification of the CPAP level that is effective over only one night, ignoring the possibility of nightly variation in therapeutic requirements, while incurring the attendant costs and inconveniences.

Two recent studies evaluated the benefits of automatic CPAP therapy used at home for several months. In the study of Boudewyns et al. (99), 15 patients previously treated by fixed CPAP were shifted to auto CPAP (REM + Auto) at home for 2 months using a 2–15 cmH_2O pressure range. No peculiar side effects were reported. The respiratory disturbance and arousal indices measured at the end of the study with the automatic CPAP machine were normal. The mean CPAP level during home auto-CPAP therapy was 5.2 cmH_2O (95% CI 4.9–6.8), while the effective pressure level determined during manual titration was 8.0 (95% CI 5.0–8.0). The effective auto-CPAP use was 6.3 hours per night (95% CI 5.1–6.7), but no comparison was made with previous fixed CPAP treatment. In a study by Konermann and colleagues (100), the AutoAdjust apparatus was used in a parallel group design comparing fixed CPAP following manual titration to auto-CPAP therapy at home for a 3- to 6-month period. Two dropouts were reported in the fixed CPAP group due to pressure intolerance. The two CPAP modes were as effective in normalizing nocturnal respiratory disturbances and sleep fragmentation. The percentage of total sleep time spent in slow-wave sleep was significantly higher at control in the auto-CPAP group. Importantly, the number of days the machine was used per week was significantly less in the fixed CPAP group than in the auto-CPAP group (5.7 ± 0.7 and 6.5 ± 0.4, respectively). It is important to mention that in these two studies, auto-CPAP was not initiated directly at home but after its accuracy had been evaluted during a conventional in-laboratory recording.

IX. Issues in Practical Application of Automatic CPAP Therapy

From our experience (Sériès), automatic CPAP therapy does not reduce side effects such as nasal dryness and stuffiness, and in our previous clinical studies, the use of a heated humidifier was similarly required during fixed and automatic CPAP therapy. With the Morphèe Plus machine, the use of an humidifier required a +1 cmH_2O rise in the reference pressure to compensate for the pressure drop, but it did not alter machine efficacy. This point may be very important, since introducing a humidifier into an automatic CPAP machine breathing circuit can perturb the airflow signal upon which the sensing algorithm may be dependent, thus potentially altering the adequacy of pressure behavior.

As previously detailed, automatic CPAP therapy should be useful to continuously adapt the positive pressure level to the required needs. This may simply be the case during one night depending on body position and sleep stages, but also in circumstances that worsen sleep-related breathing abnormalities. Two classical situations that may alter the therapeutic pressure requirements include alcohol consumption and variations in nasal resistance.

The effect of alcohol intake on automatic CPAP behavior has been evaluated with the AutoSet machine (101). No difference was found in the pressure requirement between the control and the postalcohol sleep studies for the whole night (11.9 ± 0.9 and 12.5 ± 0.9 cmH_2O) and for the first 2 hours following alcohol intake. It was not mentioned, however, if sleep position was the same in these two conditions. These results are in accordance with those previously published by Berry et al. (102) with fixed CPAP therapy. Both positive pressure therapy and alcohol ingestion decrease airway dilator muscle activity (102) and, as a consequence, increase upper airway collapsibility (103). Since CPAP acts as a pneumatic splint of upper airway structures, this effect should not be altered by the depressive effect of alcohol on upper airway muscle tone, and CPAP efficiency should remain unchanged. However, different results could be observed if alcohol ingestion leads to pharyngeal and nasal congestion that could alter the transmission of positive pressure into the collapsible segment of upper airway and increase upper airway critical pressure. In this situation, automatic CPAP therapy should be of benefit if it could counterbalance such mechanical effects of alcohol.

Lafond et al. (104) evaluated the behavior of two different automatic CPAP devices (AutoAdjust and Morphèe Plus) during histamine-induced automentation of nasal resistance in sleeping sleep apnea patients. The mean increase in nasal resistance was 126 ± 46% above baseline, while minute ventilation did not initially change. Employing the Morphèe Plus machine, a paradoxical decrease in the positive pressure level was observed following histamine application and in half of the cases a late increase of mask pressure occurred in response to a decrease in minute ventilation. This increase, however, not sufficient to abolish episodes of flow limitation and recurrent arousals. With the AutoAdjust® apparatus, mask pressure did not change in conjunction with increased nasal resistance, thus not preventing the occurrence of episodes of flow limitation with increased respiratory efforts and sleep fragmentation following histamine instillation. These results suggest that under experimental conditions, the two machines had inadequate pressure responses to acute nasal obstruction.

It could be asked to what extent automatic CPAP could replace fixed CPAP in the future. One of the main issues remaining to be explored is the optimal means of identifying those patients who would benefit most from automatic CPAP compared with conventional CPAP therapy. Sériès et al. (105) examined CPAP compliance in the 40 newly treated OSA/H patients who participated in the recently published data on home automatic CPAP therapy. Patients were randomly allocated to fixed ($n = 20$) or automatic CPAP ($n = 20$) therapy using the same machine for 3 weeks after P_{eff} had been determined during a conventional titration night. The investigators found that in the fixed pressure group, the positive pressure time was less in patients whose breathing abnormalities were position and sleep stage dependent than in the patients with abnormalities unrelated to body position and/or sleep stage. This difference in treatment compliance was accompanied by a lesser improvement in daytime somnolence with CPAP therapy in the former group. These differences in CPAP compliance were not found in the automatic CPAP group, suggesting that automatic CPAP may improve treatment compliance in patients who demonstrate the substantial body position and sleep stage–related variability in nocturnal breathing disturbances.

X. Conclusions

A goal that is frequently invoked to justify automatic CPAP therapy is to maintain the lowest possible pressure in order to improve patient comfort and improve compliance. Even if published data support this hypothesis (76), we believe that the advantages of these machine rely on their capacity not only to decrease the mean nightime pressure level, but also to transiently increase the pressure setting. It is remarkable to observe that patients whose effective pressure has been optimally determined may spend 10–15% of their CPAP time at a pressure level higher than the one that should be prescribed according to the sleep titration night. The paucity of clinical studies conducted to date in this field do not allow any conclusion regarding the degree of patient benefit that is conferred by a lower average overnight level of CPAP when using automatic CPAP technology. There are presently no data suggesting that there would be a reduction in the frequency or severity of side effects accompanying the use of systems that allow the greatest reduction in pressure relative to conventional fixed CPAP.

Accurate automatic titration may have significant practical repercussions on clinical practice patterns and sleep laboratory activities, potentially reducing treatment delays, avoiding systematic in-laboratory CPAP titration nights, and allowing additional time for diagnostic polysomnographic studies. In this new strategy of CPAP adjustment, we believe that determining the effective pressure level during a home CPAP trial rather than a partially attended recording in the hospital should allow a more physiological evaluation of the patients needs based on results obtained in their own environment for several days. Since this titration strategy has not been extensively evaluated in the literature, the consequences of the loss of any technician interaction in this setting remain to be evaluated.

Caution should be taken with the introduction of automatic CPAP machines. This mode of CPAP therapy should not simply be considered as an easy treatment in these times when the tendency is to simplify diagnostic procedures with the use of screening tests that may be very helpful in expert hands but whose diagnostic value has rarely been evaluated outside sleep laboratories. Therefore, the increased accessibility to CPAP therapy should help in the management of sleep disorders but should not lead to an inadequate rise in CPAP prescription. Furthermore, it can be anticipated that the use of automatic CPAP machines would further justify the need for an early clinical follow-up of these patients.

In view of the paucity of clinical investigations conducted with automatic CPAP machines, the variety of algorithms and experimental conditions that have been employed and especially the small patient populations and limited follow-up, auto-titrating and automatic CPAP can be considered today as promising but in development as a technology. Further studies are also required to examine the accuracy of these devices in OSA/H patients with associated lung and chest wall disease, massive obesity, left cardiac dysfunction, or chronic obstructive pulmonary disease.

References

1. Sullivan CE, Issa FG, Berthon-Jones M, et al. Reversal of obstructive sleep apnoea by continuous positive airway pressure applied through the nares. Lancet 1981; 1:862–865.
2. Sullivan CE, Issa FG, Berthon-Jones M, et al. Home treatment of obstructive sleep apnoea with continuous positive airway pressure applied through a nose mask. Bull Eur Physiopathol Respir 1984; 20:49–54.
3. Sullivan CE, Grunstein RR. Continuous positive airways pressure in sleep-disordered breathing. In: Kryger MH, Rother T, Dement WC, eds. Principles and Practice of Sleep Medicine, 1989:559–570.

4. Sanders MH, Moore SE, Evaslage J. CPAP via nasal mask: A treatment for occlusive sleep apnea. Chest 1983; 83:144–145.
5. Sanders MH. Nasal CPAP effect on patterns of sleep apnea. Chest 1984; 86:839–844.
6. Rapoport DM, Sorkin B, Garay SM, et al. Reversal of the "pickwickian syndrome" by long-term use of nocturnal airway pressure. N Engl J Med 1982; 307:931–933.
7. Frith RW, Cant BR. Severe obstructive sleep apnoea treated with long term nasal continuous positive airway pressure. Thorax 1985; 40:45–50.
8. Mayer LS, Kerby GR, Whitman RA, et al. Continued evaluation of a new nasal device for administration of continuous positive airway pressure. Am Rev Respir Dis 1990; 141:A684.
9. McEvoy RD, Thornton AT. Treatment of obstructive sleep apnea syndrome with nasal continuous positive airway pressure. Sleep 1984; 7:313–325.
10. Hoffstein V, Viner S, Mateika S, Conway J. Treatment of obstructive sleep apnea with nasal continuous positive airway pressure. Patient compliance, perception of benefits, and side effects. Am Rev Respir Dis 1992; 145:841–845.
11. Smith PL, Hudgel DW, Olson LG, et al. Indications and standards for use of nasal continuous positive airway pressure (CPAP) in sleep apnea syndromes. Am J Respir Crit Care Med 1994; 150:1738–1745.
12. Sériès F, Cormier Y, Couture J, et al. Changes in upper airway resistance with lung inflation and positive airway pressure. J Appl Physiol 1990; 68:1075–1079.
13. Sforza E, Lugaresi E. Daytime sleepiness and nasal continuous positive airway pressure in obstructive sleep apnea patients: effects of chronic treatment and 1 night therapy withdrawal. Sleep 1995; 18:195–201.
14. Lamphere J, Roehrs T, Wittig R, et al. Recovery of alertness of CPAP in apnea. Chest 1989; 96:1364–1367.
15. Rajagopal KR, Bennett LL, Dillard TA. Overnight nasal CPAP improves hypersomnolence in sleep apnea. Chest 1986; 90:172–176.
16. Kribbs NB, Pack AI, Kline LR, et al. Effects of one night without nasal CPAP treatment on sleep and sleepiness in patients with obstructive sleep apnea. Am Rev Respir Dis 1993; 147:1162–1168.
17. Engleman HM, Martin SE, Deary IJ, Douglas NJ. Effect of continuous positive airway pressure treatment on daytime function in sleep apnea/hypopnea syndrome. Lancet 1994; 343:572–575.
18. Engleman H. Self-reported use of CPAP and benefits of CPAP therapy. A patient survey. Chest 1996; 109:1470–1476.
19. Kribbs NB, Pack AI, Kline LR, et al. Objective measurement of patterns of nasal CPAP use by patients with obstructive sleep apnea. Am Rev Respir Dis 1993; 147: 887–895.
20. Meurice JC, Dore P, Paquereau J, et al. Predictive factors of long-term compliance with nasal continous positive airway pressure treatment in sleep apnea syndrome. Chest 1994; 105:429–433.
21. Rauscher H, Popp W, Wanke T, Zwick H. Acceptance of CPAP therapy for sleep apnea. Chest 1991; 100:1019–1023.
22. Reeves-Hochè MK, Meck R, Zwillich CW. Nasal CPAP: an objective evaluation of patient compliance. Am J Respir Crit Care Med 1994; 149:149–154.
23. Waldhorn RE, Herrick TW, Nguyen MC, O'Donnell AE, Sodero J, Potolicchio SJ. Long-term compliance with nasal continuous positive airway pressure therapy of obstructive sleep apnea. Chest 1990; 97:33–38.

24. Weaver TE, Chugh DK, Maislin G, et al. Comparison of CPAP nightly duration to nocturnal sleep time. Am J Respir Crit Care Med 1997; 155:A304.
25. Chervin RD, Theut S, Bassetti C, Aldrich MS. Compliance with nasal CPAP can be improved by simple interventions. Sleep 1997; 20:284–289.
26. Remmers JE, Sterling JA, Thorasinsson B, et al. Nasal airway positive pressure in patients with occlusive sleep apnea: Methods and feasibility. Am Rev Respir Dis 1984; 130:1152–1155.
27. Pépin JL, Leger P, Veale D, Langevin B, Robert D, Lévy P. Side effects of nasal continuous positive airway pressure in sleep apnea syndrome. Chest 1995; 107:375–381.
28. Mayer LS, Kerby GR, Whitman RA. Evaluation of a new nasal device for administration of continuous positive airway pressure for obstruction sleep apnea. Am Rev Respir Dis 1989; 139:A114.
29. Harris C, Daniels B, Herold D, Peterson R, Shepard J. Comparison of cannula and mask systems for administration of nasal continuous positive airway pressure for treatment of obstructive sleep apnea (abstr). Sleep Res 1990; 19:233.
30. Sanders MH, Kern NB, Costantino J, et al. Adequacy of prescribing positive airway pressure therapy by mask for sleep apnea on the basis of a partial-night trial. Am Rev Respir Dis 1992; 147:1169–1174.
31. Strohl KP, Redline S. Nasal CPAP therapy, upper airway activation, and obstructive sleep apnea. Am Rev Respir Dis 1986; 134:555–558.
32. American Thoracic Society. Official statement. Indications and standards for use of nasal continuous positive airway pressure (CPAP) in sleep apnea syndromes. Am J Respir Crit Care Med 1995; 151:1738–1745.
33. Kuna ST, Remmers JE. Neural and anatomic factors related to upper airway occlusion during sleep. Med Clin North Am 1985; 69:1221–1242.
34. Mortimore IL, Bradley PA, Murray JA, Douglas NJ. Uvulopalatopharyngoplasty may compromise nasal CPAP therapy in sleep apnea syndrome. Am J Respir Crit Care Med 1996; 154:1759–1762.
35. Meyer TJ, Pressman MR, Benditt J, McCool FD, Millman RP, Naterajan R, Hill NS. Air leaking through the mouth during nocturnal nasal ventilation: effect on sleep quality. Sleep 1997; 20:561–569.
36. Bach JR, Robert D, Leger P, Langevin B. Sleep fragmentation in kyphoscoliotic individuals with alveolar hypoventilation treated by nasal IPPV. Chest 1995; 107:1552–1558.
37. Sanders MH, Kern NB, Stiller RA. Use of an oro-nasal interface in the positive pressure therapy of sleep apnea. Chest 1994; 106:774–779.
38. Prosise GL, Berry RB. Oral-nasal continuous positive airway pressure as a treatment for obstructive sleep apnea. Chest 1994; 106:180–186.
39. Mortimore IL, Whittle AT, Douglas NJ. Comparison of nose and face mask CPAP therapy for sleep apnoea. Thorax 1998; 53:290–292.
40. Bach JR. Obstructive sleep apnea. Oral-nasal CPAP or lipseal CPAP (letter). Chest 1995; 107:1180–1181.
41. Bach JR, Alba AS, Saporito LR. Intermittent positive pressure ventilation via the mouth as an alternative to tracheostomy for 257 ventilator users. Chest 1993; 103: 174–182.
42. Bach JR, Sorter SM, Saporito LR. Interfaces for non-invasive intermittent positive pressure ventilatory support in North America. Eur Respir Rev 1993; 3:254–259.
43. Pressman MR, Peterson DD, Meyer TJ, Harkins JP, Gurijala L. Ramp Abuse. A novel

form of patient noncompliance to administration of nasal continuous positive airway pressure treatment of obstructive sleep apnea. Am J Respir Crit Care Med 1995; 151: 1632–1634.

44. Richards GN, Cistulli PA, Ungar RG, Berthon-Jones M, Sullivan CE. Mouth leak with nasal continuous positive airway pressure increases nasal airway resistance. Am J Respir Crit Care Med 1996; 154:182–186.
45. Massie CA, Hart RW, Peralez K, Richard GN. Effects of humidification on nasal symptoms and compliance in sleep apnea patients using continuous positive airway pressure. Chest 1999; 116:403–408.
46. Martins de Araujo MT, Vieira SB, Vasquez EC, FLeury B. Heated humidification or face mask to prevent upper airway dryness during continuous positive airway pressure therapy. Chest 2000; 117:142–147.
47. Sanders MH, Rogers RM, Pennock BE. Prolonged expiratory phase in sleep apnea: a unifying hypothesis. Am Rev Respir Dis 1985; 131:401–408.
48. Schwab RJ, Gefter WB, Pack AI, Hoffman EA. Dynamic imaging of the upper airway during respiration in normal subjects. J Appl Physiol 1993; 74:1504–1514.
49. Schwab RJ, Pack AI, Gupta KB, et al. Upper airway and soft tissue structural changes induced by CPAP in normal subjects. Am J Respir Crit Care Med 1996; 154:1106–1116.
50. Schwartz AR, Smith PL, Wise RA, et al. Induction of upper airway occlusion in sleeping individuals with subatmospheric nasal pressure. J Appl Physiol 1988; 64:535–542.
51. Smith PL, Wise RA, Gold AR, Schwartz AR, Permutt S. Upper airway pressure-flow relationships in obstructive apnea. J Appl Physiol 1988; 64:789–795.
52. Sanders MH, Kern N. Treatment of obstructive sleep apnea by using independently adjusted inspiratory and expiratory positive pressure via nasal mask. Physiologic and clinical implications. Chest 1990; 98:317–324.
53. Reeves-Hochè MK, Hudgel D, Meck R, Zwillich CW. Continuous versus bilevel positive airway pressure for obstructive sleep apnea. Am J Respir Crit Care Med 1995; 151:443–449.
54. Resta O, Guido P, Picca V, Sabato R, Rizzi M, Scarpelli F, Sergi M. Prescription of nCPAP and nBiPAP in obstructive sleep apnoea syndrome: Italian experience in 105 subjects. A prospective two centre study. Respir Med 1998; 92:820–827.
55. Piper AJ, Sullivan CE. Effects of short-term NIPPV in the treatment of patients with severe obstructive sleep apnea and hypercapnia. Chest 1994; 105:434–440.
56. Abboud N, Rehder K, Rodarte JR, Hyatt RE, Lung volumes and the closing capacity with continuous positive airway pressure. Anesthesiology 1975; 42:138–142.
57. Issa FG, Sullivan CE. Reversal of central sleep apnea using nasal CPAP. Chest 1986; 90:165–171.
58. Delguste P, Aubert-Tulkens G, Rodenstein DO. Upper airway obstruction during nasal intermittent positive-pressure hyperventilation during sleep. Lancet 1991; 338:1295–1297.
59. Jounieaux V, Aubert G, Dury M, Delguste P, Rodenstein DO. Effects of nasal positive-pressure hyperventilation on the glottis in normal awake subjects. J Appl Physiol 1995; 79:176–185.
60. Jounieaux V, Aubert G, Dury M, et al. Effects of nasal positive-pressure hyperventilation on the glottis in normal sleeping subjects. J Appl Physiol 1995; 79:186–193.
61. Badr MS, Toiber F, Skatrud JB, Dempsey J. Pharyngeal narrowing/occlusion during central sleep apnea. J Appl Physiol 1995; 78:1806–1815.

62. Morrell MJ, Badr MS, Harms CA, Dempsey JA. The assessment of upper airway patency during apnea using cardiogenic oscillations in the airflow signal. Sleep 1995; 18:651–658.
63. Hommura F, Nishimura M, Oguri M, et al. Continuous versus bilevel positive airway pressure in a patient with idiopathic central sleep apnea. Am J Respir Crit Care Med 1997; 155:1482–1485.
64. Gislason T, Benediktsdottir B. Snoring, apneic episodes, and nocturnal hypoxemia among children 6 months to 6 years old. An epidemiologic study of lower limit of prevalence. Chest 1995; 107:963–966.
65. Rosen GM, RP M, Mahowald MW, Goding GS, Ullevig C. Postoperative respiratory compromise in children with obstructive sleep apnea syndrome: Can it be anticipated? Pediatrics 1994; 93:784–788.
66. Gonsalez S, Thompson D, Hayward R, Lane R. Treatment of obstructive sleep apnoea using nasal CPAP in children with craniofacial dysostoses. Child Nerv Syst 1996; 12: 713–719.
67. Jarund M, Lauritzen C. Craniofacial dysostosis: airway obstruction and craniofacial surgery. Scand J Plast Reconstr Surg Hand Surg 1996; 30:275–279.
68. Waters KA, Everett FM, Bruderer JW, Sullivan CE. Obstructive sleep apnea: the use of nasal CPAP in 80 children. Am J Respir Crit Care Med 1995; 152:780–785.
69. Guilleminault C, Nino-Murcier G, Held G, Baldwin R, Hutchinson D. Alternative treatment to tracheostomy in obstructive sleep apnea syndrome: nasal continuous positive airway pressure in young children. Pediatrics 1986; 78:797–802.
70. Farrè R, Peslin R, Montserrat JM, Rotger M, Navajas D. Flow dependent positive airway pressure to maintain airway patency in sleep apnea-hypopnea syndrome. Am J Respir Crit Care Med 1998; 157:1855–1863.
71. Montserrat JM. Forth International Symposium on Sleep and Breathing, Edinburgh, Scotland, 1997.
72. Younes M. Proportional assist ventilation, a new approach to ventilatory support. Am Rev Respir Dis 1992; 145:114–120.
73. Issa FG, Sullivan CE. Upper airway closing pressures in obstructive sleep apnea. J Appl Physiol 1984; 57:520–527.
74. Thut DC, Schwartz AR, Roach D, Wise RA, Permutt S, Smith PL. Tracheal and neck position influence upper airway airflow dynamics by altering airway length. J Appl Physiol 1993; 75:2084–2090.
75. Wasicko MJ, Hutt DA, Parisi RA, Neubaeur JA, Mezrich R, Edelman NH. The role of vascular tone in the control of upper airway collapsibility. Am Rev Respir Dis 1990; 141:1569–1577.
76. Meurice JC, Marc I, Sériès F. Efficiency of auto-CPAP in the treatment of obstructive sleep apnea/hypopnea syndrome. Am J Respir Crit Care Med 1996; 153:794–798.
77. Condos R, Norman RG, Krisnasamy I, Peduzzi N, Goldring RM, Rapoport DM. Flow-limitation as a noninvasive assessment of residual upper-airway resistance during continuous positive airway pressure therapy of obstructive sleep apnea. Am J Crit Care Med 1994; 150:475–480.
78. Sériès F, Marc I, Cormier Y, La Forge J. Required levels of nasal continuous positive airway pressure during treatment of obstructive sleep apnoea. Eur Respir J 1994; 7: 1776–1781.
79. Schwartz AR, Gold AR, Schubert, N, et al. Effect of weight loss on upper airway collapsibility in obstructive sleep apnea. Am Rev Respir Dis 1991; 144:494–498.

80. Montserrat JM, Ballester E, Olivi H, et al. Time course of stepwise CPAP titration. Am J Respir Crit Care Med 1995; 152:1854–1859.
81. Montserrat JM, Allarcon A, Lloberes P, Ballester E, Fornas C, Rodriguez-Voisin R. Adequacy of prescribing nasal continuous positive airway pressure therapy on the sleep apnoea/hypopnoea syndrome on the basis of night time respiratory recording variables. Thorax 1995; 50:969–971.
82. Farrè R, Peslin R, Rotger M, Navaja D. Inspiratory dynamic obstruction detected by forced oscillation during CPAP. Am J Respir Crit Care Med 1997; 155:952–956.
83. Navajas D, Farrè R, Rotger M, Badia R, Puig-de-Morales M, Montserrat JM. Assessment of airway obstruction during CPAP by means of forced oscillation technique in patients with SAS. Am J Respir Crit Care Med 1998; 157:1526–1530.
84. Teschler H, Berthon-Jones M, Thompson AB, Henkel A, Henry J, Konietzko N. Automated continuous positive airway pressure titration for obstructive sleep apnea syndrome. Am J Respir Crit Care Med 1996; 154:734–740.
85. Behbehani K, Yen F-C, Burk JR, Lucas EA, Axe JR. Automatic control of airway pressure for treatment of obstructive sleep apnea. IEEE Trans Biomed Eng 1995; 42: 1007–1016.
86. Lloberes P, Ballester E, Montserrat JM, et al. Comparison of manual and automatic CPAP titration in patients with sleep apnea/hypopnea syndrome. Am J Respir Crit Care Med 1996; 154:1755–1758.
87. Teschler H, Farhat AA, Exner V, Konietzko N, Berthon Jones M. AutoSet? nasal CPAP titration: constancy of pressure, compliance and effectiveness at 8 month follow-up. Eur Respir J 1997; 10:2073–2078.
88. Stradling JR, Barbour C, Pitson DJ, Davies RJ. Automatic nasal continuous positive airway pressure titration in the laboratory: patient outcomes. Thorax 1997; 52:72–75.
89. Juhasz J, Schillen J, Urbigkeit A, Ploch T, Penzel T, Peter JH. Unattended continuous positive airway pressure titration. Clinical relevance and cardiorespiratory hazards of the method. Am J Respir Crit Care Med 1996; 154:359–365.
90. Randerath WJ, Parys K, Feldmeyer F, Sanner B, Rühle KH. Self-adjusting nasal continuous positive airway pressure therapy based on measurement of impedance. Chest 1999; 116:991–999.
91. Scharf MB, Brannen DE, McDannold MD, Berkowitz DV. Computerized adjustable versus fixed NCPAP treatment of obstructive sleep apnea. Sleep 1996; 19:491–496.
92. Sharma S, Wali S, Pouliot Z, Peters M, Neufeld H, Kryger M. Treatment of obstructive sleep apnea with self-titrating continuous positive airway pressure system. Sleep 1996; 19:497–501.
93. Lofaso F, Lorino AM, Duizabo D, et al. Evaluation of an auto-CPAP device based on snoring detection. Eur Respir J 1996; 9:1795–1800.
94. Berthon-Jones M, Lawrence S, Sullivan CE, Grunstein R. Nasal continuous positive airway pressure treatment: current realities and future. Sleep 1996; 19:S131–S135.
95. Miljeteig H, Hoffstein V. Determinants of continuous positive airway pressure level for treatment of obstructive sleep apnea. Am Rev Respir Dis 1993; 147:1526–1530.
96. Sériès F, Marc I. Efficacy of automatic continuous positive airway pressure that uses an estimated required pressure level in the treatment of obstructive sleep apnea syndrome. Ann Intern Med 1997; 8:588–595.
97. Sériès F, Marc I. Efficiency of auto CPAP without titration night in the treatment of sleep apnea hypopnea syndrome. Am J Respir Crit Care Med 1997; 155:A301.

98. Sériès F. Accuracy of an unattended home CPAP titration in the treatment of obstructive sleep apnea. Am J Respir Crit Care Med 2000; 162:94–97.
99. Boudewyns A, Grillier-Lanoir V, Willemen MJ, De Cock WA, Van de Heyning PH, De Backer WA. Two months follow up of auto-CPAP treatment in patients with obstructive sleep apnoea. Thorax 1999; 54:147–149.
100. Konermann M, Sanner BM, Vyleda M, Laschewki F, Groetz J, Sturn A, Zideck W. Use of conventional and self-adjusting nasal continuous positive airway pressure for treatment of severe obstructive sleep apnea syndrome. Chest 1998; 113:714–718.
101. Teschler H, Berthon-Jones M, Wessendorf T, Meyer HJ, Konietzko N. Influence of moderate alcohol consumption on obstructive sleep apnoea with and without AutoSet nasal CPAP system. Eur Respir J 1996; 9:2371–2377.
102. Berry RT, Desa MM, Light RW. Effect of ethanol on the efficacy of nasal continuous positive airway pressure as a treatment of obstructive sleep apnea. Chest 1991; 99: 339–343.
103. Schwartz AR, Smith PL, Wise RA, Bankman I, Permutt S. Effect of positive nasal pressure on upper airway pressure-flow relationships. J Appl Physiol 1989; 66:1626–1634.
104. Lafond C, Series F. Influence of nasal obstruction on auto-CPAP behavior during sleep in sleep apnea/hypopnea syndrome. Thorax 1998; 53:780–783.
105. Sériès F, Marc I. Importance of sleep stage and body position-dependence of sleep apnea in determining benefits in auto-CPAP therapy. Eur Respir J. In press.
106. Li K, Riley RW, Guilleminault C. An unreported risk in the use of home nasal continuous positive airway pressure and home nasal ventilation in children: mid-face hypoplasia. Chest 2000; 117:916–918.

18

Adherence to Continuous Positive Airway Pressure Treatment and Functional Status in Adult Obstructive Sleep Apnea

TERRI E. WEAVER

University of Pennsylvania School of Nursing
Philadelphia, Pennsylvania

I. Introduction

Since its initial description (1,2), nasal continuous positive airway pressure (CPAP) has proven to be an effective treatment for the reduction of obstructive sleep apnea (OSA)–related respiratory disturbances (1–10). Gains achieved with CPAP treatment include amelioration of sleep architecture and arousals (3,7,9,11), improved alertness (11–21), neurobehavioral performance (11–13,15,20,22), and daily functioning (11–13,15–18,23–34). Although it was previously believed that patients could occasionally take treatment holidays (10,35–37), contrary evidence indicated the importance of nightly adherence to treatment (20). Indeed, missing just one night of CPAP treatment induced the return of daytime sleepiness and disturbed sleep (20). Chronic treatment abstinence has been associated with heightened risks of cardiovascular morbidity (38–49), automobile accidents (4,12,50–62), and problems in many other areas of life (27,32,63–68), thus, the demonstrated need to apply CPAP nightly has made CPAP nonadherence one of the foremost clinical issues in the management of OSA.

The growing emphasis on adherence to CPAP and associated outcomes currently found in the literature is in response to the demand by insurance companies, accrediting bodies, regulatory agencies, and savvy consumers to demonstrate the clinical effectiveness of this treatment (69). Clinical effectiveness, unlike clinical efficacy that is evaluated within the context of clinical trials, examines the results of treatment delivered by routine clinical practice (69,70). Accordingly, the extent to which a treatment is accepted by patients is integral to the determination of clinical effectiveness. Indeed, it is essential to consider patient and family perception of treatment, their preferences, and decision-making proclivities (69). Therefore, this chapter will review the literature regarding the nature of adherence to CPAP and examine potential contributing factors and the success of interventions designed to promote CPAP use. The impact of OSA on the patient-centered clinical outcome of functional status will also be considered as well as the effect of CPAP treatment on this significant variable.

II. Nature of CPAP Adherence

A. Acceptance of CPAP and Self-Reported Use

The majority of initial studies exploring the extent to which patients use their CPAP were retrospective, relying predominately on self-report (71–78). In these studies nonadherence to CPAP was characterized as the percentage of patients who refused to initiate CPAP treatment or who abandoned this modality after treatment had commenced (72–76,78). From this perspective, CPAP adherence seemed quite effective with acceptance rates ranging from 64 to 93% (72–76,78–80). When the operational definition of adherence went beyond intention to treat to the more clinically relevant self-reported daily nocturnal use, the level of adherence ranged from 67 to 96% (29,72,73,75,78,80). The exception to this was the early study by McEvoy and colleagues (79) in a small group of OSA patients in which only four of seven (57.1%) patients reported that they used CPAP nightly.

The limitation in relying solely upon self-reported use became evident when studies employed new technology that could monitor actual duration of therapeutic pressure (mask-on time). Covertly monitoring mask-on time, Kribbs and colleagues (19) uniquely demonstrated that the majority of their subjects (66%) overestimated their duration of use by 69 ± 110 min (mean ± standard deviation), and 60% claimed that they used their CPAP nightly when this was accurate for only 46%. Subsequent studies also documented the inaccuracy of patient self-reported treatment time where patient reports were 5–30% over CPAP machine-on time (71,80–85), averaging 1 h more than actual use (19,71,80,81). It became evident that evaluating the clinical effectiveness of CPAP only on the basis of patient self-report was insufficient and, with the advent of manufacturer-installed devices capable of monitoring nightly use, that more objective techniques were essential.

B. Objectively Monitored CPAP Use

As indicated in the display of published reports of CPAP use shown in Table 1, the mean nightly duration of CPAP machine-on time was 5.39 h with a range of 3.2–7.29 h (12,14,17–19,24,29,31,33,71,77,78,81–102). However, it has been shown that machine-on and mask-on time, the duration of the effective delivery of therapeutic pressure, differ by 10% (19). Adjusting each of the mean machine-on times to reflect mask-on time, collectively the average reported duration of nightly CPAP use reported in the literature reviewed was 4.97 h (range 2.80–6.90 h) (12,14, 17–19,24,29,31,33,34,71,77,78,80–105), remarkably consistent with the seminal findings of Kribbs and colleagues (19) of 4.88 ± 1.97 h.

Evaluating the clinical significance of a single daily mean of CPAP use is difficult as it is confounded by both night-to-night variability and differences in duration of use within nights (96). It also coalesces the pattern of use of consistent users with those who use CPAP intermittently (96). In their examination of the night-to-night variability of CPAP use, Weaver and coworkers (96) plotted the proportion of subjects ($n = 32$) who skipped CPAP zero, 1–3, 4–6, or 7 nights per week for the first 9 weeks of treatment. As shown in Figure 1, there was a bimodal distribution of frequency of CPAP use. Approximately half of the subjects (53%), termed "consistent users," applied CPAP >90% of the nights for an average of 6.21 ± 1.21 h per night. Daily use by the half (47%), termed "intermittent users," varied greatly (2–79% of days) with a mean nightly hourly use when CPAP was applied of 3.45 ± 1.94 h per night. These empirical data suggested that the average of 4.97 h of CPAP use derived from previous reports (12,14,17–19,24,29,31,33, 34,71,77,78,80–105) reflected two distinct and significantly different patterns of CPAP use. Moreover, it also illustrated that there are some patients who are indeed highly compliant, using their CPAP daily for most of their nocturnal sleep time.

It appears that using CPAP for less than 4 h per night is a hallmark for eventual nonadherence and rejection of this treatment modality (76,77,79). For example, Krieger (77) found that the nightly CPAP duration of those who eventually abandoned CPAP (10.3% of 214 patients) was 2.4 ± 0.6 h versus 5.6 ± 0.1 h (84% of the sample) for those who continued treatment. The minimum duration CPAP should be applied each night to achieve maximum benefit remains undetermined. However, we do know that skipping just one night of CPAP results in negative outcomes, indicating that night-to-night consistency may be a critical dimension in the evaluation of CPAP adherence (20). After consistent use (defined as at least 4 h of objectively monitored use per night on 80% of the days), withdrawing CPAP for only one night resulted in the return of objectively and subjectively measured daytime somnolence and nocturnal respiratory disturbances to almost pretreatment levels (20). These provocative findings underscore the necessity of wearing CPAP every night and call into question the therapeutic value of CPAP in those patients who skip nights of treatment. Considering the negative consequences associated with nonadherence, Weaver and colleagues (96) attempted to determine whether frequency or nightly duration of CPAP use should be the metric to use when evaluating adherence to treatment. Not surprising, these two behaviors were highly related (rho = −0.73); those who skipped nights of CPAP use also used CPAP for shorter nightly durations.

Empirical evidence suggests that acceptance or rejection of CPAP occurs very early in treatment. Of those studies that have documented when patients have

Table 1 Studies Reporting Use of CPAP Therapy

Study	N	Pre-CPAP avg. RDI	Metric of CPAP use	Avg. CPAP pressure (cmH_2O)	Avg. time on CPAP at time of assessment	% meeting definition of CPAP use	Mean h/day machine-on time	Mean h/day mask-on time[a]
McEvoy et al. (79)	11	35.9	Self-reported use	NR	9.7 mo	64	NR	NR
Sanders et al. (72)	20	51	Self reported use	10.1 ± 3	10.3 ± 8 mo	90	NR	NR
Krieger and Kurtz (81)	45	55.2 ± 1.7	Machine-on time	NR	298 ± 43 days	90.9–93.2	5.14 ± 0.31	4.63
Nino-Murcia et al. (73)	139	80.8 ± 38.8	On CPAP/abandoned or refused CPAP	9.9 ± 14.3	≥2 mo	96	NR	NR
Waldhorn et al. (74)	96	57.2 ± 26.9	NR	10.6 ± 2.6	≥6.2 ± 7.1 mo	76	NR	NR
Rolfe et al. (75)	168	NR	On CPAP/abandoned or refused CPAP	NR	~18.2 mo	64	NR	NR
Hoffstein et al. (76)	96	54 ± 31	On CPAP/abandoned or refused CPAP	9 ± 3	17 ± 11 mo	82	NR	NR
Krieger (77)	214	82 ± 2	On CPAP/abandoned or refused	9.6 ± 0.2	NR	84	5.3 ± 0.2	4.77
Kribbs et al. (19)	35	65.1 ± 31.5	Mask-on time ≥ 4 h 70% nights	12.9 ± 3.5	106.9 ± 55.4 days	46	4.88 ± 1.97	4.88 ± 1.97
Rauscher et al. (82)	63	50.8 ± 2.9	Machine-on time ≥ 4 h per night	10.3 ± 0.3	18 ± 1 mo	71	4.9 ± 0.3	4.41
Engleman et al. (89)	54	36	Machine-on time	NR	1–3 mo	NR	4.7 ± 0.4	4.23
Reeves-Hoché et al. (83)	44	56.30	Mask-on time	8.72	6 mo	68	4.28 ± 1.03	4.28 ± 1.03
Fleury et al. (94)	20	64 ± 20	Machine-on time	11 ± 2	≥5 mo	78	6.7 ± 1.5	6.03
Meurice et al. (84)	44	52 ± 24	Machine-on time > 5 h and self-reported regular use all night q night	9.68 ± 2.68	14 mo	68	6.02 ± 2.48	5.42
Reeves-Hoché et al. (93)	62	NR	Machine-on time	NR	1 year	NR	5.0 ± 0.12	4.5
Pépin et al. (90)	193	53 ± 25	Machine-on time	11 ± 2	19 ± 17 mo	NR	6.5 ± 3	5.85
Lojander et al. (109)	21	NR	On CPAP/abandoned or refused CPAP	10	1 year	62	≥4	NR
Pieters et al. (78)	95	66 ± 23	Machine-on time	10 ± 2	784 days	74 > 4 h/day	5 ± 1.8	4.5
Krieger et al. (91)	575	74.0 ± 1.5	On CPAP/abandoned or refused CPAP	9.2 ± 0.1	1190 ± 38 days	85.5	5.3	5.1
Fleury et al. (95)	17	44.3 ± 21.2	Mask-on time	9.5 ± 1.6	820 ± 262 days	76	6.9 ± 1.3	6.9 ± 1.3
Engleman et al. (71)	215	47 ± 38	Machine-on time	NR	632 days	95	5.1 ± 2.5 (n = 62)	4.59
Weaver et al. (96)	32	66 ± 31.66	Mask-on time	NR	1 wk	53 used CPAP >90 nights	Consistent users: 6.21 ± 1.21 Intermittent users: 3.45 ± 1.94	Consistent users: 6.21 ± 1.21 Intermittent users: 3.45 ± 1.94

Lévy et al. (92)	547	59.8 ± 25.8	Machine-on time	NR	3 mo	6.6 <3 h/night	6.8	6.12
Likar et al. (85)	34	34	Machine-on time	12 ± 1	1,151 ± 75 days	NR	5.2	4.68
Chervin et al. (97)	33	49.4 ± 38.9	Machine-on time (29), mask-on time (4)	8.8 ± 3.7	40.8 ± 11.9 days	64 >6 h/night	6.0 ± 2.5	5.4
Engleman et al. (14)	16	11	Mask-on time	NR	4 wk	NR	3.2 ± 2.8	2.8 ± 2.4
Engleman et al. (50)	99	29	Self-report	NR	22 wk	NR	NR	NR
Kiely and McNicholas (33)	91	48 ± 22.2	Machine-on time	9.3 ± 2.5	178 ± 103 days	86	5.4 ± 2.4	4.86
Tiihonen and Fartinen (98)	10	NR	Machine-on time	8.3	56 days	NR	3.8	3.42
Jokic et al. (99)	10	99 ± 31	Machine-on time	12	2 wk	NR	6.6 ± 0.5 (2 wk) 6.5 ± 0.4 (4 wk)	5.94 (2 wk) 5.85 (4 wk)
Engleman et al. (100)	23	43 ± 37	Mask-on time	NR	4 wk	NR	3.2 ± 1.9	2.8 ± 2.0
Meslier et al. (29)	3,225	NR	Machine-on time	9.9 ± 2.4	78% > 1 yr 9% > 4 yr	73%	6.6 ± 2.25	5.94
Meurice et al. (101)	18	58.7 ± 21.7	Machine-on time	10.42 ± (eliminate airflow limitation—$n = 9$) 8.9 ± 2.6 (eliminate apneas, hypopneas, snoring—$n = 9$)	3 wk	NR	7.29 ± 0.95 6.01 ± 0.94	6.56 5.41
Konermann et al. (103)	23	38.3 ± 13.9	Mask-on time	8.1 ± 2.5	3–6 mo	NR	NR	5.6 ± 2.5
Pépin et al. (38)	114	>50	Mask-on time	8.7 ± 2.6	3 mo	74	5.72 ± 2[b] 4.95 ± 2.23	5.15 4.45
Yu et al. (104)	20	49.9 ± 27.7	Mask-on time	NR	1 wk	NR	NR	5.6 ± 1.1
Ballester et al. (17)	68	55 ± 2.7	Machine-on time	9.1 ± 2	3 mo	73	5.2 ± 2	4.68
Bennett et al. (105)	51	25	Mask-on time	NR	4 wk	NR	NR	5.0
McArdle et al. (86)	1103	31	Machine-on time	8	22 mo	76	5.6	5.04
D'Ambrosic et al. (31)	29	77 ± 9	Self-report	9.4 ± 0.7	8 wk	NR	6.0 ± 1.6	5.4
Jenkinson et al. (18)	52	NR	Machine-on time	9.0	4 wk	NR	5.4	4.86
Kingshott et al. (34)	62	62 ± 33	Mask-on time	NR	6 mo	NR	NR	4.8 ± 2.4
Findley et al. (24)	50	37 ± 3.8	Self-report	NR	2 yr	72	7.2 ± 0.3	6.48
Hack et al. (102)	26	NR	Machine-on time	NR	4 wk	NR	5.6	5.04
Hui et al. (30)	54	52 ± 3	Mask-on time	9.5 ± 0.2	12 wk	71 ± 4	NR	5.3 ± 0.2 (wk 4) 5.3 ± 0.3 (wk 12)

[a] For those studies reporting only machine-on time, mask-on time was calculated by subtracting 10% of the mean machine-on time, the difference suggested by the work of Kribbs et al. (19).

[b] Machine-on time in devices with and without capability to measure mask-on time.

NR = Not reported.

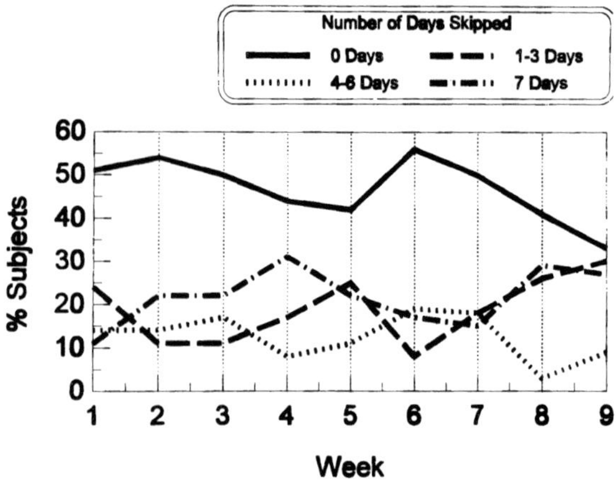

Figure 1 The percentage of subjects who skipped CPAP for varying numbers of days each week across the 9 weeks of treatment. (From Ref. 96.)

stopped using CPAP, all found that this occurred within the first 3 months of treatment (74–77,83,86,96). Kribbs and colleagues (19) and Engleman and associates (89) established that CPAP use during the first month of treatment predicted subsequent use. Reeves-Hoché and coworkers (83) showed a decrease in mean hourly use over the first 9 weeks of treatment, while Weaver and colleagues (96) documented that this decline occurred much earlier, during the first 14 days of CPAP use. Although these studies describe the relatively early deterioration of CPAP use, they examine the combined trends of consistent and intermittent users and, thus, fail to provide information regarding the temporal differences in the behavioral intention to use CPAP displayed by these two groups. To more clearly characterize that point in time when the pattern of nonuse was established, Weaver and coworkers (96) compared the pattern of CPAP use for the first 9 days of treatment of the consistent relative to the intermittent user. As clearly illustrated in Figure 2, although both types of users (88% consistent users and 67% intermittent users) apply CPAP for more than 6 hours on the first night of use, there is a sharp decline in nightly duration of CPAP use over the next 3 days of treatment with proportionately more inconsistent users skipping nights of treatment. By the fourth day of treatment, there were significantly reliable differences in duration of use (of those who used CPAP on a given night) between the two groups. These patterns of use also appeared to be very stable. With the exception of days 7 and 8 (when 40% or fewer intermittent users actually used CPAP), the significant differences between these two groups were sustained or approached significance over the remaining 5 days. This decline in CPAP use over the first week of treatment was subsequently confirmed by Rosenthal and associates (106), who documented a statistically meaningful decrease in mean hours of nightly use from 4.7 ± 2 on night 1 to 4.1 ± 3 on night 7. Thus, these

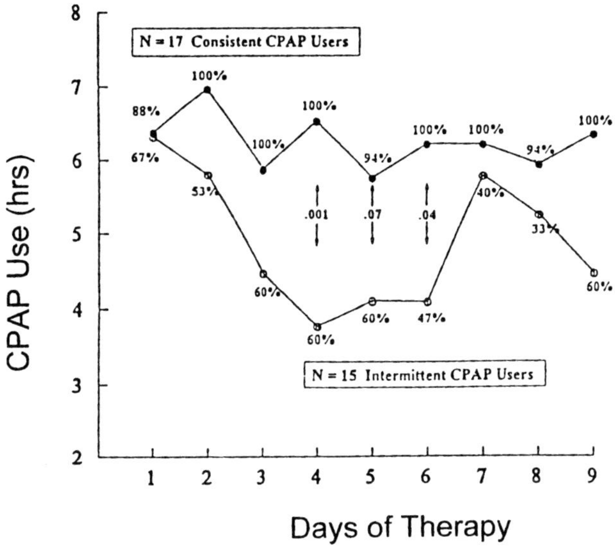

Figure 2 Mean hours of CPAP use for the first nine nights of treatment for two groups of subjects. Consistent users were those who used CPAP on 90% or more of nights during a 63-day period, while inconsistent users were those who used CPAP on 79% or fewer of the nights. The figure shows the percent of subjects in each group who used CPAP on a given day of therapy and the mean duration of that CPAP use only for that proportion of subjects who used CPAP that day. Probabilities indicating differences in mean nightly duration of CPAP use between the two groups are shown in the middle of the figure. (From Ref. 96.)

data suggest that nonadherence to treatment occurs very early and that to change this behavior intervention must occur, ideally, during the first week of therapy. The pattern of skipped days and decreased nocturnal hourly use displayed by the intermittent user group places them at high risk for the return of OSA symptoms. It is speculated that the immediate reappearance of symptoms that has been documented with even one night of nonuse could reinforce the patient's potential perception that this treatment is ineffective, further promoting nonadherence. However, for those who are able to use CPAP treatment for at least 3 months, long-term use is likely (86). The stability of long-term use has been documented by several studies, with 62–97% remaining on CPAP treatment greater than 1 year (78,83,84,86,88,91,94,95, 107–110).

Whether adherence to treatment is affected, either positively or negatively, by modalities such as bi-level pressure or auto-titration devices has received only limited consideration. Reeves-Hoché and associates (93) tested the postulate that the reduction in expiratory pressure that occurs with bi-level pressure devices would promote adherence to CPAP. This group of researchers found no significant differences in nightly hourly use or percent of mask-on time in subjects randomly assigned to either bi-level or continuous pressure devices. Mean duration of machine on time

Table 2 Studies of Variables Associated with CPAP Adherence

			Demographics			CPAP side effects						Pretreatment objective disease severity					
Study	Avg. time on CPAP	Metric of adherence	Age	Gender	Education	Noise	Mask discomfort	Rhinitis/ mucosal drying	Eye problems	Air swallowing	Claustrophobia	RDI	BMI	SaO_2	MSLT	CPAP pressure (cmH_2O)	EDS
Nino-Murcia et al. (73)	~11 mo	Record of being on CPAP	N	N	Y*							N	Y*	Y*		N	
Waldhorn et al. (74)	14.5 ± 10.7 mo	Record of being on CPAP	N	N		N	N	N	N	N		N		N		N	Y*
Fletcher and Luckett (118)	~6 mo	Machine-on time					No differences in overall side effects					N					N
Rolfe et al. (75)	~18.2 mo	Record of being on CPAP	N	N								N		Y*			Y*
Hoffstein et al. (76)	17 ± 11 mo	Persistent use	N				No differences in overall side effects				N	N	Y*	N		N	
Engleman et al. (71)	≥2 wk	Self-reported use				Y*	Y*					N		N			
Krieger (77)	29.13 ± 1.6 mo	Machine-on time	N									Y*	N	Y*		N	
Rauscher et al. (82)	18 ± 1 mo	> 4 hr: adherent < 1.5 hr. nonadherent					No differences in overall side effects					Y*	N	Y*		N	
Kribbs et al. (19)	1 mo	>4 h mask-on time 70% nights	N		Y*		No differences in overall side effects				Y*	N	N	N	N	N	Y*
Reeves-Hoché et al. (83)	6 mo	Machine-on time	N	N	N							Y*	N				N
Edinger et al. (107)	6 mo	Self-reported use	N									N	Y	N			Y*

Meurice et al. (84)	14 mo	Machine-on time > 5 h/night & self-reported use q night		N				No differences in overall side effects			Y*					
Engleman et al. (89)	1–3 mo	Machine-on time				Y*		Overall side effects			N	N		N		
Pépin et al. (90)	~19 mo	Machine-on time						No differences in overall side effects			N	N		N		
Reeves-Hoché et al. (93)	1 yr	Machine-on time									Y*					
Pieters et al. (78)	~26 mo	Machine-on time	Y								N					
Krieger et al. (91)	1,190 ± 38 days	Machine-on time	Y*								Y*	Y*		Y*	Y*	
Strollo et al. (111)	4–6 wk	Machine-on time									N				N	N
Engleman et al. (14)	4 wk	Machine-on time									Y*		N	N		N
Rosenthal et al. (106)	1 wk	Mask-on time									N	N	N	N		N
Weaver et al. (96)	1 mo	Mask-on time	N	N	N	N	Y* for users	N	N	N	N	N	N	N	N	N
McArdle et al. (86)	22 mo	Machine-on time	Y*	Y*							Y*	Y*			Y*	Y*
Janson et al. (117)	3 mo–10 yr	Persistent use	Y*	N								Y*	Y*		Y*	Y*
Sanders et al. (120)	1–2 mo	Machine-on time	N								N		N			N

[a] Nonadherent patients had greater subjective daytime sleepiness.

* $p \leq 0.05$ for either analysis of differences in CPAP use between adherent and nonadherent users or correlation between variable and CPAP use.

was 5.0 ± 0.19 (SEM) for CPAP and 4.9 ± 0.23 (SEM) for bi-level therapy. However, the dropout rate was significantly higher for those using CPAP compared to the bi-level group. The authors suggested that perhaps bi-level pressure should be recommended to those intolerant of conventional CPAP devices.

One reason for the development of auto-titrating (auto-CPAP) or ''intelligent'' CPAP devices was to provide a method for home titration and promote adherence by reducing the potentially intolerable mean pressure associated with CPAP therapy during nonapneic portions of the night. However, the premise that the level of pressure is a deterrent to CPAP use has not been supported (see Table 2) (19,73,74, 76,77,96,111). Documented nightly use on auto-CPAP devices is comparable to values reported for CPAP, ranging from 4.9 to 6.5 h (103,112–116). Patients have also experienced similar outcomes with regard to daytime sleepiness and side effects compared with traditional CPAP (112). A few studies indicate better patient acceptance of the auto-CPAP compared to conventional CPAP (103,115,116). For example, Teschler and coworkers (115) showed that although the difference in use between auto-CPAP and conventional CPAP was only 0.2 ± 0.4 h, after 3 months of using an auto-titrating device, all of the 20 subjects reported continued use compared to a 10% yearly dropout rate of their historical controls. Randomly assigning 16 subjects to either auto-CPAP or conventional CPAP, after 3 weeks of use Meurice and fellow investigators (116) reported significant differences in mask-on time, the auto-CPAP group using the device for a slightly longer duration (7.1 ± 1.0 h vs. 5.7 ± 1.1 h). Although Konermann and associates (103) found no difference in nightly duration of use in randomly assigned patients to either traditional CPAP or auto-CPAP, those patients assigned to auto-CPAP used their device more days per week. Whether these technological advances will have the intended impact on adherence will continue to require examination.

C. Why Do Patients Abandon CPAP Treatment?

The realization that approximately half of treated sleep apnea patients are nonadherent to treatment has fostered considerable speculation regarding the cause. Displayed in Table 2 are potential operating factors that have been explored in the literature, including demographic characteristics, objective and subjective disease severity, claustrophobic tendencies, and problems with the technological interface. Only a few studies have documented the impact of age (78,86,91,117) and education (19,73) on adherence to CPAP. Although it seems logical that severity of illness would dictate level of adherence, no singular physiological parameter has consistently emerged from the literature as being the predictive factor. Of the physiological correlates that have been examined (see Table 2), respiratory disturbance index (RDI) has naturally received the greatest attention (14,19,71,73–78,82–84,86,89–91,93,96,106,107,111,117–120). Several studies have found significant, but low, correlations between RDI and level of adherence (77,83,84,91,93), and others have found it to be a discriminating factor (14,82,86). However, as shown in Table 2, the majority of studies have not supported this relationship (71,73–76,78,89,90,96, 106,107,111,118,120). Additional physiological characteristics that have also received considerable exploration include body mass index (BMI) (19,73,76,82,83,86, 89–91,96,106,107,117), nocturnal Sa_{O_2} (14,19,71,73–76,82,96,106,117,119), and multiple sleep latency test (MSLT) (14,19,89–91,96,106). As with RDI, only a small portion of the studies reviewed found BMI (73,76,91,107,117) or nocturnal Sa_{O_2} (73,75,77,82,117,119) to be factors influencing CPAP use. Also noteworthy is the lack of evidence indicating pretreatment physiological sleepiness, as measured by the MSLT, as a key factor affecting adherence (14,19,89,90,96,106), with more data implicating pretreatment subjective daytime sleepiness (19,74,75, 86,107,117).

Problems with the technological interface associated with CPAP use predominate as reasons frequently cited for nonadherence (19,71,72,74,76,78,82–84,89,90,117,118,121). As would be expected, mask discomfort is the most frequently reported side effect associated with CPAP use, with an average reported occurrence across studies of 37% (see Table 3) (19,72–74,76,79,82,93,109,117,121). Engleman and associates (71) characterized the problems associated with CPAP use as clustering into three components: nuisance factors (frequent awakening, noise, sore eyes), mask problems (leaking mask, mask rubbing), and side effects (dry throat, nasal stuffiness). Subjectively reported CPAP use declined with the increased presence of nuisance factors, but use was greater in those with mask-related problems. Weaver and colleagues (96) also noted that those reporting mask problems had significantly higher use. They concluded that those who used CPAP more often would most likely experience this side effect. Kribbs and coworkers (19) found that retrospectively nonadherent patients reported significantly more claustrophobic tendencies. It is unclear whether claustrophobia contributes to nonadherence or whether the failure to use the therapy is attributed to claustrophobia when, in actuality, no causal relationship exists. Moreover, Massie and colleagues (122) reported significantly greater CPAP use and decreased incidence of dry mouth or throat and dry nose with the use of heated humidification compared to cold or no humidification.

Other self-reported side effects (Table 2) have not been found to distinguish those who do and those who do not embrace CPAP as a treatment (19,74,76, 82,84,90,96,118). Indeed, of the studies that have examined the contribution of CPAP side effects to adherence (19,71,74,76,82,84,89,90,96,118), only the work by the Edinburgh group (71,89) produced evidence supporting the role of these factors in deterring CPAP use.

Several investigators have attempted to characterize who might be at risk for abandoning CPAP therapy by examining potential predictors of CPAP use (78,86,91,93,107,118,120). When Fletcher and Luckett (118) explored the relationship between hourly CPAP use and level of baseline symptoms, perceived improvement, perceived side effects, apnea index, mean desaturation level, mean apnea duration, and CPAP pressure, no significant associations were found. Moreover, the outcome of regression analysis also failed to produce related variables that collectively correlated with nightly CPAP duration. However, baseline symptoms were

Table 3 Percentage of Reported CPAP Side Effects

Study	N	Mask discomfort	Nasal/ throat dryness	Sinus congestion or rhinorrhea	Skin irritation	Noise of machine	Chest discomfort	Air swallowing	Pressure sensation nasopharynx	Eye irritation	Headache	Intimacy	Claustrophobia	Sleep poorly
Sanders et al. (72)	20	74	68	10	NR	25	10	NR	NR	NR	NR	NR	NR	NR
Nino-Murcia et al. (73)	90	6	52	14	NR	NR	NR	NR	NR	30	16	NR	NR	NR
Waldhorn et al. (74)	96	54	36	40	20	15	8	7	NR	18	NR	NR	NR	NR
Hoffstein et al. (76)	96	65	44	16	38	47	4	24	NR	1	NR	1	10	NR
Kribbs et al. (19)	35	28.1	<25	46.9	<25	<25	<25	NR	NR	<25	<25	31.3	28.1	32.2
Rauscher et al. (82)	63	48	30	29	NR	NR	3	NR	NR	21	0	NR	NR	6
McEvoy et al. (79)	7	28.6	14.3	28.6	NR	14.3	NR	NR	NR	NR	NR	NR	NR	NR
Engleman et al. (89)	32	NR	6	28	NR	NR	NR	NR	16	NR	NR	NR	NR	NR
Meurice et al. (84)	44	NR	NR	14	52	20	14	NR	NR	NR	NR	NR	NR	NR
Meecham Jones et al. (121)	66	53	NR	NR	NR	NR	NR	NR	NR	NR	NR	NR	NR	NR
Reeves-Hoché et al. (93)	62	24	32	5	NR	NR	NR	NR	NR	NR	NR	2	0	NR
Lojander et al. (109)	13	15	15	54	NR	8	NR	NR	NR	NR	NR	NR	NR	NR
Fleury et al. (95)	17	NR	35.29	35.29	11.76	NR	NR	NR	NR	NR	NR	NR	NR	NR
Engleman et al. (71)	253	NR	62	64	41	41	21	37	NR	31	NR	NR	NR	32
Levy et al. (92)	547	NR	50	40	NR	NR	NR	NR	NR	NR	NR	NR	NR	NR
Meslier et al. (29)	3,225	NR	52.2	26	NR	47	NR	NR	NR	28	NR	NR	NR	NR
Janson et al. (117)	40	7.5	NR	35	NR	12.5	NR	NR	NR	NR	NR	NR	20	NR

NR = Not reported.

strongly related to perceived improvement. Sanders and coworkers (120) also found no association between polysomnographic variables or changes in these variables with treatment and nightly duration of CPAP use. Interestingly, in addition to BMI, Edinger and investigators (107) found that those nonadherent to treatment had higher pretreatment affect, poorer subjective sleep quality, and more daytime sleepiness compared to adherent patients. They speculated that these attributes might indicate the greater negativism that is the basis of their nonacceptance of this treatment. Reeves-Hoche and colleagues (93) found that of the demographic variables explored, BMI was associated with bi-level use, but not CPAP use, age predicted CPAP, but not bi-level use, and there was no relationship between gender and hours of use on either device. Pieters and associates (78) also found that age, in addition to movement arousal index, mean non-REM sleep Sa_{O_2}, contributed to the prediction model, with age and mean non-REM sleep Sa_{O_2} being inversely associated with CPAP adherence. Examining the records of 1103 CPAP users using a model of proportional hazard, McArdle and coworkers (86) identified that an Epworth Sleepiness Scale score > 10, RDI ≥ 15, and snoring history were predictors of long-term CPAP use. The failure of these and other studies (77,84,86,106,118) to isolate similar factors operative in CPAP use after adherence patterns have been established for some time suggests that factors influencing CPAP adherence occur very early or prior to treatment. Rosenthal and colleagues (106) seeking to isolate predictors of CPAP use during the first week of treatment were unable to associate CPAP use with any indicators of disease severity. They offered the possibility that ''personality characteristics'' might be the pretreatment factors instrumental in determining CPAP adherence.

Inadequate titration could also conceivably account for the early decline in use for some patients. Incomplete resolution of symptoms could certainly discourage continued use. The growing use of split-night studies calls into question the adequacy of titration conducted under these circumstances and its contribution to nonadherence. In a survey of pulmonologists, 19% reported that their laboratories routinely performed split-night studies (123). Iber and coworkers (124) documented that an adequate CPAP prescription was produced in 78% of the split-night studies. In several studies, Yamashiro and Kryger (125), Strollo and colleagues (111), and Sanders and associates (120) showed that prescribed pressure levels obtained during split-night studies are not statistically different from those generated during full-night studies. However, differences in CPAP pressure were noted in patients with mild OSA (RDI < 20) and when the duration of CPAP titration was less than 3 h (125). As the current emphasis in the literature has been the adequacy of a split-night protocol for CPAP titration, only a few studies have examined the impact of split-night studies on level of adherence. The issue of CPAP adherence relative to titration during split-night studies was first addressed by Fleury and colleagues (94). After the reduction in RDI in 87% ($n = 31$) of the subjects to less than 10 per hour of sleep in all sleep stages following a split-night study, CPAP was accepted by 78% of the patients. Strollo and associates (111) had a slightly lower acceptance rate of 62–67%, but this percentage rose to 86% when the study was replicated by the authors employing a larger sample (120). The adherence rates reported by these studies are comparable to those found with full-night studies (72–77,81). Continued pursuit of this issue is required before concerns regarding the adequacy of titration relative to split-night protocols can be fully eradicated.

In summary, there appears to be no clear causative element that can account for the rejection of CPAP by almost half of patients initially accepting therapy (13,41). The apparent lack of consensus as to why CPAP is abandoned is due to a number of problems in the extant literature. For example, there is no consistent definition of adherence to treatment, making comparisons of study results difficult. Many of the studies did not objectively monitor CPAP use, and most solicited predictors after CPAP use, often many months following the establishment of patterns of adherence or nonadherence. Few studies had theoretical or hypothesis-driven protocols, and most relied on a post hoc statistical evaluation. The conceptual underpinning that motivated many of the studies and directed the selection of variables for analysis was not clearly evident. This issue will remain unresolved until prospective investigations concurrently explore the relative contributions of split-night studies, physiological factors, adequacy of titration and technological interface, and patient personality factors and perception in determining adherence to CPAP treatment.

III. Interventions to Promote Adherence to CPAP Therapy

Potential strategies to promote CPAP use that have been explored have primarily employed the behavioral principles of positive reinforcement and patient education (80,85,87,97,110,118,126). For example, using weekly and then monthly telephone calls that addressed OSA severity, potential complications of apnea, benefits of CPAP, and suggestions as to how to handle side effects, the study by Fletcher and Luckett (118) was the first to evaluate the role of continued reinforcement on nightly adherence. In this randomized cross-over study in which the control group were also called monthly to report meter readings, side effects, and benefits of treatment, no significant differences were found between the two groups in nightly CPAP duration, perceived improvement, or perceived side effects during reinforced and nonreinforced periods. The limited statistical power produced by the small sample size in this study could account for these findings. However, telephone calls also made little difference when Leon and colleagues (110) compared the percentage of adherent users in similar, but not statistically matched, intervention and control groups after 3 months of treatment. Intuitively, patient education would be expected to contribute to patient use of CPAP. A few studies have examined the contribution of education and acclimatization to CPAP to the promotion of adherence to treatment. A retrospective study of the effects of education on CPAP use compared objectively recorded hours of machine-on time prior to and after participation in regularly scheduled group education sessions conducted every 6 months (85). During these sessions, conducted by a pulmonary nurse practitioner, patients evaluated their duration of CPAP use, symptoms, and equipment function, CPAP meter readings were obtained, and a treatment plan was initiated for any reported problems.

Reminders were sent to encourage attendance. After the first session, there was a statistically significant increase in CPAP of 21% that was sustained for as long as 3 years. Interestingly, before attending the education sessions, those treated with supplemental oxygen had higher initial use compared to those not using oxygen. However, these results could be attributed to having more severe and potentially more symptomatic disease, as indicated by the need for oxygen, and receiving oxygen therapy could have emphasized to those patients the seriousness of OSA as an illness and thus the need for treatment. However, these subjects also received additional education through their participation in an oxygen clinic prior to the CPAP clinic. In this study, neither nadir oxygen saturation during polysomnography, nasal pillows, patients' subjective sleepiness, nor preclinic CPAP use predicted postclinic nightly CPAP duration. There were also no significant differences in age, number of visits to their physicians, or attendance at the CPAP clinic between adherent and nonadherent patients.

Applying a combination of positive reinforcement and education, Oliver and associates (126) examined the efficacy of teaching adaptation skills to both patients and their spouse prior to treatment followed by telephone calls at 2 and 6 weeks and home visits at 4 weeks in a randomized control study. Adherence was not significantly enhanced in the intervention group, although perception of well-being was improved. Hui and colleagues (80) also found that additional education, telephone support, and early review of CPAP use did not produce a statistically significant difference compared with routine management, although quality of life was enhanced in the randomized intervention group. However, Hoy and coworkers (87) produced a positive impact on adherence using a combination of intensive support and education. After one month of the intervention, consisting of home CPAP education that included the spouse, 3 nights of CPAP titration in the laboratory, and multiple home visits over 4 months in addition to usual treatment, the randomized intervention group had significantly higher nightly objectively monitored CPAP use compared to those in the other group who received usual treatment. Interestingly, adherence to CPAP was higher in those self-referred compared to referrals initiated by the partner.

It is unclear from studies applying multiple interventions, such as patient education and positive reinforcement, which of these approaches produced the desired positive behavioral response. Indeed, in addition to the independent variable, uncontrolled aspects of the protocol employed by some studies also could potentially produce changes in behavioral response. For example, Likar and colleagues (85) demonstrated a significant increase in CPAP use with group education sessions. The thrust of this research was the effect of education on CPAP use, but the effect of this intervention was confounded by the potential influence of the positive reinforcement produced by subject estimation of nightly use and the reading of CPAP time meters, as well as the problem solving and psychological support generated by patient support groups.

In a recent study, Chervin and associates (97) made a substantial contribution by attempting to determine the relative merit of positive reinforcement versus patient education on promoting CPAP adherence. Weekly telephone calls inquiring about problems with CPAP and providing encouragement were used to provide positive reinforcement, and literature that discussed sleep apnea, good sleep habits, and information on use, benefits, and potential side effects of CPAP provided the educational content. Neither of these behavioral strategies produced strong statistically reliable differences compared to a control group. Literature yielded the greatest benefit with subjects applying CPAP 2.7 h longer than the control group. New CPAP patients, subjects with lower levels of education, and those who had a relative who also used CPAP benefited most by the intervention. The failure of this study to clearly identify either positive reinforcement or literature, a proxy for patient education, as the key component that affects CPAP use after other studies have employed them successfully in combination with other techniques, seems to suggest that either multiple interventions must be applied concurrently to produce results or that the cause of nonadherence is not addressed by either of these techniques. Indeed, there has been little exploration of factors that have been postulated to influence volitional behavior, i.e., perception of social and peer expectations, attitude toward treatment, and self-efficacy (127). Testing potential interventions to promote CPAP adherence without the benefit of a well-articulated predictive model has little chance of success as witnessed by the conflicting results of the strategies previously evaluated. The reliance on retrospective analyses applied in most of this research underscores the lack of clearly identified variables to drive the study. Of the few studies that have attempted interventions to improve adherence, the majority have used some form of reinforcement, a strategy that is resource consuming and difficult to sustain. Applying similar methodologies, the mixed results produced by these studies suggest that assumptions, rather than empirical evidence regarding the cause of nonadherence, were used as their foundation. Thus, it appears as though intervention studies are premature until reliable predictors of CPAP nonadherence are developed, since it is apparent from studies to date that assumptions about certain determinants of CPAP adherence (e.g., side effects) have not proved valid.

IV. Impact of CPAP on Functional Status

The keystone of outcomes management is functional status and quality of life (128). As a component of quality of life, functional status assesses those activities performed routinely in meeting basic needs and fulfilling roles (129). One aspect of daily life that has received considerable attention in the sleep apnea literature is driving performance.

A. Driving Performance

The intrusive nature of daytime sleepiness on driving performance has been recognized by 12% of the general population and 24% of middle-aged individuals (age 35–64 years) reporting that this happens some or all of the time (130). However, in OSA, because of the pervasiveness of associated daytime hypersomnolence, driving is particularly hazardous. Indeed, there is emerging literature reporting increased accidents (4,24,51,53,54,57,59,62,71,131–133) and impaired vigilance on driving simulator tests (12,23,55,102,134,135) in this population. Findley and coworkers (51) reported that the automobile accident rate of OSA patients was almost three times that of other drivers, and Haraldsson and colleagues (133) reported that 52% of OSA patients versus 30% of controls reported that they had been involved in a car accident, taking into account risk exposure. Similar results were documented by Barbé and associates (132) who reported that the accident rate for the prior 3 years was higher (33%) for OSA patients compared to age- and gender-matched controls (18%). After adjusting for kilometers driven, those with OSA had an almost threefold risk of having one or more accidents. Indeed, in a large study comparing the driving records of control subjects with patients who have sleep apnea, George and Smiley (57) found that 5 years preceding diagnosis, OSA patients had significantly more accidents compared with the controls. The accident rate was similar for all age groups. In two studies, one involving clinic patients (131) and the other commercial truck drivers (62), those with sleep-disordered breathing (SDB) had twice as many automobile accidents than those without, although this increased incidence in commercial drivers was not significant. In studies that have controlled for factors that could also affect driving performance, such as alcohol and coffee intake, daytime nap, visual-refraction disorders, years of driving, distance of driving, work/sleep schedules, and pertinent medical illnesses, OSA patients are still more likely to experience a motor vehicle accident (53,59). Near accidents were reported by 66% of 181 men with OSA in a study by Aldrich (136), but the frequency of accidents was not significantly different than that of controls.

In a large population-based study, Young and colleagues (54) reviewed the driving records of three groups: habitual snorers (RDI < 5), OSA patients with an RDI 5–15, and OSA patients with an RDI > 15. In this study, male subjects, but not females, having sleep-disordered breathing increased the chance of having at least one accident threefold in a 5-year period, regardless of level of OSA severity. An RDI > 15 for men and women combined increased the likelihood of having multiple crashes at seven times the rate of those without EDS. These results were independent of age and average miles driven per year, with alcohol use, BMI, and education eliminated as confounders in the study. George and Smiley (57) also discovered that the increased risk of accidents was associated with more severe OSA (RDI > 40). In a case-control study, Teran-Santos and coworkers (59) found that cases (those with OSA receiving emergency treatment for a vehicular accident) with an RDI ≥ 5 were 11 times more likely (adjusted for alcohol use, visual-refraction disorders, BMI, years and distance driving, medications causing drowsiness, work and sleep schedule, hypertension) to have a traffic accident than controls (accident-free patients randomly selected from three primary health care centers); for those with an RDI ≥ 15, the odds ratio was 8.1. However, Barbé and colleagues (132) did not find an association between the number of accidents experienced by OSA patients and referred daytime sleepiness, mood, or disease severity. In addition to this study, several other studies also failed to relate daytime sleepiness to accident rate (54,59,136). However, in commercial truck drivers those complaining of subjective daytime sleepiness did have significantly more self-reported accidents (62). In this study, being obese (BMI $\geq$ 30), reporting excessive daytime sleepiness (EDS), and having sleep-disordered breathing produced a sensitivity of 76% and specificity of 35% in identifying drivers with accidents.

Attempting to characterize the contribution of vigilance to driving performance, several studies have tested reaction time and level of concentration using computerized sustained and divided attention driving tasks (55,134,135,137). There is evidence that suggests that performance on such tasks is significantly more impaired than normal controls (55,134,135,137) and similar to those impaired by alcohol (134). For example, Findley and colleagues (55,137) found that on two different devices used to assess driving performance, a driving film simulator consisting of a film projector, simulator car, and driving analyzer (137) and Steer Clear, a computerized sustained attention task (55), sleep apnea subjects did significantly worse than control subjects similar in age and sex. Moreover, performance on Steer Clear was significantly related to automobile accidents in those with sleep apnea. Using a divided attention driving task that incorporates the key components of driving, tracking and visual search, George and collaborators (134,135) found that OSA subjects had significantly more problems performing these functions compared to age-matched controls. These differences were independent of trial number or time of day.

Studies that have sought to link indicators of sleep apnea and performance on driving-related sustained or divided attention tasks have found little empirical evidence for the role of respiratory disturbances (134,135,138), severity of oxygen desaturation (138), habitual snoring (138), or subjective sleepiness (138). However, Findley and coworkers (55) found a relationship between percentage of obstacles hit on Steer Clear and level of OSA severity (mild, moderate, severe) based on degree of oxygen desaturation. In addition to modest support for the role of objective sleepiness (MSLT) (134,135), data also suggest that level of education, somnolence while driving, and cognitive impairment, as determined by performance on standard neuropsychological testing, are also significantly related to performance on driving-related attention tasks (62). The dearth of data associating RDI and subjectively and objectively measured daytime hypersomnolence in well-controlled situations makes the prospective identification of mechanisms for the increased driving accidents in this population even more enigmatic.

Improvements in self-reported driving, accident rates, and performance on computerized sustained attention driving tasks following CPAP use have been documented by several studies (23,24,52,61,71,92,96,102). Although Kribbs and colleagues (19) found that duration of nightly CPAP use did not influence the number of times patients reported that they fell asleep while driving, when these data were analyzed using frequency of nightly CPAP use (96), consistent users reported significantly fewer of these incidents than intermittent users. Engleman and associates (71) reported a reduction in sleep-related near-miss accidents from 39% to 5% after CPAP treatment and documented a significant reduction in mileage- and time-on

CPAP-adjusted incident rates for near-miss accidents. Patients reported significantly less "dozing-off" or "severe fatigue" while driving after 1 year of CPAP treatment (52). Following CPAP use, others have also observed a decline in driving accidents (24,52,61,92) in addition to reductions in home- and work-related incidents (61). These positive results must be interpreted with caution in light of the fact that the majority of these studies were based on self-report of accidents, with few studies employing a comparison group, or controlling for other variables that might also affect driving performance. The magnitude of improvement in driving-related performance after CPAP treatment may actually be greater than current reports indicate because of underreporting by patients of pretreatment driving impairment. One quarter of those who denied having difficulty with driving before treatment altered this perception, admitting problems with driving after receiving CPAP treatment (50). The legal implications associated with the disclosure of driving accidents may also affect the veracity of self-report data.

Only a few studies have provided objective evidence of the impact of CPAP on driving behaviors. Comparing the performance on Steer Clear of OSA subjects randomly treated for 4 weeks with a placebo versus CPAP, Engleman and coworkers (12) found significant differences in the number of obstacles hit in this cross-over study. Using actual driving records, Findley and colleagues (24) demonstrated in a small study a significant reduction in accident rates (2 years prediagnosis compared to 2-years postdiagnosis) in treated compared to untreated OSA patients. Although there was no change in the accident rate of the untreated group, those who used CPAP regularly had no documented traffic accidents following treatment. There were no significant differences in RDI, weight, age, or gender between these two groups. George and colleagues (23) showed improved tracking and correct responses in OSA subjects following CPAP treatment, while little change occurred in the age-matched control subjects. The reduction in tracking error was significantly related to decreased objectively measured daytime sleepiness. Compelling data were generated by Hack and associates (102), who compared performance on a driving sustained-attention task of treated patients compared to those receiving subtherapeutic CPAP (0.5–1.0 cm H_2O). In this randomized controlled trial, the treated group demonstrated significant improvement in assessments of steering performance and response to target stimuli. The decline in performance over the 30-min task that was evident pretreatment in both groups was abolished only in the treatment group, as indicated by improved ability to stay on the road and fewer off-road events. Thus, there is growing evidence that CPAP treatment alters behaviors associated with driving in patients with OSA.

B. Other Areas of Daily Functioning

In addition to driving, current research suggests that OSA affects a wide range of daily behaviors (12,18,25,29–32,63,65–68,71,96,100,139–142). Several studies have documented the negative impact of OSA on work performance (68,139), specifically difficulty with concentrating on new tasks, learning new tasks, and performing monotonous tasks (68), and on work absenteeism (139). Indeed, taking advantage of a large dataset, Grunstein and colleagues (139) noted that women with a high likelihood of having sleep apnea with perceived EDS were almost 15 times as likely to experience problems with work performance. For both genders, those with a high likelihood of OSA and EDS used, on average, 5 weeks more sick leave than those with a low likelihood of OSA and had lower pretax income. These subjects also had lower self-rated general health, more often sought psychiatric consultations, and were more likely to have experienced divorce twice. Daytime hypersomnolence was the most predictive and significantly reliable variable for increased sick leave, impaired general health, and suboptimal work performance witnessed in this sample.

Although the association between EDS and work-related accidents has been suggested (143), aside from the few studies of commercial truck drivers and the study of self-reported accidents by Krieger and associates (61) there is little empirical evidence regarding the contribution of OSA-related accidents at the work place and in the home. Consequently, there is also a dearth of information concerning the economic sacrifice, both by employer and employee, for impaired job performance and OSA-related accidents. We also have no insight into the intangible losses associated with these incidents that may be additionally experienced by patients.

Several standardized generic measures of functional status, such as the SF36 (144), Sickness Impact Profile Scale (SIP) (145), Functional Limitations Profile (32), and Nottingham Health Profile (NHP) (146), have been employed to describe the affect of sleep apnea on a variety of functional areas. Gall and colleagues (63) used a battery of generic functional status instruments and measures of psychosocial function to characterize the limitations to daily functioning imposed by OSA. These investigators compared mild OSA patients with subjects who did not differ in age or body mass, did not complain of EDS, and had a negative polysomnogram. Findings from this study indicated that even mild sleep apnea patients suffer significant difficulties with alertness, recreation, work, social functioning, and lowered sense of well-being. They were functionally more limited for physical and emotional reasons, reporting difficulties with family relationships in addition to illness-related problems in domestic, vocational, and social milieus. Indeed, it has been shown that scores of OSA patients for the physical and mental components of the SF36 are in the lowest 29% and 32%, respectively, of scores for the general population (32). In a large survey, Meslier and colleagues (29) not only found that OSA patients had difficulty with multiple daily behaviors, they also discovered that older patients (>60 years) were more impaired than younger patients.

Using the NHP to compare functional status across levels of OSA severity (RDI < 20, 20–50, >50), Fornas and colleagues (67) explored differences in functional status between OSA patients and normal control subjects. As reported by others (31,63), OSA subjects experienced significantly lower energy and had more emotional reactions and problems with sleep, social, and physical functioning than the normal controls. Interestingly, although subjects reported a broad spectrum of functional limitations, the degree of disease severity did not seem to make a difference. Bolitschek and associates (30) also showed that the physical condition, psyche, social life and everyday functioning of untreated patients were significantly impaired in these functional areas compared to treated patients and controls.

While employing generic functional status instruments in the assessment of functional status is advantageous because a broad spectrum of tasks and roles within a variety of domains are surveyed, such measures can restrict the depth of assessment in those areas most affected by the disorder under consideration (147). Consequently, variability in functional status scores achievable across a range of illness severity may be restricted and inaccurately characterize the degree of functional limitation (148). Therefore, although valuable for cross-illness and heterogeneous comparisons, they may not be as useful as the disease-specific functional status instrument in probing those behaviors most likely to be affected. Recently, two disease-specific instruments specifically designed for sleep disorders have been developed (66,140). Developed by Weaver and colleagues (66), the Functional Outcomes of Sleep Questionnaire (FOSQ) has considerable psychometric properties including concurrent validity with the SIP and SF36, test-retest reliability, and discriminant validity. Five domains (subscales)—activity level, vigilance, intimacy and sexual relationships, general productivity, and social outcome—were identified by a factor analysis of responses on the FOSQ. Weaver and associates (65,66) used the FOSQ to compare the functional status of OSA patients with a normal cohort screened for the likelihood of having sleep apnea using the validated Multivariable Apnea Index (MAP) (149). Functionally, the sleep apnea subjects experienced more limitation in their daily endeavors as indicated by significantly reliable differences in the total FOSQ score between these two groups. They also demonstrated significantly greater impairment in all of the FOSQ subscale domains indicating that sleep apnea affects a broad array of routine behaviors. The Calgary Sleep Apnea Quality of Life Index (SAQLI), developed by Flemons and Reimer (140), is a 35-item questionnaire organized into four domains: daily functioning, social interactions, emotional functioning, and symptoms, with a fifth domain, treatment-related symptoms, applicable following the initiation of treatment. This questionnaire also possesses the psychometric properties of content validity, internal consistency, and pretreatment concurrent validity with the SF36. This team has shown differences among levels of disease severity in areas that hold importance for patients and are frequently problematic.

There is meager and inconsistent empirical evidence associating specific factors with self-reported functional status in OSA. Weaver and colleagues (65) noted that neither BMI, age, nor MSLT were related to functional status as measured by the FOSQ. However, it was significantly related to Epworth Sleepiness Scale scores for both normal and sleep apnea subjects, indicating that self-reported daytime sleepiness, more so than obesity and age, may contribute to the functional impairments associated with sleep apnea. Using a generic measure of functional status, the work of Bolitschek and associates (30) indicated that among demographic variables, marital status was the only significant factor influencing satisfaction with quality of life, although these data were derived from a small sample. Bennett and coworkers (105) reported that limitations in role performance due to physical problems were weakly associated with RDI and indices of sleep fragmentation and were also weakly related to the physical summary score. The independent relationship between sleep fragmentation and physical functioning remained even after controlling for the confounding variables of BMI and FEV_1. Surprisingly, neither the RDI nor sleep fragmentation were associated with the domain expected to be most impaired by OSA, energy and vitality. However, energy and vitality, physical role limitation, and the physical and mental summary scores were moderately related to both objective and subjective sleepiness. Kingshott and associates (34) found that change in scores on the SF36 following CPAP treatment were significantly related to objective sleepiness and oxygen desaturation. There was no statistically reliable association between daily functioning and either sleep fragmentation or RDI.

C. Changes in Daily Functioning After CPAP Treatment

Self-report data seem to suggest that problems with work performance, as well as general health and work absenteeism, respond to CPAP treatment (71). In response to a mailed survey after CPAP use, 68% of the sample ($n = 204$) indicated significant improvement in concentration, 66% reported significantly enhanced work efficiency, and 32% had a significant reduction in time taken off from work. Moreover, 61% of these patients also reported improvement in general health with CPAP treatment. The extent of improvement in daytime functioning was related to greater CPAP use as well as higher levels of pretreatment EDS and decline in EDS after treatment.

In seminal work, the Edinburgh group (12,15) found significantly greater improvements in self-rating of social life, sex life, and ability to perform household tasks on the NHP in those treated with CPAP compared to placebo. In a retrospective study, Bolitschek and colleagues (30) reported that after 3 months of treatment, the daily functioning of treated patients did not differ from normal controls. Using the NHP, Ballester and colleagues (17) also demonstrated greater gains with CPAP treatment compared to those randomly assigned to receive conservative therapy. These findings have been replicated in other randomized controlled studies using the SF36 (13,16,18). For example, treatment with CPAP compared to subtherapeutic pressure had a statistically robust effect on the physical and mental summary scores as well as energy and vitality and general health perception subscales of the SF36. Enhanced daily functioning have also been documented for those with more mild disease treated with CPAP in comparison to placebo (13) and conservative treatment (16). Clinically meaningful improvements in daily behaviors following CPAP treatment have also been documented using disease-specific measures (25,80,140). For example, using the SAQLI, Hui and associates found significant improvement compared to baseline 1 and 3 months following treatment. Finally, it appears that greater nightly CPAP duration yields better functioning (13,29,150). Among these studies, it appears that CPAP produces clinically important gains in the ability to conduct multiple daily behaviors. In addition to generating changes in areas associated with daytime hypersomnolence, such as vigilance and energy level, CPAP has restored to sleep apneic patients that which is most meaningful to them—the ability to once again engage in social activities, fulfill their daily roles, and be as active as their peers. After treatment, their functional level appears to be more consistent with normal individuals (32). Although these data are self-report, it has been suggested that the "bottom line" for the appraisal of health care delivery is the patient's perspective of how treatment affects their daily life (128). Therefore, from the patient's viewpoint, CPAP is highly effective in restoring normal functioning.

V. Summary and Conclusion

There is little question that CPAP is efficacious. However, the extent to which it is effective appears to be principally determined by the degree to which patients are adherent to treatment. When applied faithfully, CPAP does enhance the quality of life in patients with OSA. The application of CPAP affects behaviors meaningful to the patient's conduct of daily life, such as improved work performance, reduced absenteeism, increased vitality, enhanced social functions, better driving performance, and improved emotional and physical health. The mechanisms for this heightened self-reported functional status and the link to neurobehavioral performance have received minimal attention and need to be addressed. Although it has been demonstrated that compared to normal controls those with OSA experience far more functional limitations, the link to OSA will remain unconfirmed until other potential comorbid causes of reduced functional status, such as depression, are excluded.

The precise prescription of CPAP in terms of minimal nocturnal duration and frequency of use is still relatively unknown. It is apparent that CPAP needs to be used daily, but the regression in vigilance and physiological parameters associated with the acute withdrawal of treatment have been shown in few studies. Moreover, the minimum nightly duration of CPAP use that will produce positive outcomes is unidentified. Because therapy in almost half of those prescribed CPAP is less than optimal, CPAP adherence must receive continued emphasis. There does not seem to be a disease-related or demographic variable that has consistently been identified as affecting adherence to CPAP therapy. The contribution of auto-CPAP devices to promoting adherence is still unclear. Although conceptually the overall reduction in positive pressure during the night would promote patient comfort, the lack of a statistically reliable relationship between level of CPAP pressure and adherence to treatment raises doubts about its ability to greatly affect the pattern of CPAP use. The lack of a theoretical base may explain the conflicting results yielded by protocols developed to enhance adherence. The sharp decline in CPAP use by those who eventually abandon treatment suggests that the explanation for nonadherence to treatment may be antecedent to therapy. The application of conceptual models of motivation for health behaviors could provide a framework for the identification of characteristics of those less adherent to CPAP. It is unlikely, without understanding the reason for nonadherence to CPAP, that intervention strategies will be successful.

Acknowledgments

The extensive evaluation on which this chapter was based was supported by SCOR grants HL42236, HL53991, and HL60287 from the National Heart, Lung, and Blood Institute, National Institutes of Health, U.S. Public Health Service. We are grateful to Deborah Tiller for her assistance with the preparation of the manuscript.

References

1. Sullivan CE, Issa FG, Berthon-Jones M, Eves L. Reversal of obstructive sleep apnoea by continuous positive airway pressure applied through the nares. Lancet 1981; 1:862–865.
2. Rapoport DM, Garay SM, Goldring RM. Nasal CPAP in obstructive sleep apnea: mechanisms of action. Bull Eur Physiopathol Respir 1983; 19:616–620.
3. Issa FG, Sullivan CE. The immediate effects of nasal continuous positive airway pressure treatment on sleep pattern in patients with obstructive sleep apnea syndrome. Electroencephalogr Clin Neurophysiol 1986; 63:10–17.
4. Sleep apnea, sleepiness, and driving risk. Am J Respir Crit Care Med 1994; 150:1463–1473.
5. Strohl KP, Redline S. Nasal CPAP therapy, upper airway muscle activation, and obstructive sleep apnea. Am Rev Respir Dis 1986; 134:555–558.
6. Remmers JE, Sterling JA, Thorarinsson B, Kuna ST. Nasal airway positive pressure in patients with occlusive sleep apnea. Methods and feasibility. Am Rev Respir Dis 1984; 130:1152–1155.
7. Sanders MH, Moore SE, Eveslage J. CPAP via nasal mask: a treatment for occlusive sleep apnea. Chest 1983; 83:144–145.
8. Schmidt-Nowara WW. Continuous positive airway pressure for long-term treatment of sleep apnea. Am J Dis Child 1984; 138:82–84.
9. Sullivan CE, Issa FG, Berthon-Jones M, McCauley VB, Costas LJ. Home treatment of obstructive sleep apnoea with continuous positive airway pressure applied through a nose-mask. Bull Eur Physiopathol Respir 1984; 20:49–54.
10. Strohl KP, Cherniack NS, Gothe B. Physiologic basis of therapy for sleep apnea. Am Rev Respir Dis 1986; 134:791–802.
11. Jokic R, Klimaszewski A, Crossley M, Sridhar G, Fitzpatrick MF. Positional treatment vs continuous positive airway pressure in patients with positional obstructive sleep apnea syndrome. Chest 1999; 115:771–781.
12. Engleman HM, Martin SE, Deary IJ, Douglas NJ. Effect of continuous positive airway pressure treatment on daytime function in sleep apnoea/hypopnoea syndrome. Lancet 1994; 343:572–575.
13. Engleman HM, Kingshott RN, Wraith PK, Mackay TW, Deary IJ, Douglas NJ. Randomized placebo-controlled crossover trial of continuous positive airway pressure for mild sleep apnea/hypopnea syndrome. Am J Respir Crit Care Med 1999; 159:461–467.
14. Engleman HM, Martin SE, Deary IJ, Douglas NJ. Effect of CPAP therapy on daytime function in patients with mild sleep apnoea/hypopnoea syndrome. Thorax 1997; 52:114–119.

15. Douglas N. Systematic review of the efficacy of nasal CPAP. Thorax 1998; 53:414–415.
16. Redline S, Adams N, Strauss ME, Roebuck T, Winters M, Rosenberg C. Improvement of mild sleep-disordered breathing with CPAP compared with conservative therapy. Am J Respir Crit Care Med 1998; 157:858–865.
17. Ballester E, Badia JR, Hernandez L, Carrasco E, de Pablo J, Fornas C, Rodriguez-Roisin R, Montserrat JM. Evidence of the effectiveness of continuous positive airway pressure in the treatment of sleep apnea/hypopnea syndrome. Am J Respir Crit Care Med 1999; 159:495–501.
18. Jenkinson C, Davies RJO, Mullins R, Stradling JR. Comparison of therapeutic and subtherapeutic nasal continuous positive airway pressure for obstructive sleep apnoea: a randomized prospective parallel trial. Lancet 1999; 353:2100–2105.
19. Kribbs NB, Pack AI, Kline LR, Smith PL, Schwartz AR, Schubert NM, Redline S, Henry JN, Getsy JE, Dinges DF. Objective measurement of patterns of nasal CPAP use by patients with obstructive sleep apnea. Am Rev Respir Dis 1993; 147:887–895.
20. Kribbs NB, Pack AI, Kline LR, Getsy JE, Schuett JS, Henry JN, Maislin G, Dinges DF. Effects of one night without nasal CPAP treatment on sleep and sleepiness in patients with obstructive sleep apnea. Am Rev Respir Dis 1993; 147:1162–1168.
21. Kribbs N, Getsy G, Dinges D. Investigation and management of daytime sleepiness in sleep apnea. In: Saunders N, Sullivan C, eds. Sleep and Breathing. New York: Marcel Dekker, Inc., 1994:575–604.
22. Naegele B, Pepin JL, Levy P, Bonnet C, Pellat J, Feuerstein C. Cognitive executive dysfunction in patients with obstructive sleep apnea syndrome (OSAS) after CPAP treatment. Sleep 1998; 21:392–397.
23. George CF, Boudreau AC, Smiley A. Effects of nasal CPAP on simulated driving performance in patients with obstructive sleep apnoea. Thorax 1997; 52:648–653.
24. Findley L, Smith C, Hooper J, Dineen M, Suratt PM. Treatment with nasal CPAP decreases automobile accidents in patients with sleep apnea. Am J Respir Crit Care Med 2000; 161:857–859.
25. Weaver T, Chugh D, Maislin G, Schwab R, Mahowald M, Kader G, Bloxham T, Greenberg H, Younger J, Pack A, Dinges D. Changes in functional status after 3 months CPAP treatment. Am J Respir Crit Care Med 1998; 157:A53.
26. Barnes M, Houston D, Worsnop CJ, Neill AM, Mykytyn IJ, Kay A, Trinder J, Saunders NA, McEvoy R, Pierce R. A randomized controlled trial of CPAP in mild obstructive sleep apnoea. 6th World Congress on Sleep Apnea, Sydney, Australia, March 12–15, 2000.
27. Facenda J, Boon N, Mackay T, Douglas N. Quality of life on and off CPAP in patients with sleep apnea/hypopnea syndrome. Am J Respir Crit Care Med 2000; 161:A714.
28. Hernandez L, Ballester E, Vilagut G, Ferrer M, Carrasco E, Farre JDR, Badia J, Montserrat J. A randomized placebo controlled study on the effectiveness of CPAP treatment. Am J Respir Crit Care Med 2000; 161:A358.
29. Meslier N, Lebrun T, Grillier-Lanoir V, Rolland N, Henderick C, Sailly JC, Racineux JL. A French survey of 3,225 patients treated with CPAP for obstructive sleep apnoea: benefits, tolerance, compliance and quality of life. Eur Respir J 1998; 12:185–192.
30. Bolitschek J, Schmeiser-Rieder A, Schobersberger R, Rosenberger A, Kunze M, Aigner K. Impact of nasal continuous positive airway pressure treatment on quality of life in patients with obstructive sleep apnoea. Eur Respir J 1998; 11:890–894.
31. D'Ambrosio C, Bowman T, Mohsenin V. Quality of life in patients with obstructive

sleep apnea: effect of nasal continuous positive airway pressure—a prospective study. Chest 1999; 115:123–129.
32. Jenkinson C, Stradling J, Petersen S. Comparison of three measures of quality of life outcome in the evaluation of continuous positive airways pressure therapy for sleep apnoea. J Sleep Res 1997; 6:199–204.
33. Kiely JL, McNicholas WT. Bed partners' assessment of nasal continuous positive airway pressure therapy in obstructive sleep apnea. Chest 1997; 111:1261–1265.
34. Kingshott RN, Vennelle M, Hoy CJ, Engleman HM, Deary IJ, Douglas NJ. Predictors of improvements in daytime function outcomes with CPAP therapy. Am J Respir Crit Care Med 2000; 161:866–871.
35. Sullivan C, Issa F, Berthon-Jones M, Saunders N. Pathophysiology of sleep apnea. In: Saunders N, Sullivan C, eds. Sleep and Breathing. New York: Marcel Dekker, 1984:299–364.
36. Sullivan CE, Issa FG. Obstructive sleep apnea. Clin Chest Med 1985; 6:633–650.
37. Sanders MH. Nasal CPAP effect on patterns of sleep apnea. Chest 1984; 86:839–844.
38. Yamashiro Y, Kryger M. Why should sleep apnea be diagnosed and treated. Clin Pulm Med 1994; 1:250–259.
39. He J, Kryger MH, Zorick FJ, Conway W, Roth T. Mortality and apnea index in obstructive sleep apnea. Experience in 385 male patients. Chest 1988; 94:9–14.
40. Partinen M, Jamieson A, Guilleminault C. Long-term outcome for obstructive sleep apnea syndrome patients. Mortality. Chest 1988; 94:1200–1204.
41. Fletcher E, Debehnke R, Lovoi M. Undiagnosed sleep apnea syndrome in patients with essential hypertension. Arch Intern Med 1988; 103:190–195.
42. Kales A, Bixler EO, Cadieux RJ, Schneck DW, Shaw LCD, Locke TW, Vela-Bueno A, Soldatos CR. Sleep apnoea in a hypertensive population. Lancet 1984; 2:1005–1008.
43. Lugaresi E, Cirignotta F, Coccagna G, Piana C. Some epidemiological data on snoring and cardiocirculatory disturbances. Sleep 1980; 3:221–224.
44. Guilleminault C, Connolly SJ, Winkle RA. Cardiac arrhythmia and conduction disturbances during sleep in 400 patients with sleep apnea syndrome. Am J Cardiol 1983; 52:490–494.
45. Bliwise DL, Bliwise NG, Partinen M, Pursley AM, Dement WC. Sleep apnea and mortality in an aged cohort. Am J Public Health 1988; 78:544–547.
46. Konkenvus M, Daprio J, Telakiri T. Snoring as a risk factor for ischemic heart disease and stroke in man. Br Med J 1987; 294:16–19.
47. Hung J, Whitford EG, Parsons RW, Hillman DR. Association of sleep apnoea with myocardial infarction in men. Lancet 1990; 336:261–264.
48. Nieto FJ, Young TB, Lind BK, Shahar E, Samet JM, Redline S, D'Agostino RB, Newman AB, Lebowitz MD, Pickering TG. Association of sleep-disordered breathing, sleep apnea, and hypertension in a large community-based study. Sleep Heart Health Study. JAMA 2000; 283:1829–1836.
49. Young T, Peppard P, Palta M, Hla KM, Finn L, Morgan B, Skatrud J. Population-based study of sleep-disordered breathing as a risk factor for hypertension. Arch Intern Med 1997; 157:1746–1752.
50. Engleman HM, Hirst WS, Douglas NJ. Under reporting of sleepiness and driving impairment in patients with sleep apnoea/hypopnoea syndrome. J Sleep Res 1997; 6: 272–275.

51. Findley LJ, Unverzagt ME, Suratt PM. Automobile accidents involving patients with obstructive sleep apnea. Am Rev Respir Dis 1988; 138:337–340.
52. Cassel W, Ploch T, Becker C, Dugnus D, Peter JH, von Wichert P. Risk of traffic accidents in patients with sleep-disordered breathing: reduction with nasal CPAP. Eur Respir J 1996; 9:2606–2611.
53. Wu H, Yan-Go F. Self-reported automobile accidents involving patients with obstructive sleep apnea. Neurology 1996; 46:1254–1257.
54. Young T, Blustein J, Finn L, Palta M. Sleep-disordered breathing and motor vehicle accidents in a population-based sample of employed adults. Sleep 1997; 20:608–613.
55. Findley L, Unverzagt M, Guchu R, Febrizio M, Buckner J, Suratt P. Vigilance and automobile accidents in patients with sleep apnea or narcolepsy. Chest 1995; 108:619–624.
56. Findley LJ, Weiss JW, Jabour ER. Drivers with untreated sleep apnea. A cause of death and serious injury. Arch Intern Med 1991; 151:1451–1452.
57. George CF, Smiley A. Sleep apnea and automobile crashes. Sleep 1999; 22:790–795.
58. McNicholas WT. Sleep apnoea and driving risk. European Respiratory Society Task Force on "Public Health and Medicolegal Implications of Sleep Apnoea." Eur Respir J 1999; 13:1225–1227.
59. Teran-Santos J, Jimenez-Gomez A, Cordero-Guevara J. The association between sleep apnea and the risk of traffic accidents. N Engl J Med 1999; 340:847–851.
60. Horstmann S, Hess CW, Bassetti C, Gugger M, Mathis J. Sleepiness-related accidents in sleep apnea patients. Sleep 2000; 23:383–389.
61. Krieger J, Meslier N, Lebrun T, Levy P, Phillip-Joet F, Sailly JC, Racineux JL. Accidents in obstructive sleep apnea patients treated with nasal continuous positive airway pressure: a prospective study. The Working Group ANTADIR, Paris and CRESGE, Lille, France. Association Nationale de Traitement a Domicile des Insuffisants Respiratoires. Chest 1997; 112:1561–1566.
62. Stoohs RA, Guilleminault C, Itoi A, Dement WC. Traffic accidents in commercial long-haul truck drivers: the influence of sleep-disordered breathing and obesity. Sleep 1994; 17:619–623.
63. Gall R, Isaac L, Kryger M. Quality of life in mild obstructive sleep apnea. Sleep 1993; 16:S59–S61.
64. Chesire K, Engleman H, Deary I, Shapiro C, Douglas NJ. Factors impairing daytime performance in patients with sleep apnea/hypopnea syndrome. Arch Intern Med 1992; 152:538–541.
65. Weaver TE, Chugh DK, Maislin G, Schwab RJ, George CFP, Kader GA, Bloxham TJ, Pack AI, Dinges DF. Impact of obstructive sleep apnea on the conduct of daily activities. Sleep Res 1997; 26:530.
66. Weaver TE, Laizner AM, Evans LK, Maislin G, Chugh DK, Lyon K, Smith PL, Schwartz AR, Redline S, Pack AI, Dinges DF. An instrument to measure functional status outcomes for disorders of excessive sleepiness. Sleep 1997; 20:835–843.
67. Fornas C, Ballester E, Arteta E, Ricou C, Diaz A, Fernandez A, Alonso J, Montserrat JM. Measurement of general health status in obstructive sleep apnea hypopnea patients. Sleep 1995; 18:876–879.
68. Ulfberg J, Carter N, Talback M, Edling C. Excessive daytime sleepiness at work and subjective work performance in the general population and among heavy snorers and patients with obstructive sleep apnea. Chest 1996; 110:659–663.

69. Jones KR, Jennings BM, Moritz P, Moss MT. Policy issues associated with analyzing outcomes of care. Image J Nurs Sch 1997; 29:261–267.
70. Iezzoni L. Adjustment for Measuring Health Outcomes. Ann Arbor, MI: Health Administration Press, 1994.
71. Engleman HM, Asgari-Jirhandeh N, McLeod AL, Ramsay CF, Deary IJ, Douglas NJ. Self-reported use of CPAP and benefits of CPAP therapy: a patient survey. Chest 1996; 109:1470–1476.
72. Sanders MH, Gruendl CA, Rogers RM. Patient compliance with nasal CPAP therapy for sleep apnea. Chest 1986; 90:330–333.
73. Nino-Murcia G, McCann CC, Bliwise DL, Guilleminault C, Dement WC. Compliance and side effects in sleep apnea patients treated with nasal continuous positive airway pressure. West J Med 1989; 150:165–169.
74. Waldhorn RE, Herrick TW, Nguyen MC, O'Donnell AE, Sodero J, Potolicchio SJ. Long-term compliance with nasal continuous positive airway pressure therapy of obstructive sleep apnea. Chest 1990; 97:33–38.
75. Rolfe I, Olson LG, Saunders NA. Long-term acceptance of continuous positive airway pressure in obstructive sleep apnea. Am Rev Respir Dis 1991; 144:1130–1133.
76. Hoffstein V, Viner S, Mateika S, Conway J. Treatment of obstructive sleep apnea with nasal continuous positive airway pressure. Patient compliance, perception of benefits, and side effects. Am Rev Respir Dis 1992; 145:841–845.
77. Krieger J. Long-term compliance with nasal continuous positive airway pressure (CPAP) in obstructive sleep apnea patients and nonapneic snorers. Sleep 1992; 15: S42–S46.
78. Pieters T, Collard P, Aubert G, Dury M, Delguste P, Rodenstein DO. Acceptance and long-term compliance with nCPAP in patients with obstructive sleep apnoea syndrome. Eur Respir J 1996; 9:939–944.
79. McEvoy RD, Thornton AT. Treatment of obstructive sleep apnea syndrome with nasal continuous positive airway pressure. Sleep 1984; 7:313–325.
80. Hui DS, Chan JK, Choy DK, Ko FW, Li TS, Leung RC, Lai CK. Effects of augmented continuous positive airway pressure education and support on compliance and outcome in a Chinese population. Chest 2000; 117:1410–1416.
81. Krieger J, Kurtz D. Objective measurement of compliance with nasal CPAP treatment for obstructive sleep apnoea syndrome. Eur Respir J 1988; 1:436–438.
82. Rauscher H, Formanek D, Popp W, Zwick H. Self-reported vs measured compliance with nasal CPAP for obstructive sleep apnea. Chest 1993; 103:1675–1680.
83. Reeves-Hoché MK, Meck R, Zwillich CW. Nasal CPAP: an objective evaluation of patient compliance. Am J Respir Crit Care Med 1994; 149:149–154.
84. Meurice JC, Dore P, Paquereau J, Neau JP, Ingrand P, Chavagnat JJ, Patte F. Predictive factors of long-term compliance with nasal continuous positive airway pressure treatment in sleep apnea syndrome. Chest 1994; 105:429–433.
85. Likar LL, Panciera TM, Erickson AD, Rounds S. Group education sessions and compliance with nasal CPAP therapy. Chest 1997; 111:1273–1277.
86. McArdle N, Devereux G, Heidarnejad H, Engleman HM, Mackay TW, Douglas NJ. Long-term use of CPAP therapy for sleep apnea/hypopnea syndrome. Am J Respir Crit Care Med 1999; 159:1108–1114.
87. Hoy CJ, Vennelle M, Kingshott RN, Engleman HM, Douglas NJ. Can intensive support improve continuous positive airway pressure use in patients with the sleep apnea/hypopnea syndrome? Am J Respir Crit Care Med 1999; 159:1096–1100.

88. Pépin JL, Krieger J, Rodenstein D, Cornette A, Sforza E, Delguste P, Deschaux C, Grillier V, Levy P. Effective compliance during the first 3 months of continuous positive airway pressure. A European prospective study of 121 patients. Am J Respir Crit Care Med 1999; 160:1124–1129.
89. Engleman HM, Martin SE, Douglas NJ. Compliance with CPAP therapy in patients with the sleep apnoea/hypopnoea syndrome. Thorax 1994; 49:263–266.
90. Pepin JL, Leger P, Veale D, Langevin B, Robert D, Levy P. Side effects of nasal continuous positive airway pressure in sleep apnea syndrome. Study of 193 patients in two French sleep centers. Chest 1995; 107:375–381.
91. Krieger J, Kurtz D, Petiau C, Sforza E, Trautmann D. Long-term compliance with CPAP therapy in obstructive sleep apnea patients and in snorers. Sleep 1996; 19:S136–S143.
92. Lévy P, Labrun T, Meslier N, Cornette A, Reybet-Degat O, Phillip-Joet F, Krieger J, Pepin J, Fleury B, Sailly J, Racineux J. Multicentre survey of CPAP therapy for OSA in France. Am J Respir Crit Care Med 1997; 155:A847.
93. Reeves-Hoche MK, Hudgel DW, Meck R, Witteman R, Ross A, Zwillich CW. Continuous versus bilevel positive airway pressure for obstructive sleep apnea. Am J Respir Crit Care Med 1995; 151:443–449.
94. Fleury B, Rakotonanahary D, Tehindrazanarivelo AD, Hausser-Hauw C, Lebeau B. Long-term compliance to continuous positive airway pressure therapy (nCPAP) set up during a split-night polysomnography. Sleep 1994; 17:512–515.
95. Fleury B, Rakotonanahary D, Hausser-Hauw C, Lebeau B, Guilleminault C. Objective patient compliance in long-term use of nCPAP. Eur Respir J 1996; 9:2356–2359.
96. Weaver TE, Kribbs NB, Pack AI, Kline LR, Chugh DK, Maislin G, Smith PL, Schwartz AR, Schubert NM, Gillen KA, Dinges DF. Night-to-night variability in CPAP use over the first three months of treatment. Sleep 1997; 20:278–283.
97. Chervin RD, Theut S, Bassetti C, Aldrich MS. Compliance with nasal CPAP can be improved by simple interventions. Sleep 1997; 20:284–289.
98. Tiihonen M, Partinen M. Polysomnography and maintenance of wakefulness test as predictors of CPAP effectiveness in obstructive sleep apnea. Electroencephalogr Clin Neurophysiol 1998; 107:383–386.
99. Jokic R, Klimaszewski A, Sridhar G, Fitzpatrick MF. Continuous positive airway pressure requirement during the first month of treatment in patients with severe obstructive sleep apnea. Chest 1998; 114:1061–1069.
100. Engleman HM, Martin SE, Kingshott RN, Mackay TW, Deary IJ, Douglas NJ. Randomized placebo controlled trial of daytime function after continuous positive airway pressure (CPAP) therapy for the sleep apnoea/hypopnoea syndrome. Thorax 1998; 53: 341–345.
101. Meurice JC, Paquereau J, Denjean A, Patte F, Series F. Influence of correction of flow limitation on continuous positive airway pressure efficiency in sleep apnoea/hypopnoea syndrome. Eur Respir J 1998; 11:1121–1127.
102. Hack M, Davies RJ, Mullins R, Choi SJ, Ramdassingh-Dow S, Jenkinson C, Stradling JR. Randomized prospective parallel trial of therapeutic versus subtherapeutic nasal continuous positive airway pressure on simulated steering performance in patients with obstructive sleep apnoea. Thorax 2000; 55:224–231.
103. Konermann M, Sanner BM, Vyleta M, Laschewski F, Groetz J, Sturm A, Zidek W. Use of conventional and self-adjusting nasal continuous positive airway pressure for

treatment of severe obstructive sleep apnea syndrome: a comparative study. Chest 1998; 113:714–718.

104. Yu BH, Ancoli-Israel S, Dimsdale JE. Effect of CPAP treatment on mood states in patients with sleep apnea. J Psychiatr Res 1999; 33:427–432.

105. Bennett LS, Barbour C, Langford B, Stradling JR, Davies RJ. Health status in obstructive sleep apnea: relationship with sleep fragmentation and daytime sleepiness, and effects of continuous positive airway pressure treatment. Am J Respir Crit Care Med 1999; 159:1884–1890.

106. Rosenthal L, Nykamp K, Guido P, Syron M, Day R, Fortier J, Bishop C, Rice F, Roehrs T, Roth T. Compliance with CPAP during the first week of treatment. Sleep Res 1997; 26:489.

107. Edinger JD, Carwile S, Miller P, Hope V, Mayti C. Psychological status, syndromatic measures, and compliance with nasal CPAP therapy for sleep apnea. Percept Mot Skills 1994; 78:1116–1118.

108. Meurice JC, Paquereau J, Neau JP, Caron F, Dore P, Ingrand P, Patte F. Long-term evolution of daytime somnolence in patients with sleep apnea/hypopnea syndrome treated by continuous positive airway pressure. Sleep 1997; 20:1162–1166.

109. Lojander J, Maasilta P, Partinen M, Brander PE, Salmi T, Lehtonen H. Nasal-CPAP, surgery, and conservative management for treatment of obstructive sleep apnea syndrome. A randomized study. Chest 1996; 110:114–119.

110. Leon C, Ballester E, Lloberes P, Alarcon A, Rodriguez-Roisin R, Montserrat J. More about the acceptable CPAP compliance in patients with sleep apnea hypopnea syndrome (SAHS). Am J Crit Care Med 1997; 155:A305.

111. Strollo PJ, Jr., Sanders MH, Costantino JP, Walsh SK, Stiller RA, Atwood CW, Jr. Split-night studies for the diagnosis and treatment of sleep-disordered breathing. Sleep 1996; 19:S255–S259.

112. Boudewyns A, Grillier-Lanoir V, Willemen MJ, De Cock WA, Van de Heyning PH, De Backer WA. Two months follow up of auto-CPAP treatment in patients with obstructive sleep apnoea. Thorax 1999; 54:147–149.

113. Teschler H, Farhat AA, Exner V, Konietzko N, Berthon-Jones M. AutoSet nasal CPAP titration: constancy of pressure, compliance and effectiveness at 8 month follow-up. Eur Respir J 1997; 10:2073–2078.

114. Gagnadoux F, Rakotonanahary D, Martins de Araujo MT, Barros-Vieira S, Fleury B. Long-term efficacy of fixed CPAP recommended by Autoset for OSAS. Sleep 1999; 22:1095–1099.

115. Teschler H, Berthon-Jones M, Thompson AB, Henkel A, Henry J, Konietzko N. Automated continuous positive airway pressure titration for obstructive sleep apnea syndrome. Am J Respir Crit Care Med 1996; 154:734–740.

116. Meurice JC, Marc I, Series F. Efficacy of auto-CPAP in the treatment of obstructive sleep apnea/hypopnea syndrome. Am J Respir Crit Care Med 1996; 153:794–798.

117. Janson C, Noges E, Svedberg-Randt S, Lindberg E. What characterizes patients who are unable to tolerate continuous positive airway pressure (CPAP) treatment? Respir Med 2000; 94:145–149.

118. Fletcher EC, Luckett RA. The effect of positive reinforcement on hourly compliance in nasal continuous positive airway pressure users with obstructive sleep apnea. Am Rev Respir Dis 1991; 143:936–941.

119. Noseda A, Jann E, Hoffmann G, Linkowski P, Kerkhofs M. Compliance with nasal

continuous positive airway pressure assessed with a pressure monitor: pattern of use and influence of sleep habits. Respir Med 2000; 94:76–81.

120. Sanders M, Costantino J, Strollo P, Studnicki K, Atwood C. The impact of split-night polysomnography for diagnosis and positive pressure therapy titration on treatment acceptance and adherence in sleep apnea/hypopnea. Sleep 2000; 23:17–24.
121. Meecham Jones DJ, Paul EA, Grahame-Clarke C, Wedzicha JA. Nasal ventilation in acute exacerbations of chronic obstructive pulmonary disease: effect of ventilator mode on arterial blood gas tensions. Thorax 1994; 49:1222–1224.
122. Massie CA, Hart RW, Peralez K, Richards GN. Effects of humidification on nasal symptoms and compliance in sleep apnea patients using continuous positive airway pressure. Chest 1999; 116:403–408.
123. Phillips B, Collop N, Strollo P. Controversies in sleep disorders medicine. Pulmonologists respond! Chest 1996; 110:1597–1602.
124. Iber C, O'Brien C, Schluter J, Davies S, Leatherman J, Mahowald M. Single night studies in obstructive sleep apnea. Sleep 1991; 14:383–385.
125. Yamashiro Y, Kryger MH. CPAP titration for sleep apnea using a split-night protocol. Chest 1995; 107:62–66.
126. Oliver C, Flaherty M, Levy R, Tousignant P, Pepler C, Kimoff R. Effects of nursing intervention on patient and spouse well-being and CPAP compliance in obstructive sleep apnea (OSA). Am J Respir Crit Care Med 1997; 155:A305.
127. Conner M, Sparks P. The theory planned behaviour and health behaviours. In: Conner M, Norman P, eds. Predicting Health Behaviour. Research and Practice with Social Cognition Models. Philadelphia: Open University Press, 1996:121–162.
128. Ellwood PM. Shattuck lecture—outcomes management. A technology of patient experience. N Engl J Med 1988; 318:1549–1556.
129. Leidy N. Functional status and the forward progress of merry-go-rounds: toward a coherent analytical framework. Nurs Res 1994; 43:196–202.
130. Sleepiness in America. Princeton, NJ: The Gallup Organization, 1997.
131. George CF, Nickerson PW, Hanly PJ, Millar TW, Kryger MH. Sleep apnoea patients have more automobile accidents. Lancet 1987; 2:447.
132. Barbé F, Pericás J, Muñoz A, Findley L, Antó JM, Agustí AGN, Hoan MdL. Automobile accidents in patients with sleep apnea syndrome: an epidemiological and mechanistic study. Am J Respir Crit Care Med 1998; 158:18–22.
133. Haraldsson PO, Carenfelt C, Diderichsen F, Nygren A, Tingvall C. Clinical symptoms of sleep apnea syndrome and automobile accidents. J Otorhinolaryngol Relat Spec 1990; 52:57–62.
134. George CF, Boudreau AC, Smiley A. Simulated driving performance in patients with obstructive sleep apnea. Am J Respir Crit Care Med 1996; 154:175–181.
135. George CFP, Boudreau AC, Smiley A. Comparison of simulated driving performance in narcolepsy and sleep apnea patients. Sleep 1996; 19:711–717.
136. Aldrich MS. Automobile accidents in patients with sleep disorders. Sleep 1989; 12: 487–494.
137. Findley LJ, Fabrizio MJ, Knight H, Norcross BB, LaForte AJ, Suratt PM. Driving simulator performance in patients with sleep apnea. Am Rev Respir Dis 1989; 140: 529–530.
138. Flemons W, Remmers J, Whitelaw W. The correlation of a computer simulated driving program with polysomnographic indices and neuropsychological tests in consecutively referred patients for assessment of sleep apnea. Sleep 1993; 16:S71.

139. Grunstein RR, Stenlof K, Hedner JA, Sjostrom L. Impact of self-reported sleep-breathing disturbances on psychosocial performance in the Swedish Obese Subjects (SOS) study. Sleep 1995; 18:635–643.
140. Flemons WW, Reimer MA. Development of a disease-specific health-related quality of life questionnaire for sleep apnea. Am J Respir Crit Care Med 1998; 158:494–503.
141. Flemons WW, Tsai W. Quality of life consequences of sleep-disordered breathing. J Allergy Clin Immunol 1997; 99:S750–S756.
142. Flemons WW. Measuring health related quality of life in sleep apnea. Sleep 2000; 23(suppl 4):S109–S114.
143. Mitler MM, Carskadon MA, Czeisler CA, Dement WC, Dinges DF, Graeber RC. Catastrophes, sleep, and public policy: consensus report. Sleep 1988; 11:100–109.
144. Ware J, Snow K, Kosinski M, et al. SF 36 Health Survey. Manual and Interpretation Guide. Boston: The Health Institute, New England Medical Center, 1990.
145. Bergner M, Bobbitt R, Carter W, Gilson B. The Sickness Impact Profile: development and final revision of a health status measure. Med Care 1981; 19:787–805.
146. Hunt S, McEwen J, McKenna S. Perceived health; age and sex comparisons in a community. J Epidemiol Commun Health 1984; 38:156–160.
147. Schwartz J, Lurie N. Assessment of medical outcomes. Int J Technol Assess Health Care 1990; 6:333–339.
148. Kane R. Functional assessment questionnaire for geriatric patients—or the clinical Swiss army knife. J Chron Dis 1987; 40:95S–98S.
149. Maislin G, Pack AI, Kribbs NB, Smith PL, Schwartz AR, Kline LR, Schwab RJ, Dinges DF. A survey screen for prediction of apnea. Sleep 1995; 18:158–166.
150. Weaver T, Maislin G, Pack A, Dinges D, Group MOS. Improvements in OSA outcomes relative to hours of nightly CPAP use. Sleep 2000; 23:A81.

19

Oral Appliance Therapy for Snoring and Sleep Apnea

ALAN A. LOWE

University of British Columbia
Vancouver, British Columbia, Canada

WOLFGANG W. SCHMIDT-NOWARA

University of New Mexico
Albuquerque, New Mexico
Sleep Medicine Institute
Dallas, Texas

I. Introduction

The development of clinical activity in obstructive sleep apnea (OSA) syndromes has been influenced by two basic themes: prevalence and treatment. Upper airway obstruction during sleep is widely prevalent in adults (1), remarkably so in view of the fact that the modern recognition of this problem began in 1965 (2), and as recently as 1978 sleep apnea was still considered a new and curious entity (3). OSA produces a spectrum of clinical effects: most subjects have symptoms, many have obvious disability and morbidity, and mortality is increased, although the relation of the increase to sleep apnea is controversial (4). At the same time it should be emphasized that most persons with OSA have a mild version of the condition. Using an Apnea/Hypopnea Index (AHI) of <30 to describe mild, more than 50% of persons with AHI >5 in the Madison study are classified as being in this category (1).

Treatment for OSA has been available since shortly after its original description (5), but every therapy devised is either limited in efficacy or requires trade-offs in comfort, convenience, and lifestyle. Acceptance and compliance with therapy have been a major challenge. The search for a therapy with a suitable profile of efficacy, safety, patient acceptance, and reasonable cost has been wide and often ingenious, and it still goes on.

In this setting, oral appliances (OA) have emerged as an increasingly popular alternative to more established therapies, including nasal continuous positive airway pressure (nCPAP) and various surgeries. For this discussion, OA are devices worn in the mouth during sleep in order to modify the upper airway so as to relieve upper airway obstruction. Clinical research of this therapy is increasing. The early literature consisted of case reports and a number of small case series. More recently, controlled studies have appeared. A number of reviews have documented the growing literature (6–8) and practice guidelines have been developed (9). In this chapter, the scientific basis of oral appliance therapy for upper airway obstruction during sleep will be reviewed. The emphasis will be on experimental observations and on clinical studies published after 1994, since earlier studies have been adequately reviewed (7,8).

II. DEVELOPMENT OF OA FOR SNORING AND OSA

A. Historical Development

The concept of moving the tongue and jaw forward to correct a compromised airway has been effectively used for many decades in anesthesiology and orthodontics. Pierre Robin treated tongue obstruction (glossoptosis) with a mandibular repositioning appliance as early as 1934 (10). Since that time, numerous appliances have been used to change airway size, affect craniofacial growth, alter the dentition, and modify snoring and OSA (7). The treatment of OSA in a child with an oral appliance was first described by Boraz et al. in 1979 (11). Meier-Ewert et al. used a mandibular repositioner (12), and Cartwright and Samelson described successes with a tongue-retaining device in adult OSA cases (13).

Since the last major overview of oral appliance design when only 13 appliances were commercially available (7), and since the American Sleep Disorders Association (ASDA) position paper (9), two significant advances have occurred. The first is the concept of an adjustable appliance allowing titration of the mandibular position over time. The second is the use of materials and designs that have significantly improved retention. Of the more than 40 oral appliances currently on the market, fewer than 5 are fully adjustable, and only 3 have undergone any form of controlled or randomized clinical trial. Dentists realized early on that determining the correct jaw position was the most difficult step when using oral appliances successfully. Considerable variations in the initial comfortable range of the anteroposterior movement of the mandible and differences in the speed and the amount of forward jaw position that any given patient could tolerate were found. Single jaw position appliances often need to be remade if the initial jaw position proves to be inadequate. Gradual titration forward of the mandible without the necessity of making a new appliance each time became the objective, and adjustable appliances were invented and marketed. It was also observed that a subgroup of patients, particularly those who suffered from sleep bruxism (14), often experienced a considerable amount of jaw discomfort in the morning after wearing a rigid hard acrylic single jaw position OA. A need to develop an OA that could allow for lateral jaw movement as well as some degree of vertical jaw opening was identified. At the same time, major advances in dental materials significantly improved the flexibility and strength of thermosensitive acrylic resin materials. Appliances made of temperature-sensitive material that the patient could heat in hot water before insertion that would cool and harden somewhat intraorally were found to have considerably more retention than traditionally designed cold cure acrylic appliances. The combination of adjustability, lateral and vertical jaw movement, increased retention, and better defined titration protocols appear to have significantly improved the effectiveness of OA since they were last reviewed.

B. Cephalometric Morphology

The use of cephalometric radiographs to evaluate both hard and soft tissues in snorers and OSA subjects has significantly increased in the last decade as clinicians search out inexpensive technology to evaluate airway size and/or predict severity of disease. One of the major deficiencies of cephalometrics is that it only evaluates structures in the anteroposterior plane and does not detect lateral dimensional structures. Racial cephalometric differences have been documented for OSA patients (15), and skeletal type appears to be of importance (16). OSA patients may have more upper airway abnormalities than snorers (17). Battagel and L'Estrange, in a sample of adult OSA subjects, found a narrower oropharynx in the retropalatal area and a larger cross-sectional area of the soft palate (18). Similarly, Solow et al. identified a 50% reduction in airway size behind the soft palate in adult OSA patients when compared to controls (19). A large craniocervical angle has been reported by several investigators (20–22). Cephalometric scores to differentiate snorers from OSA patients (23) and cephalometric predictors for the success of OA therapy have been reported.

The analysis of cephalometric predictors for OA use is seriously complicated by the gender, age, and skeletal type differences, which have not been accounted for by several authors. Lowe et al. used cephalometric comparisons in both the upright and the supine positions in subjects with and without OSA, who were then grouped according to their craniofacial skeletal type and gender (16). OSA patients and control subjects were divided into male and female groups and then classified into Class I (CI—well-related maxilla and mandible); Class II, Division 1 (CII/1—forward-positioned maxilla with protruding upper teeth); Class II, Division 2 (CII/2—forward maxilla and upright central incisors); and Class III (CIII—forward-positioned mandible) skeletal subtypes. In the upright position, the most atypical craniofacial and upper airway structure was shown in male patients with CI OSA. In the supine position, the most atypical craniofacial and upper airway structure was also shown in male patients with CI OSA; there were no significant differences between male patients with CII/2 OSA and control subjects or between female patients with CI OSA and control subjects. With a change in body position from upright to supine, distinctive changes in the upper airway structure in both OSA patients and control subjects occurred according to skeletal subtype and gender. Lowe et al. evaluated male OSA patients and male nonapneic snorers and found that the predictive powers of obesity and neck size variables for OSA severity were higher than the cephalometric variables (24). Compared with other cephalometric characteristics, an extended and forward natural head posture, lower hyoid bone position, increased soft palate and tongue dimensions, and decreased nasopharyngeal and velopharyngeal airway dimensions had relatively higher associations with OSA severity. The AHI was the OSA outcome variable that was best explained by the demographic and cephalometric predictor variables.

Cephalometric quantification of tongue posture in snorers and OSA patients has also intrigued researchers. Tangugsorn et al. reported larger and more upright tongue postures in OSA subjects (25). Miyamoto et al. undertook detailed measurements of tongue posture from upright and supine lateral cephalograms in OSA male patients and males with nonapneic snoring matched for age, body mass index (BMI), and craniofacial skeletal pattern (26). Patients with OSA had an AHI of >50/h while nonapneic snorers had an AHI of <10/h. In nonapneic snorers, the tongue depth measurements for the superior-posterior portion of the tongue were larger in the supine than in the upright position. There was no significant difference in tongue depth measurements between the upright and the supine position in the patients with OSA. When awake patients with OSA move from the upright to the supine position, they maintain their upright tongue posture, which may tend to protect against upper airway collapse secondary to the increased gravitational load on the tongue. In contrast, when awake nonapneic snorers move from the upright to the supine position, a significant dorsal movement in the superior-posterior portion of the tongue is observed.

The clinical role of cephalometry in OA therapy continues to be controversial. Menn et al. found that cephalometric radiographic measurements were not good predictors of OA treatment outcomes (27). Eveloff et al. claimed that both the vertical position of the hyoid bone and the length of the soft palate were less in subjects who responded well to OA therapy (28). Mayer and Meier-Ewert identified better treatment success in those subjects with a short oral height and soft palate and a narrow oropharynx (29). Liu et al. (30), based on a stepwise regression analysis, found that OSA subjects had a better response with the Klearway™ appliance if they were younger, had a lower BMI, a longer maxilla, a smaller oropharynx, a smaller overjet, less erupted maxillary molars, and a larger ratio of airway length to the cross-sectional area of the soft palate. Based on a supine cephalometric evaluation and another sample of OSA subjects, Liu et al. (31) identified that good responders to the Klearway appliance had less prominent chins, larger tongue heights, and an increase in hypopharyngeal cross-sectional area after appliance insertion.

In summary, cephalometric studies have documented the importance of both skeletal type and gender when comparing differences between groups of patients. The base of tongue appears to fall back only in nonapneic snorers when they move from the upright to the supine body position. Neck size and weight appear to be better predictors of OSA severity than cephalometric measurements. Additional studies of craniofacial form and tongue posture obtained from large population samples are required before reliable cephalometric predictors of OA success can be applied with confidence to a specific case.

III. Mechanisms of Action

Although OA are designed to increase the upper airway lumen, it is presently not known whether this is the mechanism of their effect. The principal obstacle to a better understanding is the absence of direct observations during sleep. A number of studies have confirmed that OA modify the size and shape of the airway in awake subjects, and these will be reviewed in this section. However, it is unknown whether these airway effects persist with the change in sleep stage or whether other factors related to OA use may be important.

The effect of OA on the upper airway has been studied in awake patients with radiographic imaging and with videoendoscopy (Table 1). Each study has shown an increase in upper airway cross-sectional area at different levels. Significant group effects were found in the retropalatal area (32,33) and in the retroglossal area (27,34–36). Soft tissue effects have included a shortening of the soft palate (27,28) and a change in tongue shape (33). Eveloff et al. have also reported a reduction in the mandibular plane-hyoid distance, which may also indicate a change in tongue shape or position (28). Perhaps the most consistent finding was the variation among individual patients. Each of these studies was performed with a mandibular advancement type of OA. Other types of OA have not been investigated in this manner. However, Ferguson et al. have shown that active tongue protrusion produces significant increase in the upper airway lumen extending from the retropalatal to the hypopharyngeal region (37); this observation may explain one of the effects of tongue-retaining appliances.

Table 1 The Effect of Mandibular Repositioners on the Upper Airway in Awake Patients

Patients	Technique	Airway effects	Soft tissue effects	Ref.
23	Cephalometrics	↑ PAS	Less hyoid displacement	27
19	Cephalometrics	NS	Less hyoid displacement	28
12	Cephalometrics	↑ SAS	None described	32
1	CT	↑ SAS, PAS	Tongue shape	33
61	Cephalometrics	↑ PAS	None described	34
10	Cephalometrics	↑ PAS	None described	35
9	Videoendoscopy	↑ SAS	—	36

NS = Not significant; SAS = superior airway space; PAS = posterior airway space.

Two studies with MR of the upper airway and the effects of OA have been reported. Tomographic studies have the advantage over cephalometry since they examine the airway in three dimensions and can describe changes in airway shape in addition to the position of adjacent structures. Schmidt-Nowara et al. described an increase in the retropalatal and retroglossal airspace with OA in 13 patients studied awake and supine without and with a Snore Guard or Thera Snore OA in place (38). Schwab et al. reevaluated the same data and found that the increase in cross-sectional area with OA was related to a reduction in the thickness of the lateral pharyngeal walls (39).

Oral appliances may modify upper airway function separate from an effect on airway anatomy. Lowe et al. showed that tongue EMG increased with OA insertion, suggesting that muscle tone and perhaps airway compliance might be modified by this intervention (33). Another possible mechanism independent of airway size may be stabilization of mandibular posture. Two recent publications describe downward rotation and retrusion of the mandible with sleep in seven normal subjects (40) and with sleep apnea in seven OSA patients (41). The percentage of total sleep time spent with the mandible open more than 5.0 mm was significantly larger in OSA patients (69.3%) than in healthy adults (11.1%). If these observations are generally applicable to OSA, then the prevention of mandibular rotation during sleep might be an important element in the treatment effect of OA. This concept could explain why some patients seem to derive benefit with relatively little mandibular advancement and without manifest change in airway size during wakefulness.

IV. Evidence of Effectiveness

Since the earliest reports, it has been clear that OA are capable of relieving OSA and also that they are not effective in every patient. The important questions then are what is the expected rate of treatment success and what factors account for success or failure. Considerable caution must be exercised in the interpretation of treatment success since different studies use different values for success such as a 50% or some other percent reduction of initial AHI, an AHI of less than 10 or 15 after treatment, and/or the inclusion of symptomatic improvement. In this review, an attempt has been made to provide criteria for success for each set of data presented. In a 1995 review of 19 published case series encompassing 304 patients, 70% of the patients had a 50% reduction of the AHI, and in 51% the AHI was reduced to 10 or less (8). Despite considerable variety in appliance design, the success rate was remarkably consistent. In eight case series published since that review, the success rates are similar to this earlier report (Table 2) (8,27,36,42–45). Another consistent finding is a significant failure rate as indicated by the proportion of patients with AHI > 20 after initial treatment; every case series includes treatment failures, the proportion ranging between 11 and 42% (8) (Table 2).

Treatment success appears to be related to sleep apnea severity. In all large case series, patients with higher AHI, defined as >30 (36), >50 (34), or >60 (46),

Table 2 Efficacy of OA Therapy in OSA

Patients	Appliance type	AHI without/ with OA	Treatment response[a] (%)			Lowest O_2 Sat% without/ with OA	Ref.
			<a	<b	>c		
304	MRD and tongue device, not adjustable	42.6/18.8	70	51	39		8
23	MRD, adjustable	37/18	70	52	22		27
38	MRD, adjustable	33/12	68	55	23		36
19	MRD, not adjustable	20/10	32	57	11	83/84	42
19	MRD, adjustable	25/14	42	42	16	79/76	43
21	MRD, not adjustable	34/20	38	14	42	84/90	44
44	MRD, not adjustable	—	52	64	—		45

All values are group means.
MRD = mandible repositioning device.
[a] a: 50% of initial AHI; b: AHI < 10; c: AHI > 20.

show a lower portion of treatment success compared with less severe patients. In another study of 44 patients, treatment success was inversely related to OSA severity graded as mild (AHI < 20), moderate (AHI 20–39), and severe (AHI 40+) (45). Although most case series consist of patients with mild to moderate disease, a sufficient number of severe cases have been described to support the conclusion that treatment success can be expected to be lower in such patients.

Several authors have examined the use of cephalometric parameters to predict treatment success. Mayer et al. correlated cephalograms in 30 OSA patients with response to OA treatment as indicated by polysomnography (17,29). Although several skeletal and soft tissue features could be associated with treatment success, the overlap between good and poor treatment response was substantial. Eveloff et al. included mandibular-hyoid distance, posterior airway space, and two skeletal parameters in a prediction formula that also included apnea/hypopnea frequency (28). The correlation between predicted and measured AHI was strong ($r = 0.86$). Both studies indicate a relation between upper airway anatomy and OA treatment success. What remains to be determined is whether and how these associations can be converted to a clinically useful rule.

Can appliance design be related to treatment success? Five of 19 papers before 1995 reported on one tongue appliance, the TRD; the remainder described the effect of various single jaw position mandible repositioners (MRD) (8). Two more recent studies have used an adjustable MRD appliance (36,43). When examined by several criteria of success or failure, no consistent difference appears among appliances classified in this manner. An exception may be the recently introduced adjustable appliances, which vary not only by appliance design but also the titration protocol. A more aggressive treatment protocol may result in a better success rate. An example may be a report of the Klearway appliance in which oximetry monitoring, together with snoring reduction and symptom improvement, were used to define the endpoint of appliance adjustment (36). In this study, treatment success (after treatment AHI < 15) was achieved in 80% of mild (AHI < 30) cases and in 61% of more severe (AHI 30+) cases. It is noteworthy that most earlier OA titration protocols used clinical symptoms as the endpoint, and this may account for an apparently higher proportion of treatment failures.

The effect of OA on oxygenation is less well studied, but it appears that the effect is less robust than the effect on the AHI (Table 2). Of particular interest are the several recent comparisons between OA and nCPAP in which minimum oxygen saturation and desaturation frequency were improved less with OA than with nCPAP (42,43). The effect of OA on sleep and sleepiness has also seen limited study. The evidence indicates, not surprisingly, that improvement in sleep parameters parallels the effect on AHI. Improvement in polygraphic sleep parameters was reported in the 1995 review and also in several of the more recent publications (27,43,45). Various ways are used to express the improvement including improved sleep efficiency, reduced proportion of stage 1 sleep, and increase in slow-wave and/or rapid eye movement (REM) sleep. Objectively measured sleepiness, by MWT, was improved in one study (27). Subjective sleepiness assessed by a validated symptom scale was improved in another study (43). Eight of 21 papers of the 1995 review evaluated sleepiness by patient report and found it to be reduced (8).

The effect of OA on snoring is excellent, with a substantially higher proportion of patients indicating a satisfactory result compared to the effect on AHI. In the 1995 review, each of nine papers reported improvement in the majority of patients, with six papers reporting some improvement in 100% of patients (8). For example, in 68 patients followed for an average of 7 months, all but one reported less snoring and 50% said it was totally relieved (34). In another study of 51 patients, objective recording documented reduced frequency and intensity of snoring (46). In that study, 44 of 48 patients had a more than minor effect on snoring and 15 of 23 couples who had slept apart for snoring resumed sleeping together.

Snoring can be associated with sleep disturbance in the absence of measurable apneas or hypopneas, the so-called upper airway resistance syndrome (47). The good effect of OA on snoring suggests that OA may be effective in this condition. A carefully documented case report of one patient demonstrated an improvement in inspiratory esophageal pressure with OA use (48). Further studies are needed in this area.

Limited data suggest that compliance with OA therapy is not perfect. To date, only data on patient reported compliance have been published (Table 3). However, experience with nCPAP suggests that patient reports tend to overestimate the actual use (49). Ferguson et al. revealed a 24% compliance failure rate with a single jaw appliance and a 5% compliance failure rate with a partially adjustable appliance (42,44). Based on a miniaturized covert compliance monitor embedded in the OA, Lowe et al. (36) reported compliance data from eight OSA subjects using the Klearway appliance and found that it was worn for a mean of 6.8 h per night with a range

Table 3 Compliance with OA Therapy in OSA

Patients	Appliance type	Follow-up duration (months)	Use %	Ref.
233	MRD and tongue, fixed	3–36+	100–50	8
23	MRD, adjustable	41	70	27
25	MRD, adjustable	4	76	42
20	MRD, adjustable	4	95	43
21	MRD, fixed	3–10	81	44

of 5.6–7.5 h. The reasons for limited compliance are not well defined, but several authors (8) have implicated variable efficacy and discomfort, especially with single jaw position appliances.

The safety of OA therapy has not been systematically studied. The potential for injury to the temporomandibular joint (TMJ) and to teeth is one consideration. Stress on these structures defines the limits of maximal mandibular repositioning. Experience with nonadjustable appliances, particularly in the setting of clinical studies, has been good, with infrequent occurrence of pain or occlusive changes. Nevertheless, both problems have been cited as reasons for treatment failure (8). For example, dental or jaw ''discomfort'' was reported with nonadjustable OAs in 48% and 67% of two large series (34,46). The more aggressive treatment protocols associated with adjustable appliances might be expected to produce a greater incidence of complications, but experience to date has not found this to be the case (34). The importance of supervision and long-term follow-up has not been investigated, although these are essential elements of a practice guideline because of concern of injury (9).

V. Commonly Used Appliances

Appliance design variations may have a direct effect on treatment outcome for any specific patient, and the advantages and disadvantages of each design vary considerably. For this review, three appliances which are in most common usage will be reviewed in depth—the Snore Guard, the Tongue Retaining Device, and the Klearway. For more complete overviews of the range of appliances currently used, the reader is directed to three previously published reviews (7,8,50). Many but not all currently marketed appliances have obtained Federal Drug Administration (FDA) marketing clearance for snoring and/or OSA. This process does not require proof of clinical efficacy, but it does assure some level of review for safety, which may be important in a therapy with a potential for injury if improperly used.

The Snore Guard appliance is a prefabricated OA lined with a soft thermosensitive material that allows molding to the patient's teeth (Fig. 1). The Snore Guard engages the mandible mainly at the incisors and, therefore, applies the force of ad-

Snore Guard

Tongue Retaining Device

Klearway

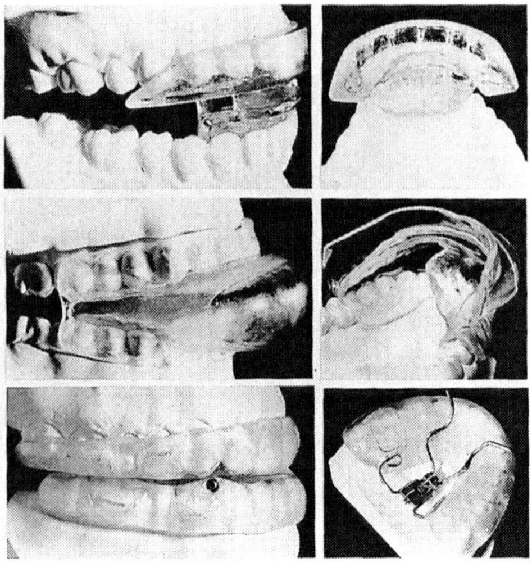

Figure 1 Lateral and single arch views of the Snore Guard, Tongue Retaining Device, and Klearway™ appliances.

vancement to fewer teeth than appliances with full occlusal coverage. Several reports have documented its usefulness in the treatment of snoring and OSA (34,51–53). Ferguson et al. compared the efficacy, side effects, patient compliance, and preference between 4 months of Snore Guard and nCPAP therapies in a randomized, prospective crossover study in patients with mild-to-moderate OSA (42). The AHI was lower with nCPAP (3.5 ± 1.6) than with the OA (9.7 ± 7.3). Some 48% of the patients who used the Snore Guard were treatment successes (reduction of AHI to <10/h and relief of symptoms), 24% were compliance failures (unable or unwilling to use the treatment), and 28% were treatment failures (failure to reduce AHI to <10/h and/or failure to relieve symptoms). Four people refused to use nCPAP after using the Snore Guard. Some 62% of the patients who used nCPAP were overall treatment successes, 38% were compliance failures, and there were no treatment failures. Side effects were more common and the patients were less satisfied with nCPAP. Seven patients were treatment successes with both treatments; six of these patients preferred Snore Guard and one preferred nCPAP as a long-term treatment. The Snore Guard is an effective treatment in some patients with mild-to-moderate OSA and is associated with fewer side effects and greater patient satisfaction than nCPAP. The advantages of the Snore Guard are its relatively low cost and reduced chair time. However, it is nonadjustable, it may apply excessive pressure to the lower anterior teeth in some patients, and retention problems may develop over time.

The Tongue Retaining Device (TRD) is a custom-made appliance with an anterior bulb (Fig. 1) that holds the tongue by means of negative pressure in a forward position during sleep (54). The TRD has been evaluated in various sleep positions and in conjunction with other forms of treatment (55,56). The TRD has different effects on the awake genioglossus muscle activity in control subjects and patients with OSA (57). The TRD reduces the AHI, normalizes the genioglossus muscle time lag before an apneic event, and counteracts fluctuating genioglossus EMG activity observed when no bulb is present (58). In summary, the TRD reduces genioglossus muscle activity in awake OSA patients and corrects the delayed timing of the muscle before an apneic period during sleep. Currently, the TRD appears to be the appliance of choice for patients who have limited or no teeth and in those subjects who have large tongues. In addition, the TRD is a good appliance for those patients who cannot adequately advance their mandible for whatever reason. Its disadvantages are that it is more difficult for both clinicians and patients to use on a regular basis, it poses problems for patients who cannot breathe through their nose, and it is a single jaw and tongue position appliance, i.e., it is not adjustable.

With increasing clinical experience, clinicians soon identified a need for an OA that could be adjusted and did not require a series of remakes if the initial jaw position was not adequately positioned forward. In addition, the need to develop an appliance with greater retention, which allowed both vertical and lateral jaw movements during sleep, was apparent. The Herbst appliance (6) holds the mandible in a forward position by means of a plunger-like mechanism. Eveloff et al. (28) documented a decrease in the mean AHI from 34.7 to 12.9 with the Herbst appliance. In a crossover study, Clark et al. (44) found that the mean pretreatment AHI decreased 38.9% with the Herbst appliance and 59.5% with nCPAP. The Silencer, an adjustable appliance with a hinge positioned lingual to the lower incisors that allows progressive advancement of the mandible, was evaluated by Ferguson et al. (43). A prospective, crossover study was designed to compare efficacy, side effects, patient compliance, and preference between 4 months of wear of the Silencer and nCPAP in patients with symptomatic mild to moderate OSA. The AHI was lower with nCPAP (4.2/h) than with the adjustable OA (13.6/h). Of the patients who used the adjustable OA, 55% were treatment successes (reduction of AHI to ≤10/h and relief of symptoms), 5% were a compliance failure (unable or unwilling to use the treatment), and 40% were treatment failures (failure to reduce AHI to ≤10/h and/or failure to relieve symptoms). Some 70% of the patients who used nCPAP were treatment successes, 30% were compliance failures, and there were no treatment failures. Adjustable OAs are an effective treatment in some patients with mild to moderate OSA and are associated with greater patient satisfaction than nCPAP.

The Klearway appliance (Fig. 1) was designed to remove the hinge apparatus from behind the lower incisors (so as to not encroach on tongue space) and to incorporate a total of 44 0.25 mm increments of mandibular advancement to improve patient tolerance.* In addition, the material was changed to a temperature-sensitive

---

* The Klearway appliance was invented by Alan A. Lowe at The University of British Columbia. International patents have been obtained by the university, and specific licensees are assigned the rights to manufacture and distribute the appliance worldwide.

acrylic resin to increase retention particularly in those patients who did not have a full complement of teeth or who had teeth without natural undercuts. Lowe et al. have evaluated the effect of the Klearway appliance on the AHI and airway size in a series of 38 OSA patients recruited at three sites across Canada (36). The mean AHI before treatment was 32.6, and after the insertion of the Klearway appliance the AHI was reduced to 12.1. AHI was reduced to less than 15 in 80% of a group of moderate OSA patients (AHI 15–30) and in 61% of a group of severe OSA patients (AHI>30). Lui et al. (31) identified a reduction in the mean AHI from 33.4 to 11.2 in a sample of OSA patients and found a better response in younger subjects. In another report, Liu et al. (31) divided subjects into three groups based on the degree of change in the AHI after insertion of the Klearway appliance; good responders (13/47) had more than a 75% decrease in AHI, moderate responders (25/47) had a 25–75% decrease in AHI, and poor responders (9/47) had a <25% decrease in AHI. Good responders were found to be younger and have smaller upper airways. Using awake videoendoscopy at end-tidal expiration during quiet nasal breathing in the supine position, Ryan et al. documented that the size of the velopharynx and hypopharynx increased with the Klearway appliance in place, but no significant differences in the oropharynx could be identified (59). The lateral diameter of the velopharynx increased more than the anteroposterior dimension. In conclusion, the Klearway adjustable anterior mandibular advancement appliance significantly reduces the AHI in a cross section of OSA patients and directly affects airway size. It appears to reduce OSA severity by keeping the velopharynx patent especially in the lateral dimension. The advantages of the Klearway appliance are increased retention because of the thermoactive material used in its construction, the inclusion of vertical and lateral jaw movements, and the option of a significant number of mandibular positions that can be evaluated over time for adequate titration.

Although treatment success as measured by a relative decrease in AHI or an improvement in oxygen saturation appears to be better with nCPAP than with OA (Table 4), patients when offered either therapy after having used both in a controlled study have clearly chosen an OA. The total number of patients who chose either nCPAP or an OA in Table 4 does not equal the initial number of participants because of dropouts. The preference for OA therapy may be for several reasons—convenience, sound, power supply needs, claustrophobia, and airway irritation. Ferguson et al. found with the Snore Guard (42) and the Silencer (43) that the majority of

Table 4 Comparison of nCPAP and OA Effectiveness and Patient Preference in OSA

Appliance	Patients (N)	Baseline AHI	Therapy AHI nCPAP	Therapy AHI OA	Preference nCPAP	Preference OA	Ref.
Snore Guard	25	19.7	3.6	9.7	3	17	42
Silencer	20	25.3	4.0	14.2	6	11	43
Herbst	23	33.8	13.7	20.7	1	19	44

patients chose an OA. Clark et al. found a similar OA preference with the Herbst appliance (44). Strong preferences for OA have been identified in all three studies where patients have experienced both forms of therapy.

VI. Protocol for OA Use

The American Academy of Sleep Medicine (AASM) has developed practice guidelines for OA use for the treatment of snoring and OSA (9). Based on a contemporaneous review of the literature (8), these guidelines state that all patients considered for OA therapy should have a competent medical evaluation for OSA. Comparison of the risk and benefit of OA therapy with the other available treatments suggests that OA present a useful alternative to nCPAP, especially for patients with simple snoring and patients with OSA who cannot tolerate nCPAP therapy. The ASDA recommended that OA should be used for primary snoring or mild OSA for patients where behavioral measures such as weight control or sleep position are or have been ineffective. Nasal CPAP should be tried first in patients with moderate to severe OSA, but OA are indicated for these patients if nCPAP or surgery is refused or found not to be successful. Follow-up polysomnography or another objective measurement of respiration during sleep with the OA in place should be undertaken in moderate and severe OSA patients. Follow-up care by both the sleep physician and the dentist to monitor success and evaluate the development of any complications was also recommended.

The Academy of Dental Sleep Medicine (ADSM), a group of dentists with special interest in OA therapy, have produced a protocol that is very similar but provides greater detail regarding the initial dental examination and the process of appliance selection, fabrication, and adjustment. A medical assessment by the attending physician or a sleep specialist occurs before a written report/prescription and diagnostic report is sent to the dentist. A dental examination would consist of a medical and dental history, a soft tissue and intraoral assessment, a periodontal evaluation, a temporomandibular joint and occlusal examination, an intraoral habit/parafunction assessment, a detailed examination of the teeth and all restorations, and the collection of radiographs and models as required. An oral appliance is selected that, in the opinion of the clinician, is best suited for that particular patient. No one appliance can be used for all patients and attempts to implement therapy may on occasion require more than one appliance in the same patient. The selected appliance is designed, constructed by a dental laboratory, and fitted for the patient. Patient instructions are given at the time of insertion, and the appliance is adjusted for adequate retention and comfort. When the patient has accommodated to the appliance, gradual titration (forward mandibular positioning) over several months may be required to advance the mandible to an advanced forward position, which is comfortable for the patient and adequate to relieve the snoring and/or sleep apnea. Reports from the bed partner as to changes in the frequency or level of snoring are often used to evaluate the effectiveness of the appliance at this stage. If the patient also feels more rested, the dentist will refer him or her back to the attending physician or sleep specialist for assessment. A possible redesign, modification, or remake of the OA may be required for some patients depending on the physician's assessment of the success of the initial OA treatment. OA patients should be seen on a regular basis over the first 12 months of OA wear to ensure adequate retention and comfort of the appliance.

Neither the ASDA nor the SDDS guidelines address the complex issue of the titration of mandibular position to the extent now possible with modern adjustable appliances. Although no studies have evaluated how this should be done, a developing consensus among practitioners is that optimal treatment, in conjunction with the reduction of snoring and an improvement in symptoms, requires that titration be monitored with objective measures of OSA. Since it is impractical to perform polysomnography repeatedly for this purpose, a home monitor, such as oximetry or more complex systems, seems more suitable. In addition, several investigators have reported preliminary experience with titration of optimal mandibular advancement in the sleep laboratory. Although this is technically feasible, the way that this information might be fully incorporated into a treatment protocol remains to be clarified.

VII. Future Studies

Although OA usage and effectiveness have both greatly increased in the last 5 years, many clinical and research questions remain unanswered. If it were possible to determine the correct jaw position required to adequately open the airway prior to the insertion of the appliance, titration procedures would be greatly simplified. Currently, determining the correct jaw position for mandibular repositioners and the correct tongue posture for TRD appliances is highly subjective and varies a great deal between clinicians. Part of this variability is due to the inability to accurately determine clinically where the airway obstruction(s) is/are located. Although traditional cephalometry can predict with some accuracy the volume of the tongue, soft palate, and nasopharynx, it is not a reliable indicator of oropharynx or hypopharynx size (60). Because the airway obstruction is most commonly seen in the collapsible oropharynx, computed tomography (CT) or magnetic resonance imaging techniques appear superior to two-dimensional cephalometry for this structure (61,62). Three-dimensional evaluations of tongue, soft palate, and airway may be of significant clinical usefulness in the differential diagnosis of patients with OSA. If the obstruction is in the oropharynx and a large soft palate volume is observed, uvulopalatopharyngoplasty may be useful. If a small oropharynx is observed, any appliance that could enlarge the airway by either advancing the tongue alone or advancing the mandible and the tongue together could be useful. If a disproportionately large tongue is seen, a TRD could be effective. The TRD is even more effective if it is used in conjunction with behavioral modifications. Several mandibular advancement appliances are effective in changing the three-dimensional size of the airway tube. OA have an effect on the tongue muscle by advancing the mandible, holding the tongue forward, or altering the vertical dimension and thus affecting baseline tongue activity (33,63).

Other more general areas warrant further study. Questions of OA compliance remain to be answered. How many hours per night does the average patient wear the appliance? How many nights per week/per month are the appliances worn? What treatment response factors determine compliance? Are adjustability and retention important? Is the initial OSA severity an important factor? How does OA compliance compare to nCPAP? The combined effects of UPP surgery, nCPAP, weight loss, and OA wear are unknown, although many patients have tried all or some combination of these treatment modalities. A careful designed clinical trial to evaluate the effects of combination therapy is required. Finally, a long-term follow-up study of the effects of OA use on the dentition and the temporomandibular joint is indicated.

VIII. Summary

OA are effective in varying degrees and appear to work because of an increase in airway space, the provision of a stable anterior position of the mandible, the advancement of the tongue or soft palate, and possibly a change in genioglossus muscle activity. OA therapy for snoring and OSA is simple, reversible, and quiet and may be indicated in patients who are unable to tolerate nCPAP or who are poor surgical risks. The appliance should be used during sleep for life, must be comfortable for the patient, and ideally should have full occlusal coverage to prevent vertical changes to the dentition over time. The attending physician must always make the selection of which patients are potentially suitable for dental appliance therapy. The dentist then selects which dental appliance to use and titrates the OA over time before follow-up by the attending sleep physician. With the currently available adjustable appliances, gradual titration over several weeks and/or months may be required for some subjects. Increased retention with temperature-sensitive acrylic materials and the ability to move the lower jaw laterally and vertically has significantly increased patient comfort and cooperation and the effectiveness of treatment.

References

1. Young T, Palta M, Dempsey J, Skatrud J, Weber S, Badr S. The occurrence of sleep-disordered breathing among middle-aged adults. N Engl J Med 1993; 328:1230–1235.
2. Gastaut H, Tassinari CA, Duron B. Etude polygraphique des manifestations episodiques (hypniques et respiratoires), diurnes et nocturnes, du syndrome de Pickwick. Rev Neurol 1965; 115:456.
3. Guilleminault C, Dement WC, eds. Sleep Apnea Syndromes. New York: A. R. Liss, 1978.
4. Lavie P, Herer P, Peled R, Berger I, Yoffe N, Zomer J, Rubin A. Mortality in sleep apnea patients: a multivariate analysis of risk factors. Sleep 1995; 18:149–157.

5. Kuhlo W, Doll E, Frank C. Erfolgreiche Behandlung eines Pickwick Syndromes durch Dauertracheakanuele. Dtsch Med Wochenschr 1969; 94:1286–1290.
6. Clark GT, Nakano M. Dental appliances for the treatment of obstructive sleep apnea. J Am Dent Assoc 1989; 118:611–618.
7. Lowe AA. Dental appliances for the treatment of snoring and obstructive sleep apnea. In: Kryger M, Roth T, Dement W, eds. Principles and Practice of Sleep Medicine, 2d ed. Philadelphia: WB Saunders Co, 1994:722–735.
8. Schmidt-Nowara W, Lowe AA, Wiegand L, Cartwright R, Perez-Guerra F, Menn S. Oral appliances for the treatment of snoring and obstructive sleep apnea: a review. Sleep 1995; 18:501–510.
9. American Sleep Disorders Association Standards of Practice Committee. Practice parameters for the treatment of snoring and obstructive sleep apnea with oral appliances. Sleep 1995; 18:511–513.
10. Robin P. Glossoptosis due to atresia and hypotrophy of the mandible. Am J Dis Child 1934; 48:541–547.
11. Boraz R, Martin H, Michel J. Sleep apnea syndrome: report of case. J Dent Child 1979; 46:50–52.
12. Meier-Ewert K, Schafer H, Kloe W. Treatment of sleep apnea by a mandibular protracting device. Berichtsband 7th European Congress on Sleep Research. Munich, Germany, 1984, p. 217.
13. Cartwright R, Samelson C. The effects of a nonsurgical treatment for obstructive sleep apnea—the tongue-retaining device. JAMA 1982; 248:705–709.
14. Sjoholm TT, Piha S, Mantyvaara J, Lehtinen I, Polo O, Lowe AA. Spectral analysis of circulation in teethgrinders: correlation with masseter activity during sleep. J Dent Res. In press.
15. Will MJ, Ester MS, Ramirez SG, Tiner BD, McAnear JT, Epstein L. Comparison of cephalometric analysis with ethnicity in obstructive sleep apnea syndrome. Sleep 1995; 18:873–875.
16. Lowe AA, Ono T, Ferguson KA, Pae E-K, Ryan CF, Fleetham JA. Cephalometric comparisons of craniofacial and upper airway structure by skeletal subtype and gender in patients with obstructive sleep apnea. Am J Orthod Dentofac Orthop 1996; 110:653–664.
17. Mayer P, Pepin J-L, Bettega G, Veale D, Ferretti G, Deschaux C, Levy P. Relationship between body mass index, age and upper airway measurements in snorers and sleep apnoea patients. Eur Respir J 1996; 9:1801–1809.
18. Battagel JM, L'Estrange PR. The cephalometric morphology of patients with obstructive sleep apnoea (OSA). Eur J Orthod 1996; 18:557–569.
19. Solow B, Skov S, Ovesen J, Norup PW, Wildschiedtz G. Airway dimensions and head posture in obstructive sleep apnoea. Eur J Orthod 1996; 18:571–579.
20. Solow B, Ovesen J, Nielson PW, Wildschiedtz G, Tallgren A. Head posture in obstructive sleep apnoea. Eur J Orthod 1993; 15:107–114.
21. Tangugsorn V, Skatvedt O, Krogstad O, Lyberg T. Obstructive sleep apnoea: a cephalometric study. Part I. Cervico-craniofacial skeletal morphology. Eur J Orthod 1995; 17: 45–56.
22. Ozbek M, Miyamoto K, Lowe AA, Fleetham JA. Natural head posture, upper airway morphology and obstructive sleep apnea severity in adults. Eur J Orthod 1998: 20:133–143.
23. Pracharktam N, Nelson S, Hans MG, Broadbent BH, Redline S, Rosenberg C, Strohl

KP. Cephalometric assessment in obstructive sleep apnea. Am J Orthod Dentofac Orthop 1996; 109:410–419.
24. Lowe AA, Özbek MM, Miyamoto K, Pae E-K, Fleetham JA. Cephalometric and demographic characteristics of obstructive sleep apnea: an evaluation with partial least squares analysis. Angle Orthod 1997; 67:143–154.
25. Tangugsorn V, Skatvedt O, Krogstad O, Lyberg T. Obstructive sleep apnoea: a cephalometric study. Part II. Uvulo-glossopharyngeal morphology. Eur J Orthod 1995; 17:57–67.
26. Miyamoto K, Özbek MM, Lowe AA, Fleetham JA. Effect of body position on tongue posture in awake patients with obstructive sleep apnea. Thorax 1997; 52:255–259.
27. Menn SJ, Loube DI, Morgan TD, Mitler MM, Berger JS, Erman MK. The mandibular repositioning device: role in the treatment of obstructive sleep apnea. Sleep 1996; 19(10):794–800.
28. Eveloff SE, Rosenberg CL, Carlisle CC, Millman RP. Efficacy of a Herbst mandibular advancement device in obstructive sleep apnea. Am J Respir Crit Care Med 1994; 149: 905–909.
29. Mayer G, Meier-Ewert K. Cephalometric predictors for orthopaedic mandibular advancement in obstructive sleep apnoea. Eur J Orthod 1995; 17:35–43.
30. Liu Y, Lowe AA, Fleetham JA, Park Y. Cephalometric and physiological predictors of the efficacy of an adjustable oral appliance for the treatment of obstructive sleep apnea. Am J Orthod Dentofacial Orthop 2001; 120:639–647.
31. Liu Y, Park Y, Lowe AA, Fleetham JA. Supine cephalometric analysis of an adjustable oral appliance used in the treatment of obstructive sleep apnea. Sleep Breathing 2000; 4:59–66.
32. Bonham PE, Currier GF, Orr WC, Othman J, Nanda RS. The effect of a modified functional appliance on obstructive sleep apnea. Am J Orthod Dentofac Orthop 1988; 94: 384–392.
33. Lowe AA, Fleetham JA, Ryan CF, Matthews B. Effects of mandibular repositioning appliance used in the treatment of obstructive sleep apnea on tongue muscle activity. In: Suratt PM, Remmers JE, eds. Sleep and Respiration. New York: Wiley-Liss, 1990: 395–405.
34. Schmidt-Nowara W, Meade T, Hays M. Treatment of snoring and obstructive sleep apnea with a dental orthosis. Chest 1991; 99:1378–1385.
35. Johnson LM, Arnett GW, Tanborello JA, Binder A. Airway changes in relationship to mandibular posturing. Otolaryngol Head Neck Surg 1992; 106:143–148.
36. Lowe AA, Sjöholm TT, Ryan CF, Fleetham JA, Ferguson KA, Remmers JE. Treatment, airway and compliance effects of a titratable oral appliance. Sleep 2000; 23(Suppl 4): 172–178.
37. Ferguson KA, Love LL, Ryan CF. Effect of mandibular and tongue protrusion on upper airway size during wakefulness. Am Rev Respir Dis 1997; 155:1748–1754.
38. Schmidt-Nowara WW, Williamson MS, Olivera DL, Meade TE. The effect of a dental appliance for snoring on upper airway anatomy. Am Rev Respir Dis 1993; 147:682A.
39. Schwab RJ, Gupta KB, Duong D, Schmidt-Nowara WW, Pack AI, Gefter WB. Upper airway soft tissue structural changes with dental appliances in apneics. Am J Respir Crit Care Med 1996; 153:A719.
40. Miyamoto K, Ozbek M, Lowe AA, Sjoholm TT, Love LL, Fleetham JA, Ryan CF. Mandibular posture during sleep in healthy adults. Arch Oral Biol 1998; 43:269–275.

41. Miyamoto K, Ozbek M, Lowe AA, Sjoholm TT, Love LL, Fleetham JA, Ryan CF. Mandibular posture during sleep in patients with obstructive sleep apnea. Arch Oral Biol 1999; 44:657–664.
42. Ferguson KA, Ono T, Lowe AA, Keenan SP, Fleetham JA. A randomized crossover study of an oral appliance vs. nasal-continuous positive airway pressure in the treatment of mild-moderate obstructive sleep apnea. Chest 1996; 109:1269–1275.
43. Ferguson KA, Ono T, Lowe AA, Al-Majed S, Love LL, Fleetham JA. A short term controlled trial of an adjustable oral appliance for the treatment of mild-moderate obstructive sleep apnea. Thorax 1997; 52:362–368.
44. Clark GT, Blumenfeld I, Yoffe N, Peled E, Lavie P. A crossover study comparing the efficacy of continuous positive airway pressure with anterior mandibular positioning devices on patients with obstructive sleep apnea. Chest 1996; 109:1477–1483.
45. Marklund M, Franklin KA, Sahlin C, Ludgren R. The effect of a mandibular advancement device on apneas and sleep in patients with obstructive sleep apnea. Chest 1998; 113:707–713.
46. O'Sullivan RA, Hillman DR, Mateljan R, Pantin C, Finucane KE. Mandibular advancement splint: an appliance to treat snoring and obstructive sleep apnea. Am J Respir Crit Care Med 1995; 151:194–198.
47. Guilleminault C, Stoohs R, Duncan S. Snoring (I). Daytime sleepiness in regular snorers. Chest 1991; 99:40–48.
48. Loube DI, Andrada T, Shanmagum N, Singer M. Successful treatment of upper airway resistance syndrome with an oral appliance. Sleep Breathing 1997; 2:97–101.
49. Kribbs NB, Pack AI, Kline LR, et al. Objective measurement of patterns of nasal CPAP use by patients with obstructive sleep apnea. Am Rev Respir Dis 1993; 147:887–895.
50. Rogers R, Lowe AA. Oral appliances for the management of snoring and obstructive sleep apnea—a comprehensive guide for the sleep disorder dentist. Slide/Tape sequence for the Sleep Disorders Dental Society, 1997.
51. Dushell M, Baldock P, Antic R, et al. Obligatory nasal breathing: effects on snoring and sleep apnea. Med J Aust 1991; 155:83–85.
52. Menn S, Berger J, Morgan T. Efficacy of a jaw advancement device in the treatment of sleep apnea: nighttime and daytime polysomnography. Sleep Res 1992; 21:231.
53. Hans MG, Nelson S, Luks VG, Lorkovich P, Baek S-J. Comparison of two dental devices for treatment of obstructive sleep apnea syndrome (OSAS). Am J Orthod Dentofac Orthop 1997; 111:562–570.
54. Samelson C. The role of the tongue retaining device in treatment of snoring and obstructive apnea. CDS Rev 1988; October:44–47.
55. Cartwright R, Stefoski D, Caldarelli D, et al. Toward a treatment logic for sleep apnea: the place of the tongue retaining device. Behav Res Ther 1988; 26:121–126.
56. Cartwright R, Ristanovic R, Diaz F, et al. A comparative study of treatments for positional sleep apnea. Sleep 1991; 14:546–552.
57. Ono T, Lowe AA, Ferguson KA, Pae E-K, Fleetham JA. The effect of the tongue retaining device on awake genioglossus muscle activity in patients with obstructive sleep apnea. Am J Orthod Dentofac Orthop 1996; 110:28–35.
58. Onto T, Lowe AA, Ferguson KA, Fleetham JA. A tongue retaining device and sleep-state genioglossus muscle activity in patients with obstructive sleep apnea. Angle Orthod 1996; 66:273–280.
59. Ryan CF, Love LL, Peat D, Fleetham JA, Lowe AA. Mandibular advancement oral

appliance therapy for obstructive sleep apnea: effect on awake caliber of the velopharynx. Thorax 1999; 54:972–977.
60. Lowe AA, Fleetham JA. Two- and three-dimensional analysis of tongue, airway and soft palate size. In: Norton ML, Brown AC, eds. Atlas of the Difficult Airway. Chicago: Year Book Medical Publishers, 1991:74–82.
61. Lowe AA, Gionhaku N, Takeuchi K, Fleetham JA. Three dimensional CT reconstructions of tongue and airway in adult subjects with obstructive sleep apnea. Am J Orthod Dentofac Orthop 1986; 90:364–374.
62. Lowe AA, Fleetham JA, Adachi S, Ryan CF. Cephalometric and CT predictors of apnea index severity. Am J Orthod Dentofac Orthop 1995; 107:589–595.
63. Lowe AA. Neural control of tongue posture. In: Taylor A, ed. Neurophysiology of the Jaws and Teeth. London: McMillan Press Ltd, 1990:322–368.

20

Upper Airway Surgery for Obstructive Sleep Apnea

AARON E. SHER

Albany Medical College
Albany, New York

ANDREW N. GOLDBERG

University of California, San Francisco
San Francisco, California

I. Introduction

Treatment for obstructive sleep apnea syndrome (OSAS) is aimed at reducing morbidity and mortality from the consequences of sleep-disordered breathing associated with this syndrome. Obstructive sleep apnea rarely regresses and commonly progresses during the life of the patient, necessitating long-term treatment that is well tolerated and effective. In order to achieve the desired goals of improved health and quality of life for patients in the long term, it is necessary to match the suggested therapy to patient tolerance and preference.

Numerous treatment options are available for patients with OSAS. These include weight loss for obese patients, nasal continuous positive airway pressure (CPAP), dental appliances, and surgical therapy. Such treatments have been shown to be effective in certain patient populations or certain individuals and to positively impact some consequences of the disease. Clearly, patients should be made aware of these treatment options and should, with the physician, embark on a treatment plan. For example, in patients whose OSAS has its origin in obesity, weight loss represents an ideal option for treatment. It has positive impact on OSAS and on numerous other pathological processes. Unfortunately, few patients are able to lose the necessary weight and maintain the achieved ideal weight for a sustained period of time. Similarly, covert compliance data have shown that while a segment of patients with OSAS can tolerate nasal CPAP therapy, a significant percentage of patients cannot. These patients may misrepresent their noncompliance to the physician, leaving them untreated. For sustained therapy, dental appliances have been shown to be better tolerated than nasal CPAP but are not universally tolerated and are not universally effective.

Surgical therapy is minimally dependent on patient compliance for long-term success. While some incidence of recidivism exists when followed over time, the results of surgical therapy are generally lasting. Surgical therapy is not without its drawbacks, however, as it requires permanent changes to the upper aerodigestive track and can alter the appearance and function of the patient. As with all therapies, complications or untoward effects can occur. Furthermore, surgical therapy is not universally effective and may require serial procedures for effectiveness. Despite these shortcomings, many patients opt for surgical therapy and are rewarded with effective treatment that requires no ongoing maintenance.

II. Rationale and Overall Strategy for Upper Airway Surgery

Upper airway surgical treatments for OSAS either attempt to modify dysfunctional pharyngeal anatomy or bypass the pharynx (tracheotomy). Modifications to the pharynx diminish the bulk of soft tissue structures that impinge on the air column or alter the position, stiffness, or configuration of those structures creating an enlarged air column with less collapse. The former goal is achieved through removal of pharyngeal soft tissue. The latter goals are typically accomplished indirectly, by modifying the facial skeleton from which the soft tissues are suspended.

In the small percentage of patients with OSAS who possess specific space-occupying pathological lesions, surgical removal of these lesions is corrective. In the remaining patients with OSAS, the ''disproportionate anatomy'' of the upper airway and its supporting skeletal structures is likely responsible for OSAS. The configuration and dimensions of the airway are determined by the size and shape of soft tissue structures that surround the pharyngeal airway (such as faucial and lingual tonsils, tongue, soft palate), their spatial orientation and degree of mucosal overlap. That orientation is determined by the muscle planes that serve as support of the pharynx and, therefore, by the location of the origins and insertions of those muscles in the vertebral and craniofacial skeleton. The relative location of these origins and insertions is, in turn, determined by craniofacial skeletal characteristics of the patient (1–3).

The pharynx has properties that are shared with other collapsible biological conduits. Collapse occurs at a discrete ($<$1 cm) locus. Data derived from studies of the pharynx with awake endoscopy, awake endoscopy with Müller maneuver, asleep (drug-induced) endoscopy, asleep (natural and drug-induced) endoscopy with continuous positive airway pressure (CPAP), asleep fluoroscopy, computed tomo-

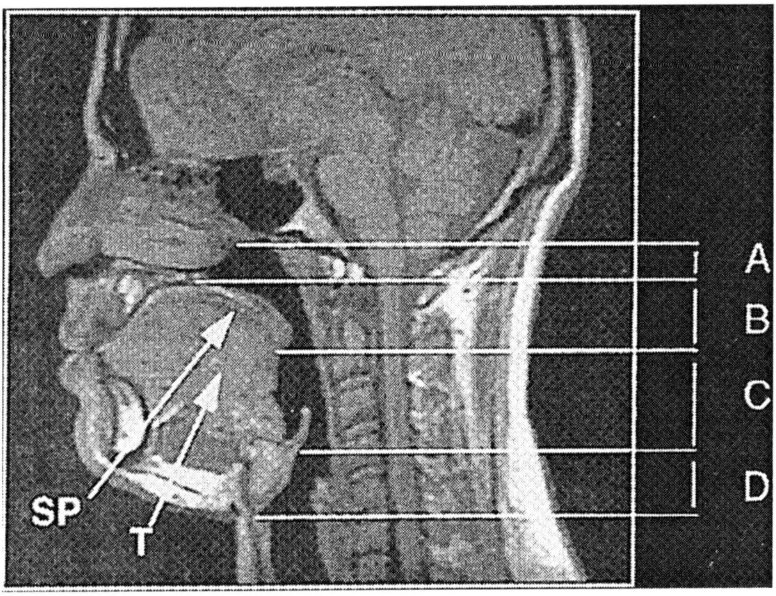

Figure 1 Sagittal MRI image of the pharynx. A—the nasopharynx; B—the retropalatal pharynx located posterior to the soft palate; C—the retrolingual pharynx located posterior to the vertical portion of the tongue; D—remainder of hypopharynx below the level of the tongue; SP—soft palate; T—tongue. (From Ref. 66.)

graphic (CT) scan, and manometry suggest that the pattern of static pharyngeal narrowing and/or dynamic pharyngeal collapse is localized and patient specific (3–5).

The pattern of pharyngeal narrowing or collapse has been demonstrated to be related to the degree of effectiveness of specific surgical procedures. This led to the division of the pharynx into two somewhat overlapping regions: (1) the retropalatal pharynx located posterior to the soft palate and (2) the retrolingual pharynx located posterior to the vertical portion of the tongue (Fig. 1). Based on this paradigm, patterns of pharyngeal narrowing or collapse are classified in the following manner. Type I narrowing or collapse involves only the retropalatal region. Type II involves both the retropalatal and retrolingual regions, and Type III is limited to the retrolingual region (6). This interpretation of the anatomical distribution of the obstructive tendency in OSAS has been fundamental to the development of contemporary surgical strategies (2,7).

III. Upper Airway Surgical Procedures

Classic otorhinolaryngological techniques to enlarge the nasal or pharyngeal airways, such as nasal septal reconstruction, turbinate mucosal cauterization and outfracture and tonsillectomy frequently fail to correct OSAS in adults (7). Several reports on highly selected use of tonsillectomy alone in adults report that in the selected population with OSAS and tonsillar hypertrophy, tonsillectomy alone is effective in reducing Respiratory Disturbance Index (RDI) and symptoms of OSAS (8–10). In one small recent series of nine patients, eight were cured of their OSAS by tonsillectomy alone (10). Because of the lack of applicability of these procedures for the vast majority of patients with OSAS, new surgical approaches were developed. Some involve extirpation of pharyngeal soft tissue, while others modify the position of pharyngeal soft tissue structures through mobilization and repositioning of the skeletal structures to which they attach.

A. Surgical Techniques Involving Extirpation of Soft Tissue

The most commonly used technique is uvulopalatopharyngoplasty (UPPP), which enlarges the retropalatal airway by excision of the tonsils if they are present, trimming and reorientation of the posterior and anterior tonsillar pillars, and excision of the uvula and posterior portion of the palate (11) (Fig. 2). This is the most common procedure performed today for obstructive sleep apnea.

Laser-assisted uvulopalatoplasty (LAUP) enlarges the retropalatal airway by ablation of the uvula and posterior margin of the soft palate with carbon dioxide laser. While tonsil ablation can be accomplished with laser, LAUP, as reported, frequently does not include tonsil ablation. Unlike other procedures described herein,

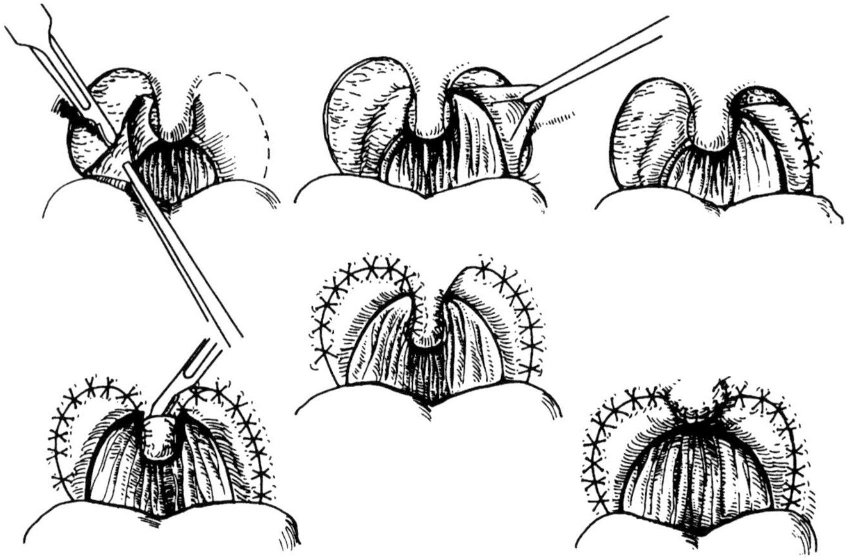

Figure 2 Technique for uvulopalatopharyngoplasty (UPPP). Redundant tissue of the soft palate and uvula are trimmed, advanced anteriorly and sutured to form an arch. (From Ref. 11.)

LAUP is generally performed under topical and local anesthesia in the setting of a physician's office (12) (Fig. 3). This procedure is commonly used for mild OSAS or primary snoring in a patient with suitable anatomy.

Uvulopalatopharyngo-glossoplasty (UPPGP) combines modified UPPP with additional limited resection of the tongue base, thereby enlarging both retropalatal and retrolingual portions of the airway (13,14) (Fig. 4). While this procedure has theoretical advantages, it has not gained wide acceptance for its use.

Laser midline glossectomy (LMG) and lingualplasty represent variations of a procedure that enlarges the retrolingual airway by laser extirpation of a 2.5 cm × 5 cm midline rectangular strip of posterior tongue. Laser lingual tonsillectomy, reduction of the aryepiglottic folds, and partial epiglottectomy are performed in selected patients. Lingualplasty differs from LMG in that additional tongue tissue is

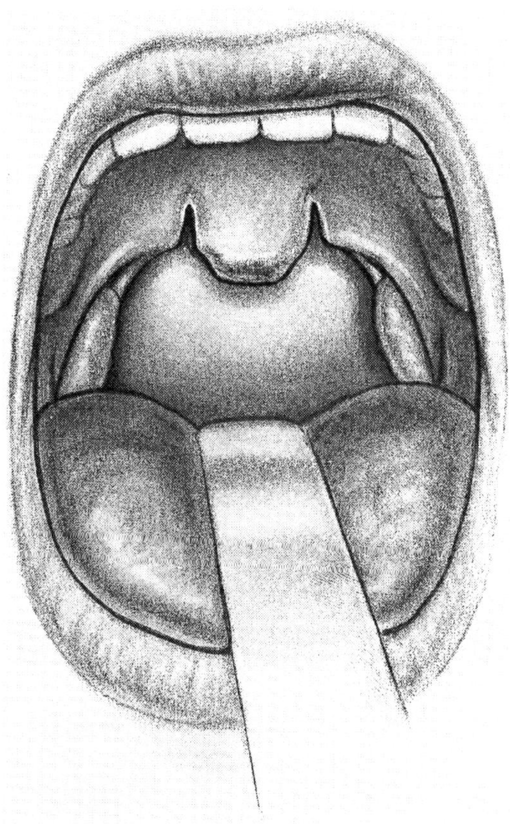

Figure 3 Laser-assisted uvulopalatoplasty (LAUP). The uvula is trimmed and trenches are made in the soft palate using a laser or other cutting instrument. Redundant tissue is removed and the level of the palate is raised. (From Ref. 67.)

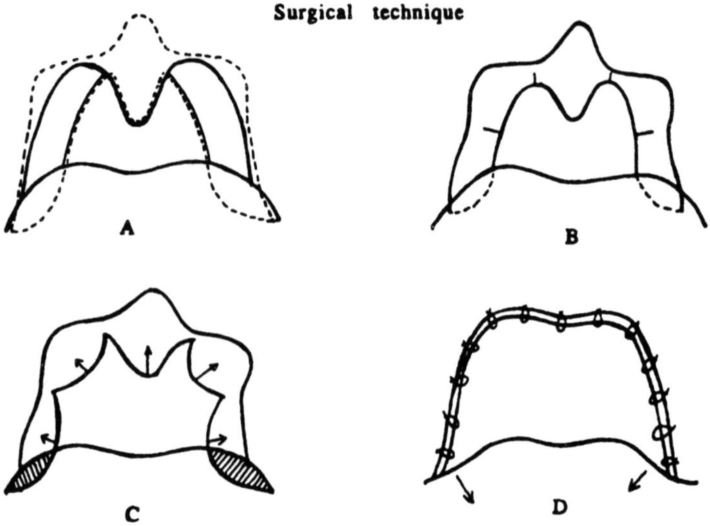

Figure 4 Uvulopalatopharyngo-glossoplasty (UPPGP). UPPP is combined with limited resection and suturing of the tongue base to address retropalatal and retrolingual collapse. A—redundant soft tissue from the palate, uvula, and lateral tongue base are resected. B—relaxing incisions are made to allow soft tissue to be advanced without tension. C—Soft tissue is advanced. D—Soft tissue of the palate, pharynx, and base of tongue are sutured to form a smooth arch enlarging the retropalatal and retrolingual airways. (From Ref. 14.)

extirpated posteriorly and laterally to that portion excised in LMG. Tracheotomy is sometimes needed for airway control in the perioperative period (15,16) (Fig. 5). Because of the need for tracheotomy in a significant percentage of these patients and the discomfort and swelling, its use is uncommon.

B. Surgical Techniques Affecting Secondary Soft Tissue Repositioning Through Primary Skeletal Mobilization

Transpalatal advancement pharyngoplasty (TPAP) enlarges the retropalatal airway by resection of the posterior hard palate with advancement of the soft palate in an anterior direction into the bony defect (17) (Fig. 6). This procedure is used for retropalatal obstruction that persists after UPPP, but has technical challenges associated with its use and lack of experience with the technique. Its place in the surgical armamentarium has yet to be fully elucidated.

Mandibular advancement (MA) enlarges the retrolingual airway, utilizing sagittal mandibular osteotomies to effect anterior mobilization of the tongue by advancing the insertion at the genioid tubercle. For this procedure, there must be significant antecedent mandibular deficiency and dental malocclusion to permit the

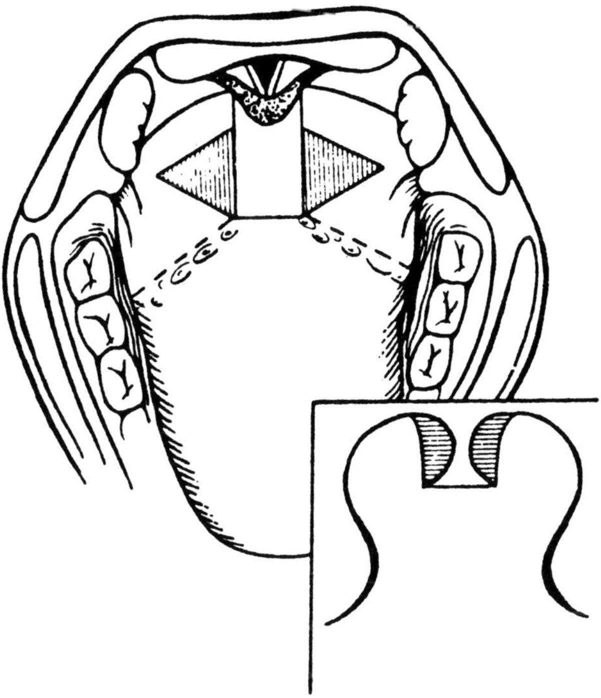

Figure 5 Laser midline glossectomy (LMG) and lingualplasty. Resection of areas in the central tongue is performed to improve tongue obstruction during sleep. Prolapsing tissue from the lateral portions of the incision are excised in a wedge (inset). (From Ref. 16.)

requisite degree of anterior movement of the mandible and mandibular teeth (18) (Fig. 7). This procedure is beneficial for a small group of patients with Class II dental occlusion and anatomy as described.

Maxillo-mandibular advancement (MMA) provides maximal enlargement of the retrolingual airway and some enlargement of the retropalatal airway. The maxilla and mandible are advanced simultaneously by means of LeFort I maxillary and sagittal-split mandibular osteotomies. This permits a greater degree of mandibular advancement, which is frequently required to treat OSAS successfully. The requisite degree of mandibular advancement, in the absence of maxillary advancement, would typically result in mandibular prognathism and dental malocclusion. Details of the procedure performed vary depending on the patient's initial occlusion (19) (Fig. 8). This procedure permanently and effectively enlarges the airway, but the magnitude of the procedure and expertise needed to perform it in this patient population limits more widespread use.

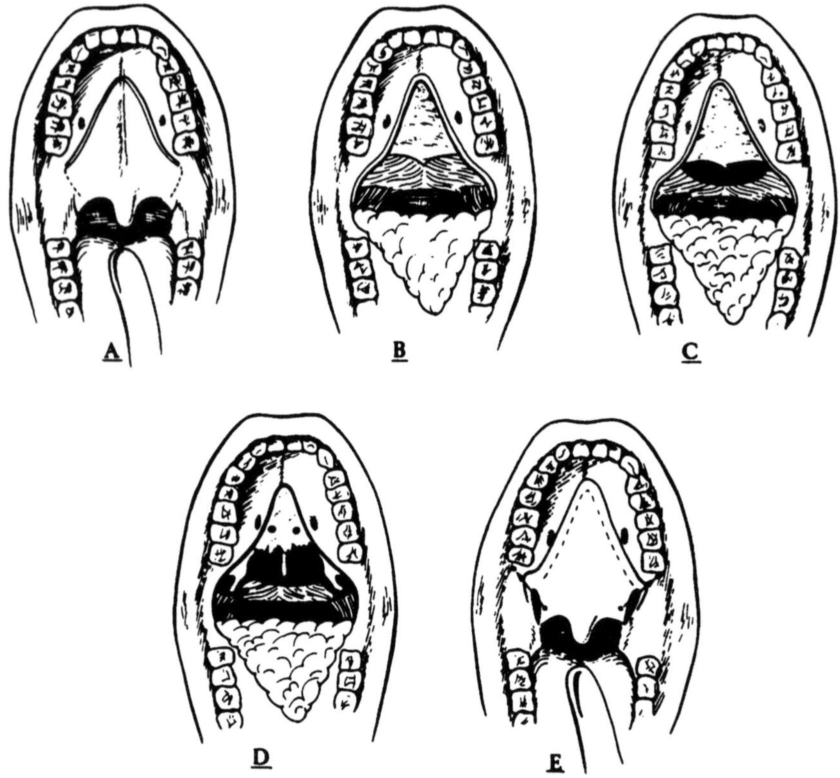

Figure 6 Transpalatal advancement pharyngoplasty (TPAP). Resection of the posterior hard palate is performed and the soft palate is advanced anteriorly into the bony defect. A—Site of incision outlined from posterior alveolus to palatoglossal fold. B—Flap elevated. C—Soft and hard palate are separated exposing the nasopharynx. D—Hamulus exposed and fractured and posterior hard palate removed. E—Redundancy of palate mucosa shown (dashed line) and lateral flaps are advanced and sutured to mucoperiosteum. (From Ref. 17.)

Genioglossal advancement (GA) enlarges the retrolingual airway by anterior advancement of the genioid tubercle of the mandible by means of a limited parasagittal mandibular osteotomy. This tends to advance the tongue in an anterior direction without altering dental occlusion (20) (Fig. 9). For patients with retroglossal collapse, GA is a commonly performed intervention.

Hyoid myotomy and suspension (two variations, HM-1 and HM-2) enlarge the retrolingual airway by anterior advancement of the tongue, hyoid, and suprahyoid musculature, with suspension of the hyoid by one of two techniques: from the mandible by a fascial strip (HM-1) or from the superior margin of the thyroid

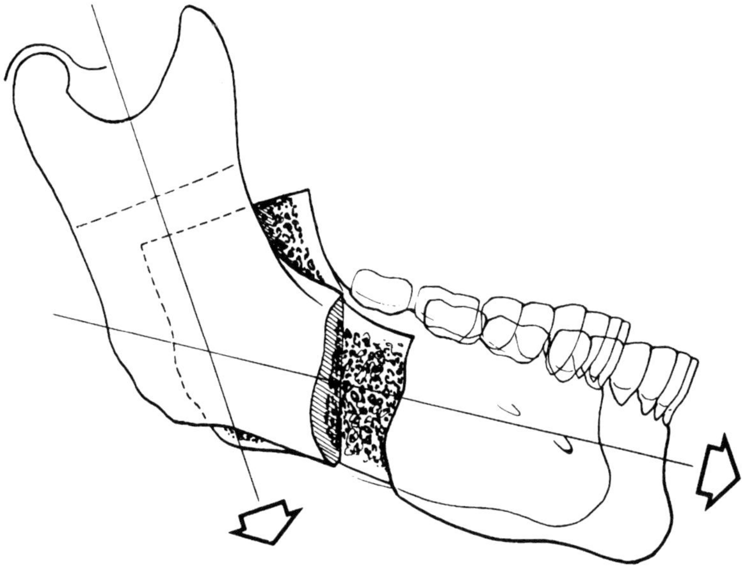

Figure 7 Mandibular advancement (MA). A sagittal split osteotomy of the mandible is performed and the mandible and associated dentition are advanced anteriorly. (From Ref. 68.)

cartilage by permanent suture (HM-2) (20,21) (Figs. 9 and 10). It is commonly performed in conjunction with GA for patients with retroglossal collapse.

C. Surgical Technique That By-Passes the Pharyngeal Airway

Tracheotomy creates a percutaneous opening into the trachea. The tracheostomy is usually stented and maintained by inserting a rigid or semi-rigid hollow tube that extends to the body surface. The patient breathes through the tube when the external end is unplugged. Since the tracheostomy enters the airway distal to the pharynx, it bypasses the region of collapse. When the patient is awake, the external end of the tube is plugged, redirecting the flow of air through the nose or mouth, pharynx, and larynx. The tracheostomy tube is of sufficiently small diameter that, when plugged, it permits air entering the trachea from the pharynx and larynx to pass around the tube into the distal trachea and lungs. Alternatively, a tracheostomy cannula can be used, which is held in place with a flange on the anterior tracheal wall and the skin, or a stomal plug can be utilized instead of cannula (22) (Fig. 11). This procedure is easy to perform and effective for OSAS treatment, but the inconvenience and hygiene issues preclude more widespread use in the typical patient with OSAS.

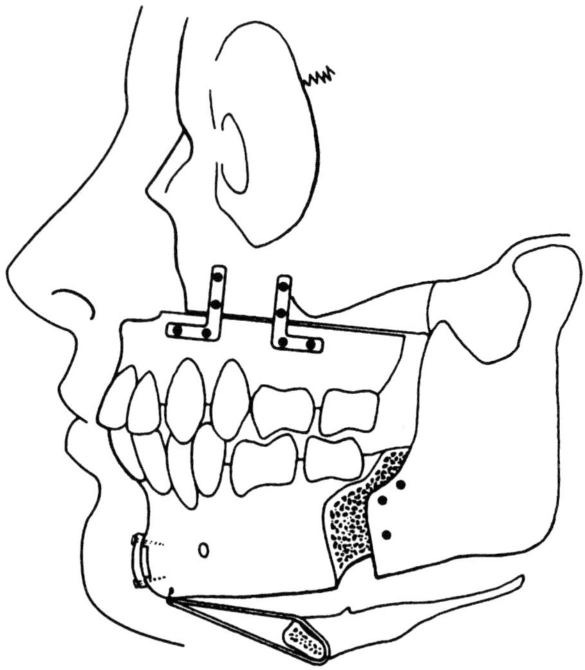

Figure 8 Maxillo-mandibular advancement (MMA) shown here with genioglossus advancement and hyoid suspension. The maxilla is advanced with a LeFort I osteotomy and the mandible is advanced with a sagittal split osteotomy. They are advanced anteriorly approximately 12 mm and fixed into place. (From Ref. 19.)

IV. Outcomes Data for Upper Airway Surgical Procedures

A. Uvulopalatopharyngoplasty

Short-term mean outcomes data for UPPP have been derived by meta-analysis of 37 papers on UPPP, each of which reported on at least nine surgical subjects and assessed surgical outcomes through clear and unambiguous outcome measures, i.e., a pre- and postoperative polysomnogram (7). The mean decrease in apnea index (AI) in more than 500 patients was 55% from a mean preoperative AI of 45 apneas per hour. The mean decrease in RDI in approximately 500 patients was 38% from a mean preoperative RDI of 60 apneas and hypopneas per hour. In 14 papers defining surgical response as 50% decrease in AI, the response rate for 352 patients was 65%. In 16 papers defining surgical response as 50% decrease in RDI, the response rate for 375 patients was 53%. There was no significant preoperative difference between responders and nonresponders in terms of age, AI, RDI, minimum oxygen saturation, or body weight (7).

The preoperative pattern of pharyngeal narrowing or collapse was specified

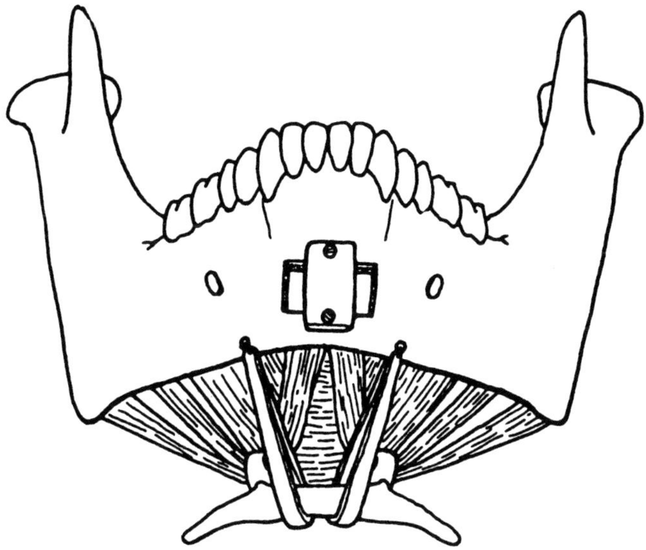

Figure 9 Genioglossal advancement shown here with hyoid myotomy and suspension from the mandible (HM-1). The attachment of the genioglossus muscle is advanced anteriorly and the hyoid bone is suspended from the mandible to advance the tongue and improve the retroglossal airway. (From Ref. 20.)

to be Type I, II, or III in each of 168 patients subjected to UPPP and reported in nine papers (7). In these patients, pharyngeal typing was determined by one of the following techniques: awake fiberoptic endoscopy with or without Müller maneuver, asleep endoscopy with nasal-CPAP, lateral cephalometry, airway manometry, or pharyngeal CT scan. The mean percent decrease in AI for Type I patients was 75% (from a mean preoperative AI of 39 apneas per hour). For Types II or III, the mean percent decrease in AI was 23% (from a mean preoperative AI of 60 apneas per hour). The mean decrease in RDI for Type I patients was 33% (from a mean preoperative RDI of 57 apneas and hypopneas per hour). For Types II and III, the mean percent decrease in RDI was 7% (from a mean preoperative RDI of 65 apneas and hypopneas per hour). The percentage of patients who attained at least 50% decrease in RDI to a postoperative RDI of less than 20 apneas and hypopneas per hour (or at least 50% decrease in AI to a postoperative AI of less than 10 apneas per hour, if that criterion of success was applied) was 52% for Type I patients and 5% for Type II or Type III patients (7).

If all patients (Types I, II, and III) are combined, 43% (79/185) achieved at least a 50% decrease in AI and a postoperative AI less than 10 apneas per hour, and 39% (74/189) achieved at least a 50% decrease in RDI and a postoperative RDI of less than 20 apneas and hypopneas per hour. If achievement of either of these criteria defines surgical success, 41% (137/337) of patients responded to UPPP (7).

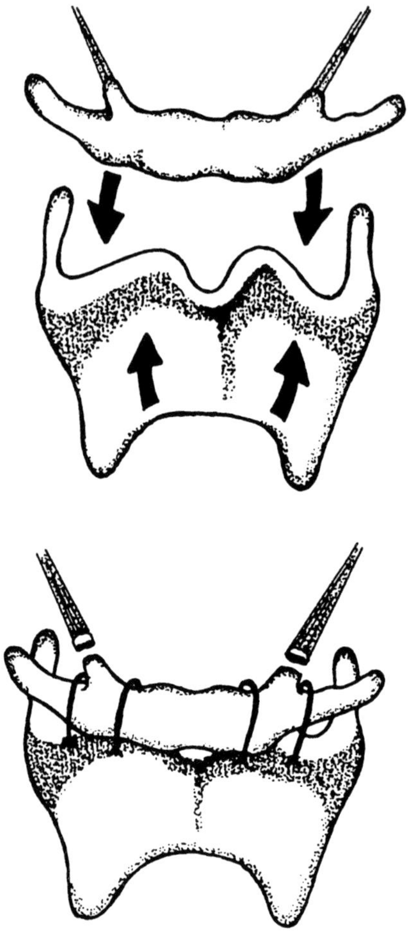

Figure 10 Hyoid myotomy and suspension from the superior margin of the thyroid cartilage by permanent suture (HM-2). Top—Hyoid bone is advanced anteriorly and inferiorly to meet the thyroid cartilage. Bottom—Hyoid bone is permanently sutured to the thyroid cartilage after the stylohyoid ligament is released. (From Ref. 21.)

Surgical complications described in the 37 papers include velopharyngeal insufficiency (VPI) for greater than 1 month (14/640), postoperative bleeding (7/640), nasopharyngeal stenosis (5/640), voice change (4/640), vague foreign body sensation (1/640), successfully managed perioperative upper airway obstruction (2/640), and death secondary to upper airway obstruction (1/640). However, since more than half of the papers did not comment on the presence or absence of postoperative complications, it is impossible to determine the true incidence of complications in the entire population (7). In two series focusing on UPPP complications, the death

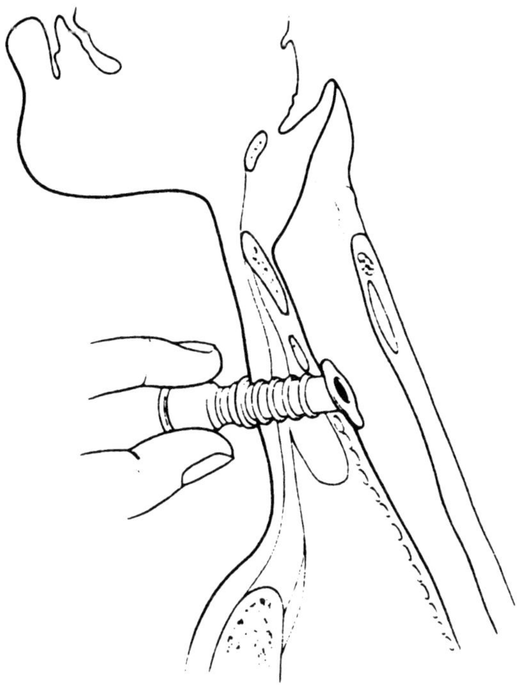

Figure 11 Tracheotomy cannula held in place with a flange on the anterior tracheal wall and the skin. (From Ref. 69.)

rate from unsuccessfully managed upper airway obstruction was approximately 1% (23,24). The incidence of postoperative VPI was shown to be heavily dependent on the definition of VPI applied (25). Its incidence in 71 patients 2 years after UPPP varied from 39% to 3% (39% with subclinical reflux of liquids, apparent only on nasal endoscopy; 16% with nasal reflux when the patient bent over a water fountain to drink water; 7% with subclinical nasal regurgitation, i.e., patients feeling bubbles in the nose after drinking gaseous drinks; and 3% with mild nasal reflux for liquids) (25). One series reported that 31% (28/91) of patients complained of dry throat and 10% (9/91) complained of swallowing abnormalities at 1 year (24).

Long-term follow-up after UPPP is limited. Fifty patients were followed for a mean of 46 months after UPPP. At 6 months postoperatively, 60% were considered to be responders (response rate defined by 50% reduction to a postoperative RDI of less than 20). At 21 months postoperatively, 39% patients were considered to be responders. Patients in whom OSAS had relapsed had sustained significant weight gain. At 46 months postoperatively, 50% were deemed responders. Weight loss, abstinence from alcohol, and positional conditioning were cited in some of those patients who sustained late improvement (26). In another study, 25 patients who underwent UPPP had a 6-month postoperative response rate of 64% (response defined by 50% decrease to postoperative RDI of less than 10). At long-term follow-up (4–8 years postoperatively), the response rate was 48%. No difference in preoperative apnea/hypopnea index (AHI), body mass index (BMI), or change in BMI was found between long-term responders and nonresponders (27). In another study, patients had UPPP, with early response rate of 67% at 3–6 months (response defined by greater than 50% reduction in RDI). At long-term evaluation (more than 5 years postoperatively, mean 88 months), the response rate was 33% (28). Thus, all studies show that response rate declines over time following the surgery.

B. Laser-Assisted Uvulopalatoplasty

Only a few studies have published postoperative polysomnographic data for patients with OSAS treated by LAUP. Sixty-three patients had a response rate of 87% (55/63) (response defined as 50% decrease in RDI). Mean preoperative RDI of 41 decreased to a mean postoperative RDI of 20 apneas and hypopneas per hour. For the responder population (mean BMI 29), the mean preoperative RDI of 42 decreased to a mean postoperative RDI of 17 apneas and hypopneas per hour (29). Forty-three polysomnography-documented ''moderate to severe OSAS'' patients treated by LAUP ''failed to show any changes in the sleep parameters that were statistically significant'' (30). Little substantiating data were given. Of 65 polysomnography-documented OSAS patients subjected to LAUP (mean preoperative RDI 29 apneas and hypopneas per hour), 51% (33/65) underwent postoperative polysomnography (31). Of those who underwent postoperative polysomnography, 21% (7/33) were worse; 15% (5/33) had no change; 64% (21/33) achieved a 50% decrease in RDI; and 48% (16/33), defined as ''responders,'' achieved a 50% decrease in RDI and a postoperative RDI less than 10 apneas and hypopneas per hour. The ''responders'' (mean preoperative RDI 25 apneas and hypopneas per hour, mean BMI 31 kg/m^2), achieved a mean postoperative RDI of 3 apneas and hypopneas per hour. The nonresponders (mean preoperative RDI 40 apneas and hypopneas per hour, mean BMI 31 kg/m^2) did not change after LAUP (31). Of 34 OSAS patients subjected to LAUP, 38% (13/34) had postoperative polysomnography (mean preoperative RDI of 31 apneas and hypopneas per hour and mean preoperative BMI of 30 kg/m^2). The mean postoperative RDI was 16, and 54% (7/13) achieved a 50% decrease in RDI, while 39% (5/13) achieved a 50% decrease in RDI and a postoperative RDI less than 10 apneas and hypopneas per hour (32).

When 41 OSAS patients treated with UPPP and 38 OSAS patients treated with LAUP were compared, the response rates reported were 51% and 47% (response defined by at least 50% reduction in RDI) (33). However, RDI was reduced by a mean of 51% in patients treated with UPPP and by a mean of 27% in patients treated with LAUP. Postoperative polysomnograms were available for only 50% of treated patients calling into question the issue of bias in the results. Furthermore, the two patient groups were not matched for OSAS severity, patients treated with UPPP having a statistically significantly higher mean preoperative RDI than patients treated with LAUP (52 vs. 30 apneas and hypopneas per hour) and a significantly higher BMI (32 vs. 30 kg/m^2). While the author compares the reported 47% LAUP success rate with the 41% success rate for UPPP described in a meta-analysis on UPPP (34), two significant differences between the report on LAUP and the meta-analysis on UPPP are omitted. The criterion for success in the report on LAUP (50% decrease in RDI) is not comparable to the more restrictive criterion for success in the meta-analysis on UPPP (50% decrease in postoperative RDI or AI and RDI less than 20 apneas and hypopneas per hour or AI less than 10 apneas per hour). The population in the report on LAUP is not comparable to the more severely affected population in the meta-analysis on UPPP (mean preoperative RDI of 30 vs. 55 apneas and hypopneas per hour, and mean AI of 20 vs. 45 apneas per hour, respectively) (7,33).

LAUP patients studied by polysomnography, videoendoscopy and MRI within 3 days after surgery demonstrated exacerbation of OSAS severity in the early postoperative period. In seven patients having polysomnography at 48–72 h after surgery, the mean preoperative RDI of 11 doubled to 22 apneas and hypopneas per hour, and the mean preoperative AI of three was multiplied by a factor of more than four, to 14 apneas per hour. The pharyngeal cross-sectional area at 72 h postoperatively revealed a 48% decrease from the preoperative cross-sectional area. The authors emphasize the risk of postoperative airway compromise (35).

The dimensions and configuration of the pharynx before and after LAUP and UPPP were analyzed in 10 patients by peroral photography of the oropharynx, nasopharyngoscopy of the velopharyngeal region, and lateral and frontal cephalometry with contrast enhancement. While UPPP resulted in enlargement of the velopharyngeal space, LAUP resulted in diminished velopharyngeal space. The authors express concern that LAUP may, therefore, prove inferior to UPPP and may actually prove deleterious for at least some OSAS patients (36). In review of this paper, however, questions remain concerning individual anatomical variations, surgical technique, and the generalizability of the conclusions, and further study is needed if conclusions from these comparisons are to be made.

Finally, it appears that LAUP can improve OSAS in selected patients, but there is no reliable evidence that LAUP and UPPP are interchangeable in any given patient.

C. Uvulopalatopharyngo-glossoplasty

Twenty patients underwent UPPGP with a 43% decrease in mean RDI at 9 months postoperatively (mean preoperative RDI 54, mean postoperative RDI 31 apneas and hypopneas per hour). Fifty percent (10/20) had at least a 50% postoperative decrease in RDI (13). When 19 patients were treated with UPPGP, the response rate (response defined as a 50% reduction in AI) was 67% at 6 months postoperatively (14).

D. Laser Midline Glossectomy and Lingualplasty

Twelve patients who underwent LMG had significant preoperative retrolingual narrowing on physical examination and dynamic cephalometric radiographs. Fiberoptic endoscopy with Müller maneuver demonstrated greater than 75% retrolingual airway collapse. Eleven of the patients had undergone previous UPPP, which had failed. The twelfth patient had primary LMG. The response rate (response defined as a reduction in RDI of at least 50%) was 42% (5/12). For the responder group, the RDI decreased from 61 to 15 apneas and hypopneas per hour. Nonresponders were significantly more obese than responders (BMI 38 vs. 31 kg/m^2) (15). Twenty-two patients were treated by lingualplasty, a modification of LMG. Fourteen had prior unsuccessful UPPP, and 8 had synchronous UPPP and lingualplasty. Response rate (response defined by 50% reduction to a postoperative RDI less than 20 apneas and hypopneas per hour) was 77% (17/22). The mean RDI in the responder group decreased from 59 to 9 apneas and hypopneas per hour. For the group that had previously undergone unsuccessful UPPP, the response (i.e. salvage) rate was 79% (11/14), and the mean preoperative RDI of 50 decreased to a mean postoperative RDI of 9 apneas and hypopneas per hour. No permanent complications resulted from LMG (16).

E. Transpalatal Advancement Pharyngoplasty

Six patients underwent UPPP and TPAP, in that order, in one surgical session (37). Intraoperative measurements of retropalatal cross-sectional area and pharyngeal collapsibility were made upon completion of the UPPP and repeated upon completion of TPAP. Transpalatal pharyngoplasty further increased cross-sectional area and decreased pharyngeal collapsibility compared to the post-UPPP measurements. When six patients (mean preoperative RDI 70 apneas and hypopneas per hour) underwent both UPPP and TPAP, 67% (4/6) responded (response defined by 50% decrease to a postoperative RDI less than 20 apneas and hypopneas per hour) (17,37).

F. Mandibular Advancement

Individual case reports describe successful treatment of OSAS by mandibular advancement (MA) in patients with severe mandibular micrognathia, or retrognathia resulting from developmental or posttraumatic mandibular deformity or from temporomandibular joint ankylosis (18,38). These patients, described as having ''birdlike'' facial profiles, have a major degree of mandibular deficiency in the absence of significant maxillary deficiency. While few in number, these reports are of historical significance for demonstrating that mandibular deficiency can result in OSAS and that skeletal correction results in resolution of OSAS through enlargement of the retrolingual airway by anterior tongue movement.

G. Maxillo-Mandibular Advancement

Maxillo-mandibular advancement (MMA) was applied as a primary approach in 38 OSAS patients selected for maxillo-mandibular deficiency, dolichofacial characteristics, and a narrow retrolingual airway space. Morbidly obese subjects were excluded, and only two patients had a BMI greater than 32 kg/m^2. Ninety-five percent (36/38) responded (response defined as 50% decrease in RDI to less than 10 apneas and hypopneas per hour). The mean preoperative RDI of 47 apneas and hypopneas per hour was diminished to a mean postoperative RDI of three apneas and hypopneas per hour. The two nonresponders had retropalatal narrowing and were subsequently successfully treated with UPPP and TPAP (39). In a subsequent study, MMA was applied as a primary approach in seven OSAS patients selected for severe facial skeletal deformity and/or dental malocclusion. The rate of response was 100% (7/7) (response defined as 50% decrease in RDI to less than 20 apneas and hypopneas per hour) (40). In another study, five OSAS patients treated with MMA had a response rate of 65% when treated primarily with MMA (41). These patients did not have previous OSAS surgery to the palate, uvula, tonsils, or jaw and were primarily treated with MMA. This implies that surgical treatment of palatal and base of tongue obstruction is needed in some patients to maximize treatment outcome from MMA. It is results like these that advance the idea of a phased surgical approach to OSAS, as outlined in the Stanford Protocol described later in this chapter.

H. Genioglossal Advancement

There are no reports of genioglossal advancement (GA) performed as a sole surgical procedure.

I. Hyoid Myotomy and Suspension

There are no reports of hyoid myotomy and suspension (HM-1 or HM-2) performed as a sole surgical maneuver.

V. Outcomes Data for Upper Airway Surgical Procedures Performed in Combination

UPPP, GA, HM-1, HM-2, and MMA have been performed in various combinations, either contemporaneously (in one surgical episode) or sequentially (in different surgical episodes), as follows:

GA and HM-1
GA and HM-2
UPPP and GA
UPPP and GA and HM-1
UPPP and GA and HM-2
UPPP and GA and HM-1 and MMA
GA and HM-1 and MMA
UPPP and MMA

In these patients, UPPP was applied to address retropalatal narrowing, and all other procedures were applied to address retrolingual narrowing.

A. Genioglossal Advancement and Hyoid Myotomy and Suspension-1

GA and HM-1 was performed in six patients identified to have retrolingual collapse in the absence of retropalatal collapse. The response rate was 66% (4/6) (response defined as 50% decrease to postoperative RDI less than 20 apneas and hypopneas per hour). Note that these 6 patients were the only ones in a series of 239 OSAS patients (2.5%) who demonstrated retrolingual collapse in the absence of retropalatal collapse (determined cephalometrically and endoscopically) (40).

B. Genioglossal Advancement and Hyoid Myotomy-2

Three patients with retrolingual narrowing in the absence of retropalatal narrowing had GA and HM-2 as an isolated surgical procedure with a response rate of 100% (3/3) (response defined as 50% decrease to postoperative RDI less than 20 apneas and hypopneas per hour). The mean preoperative RDI was 55, and the mean preoperative BMI was 25 kg/m^2.

C. Uvulopalatopharyngoplasty and Genioglossal Advancement

Nine patients underwent UPPP and GA, with a response rate of 78% (7/9) (response defined as 50% decrease to postoperative RDI less than 10 apneas and hypopneas per hour). The mean preoperative BMI was 33 kg/m^2, and the mean preoperative RDI was 58 (42). Other studies as outlined below combine UPPP, GA, and other procedures, such as hyoid myotomy making the specific role of UPPP and GA more difficult to define.

D. Uvulopalatopharyngoplasty and Genioglossal Advancement and Hyoid Myotomy and Suspension-1

Of 233 patients subjected to UPPP and GA and HM-1, 57% (133/233) were responders (response defined as decrease by 50% to RDI less than 20 apneas and hypopneas per hour). For patients with mild and moderate OSAS (defined as preoperative RDI less than 60 apneas and hypopneas per hour and preoperative mean lowest oxygen saturation greater than 70%) the rate of success was 75% (101/135), while for patients with severe OSAS (defined as preoperative RDI greater than 60 apneas and hypopneas per hour and preoperative mean lowest oxygen saturation less than 70%) the success rate was 42% (44/104) (40). In 12 obese patients (mean BMI 35 kg/m^2, mean preoperative RDI 49 apneas and hypopneas per hour) subjected to UPPP and GA and HM-1, the success rate was 42% (5/12) (response defined as decrease by 50% to postoperative RDI less than 20 apneas and hypopneas per hour) (43).

E. Uvulopalatopharyngoplasty and Genioglossal Advancement and Hyoid Myotomy and Suspension-2

Eleven patients (mean preoperative RDI 80 apneas and hypopneas per hour; mean preoperative BMI 31 kg/m^2) had UPPP and GA and HM-2, with a response rate of 73% (8/11) (response defined as 50% decrease to postoperative RDI less than 20 apneas and hypopneas per hour) (21). In another study, 32 patients (mean preoperative RDI 47 apneas and hypopneas per hour) were subjected to UPPP and GA and HM-2, and 44% (14/32) were studied postoperatively with either polysomnography or cardiorespiratory study with estimation of sleep by movement assessment. The success rate was 57% (8/14) (success defined as 50% decrease to postoperative RDI less than 20 apneas and hypopneas per hour) (44).

F. Maxillo-Mandibular Advancement with Uvulopalatopharyngoplasty and/or Genioglossal Advancement and Hyoid Myotomy and Suspension-1 or Suspension-2

One hundred and sixty-four patients completed MMA after failed UPPP and/or GA and HM-1 or HM-2, with a success rate of 95% (156/164) (success defined as 50% decrease to postoperative RDI less than 20 apneas and hypopneas per hour). The mean preoperative RDI of 72 apneas and hypopneas per hour was decreased to a mean postoperative RDI of eight apneas and hypopneas per hour (45). A series of 23 patients was treated with MMA, and the following adjunctive procedures performed when indicated on the basis of preoperative endoscopic and cephalometric assessment: sliding horizontal geniotomy (15/23), partial glossectomy (8/23), and UPPP (7/23). Seventy-eight percent (18/23) had at least one adjunctive procedure, and 53% (12/23) had two adjunctive procedures. Response was defined as postoperative RDI less than 10 apneas and hypopneas per hour. The mean preoperative and postoperative RDI for each group were as follows: MMA without ancillary procedures: 56, 18 apneas and hypopneas per hour; MMA and at least one ancillary procedure: 65, 14 apneas and hypopneas per hour; MMA and UPPP: 67, five apneas and hypopneas per hour. The response rate for the group that had MMA with no adjunctive procedure was 20% (1/5). The response rate for patients having MMA and at least one adjunctive procedure was 78% (14/18). The response rate for the patients who had MMA and UPPP as their only adjunctive procedure or as one of two adjunctive procedures was 100% (7/7). If response had been defined as 50% decrease to postoperative RDI less than 20 apneas and hypopneas per hour (instead of less than 10 apneas and hypopneas per hour), the success rate for MMA alone would be 40% (2/5), for MMA plus UPPP would be 100% (7/7), and for MMA plus at least one adjunctive procedure would be 78% (14/18) (41).

G. Tracheotomy

In one series of 11 patients who had tracheotomy, the indications were cor pulmonale (4/11), chronic alveolar hypoventilation (5/11), nocturnal cardiac arrhythmia (4/11), and disabling daytime sleepiness (9/11). During the mean 17-month postoperative follow-up period, excessive daytime sleepiness resolved in 82% (9/11). Central apnea and alcohol or drug abuse accounted for persistence in the remaining patients. Chronic hypercapnia resolved in 100% (5/5). Cor pulmonale resolved in 100% (4/4), but recurred in one. Cardiac arrhythmias resolved or improved in 100% (4/4).

Hypertension resolved in 40% (2/5). Patients who lost weight initially after tracheotomy gained it back within 6 months. Complications included psychosocial problems resulting from having a tracheotomy in 90% (10/11), granulation tissue formation resulting in hemoptysis or obstruction in 82% (9/11), and recurrent bronchitis in 55% (6/11). The number of patients who were unable to work increased from two to seven after tracheotomy, generally as the result of employer concern regarding liability (46).

In another series of 50 patients who were followed for a mean of 32 months after tracheotomy, indications for tracheotomy were disabling daytime sleepiness, severe cardiac arrhythmias, apnea index greater than 60 apneas per hour, and minimum oxygen saturation less than 40%. Thirty patients were hypertensive and 25 were taking antihypertensive medications. Polysomnography was conducted within 6 days postoperatively in 60% (30/50). Resolution of OSAS was demonstrated in 83% (25/30), and these patients were free of excessive daytime sleepiness. Ultimately, all patients had resolution of excessive daytime sleepiness. Only 7% (2/30) of hypertensive patients became normotensive postoperatively. However, of the 25 patients previously taking antihypertensive medications, 40% (10/25) required less vigorous medical therapy for their hypertension. Return to work or school was achieved by 94% (47/50) of patients. All patients eventually achieved an AI of less than five apneas per hour. Central apnea that appeared shortly after the performance of tracheotomy resolved over time. Sleep architecture became normal. All attempts at tracheotomy closure resulted in reappearance of the OSAS. Granulation tissue developed at the tracheotomy site in 42% (21/50) (47).

In another series of 38 patients subjected to tracheotomy, 26% (10/38) had preoperative and postoperative polysomnography. All patients were overweight and hypertensive. Indications for tracheotomy included severe excessive daytime sleepiness, serious cardiac arrhythmias, past history of cardiac or cerebrovascular disease, and systemic hypertension. Excessive daytime sleepiness resolved in all patients within 48 h postoperatively. Polysomnography performed postoperatively (within 9 days in nine patients and on the forty-first day in the tenth) revealed that the number of mixed and obstructive apneas diminished to normal, but the number of central events and hypopneas increased. Tracheotomy could be closed in only one patient who had lost a considerable amount of weight (22).

While it is difficult to outline precise criteria for tracheotomy, tracheotomy continues to play a valuable role in surgical treatment of OSAS. Primary candidates for tracheotomy include OSAS patients with severe OSAS, morbid obesity, Pickwickian syndrome, cor pulmonale, cardiac arrhythmias, coronary artery disease with desaturation, severe daytime sleepiness, or other cardiovascular or medical comorbidities exacerbated by OSAS. Tracheotomy in the perioperative period should be considered in patients who meet the above criteria and who cannot tolerate worsening of their OSAS in the perioperative period. This is especially important in those who cannot tolerate CPAP and patients in whom further control of the postoperative airway may be needed.

H. The Stanford Protocol

The Stanford Protocol was developed to systematically approach reconstruction of the upper airway based on the hypothesis that pharyngeal classification into Types I, II, and III could serve as an effective basis for establishing a treatment plan for each patient (see protocol outline in Fig. 12). The goal was to apply limited but regionally specific anatomical modification as Phase 1 of surgical therapy (UPPP, GA, HM). The specific procedure(s) performed are selected in accordance with the pharyngeal classification into Type I, II, or III based on fiberoptic endoscopy and lateral cephalometry. Patients who were Type I underwent UPPP. Patients who were Type III underwent GA and HM. Patients who were Type II underwent UPPP, GA, and HM. Nasal surgery was performed as part of Phase I if indicated by the clinical finding of nasal obstruction. Patients were then studied with polysomnograms. If they demonstrated significant residual OSAS and elected to complete the surgical protocol, they were treated with Phase II of the protocol: MMA. Exceptions were made for patients who, on initial presentation, demonstrated severe maxillo-mandibular disproportion with sequelae in addition to OSAS (such as dental malocclusion, temporomandibular joint syndrome, or cosmetic concerns). These patients were allowed to enter the protocol at Phase II instead of Phase I. The goal of the protocol was to strive for universal cure of OSAS, while minimizing the degree of surgical modification necessary to achieve the goal in each case. Response was defined as 50% decrease to postoperative RDI less than 20 apneas and hypopneas per hour. The response rate for Phase I surgery was approximately 60% (75% for patients with mild and moderate OSAS and 40% for patients with severe OSAS). The response rate for those patients who went on to Phase II after failing Phase I surgery was 95%. The response rate for those with severe skeletal deformity entering Phase

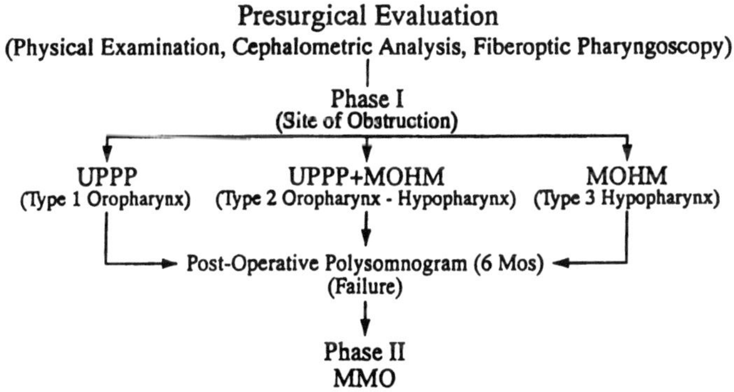

Figure 12 The Stanford Protocol for surgical treatment of OSAS. UPPP—uvulopalatopharyngoplasty, MOHM—mandibular osteotomy with hyoid myotomy (same as genioglossus advancement with hyoid myotomy); MMO—maxillo-mandibular osteotomy. (From Ref. 21.)

II without Phase I was 91% (45). Even obese patients have had good success with this protocol (48). A group of 21 morbidly obese patients with a mean BMI of 45 had an 81% response rate (RDI < 20, oxygen nadir $> 90\%$) (48). Others who have applied this protocol have enjoyed similar success overall, but with less success after Phase I than is noted above (49). The systematic approach of this protocol is generally accepted as the standard for evaluation of patients with OSAS and selection of operative procedures.

VI. Summary of Surgical Treatment

The role of upper airway surgery for obstructive sleep apnea is in evolution. The complex etiology of sleep apnea has resulted in an array of differing treatment options, each with inherent advantages and disadvantages. These modalities include behavioral approaches (weight reduction, postural conditioning), application of devices (intraoral devices, positive airway pressure devices), and surgical approaches (upper airway modification, tracheostomy). Etiological variability, differences in severity, comorbidity, and patient preference make each patient a relatively unique clinical entity around which to customize a treatment strategy by choosing from and possibly combining treatment options. While behavioral measures remain an integral part of the treatment program, patient ability to lose weight or permanently alter sleep position is generally limited. Nasal CPAP is highly effective when applied under laboratory conditions, but the considerable issue of patient noncompliance was underestimated until the development of technology capable of objective assessment (50). Intraoral devices appear to have efficacy in some cases, and there is ongoing research into the objective assessment of patient compliance with these devices (51). There is clearly a group of patients who fail nonsurgical therapies leaving their apnea untreated.

Uvulopalatopharyngoplasty was introduced in 1981 as the first surgical procedure specifically designed to treat sleep apnea. After an initial period of enthusiasm, UPPP fell into disfavor because of a failure rate exceeding 50%. However, partly through analysis of UPPP success and failure, it became clear that sleep apnea results from anatomical compromise at different sites in the pharynx and that UPPP addresses only one of these, the upper or retropalatal pharynx. With this understanding came the introduction of new surgical procedures to modify the lower, or retrolingual, portion of the pharynx. This was approached by two alternative techniques. One of these techniques, laser ablation of a portion of the posterior tongue, actually diminished the soft tissue load in the lower pharynx. The other technique, genioglossal advancement and hyoid myotomy and suspension, resulted in anterior relocation of the tongue base, thereby enlarging the retrolingual airway. Both techniques were documented to achieve surgical ‘‘salvage’’ of some patients who were UPPP failures. Another approach was developed to move palate and tongue in an anterior direction, thus enlarging the retropalatal and retrolingual airways. This was accomplished by aggressive skeletal advancement of both upper and lower jaws, maxillomandibular osteotomy (MMO).

Powell and Riley, who were highly innovative in customizing surgical procedures to deal with sleep apnea, developed the Stanford Protocol in an effort to systematically customize the surgical approach to meet the specific anatomical needs of the patient. The rationale for the Stanford Protocol is to minimize the extent of surgery required for each patient, though striving for surgical cure in all cases. In the effort to minimize the extent of surgical intervention, patients accept that they may require more than one surgical session, and they will be monitored polysomnographically for residual apnea at the conclusion of each phase.

Application of the Protocol is based on the use of lateral cephalometry and fiberoptic endoscopy with Müller maneuver to characterize the pharynx as being most vulnerable to collapse in the retropalatal segment, retrolingual segment, or both. Uvulopalatopharyngoplasty is the surgical procedure for retropalatal compromise, and genioglossal advancement and hyoid myotomy and suspension is the procedure for retrolingual compromise. Nasal correction is done in a staged fashion, when indicated by physical findings, as part of the planned treatment. All of the above together comprise Phase I of the surgical protocol and achieves an approximate 60% cure rate in the hands of Powell and Riley. The patient who still has significant apnea after completing Phase I has the option of proceeding to Phase II, MMA, and advancement. Powell and Riley report success in well over 90% of patients who complete the Protocol.

Noting that many patients drop out of the Protocol after unsuccessful completion of Phase I, Hochban and Waite attempted to streamline the treatment process by applying MMA and advancement as the primary surgical procedure (39,41). Available data suggest that while this approach may be appropriate in a carefully selected subset of moderately severe, maxillo-mandibular-deficient, nonobese apnea patients, it, as a sole surgical procedure, has a high rate of failure if applied universally. Patient's who fail primary maxillo-mandibular advancement must then be treated for ''salvage'' by subsequent application of the bypassed Stanford Phase I procedures.

There is no limited surgical modification, short of tracheotomy, that consistently cures obstructive sleep apnea through elimination of the pathological event, transient airway obstruction. Therefore, tracheotomy probably remains the gold standard of treatment in that it assures that obstruction in the upper aerodigestive track is eliminated. However, the negative impact of tracheotomy on the patient is significant. Surgical upper airway modification has the potential advantage of elimination of sleep apnea without dependence on behavioral modification, mechanical devices, or tracheotomy. With the success of innovative application of surgical procedures, such as the Stanford Protocol, control of OSAS is possible with surgical intervention in a high percentage of cases.

A. Criteria for Success in Surgery for OSAS

Criteria for success in surgery for OSAS remain controversial. In 1981 Fujita introduced UPPP as the first specialized surgical procedure for OSAS and arbitrarily selected as the criterion defining surgical response postoperative decrease in AI of at least 50% from its preoperative value. The current understanding of OSAS mandates a more restrictive criterion for success, one that takes into account not only apneas but also hypopneas and subobstructive events that result in arousal. The definition of response must also include parameters of oxygenation, sleep architecture, and excessive daytime sleepiness. While fractional improvement may be beneficial, achievement of the threshold level of apnea severity (utilizing all of these parameters) at which there is no significant morbidity or mortality would appear to be the appropriate criterion for surgical response. Many authors have assumed that an RDI of 20 apneas and hypopneas per hour represents this threshold based on a report indicating increased mortality above this level of severity (52). However, AI equal to 20 apneas per hour, not RDI equal to 20 apneas and hypopneas per hour, was the severity threshold of increased mortality in that study. The current concept of upper airway resistance syndrome (UARS) precludes a bottom level below which RDI is clinically insignificant in sleepy patients, since UARS patients may present with excessive daytime sleepiness secondary to sleep-disordered breathing despite the total absence of apneas or hypopneas. In this case arousals resulting from increased upper airway resistance define the critical measurement (53). The definition of a severity threshold below which sleep-disordered breathing becomes inconsequential, and therefore, the criterion for surgical response, needs to be better defined.

There are frequently large discrepancies between modest postoperative success rates by polysomnographic criteria and higher "success" rates based on subjectively diminished excessive daytime sleepiness (54). These discrepancies remain inadequately explained. It has been shown that postoperative objective improvement in daytime sleepiness (as measured by the multiple sleep latency test) confirms subjective improvement in excessive daytime sleepiness only when UPPP has resulted in polysomnographically documented improvement in respiratory measures. Furthermore, subjective improvement in excessive daytime sleepiness in the absence of polysomnographic improvement is not confirmed by objective multiple sleep latency test data (55). While it has been shown that UPPP can eliminate alpha-EEG arousals in UARS patients who do not have polysomnographic evidence of OSAS (53,56), polysomnographic measures of sleep architecture are only infrequently reported in the surgical literature (7,34). It is sometimes assumed that the discrepancy between objective and subjective surgical outcome measures may reflect placebo effect. However, it is possible that the disproportionately high rate of subjective improvement in excessive daytime sleepiness brought about by UPPP might be explained by more rigorous analysis of EEG or more sophisticated data relating to the state of arousal. Further work is needed to clarify these issues (57).

B. Methodological Problems with the Surgical Literature on OSAS

Numerous methodological problems are encountered in the surgical literature that create difficulty in interpreting the optimal method for surgical intervention. These issues include the following (34):

1. There are no randomized studies and few with control groups.
2. Median sample size is low. Thus statistical power is low, and clinically important associations are routinely classified as ''not statistically significant.''
3. Papers generally do not present confidence bounds that might distinguish between statistical and clinical significance.
4. Papers generally give only short follow-up time and infrequent repeat follow-ups.
5. Bias caused by retrospective designs and nonrandom loss to follow-up raise questions about the generalizability of results.
6. Few papers associate polysomnographic data with patient-based quality-of-life measures.
7. Missing data and missing and inconsistent definitions are common.
8. Baseline measures are often biased because the same assessment is inappropriately but routinely used for both screening and baseline.

VII. New Techniques

The field of surgical treatment of OSAS is changing rapidly. As with many surgical procedures in medicine, less morbid techniques are being sought to replace or augment existing techniques. Many of these have been introduced but not proven in terms of efficacy. Further, their role in the algorithm for use in the patient with OSAS is unclear. Many of these newer procedures are focused on producing changes in the retroglossal airway. Whether they replace or augment present approaches and exactly when they should be applied will hopefully be delineated through rigorous research and clinical study. A number of these newer techniques will be outlined below.

A. Radiofrequency Volumetric Reduction of the Palate

Efforts to shrink and stiffen the palate have taken many forms, from cryosurgery to laser or electrocautery ablation of tissue. These techniques have been fraught with modest success and considerable morbidity in the way of pain for the patient. Recently another technique has been applied to patients with snoring, upper airway resistance syndrome, and mild obstructive sleep apnea, which seems to offer advantages over the previously mentioned techniques. It involves insertion of a probe into the palate and application of radiofrequency energy to heat the tissue causing coagulation necrosis, formation of scar tissue, and loss of volume (58). Patients with mild OSAS (RDI < 15), primary snoring, or upper airway resistance syndrome were selected for the initial human trial (59). The procedure was well tolerated with initial edema, minimal pain, and slight worsening of snoring and apneas. This is followed by volume loss over the course of weeks and improvement in snoring, UARS (based on esophageal pressure improvements), and slight improvements in RDI. Mean RDI changed from 3.93 to 3.4, demonstrating no statistically significant change in the mild degree of apnea in these patients. Measures of snoring and daytime sleepiness (Epworth Sleepiness Scale) improved and minimal complications occurred.

A more recent study compared the application of one lesion in the palate, as was used in the above study, to the application of three lesions for snoring and mild OSAS (60). In both groups, subjective daytime sleepiness was significantly reduced and snoring was improved after an average of three treatments or less. Ninety-six percent of the group who received three lesions had an improvement in snoring to levels that were not bothersome to the bed partner versus 79% of the one lesion group (60). While this technology is in its infancy, it represents an innovative, minimally invasive approach with less morbidity. Patient selection, which has yet to be precisely defined, will undoubtedly play an important role in optimizing results. Further studies are in progress to assess its efficacy in a larger group of patients with a greater degree of apnea.

B. Radiofrequency Volumetric Reduction of the Base of Tongue

In similar fashion, radiofrequency volumetric reduction of the base of tongue has shown some promise in treating obstruction in the retroglossal region. The original studies done in pigs demonstrated a 26% reduction in volume of the treated area (58). Subsequent studies have been done in humans resulting in FDA approval on November 5, 1998, of the Somnoplasty System for reduction of the incidence of airway obstructions in patients suffering from UARS and OSAS. In a group of 18 patients, it was shown to reduce the RDI with well tolerated serial outpatient treatment (61). An average of 5.5 treatments were used per patient with a resulting decrease in RDI from 39.5 to 17.8. Tongue volume was decreased by 17%, and posterior airway space was increased by an average of 14.6% in patients treated. Hydrocodone was used by the patients for pain for an average of 3–4 days, with one notable complication of tongue abscess, which was successfully treated. Though much more work is needed, this does represent a promising, less invasive method for treating patients with OSAS. Once again, the optimal timing and treatment sites as well as patient selection criteria have yet to be determined.

C. Tongue Suspension

In an attempt to address the problem of retroglossal collapse, suture material anchored to a bone screw has been used to suspend the tongue from the inner cortex of the anterior mandible. The suture is passed through the floor of the mouth and into the tongue, causing a triangular configuration with the point anteriorly. The suture suspends the tongue, preventing or decreasing posterior displacement. Preliminary reports on this technique demonstrate improvement in RDI, snoring, and daytime sleepiness at 3 months, though long-term results are lacking. Morbidity was low and the device was well tolerated in one study (62), while in another study evaluating outcomes, subjective improvements were incomplete and significant complications occurred (63).

D. Electrical Stimulation

In another attempt to reduce obstruction caused by retroglossal obstruction, electrical stimulation of the hypoglossal nerve has been used. Stimulation of the hypoglossal nerve was performed in humans and dogs to determine the effect on airway obstruction. Unilateral stimulation was successful in achieving 77% of maximal airflow in an experimentally induced obstruction with no histological changes to the nerve (64). Stimulation of humans below the arousal threshold was successful in improving airflow in patients with OSAS (65). Clinical trials are planned.

VIII. Conclusion

A patient's decision to pursue surgical treatment should follow full disclosure of the risks of untreated sleep apnea, the risks and benefits of nonsurgical modalities, and the risks and benefits of surgical modalities. It is prudent to suggest a preliminary trial of nonsurgical treatment in most cases, reserving surgical approaches for those who reject or undergo unsuccessful nonsurgical interventions.

The medical, financial, and psychosocial costs of effective treatment for obstructive sleep apnea will have to be compared to the cost of lack of treatment, both to the patient and to society as a whole. The relative costs of surgical and nonsurgical approaches will have to be compared with the relative benefit of each, to be defined through adequate outcomes assessment. Only in this way will the appropriate role for surgical approaches be established.

References

1. Rojewski TE, Schuller DE, Clark RW, Schmidt HS, Potts RE. Videoendoscopic determination of the mechanism of obstruction in obstructive sleep apnea. Otolaryngol Head Neck Surg 1984; 92:127–131.
2. Sher AE. Obstructive sleep apnea syndrome: a complex disorder of the upper airway. Otolaryngol Clin North Am 1990; 23:593–608.
3. Shepard JW, Jr, Thawley SE. Evaluation of the upper airway by computerized tomography in patients undergoing uvulopalatopharyngoplasty for obstructive sleep apnea. Am Rev Respir Dis 1989; 140:711–716.
4. Schwartz AR, Schubert N, Rothman W, Godley F, Marsh B, Eisele D, Nadeau J, Permutt L, Gleadhill I, Smith PL. Effect of uvulopalatopharyngoplasty on upper airway collapsibility in obstructive sleep apnea. Am Rev Respir Dis 1992; 145:527–532.
5. Launois SH, Feroah TR, Campbell WN, Issa FG, Morrison D, Whitelaw WA, Isono S, Remmers JE. Site of pharyngeal narrowing predicts outcome of surgery for obstructive sleep apnea. Am Rev Respir Dis 1993; 147:182–189.
6. Fujita S. Midline laser glossectomy with lingualplasty: A treatment of sleep apnea syndrome. Oper Tech Otolaryngol Head Neck Surg 1991; 2:127–131.
7. Sher AE, Schechtman KB, Piccirillo JF. The efficacy of surgical modifications of the upper airway in adults with obstructive sleep apnea syndrome. Sleep 1996; 19:156–177.

8. Orr WC, Martin RJ. Obstructive sleep apnea associated with tonsilar hypertrophy in adults. Arch Int Med 1981; 141:990–992.
9. Moser RJI, Rajagopal KR. Obstructive sleep apnea in adults with tonsillar hypertrophy. Arch Int Med 1987; 147:1265–1267.
10. Verse T, Kroker BA, Pirsig W, Brosch S. Tonsillectomy as a treatment of obstructive sleep apnea in adults with tonsillar hypertrophy. Laryngoscope 2000; 110:1556–1559.
11. Fujita S, Conway W, Zorick F. Surgical correction of anatomical abnormalities in obstructive sleep apnea: uvulopharyngoplasty. Otolaryngol Head Neck Surg 1981; 89: 923–934.
12. Kamami YV. Outpatient treatment of snoring with CO_2 laser: laser-assisted UPPP. J Otolaryngol 1994; 23:391–394.
13. Djupesland G, Schrader H, Lyberg T, Refsum H, Lilleas F, Godtlibsen OB. Palatopharyngoglossoplasty in the treatment of patients with obstructive sleep apnea syndrome. Acta Oto-Laryngol Suppl 1992; 492:50–54.
14. Miljeteig H, Tvinnereim M. Uvulopalatopharyngoglossoplasty (UPPGP) in the treatment of the obstructive sleep apnea syndrome. Acta Oto-Laryngol Suppl 1992; 492: 86–99.
15. Fujita S, Woodson BT, Clark JL, Wittig R. Laser midline glossectomy as a treatment for obstructive sleep apnea. Laryngoscope 1991; 101:805–809.
16. Woodson BT, Fujita S. Clinical experience with lingualplasty as part of the treatment of severe obstructive sleep apnea. Otolaryngol Head Neck Surg 1992; 107:40–48.
17. Woodson BT, Toohill RJ. Transpalatal advancement pharyngoplasty for obstructive sleep apnea. Laryngoscope 1993; 103:269–276.
18. Kuo PC, West RA, Bloomquist DS, McNeil RW. The effect of mandibular osteotomy in three patients with hypersomnia sleep apnea. Oral Surg Oral Med Oral Pathol 1979; 48:385–392.
19. Riley RW, Powell NB, Guilleminault C. Maxillofacial surgery and nasal CPAP. A comparison of treatment for obstructive sleep apnea syndrome. Chest 1990; 98:1421–1425.
20. Riley RW, Powell NB, Guilleminault C. Inferior mandibular osteotomy and hyoid myotomy suspension for obstructive sleep apnea: a review of 55 patients. J Oral Maxillofac Surg 1989; 47:159–164.
21. Riley RW, Powell NB, Guilleminault C. Obstructive sleep apnea and the hyoid: a revised surgical procedure. Otolaryngol Head Neck Surg 1994; 111:717–721.
22. Weitzman ED, Kahn E, Pollak CP. Quantitative analysis of sleep and sleep apnea before and after tracheostomy in patients with the hypersomnia-sleep apnea syndrome. Sleep 1980; 3:407–423.
23. Esclamado RM, Glenn MG, McCulloch TM, Cummings CW. Perioperative complications and risk factors in the surgical treatment of obstructive sleep apnea syndrome. Laryngoscope 1989; 99:1125–1129.
24. Haavisto L, Suonpaa J. Complications of uvulopalatopharyngoplasty. Clin Otolaryngol Allied Sci 1994; 19:243–247.
25. Zohar Y, Finkelstein Y, Talmi YP, Bar-Ilan Y. Uvulopalatopharyngoplasty: evaluation of postoperative complications, sequelae, and results. Laryngoscope 1991; 101:775–779.
26. Larsson LH, Carlsson-Nordlander B, Svanborg E. Four-year follow-up after uvulopalatopharyngoplasty in 50 unselected patients with obstructive sleep apnea syndrome. Laryngoscope 1994; 104:1362–1368.

27. Janson C, Gislason T, Bengtsson H, Eriksson G, Lindberg E, Lindholm CE, Hultcrantz E, Hetta J, Boman G. Long-term follow-up of patients with obstructive sleep apnea treated with uvulopalatopharyngoplasty. Arch Otolaryngol Head Neck Surg 1997; 123: 257–262.
28. Lu SJ, Chang SY, Shiao GM. Comparison between short-term and long-term postoperative evaluation of sleep apnoea after uvulopalatopharyngoplasty. J Laryngol Otology 1995; 109:308–312.
29. Kamami YV. Outpatient treatment of sleep apnea syndrome with CO_2 laser: laser-assisted UPPP. J Otolaryngol 1994; 23:395–398.
30. Krespi YP, Keidar AK, Khosh MM, et al. The efficacy of laser-assisted uvulopalatopharyngoplasty in the management of obstructive sleep apnea and upper airway resistance syndrome. Oper Tech Otolaryngol Head Neck Surg 1994; 5:235–243.
31. Walker RP, Grigg-Damberger MM, Gopalsami C, Totten MC. Laser-assisted uvulopalatoplasty for snoring and obstructive sleep apnea: results in 170 patients. Laryngoscope 1995; 105:938–943.
32. Mickelson SA. Laser-assisted uvulopalatoplasty for obstructive sleep apnea. Laryngoscope 1996; 106:10–13.
33. Walker RP, Grigg-Damberger MM, Gopalsami C. Uvulopalatopharyngoplasty versus laser-assisted uvulopalatoplasty for the treatment of obstructive sleep apnea. Laryngoscope 1997; 107:76–82.
34. Schechtman KB, Sher AE, Piccirillo JF. Methodological and statistical problems in sleep apnea research: the literature on uvulopalatopharyngoplasty. Sleep 1995; 18:659–666.
35. Terris DJ, Clerk AA, Norbash AM, Troell RJ. Characterization of postoperative edema following laser-assisted uvulopalatoplasty using MRI and polysomnography: implications for the outpatient treatment of obstructive sleep apnea syndrome. Laryngoscope 1996; 106:124–128.
36. Finkelstein Y, Shapiro-Feinberg M, Stein G, Ophir D. Uvulopalatopharyngoplasty vs laser-assisted uvulopalatoplasty. Anatomical considerations. Arch Otolaryngol Head Neck Surg 1997; 123:265–276.
37. Woodson BT. Retropalatal airway characteristics in uvulopalatopharyngoplasty compared with transpalatal advancement pharyngoplasty. Laryngoscope 1997; 107:735–740.
38. Bear SE, Priest JH. Sleep apnea syndrome: correction with surgical advancement of the mandible. J Oral Surg 1980; 38:543–549.
39. Hochban W, Conradt R, Brandenburg U, Heitmann J, Peter JH. Surgical maxillofacial treatment of obstructive sleep apnea. Plast Reconstr Surg 1997; 99:619–626; discussion 627–628.
40. Riley RW, Powell NB, Guilleminault C. Obstructive sleep apnea syndrome: a review of 306 consecutively treated surgical patients. Otolaryngol Head Neck Surg 1993; 108: 117–125.
41. Waite PD, Wooten V, Lachner J, Guyette RF. Maxillomandibular advancement surgery in 23 patients with obstructive sleep apnea syndrome. J Oral Maxillofac Surg 1989; 47:1256–1262.
42. Johnson NT, Chinn J. Uvulopalatopharyngoplasty and inferior sagittal mandibular osteotomy with genioglossus advancement for treatment of obstructive sleep apnea. Chest 1994; 105:278–283.
43. Ramirez SG, Loube DI. Inferior sagittal osteotomy with hyoid bone suspension for

obese patients with sleep apnea. Arch Otolaryngol Head Neck Surg 1996; 122:953–957.

44. Utley DS, Shin EJ, Clerk AA, Terris DJ. A cost-effective and rational surgical approach to patients with snoring, upper airway resistance syndrome, or obstructive sleep apnea syndrome. Laryngoscope 1997; 107:726–734.
45. Troell RJ, Powell JB, Riley RW. Hypopharyngeal airway surgery for obstructive sleep apnea syndrome. Sem Respir Crit Care Med 1998; 19:175–183.
46. Conway WA, Victor LD, Magilligan DJ Jr, Fujita S, Zorick FJ, Roth T. Adverse effects of tracheostomy for sleep apnea. JAMA 1981; 246:347–350.
47. Guilleminault C, Simmons FB, Motta J, Cummiskey J, Rosekind M, Schroeder JS, Dement WC. Obstructive sleep apnea syndrome and tracheostomy. Long-term follow-up experience. Arch Intern Med 1981; 141:985–988.
48. Li KK, Powell NB, Riley RW, Zonato A, Gervacio L, Guilleminault C. Morbidly obese patients with severe obstructive sleep apnea: Is airway reconstructive surgery a viable treatment option? Laryngoscope 2000; 110:982–987.
49. Bettega G, Pepin JL, Veale D, Deschaux C, Raphael B, Levy P. Obstructive sleep apnea syndrome. Fifty-one consecutive patients treated by maxillofacial surgery. Am J Respir Crit Care Med 2000; 162:641–649.
50. Kribbs NB, Pack AI, Kline LR, Getsy JE, Schuett JS, Henry JN, Maislin G, Dinges DF. Effects of one night without nasal CPAP treatment on sleep and sleepiness in patients with obstructive sleep apnea. Am Rev Respir Dis 1993; 147:1162–1168.
51. Ferguson KA. Oral appliance therapy for the management of sleep-disordered breathing. Sem Respir Crit Car Med 1998; 19:157–164.
52. He J, Kryger MH, Zorick FJ, Conway W, Roth T. Mortality and apnea index in obstructive sleep apnea. Experience in 385 male patients. Chest 1988; 94:9–14.
53. Guilleminault C, Stoohs R, Clerk A, Cetel M, Maistros P. A cause of excessive daytime sleepiness. The upper airway resistance syndrome. Chest 1993; 104:781–787.
54. Miljeteig H, Mateika S, Haight JS, Cole P, Hoffstein V. Subjective and objective assessment of uvulopalatopharyngoplasty for treatment of snoring and obstructive sleep apnea. Am J Respir Crit Care Med 1994; 150:1286–1290.
55. Zorick F, Roehrs T, Conway W, Fujita S, Wittig R, Roth T. Effects of uvulopalatopharyngoplasty on the daytime sleepiness associated with sleep apnea syndrome. Bull Eur Physiopathol Respir 1983; 19:600–603.
56. Boudewyns A, De Cock W, Willemen M, Wagemans M, De Backer W, Van de Heyning PH. Influence of uvulopalatopharyngoplasty on alpha-EEG arousals in nonapnoeic snorers. Eur Respir J 1997; 10:129–132.
57. Sher AE. Soft tissue surgery for obstructive sleep apnea syndrome. Sem Respir Crit Care Med 1998; 19:165–173.
58. Powell NB, Riley RW, Troell RJ, Blumen MB, Guilleminault C. Radiofrequency volumetric reduction of the tongue. A porcine pilot study for the treatment of obstructive sleep apnea syndrome. Chest 1997; 111:1348–1355.
59. Powell NB, Riley RW, Troell RJ, Li K, Blumen MB, Guilleminault C. Radiofrequency volumetric tissue reduction of the palate in subjects with sleep-disordered breathing. Chest 1998; 113:1163–1174.
60. Emery BE, Flexon PB. Radiofrequency volumetric tissue reduction of the soft palate: a new treatment for snoring. Laryngoscope 2000; 110:1092–1098.
61. Powell NB, Riley RW, Guilleminault C. Radiofrequency tongue base reduction in sleep-disordered breathing: a pilot study. Otolaryngol Head Neck Surg 1999; 120:656–664.

62. Derowe A, Gunther E, Fibbi A, Lehtimaki K, Vahatalo K, Maurer J, Ophir D. Tongue-base suspension with a soft tissue-to-bone anchor for obstructive sleep apnea: preliminary clinical results of a new minimally invasive technique. Otolaryngol Head Neck Surg 2000; 122:100–103.
63. Woodson BT, Derowe A, Hawke M, Wenig B, Ross EB Jr, Katsantonis GP, Mickelson SA, Bonham RE, Benbadis S. Pharyngeal suspension suture with repose bone screw for obstructive sleep apnea. Otolaryngol Head Neck Surg 2000; 122:395–401.
64. Goding GS Jr, Eisele DW, Testerman R, Smith PL, Roertgen K, Schwartz AR. Relief of upper airway obstruction with hypoglossal nerve stimulation in the canine. Laryngoscope 1998; 108:162–169.
65. Eisele DW, Smith PL, Alam DS, Schwartz AR. Direct hypoglossal nerve stimulation in obstructive sleep apnea. Arch Otolaryngol Head Neck Surg 1997; 123:57–61.
66. Schwab RJ, Goldberg AN. Upper airway assessment: radiographic and other imaging techniques. Otolaryngol Clin North Am 1998; 31:931–968.
67. Slatkine M, Krespi YP. Instrumentation for office laser surgery. Operative Techniques in Otolaryngol Head Neck Surg 1994; 5:211–217.
68. Spiessl B. Internal Fixation of the Mandible. Berlin: Springer-Verlag, 1989:348.
69. Maisel RH, Goding GS. Tracheostomy for obstructive sleep apnea: indications, techniques and selection of tubes. Oper Tech Otolaryngol Head Neck Surg 1991; 2:107–111.

21

Pharmacotherapeutic Trials for Sleep-Disordered Breathing

SIGRID C. VEASEY

University of Pennsylvania
Philadelphia, Pennsylvania

Recent data from the cardiovascular studies in persons with obstructive sleep-disordered breathing (OSDB) challenge us to reconsider how we define ''successful'' therapies for OSDB (1–3); at the same time, these data substantiate the need to develop novel therapies for this disease. OSDB is an independent risk factor for hypertension (1), myocardial ischemia, congestive heart failure, and stroke (2,3). The need to treat this highly prevalent disease is now more apparent than ever. Results of these studies, however, pose a great challenge to physicians caring for persons with OSDB. Specifically, the relative risk for myocardial ischemia and congestive heart failure increases sharply for persons with an apnea/hypopnea index (AHI) up to 5 events per hour and then levels off. Thus, it would seem that the target AHI after therapy should be under 5, and that lowering an AHI from severe to moderate levels, e.g., from 60 to 20 events per hour, may not reduce the relative risk of all types of cardiovascular morbidity. Certainly, follow-up studies must be performed to substantiate the above relative risks, and we must determine how effective present therapies are in reducing cardiovascular risk. In the interim, however, we are obliged to consider novel therapies.

Although many patients enjoy dramatic improvements with treatment of OSDB, it is the exceptional patient in whom we are able to fully abolish OSDB events for all of sleep. Continuous positive airway pressure (CPAP) is the most widely effective therapy for OSDB, and when properly titrated, CPAP use typically lowers the AHI to <5 events. Many persons with OSDB, however, do not tolerate CPAP well enough to wear it for a full night's sleep (4). Surgery can dramatically improve OSDB, but the fraction of patients with a long-term postoperative AHI of <5 is small (5). Oral appliances are effective in some patients, but as with surgery, few patients with moderate to severe disease can expect an AHI of <5 with use of an oral appliance (6). The goals for a pharmacotherapy for OSDB, therefore, must be safe, well-tolerated medications that fully abolish OSDB events. While such medications elude us presently, the increased understanding of neurochemical mechanisms underlying sleep apnea clearly brings us closer to effective therapies.

I. A Rationale for Treating OSDB with Medication

Research over the past two decades has substantially advanced our knowledge of the mechanisms that underlie OSDB. Persons with this syndrome have narrowed and more collapsible upper airways (7). To maintain patency of the upper airway and normal respiration, persons with OSDB rely on upper airway dilator muscle activity (8). During wakefulness, upper airway dilator muscles remain active, so that the airway is patent and respiration is normal. In sleep, upper airway dilator motor activity is reduced intermittently, coinciding with upper airway obstruction and OSDB (9). The promise that a pharmacotherapy could effectively treat OSDB is evident from the normal respiration in waking in persons with OSDB. The state dependency of this disease strongly suggests that collapsibility of the upper airway is neurally mediated, and this, in turn, suggests neurochemical changes across behavioral states that could be treated with medications.

II. Neurochemical Control of the Upper Airway Dilator Muscles

Understanding the neurochemical control of upper airway motoneurons has been a major focus in the quest to find a drug therapy for OSDB. The rationale for focusing on motoneuron control is that all changes, central or peripheral, ultimately result in a change in upper airway dilator motoneuronal control. The neurochemical control of upper airway motoneurons is complex with many distinct neurochemicals, active within motor nuclei, affecting levels of motoneuronal activity (for review, see Refs. 10,11).

Several approaches have been used to determine which neurochemicals are involved in state-dependent suppression of motoneuronal activity. The most widely used approach has been the carbachol model of rapid eye movement (REM) sleep–like postural muscle suppression. This model produces a glycinergic postsynaptic inhibition as is observed in REM sleep (12–14). Carbachol injected locally into the dorsal pontine tegmentum in an anesthetized rat produces a state of postural muscle atonia, ponto-geniculate-occipital waves, hippocampal theta synchronization, and respiratory suppression characteristic of REM sleep (15). There are differences between the REM sleep–like state and spontaneous REM sleep. First, some phasic events, e.g., ponto-geniculate-occipital waves, are more frequent and occur at regular intervals in the carbachol model (15). Second, although the muscle suppression is very similar to what happens in spontaneous REM sleep, the respiratory rate in the carbachol model is reduced, while in spontaneous REM sleep the rate frequency increases, particularly in association with phasic events. A distinct advantage with this model, however, is a controlled long-lasting REM sleep–like muscle suppression in which Pa_{CO_2}, Pa_{O_2}, lung volume, temperature, and blood pressure may be held constant. Presently, it is unclear whether the carbachol model represents the neurochemical changes for all behavioral states or exclusively REM sleep. Nonetheless, this model has begun to provide insight into neurochemical control of upper airway muscle suppression (for further discussion of results from the carbachol model, see Chap. 4). Specifically, glycine antagonists injected into the hypoglossal nucleus prevent approximately 20% of the motoneuronal suppression in the carbachol model (16). Another source of postsynaptic inhibition, $GABA_A$, has been evaluated. Like glycine, $GABA_A$ appears to contribute little to the suppression of brainstem motoneurons in the carbachol model (16). Electrophysiological studies provide further support for disfacilitation, or loss of excitatory influences in sleep, as important mechanism(s) of upper airway motoneuronal suppression in sleep.

The list of excitatory neurochemicals that modulate brainstem motoneuronal activity is large, but a focus is provided when considering which excitatory influences have state-dependent reductions in activity at motoneurons. Serotonin (5-HT) [and it co-localized neuromodulators, thyrotropin-releasing hormone (TRH) and substance P], norepinephrine (NE), and acetylcholine (Ach) are excitatory neurochemicals at one or more of their receptor subtypes within the hypoglossal nucleus (17–20), and all of these neurochemicals are likely to have reduced levels in non-REM (NREM) sleep. Levels of NE, 5-HT, and its colocalized neuromodulators are likely to be further reduced in REM sleep, while Ach levels in REM sleep would be expected to increase. Thus, much research concerning the neurochemical control of upper airway dilator muscles has focused on 5-HT, NE, and Ach. However, other neurochemicals, such as orexin, and the neuromodulators co-localized with 5-HT or NE, are likely to be involved in state-dependent changes and may represent potential additional therapeutic avenues for OSDB.

There is much evidence to support the hypothesis that state-dependent changes in 5-HT contribute to the pathogenesis of OSDB. The activity of brainstem serotonergic neurons innervating motoneuronal groups increases with motor challenges, including respiratory challenges (21) and declines in sleep (22,23). Thus, one might expect that persons with OSDB have increased serotonergic excitation in waking relative to normal individuals and that in sleep the reduction in 5-HT at upper airway motoneurons is more profound than in normals. Within the hypoglossal nucleus, extracellular levels of 5-HT decline following pontine carbachol injection (24).

The importance of 5-HT in maintenance of upper airway control has been shown in the carbachol model (25), in the spontaneously sleeping rat model (26), and also in a natural animal model of OSDB, the English bulldog (27). In the pontine carbachol model of REM atonia, pretreatment of the hypoglossal nucleus with 5-HT can largely prevent suppression of hypoglossal activity after the carbachol injection (25). In a spontaneously sleeping rat model, 5-HT microdialyzed into the hypoglossal nuclei prevents suppression of hypoglossal nerve activity in NREM sleep (26). The OSDB in the bulldog is best characterized as snores with arousals and rare hypopneas in NREM sleep, with more frequent OSDB events in REM sleep with oxyhemoglobin desaturations (27). 5-HT antagonists administered to the English bulldog in wakefulness result in collapse of the upper airway and obstructive breathing (28). Moreover, administration of broad-spectrum serotonergic drugs (trazodone and L-tryptophan) to the English bulldog prior to sleep significantly reduce the frequency of sleep-disordered breathing events in the animal model (27). Serotonergic drugs that excite upper airway motoneurons, therefore, represent a potential avenue for pharmacotherapeutics for OSDB, and a potential advantage of 5-HT pharmacology is the large number of receptor subtypes (for review see Ref. 29). This may allow very specific therapy for motoneuronal activation. A complete understanding of the 5-HT receptor subtypes involved in control of the upper airway will be important in determining the safest and most efficacious drugs for this disease. Indeed, there are inhibitory effects of 5-HT within the hypoglossal nucleus through activation of the 5-HT_{1B} receptor (30). Currently the functional significance of different 5-HT receptor subtypes within the hypoglossal nucleus is unknown.

Noradrenergic facilitation of upper airway dilator motoneurons may also contribute to patency of the upper airway (19). In a slice preparation NE in pmol concentrations powerfully excites hypoglossal motoneurons via α_1 receptors (19). The majority of dissociated single hypoglossal motoneurons express mRNA for the α_{1B} subtype receptor; very few cells express α_{1A} or α_{2B}, and no cells express α_{1D} or β subtypes (31). The α_{1D} receptor contributes to vasoconstriction (32). Thus, while possibly effective in exciting upper airway dilator motoneurons, α_{1D} antagonists are unlikely to yield safe medications for OSDB.

Acetylcholine, glutamate, substance P, and TRH may also contribute to excitation of the upper airway in OSDB. Further study is needed both to substantiate roles for each of these neurochemicals in sleep state–dependent changes in neural control of the upper airway dilators and to identify receptor subtypes to permit use of more selective, and therefore better tolerated drugs.

In summary, glycinergic and perhaps GABAergic mechanisms contribute to the profound suppression of postural muscle atonia, particularly during phasic REM sleep. But this postsynaptic inhibition alone cannot explain the suppression of hypoglossal motoneuronal activity that occurs in NREM sleep and tonic REM sleep. Indeed, available evidence suggests that postsynaptic inhibition plays a minor role (16). In normal animals, neurochemical control of upper airway motoneurons is likely affected by neurotransmitters including 5-HT, NE, glutamate, Ach, TRH, substance P, as well as other neurotransmitters. In animals and persons with OSDB, we believe it likely that the serotonergic input and effect are increased during wakefulness and that a predominant neurochemical change in sleep-related suppression of upper airway dilators is a sleep-related reduction of 5-HT delivery to upper airways motoneurons.

III. Trials of Pharmacotherapeutics in Humans with Sleep-Disordered Breathing

Initially, drugs selected for study as potential pharmacotherapeutics for sleep apnea were selected because of their respiratory stimulant properties or REM sleep–suppressant effects or were found incidentally to improve mild OSDB in patients with narcolepsy. While subsequent studies have shown that none of these drugs substantially reduced OSDB, important lessons have been learned. The results from studies with different classes of compounds are now discussed.

One of these drugs, acetazolamide, a carbonic anhydrase inhibitor, induces a metabolic acidosis, thereby stimulating respiration. The drug is effective in treating high altitude–induced SDB (33) and also improves Cheyne–Stokes respiration and other forms of ''central'' apneas (34,35). In a randomized, double-blind study of acetazolamide, in patients with obstructive sleep apnea, there was a significant reduction in the AHI from 50 $\pm$ 26 to 26 $\pm$ 20 ($p < 0.03$) (36). There were no changes in oxygenation, as measured by the oxyhemoglobin nadir and the number of desaturations ($\geq$4%). Symptomatically, these patients did not feel that sleep quality or daytime somnolence was improved. Long-term therapy with acetazolamide was tried in the three patients in whom the greatest response was seen. In two of the three patients, the drug was ultimately discontinued because of paresthesias or nocturnal enuresis. Overall, chronic administration of acetazolamide is not well tolerated, and the effects of this drug on OSBD are minimal.

Medroxyprogesterone is a respiratory stimulant that has been shown in normal adults to lower the arterial CO_2 tension (37). That OSDB is less prevalent in premenopausal females with higher levels of progesterone raises the possibility that progesterone may have a protective effect (38). There have been several clinical studies testing the effectiveness of medroxyprogesterone in treating OSDB, but these studies have shown minimal effects (39–41). In one randomized, placebo-controlled, double-blind, crossover study of 10 men, high-dose medroxyprogesterone (50 mg every 8 h) was given for 1 week, after which a polysmonography was performed, followed by an adequate washout and then the other treatment condition (39). There were no significant differences in either sleep quality, sleepiness, or in the frequency of OSDB events (39). Medroxyprogesterone has also been evaluated for its effectiveness in preventing alcohol-associated exacerbations in OSDB (39). Although the AHI did not change with progesterone, the oxyhemoglobin saturation nadir was not as low with progesterone 20 mg three times daily (40). In a third study, medroxyprogesterone administered to normocapneic patients decreased the waking arterial CO_2 tension without impacting upon OSDB (41). Based on the observation that OSDB is less common in premenopausal females than either males or postmenopausal females, medroxyprogesterone has been tested in postmenopausal women with OSDB and is again without effect (42).

Theophylline, an adenosine antagonist, is a respiratory stimulant effective in reducing central apneas in some studies (43,44). Aminophylline, a theophylline derivative, has been evaluated for effectiveness in OSDB patients in several studies (45–47). In one randomized, double-blind, crossover study with 10 subjects with OSDB, aminophylline was without effect on OSDB event frequency (44). Sleep efficiency was reduced significantly, and more sleep time was spent in light NREM sleep. Similar results were observed in two other small studies. One of these studies reported a statistically significant reduction in AHI, although the reduction was from 49 ± 9 to 40 ± 9 (47). With a narrow therapeutic window, substantial adverse effects and reduced sleep times without substantial reductions in apneas, theophylline cannot be recommended as a therapy for OSDB.

Nicotine is a central and peripheral stimulant through activation of nicotinic acetylcholine receptors throughout the nervous system. Nicotine has been shown to increase respiratory drive to the genioglossus and reduce upper airway resistance in animals (41). Consequently, nicotine was evaluated for effectiveness in treating OSDB (49). Nicotine gum was administered acutely to eight persons with obstructive sleep apnea, who were studied with polysomnography 30 mins following the last dose of gum after a total dose of 14 mg (49). Nicotine reduced the apnea index for the first 2 h of sleep. Hypopneas were not measured. Thus, it is unclear whether SDB resolved completely or apneas became hypopneas. Muscarinic Ach receptors may also impact upon respiratory drive, either at upper airway motoneurons or at respiratory neurons. Therefore, a more complete understanding of the role of both nicotinic and muscarinic receptor subtypes in control of airway motoneuronal activity, and their second messenger systems, will be an important avenue to explore for OSDB pharmaceuticals.

Doxapram is a general anesthetic with respiratory stimulant properties, and in a small study ($n = 4$) this drug reduced the severity of desaturations without affecting the AHI (50). Low-dose doxapram (0.2–1.0 mg/kg/min IV) does reduce apnea frequency in premature infants (51). Whether this would work in adult humans requires further study. This drug may only be administered intravenously, and there are safety concerns with doxapram use (51).

In general, respiratory stimulants, although effective in reducing central events, are not effective in alleviating OSDB events. Respiratory stimulants are likely to increase the respiratory drive to the diaphragm more than to the upper airway dilators. Thus, in persons with OSDB, stimulating diaphragmatic activity might actually create more negative intraluminal upper airway pressure, thereby predisposing the upper airway to collapse in sleep and obviating any benefit from increased activity of upper airway dilator muscles.

B. Drugs That Promote Stage III/IV or Slow-Wave Sleep

OSDB events occur less frequently in slow-wave sleep (stage III/IV) than in light NREM sleep or REM sleep. Thus, a second category of drugs that have been tested for effectiveness in OSDB is a collection of drugs that promote slow wave sleep.

One of these, sabeluzole, a glutamate antagonist, was tested in 13 persons with OSDB using a randomized, double-blind study design (52). No overall effect on SDB was found. It was noted, however, that individual improvement with drug correlated significantly with drug level. Thus, it is possible that with higher doses and a larger patient population, the drug may prove to be have some efficacy in treating OSDB.

Gamma-hydroxybutyrate consolidates sleep and increases the percentage of stage III/IV NREM sleep (53). This drug was administered to eight subjects with OSDB, using a study design consisting of three polysomnographies in a specific order: a control study, followed by a drug study, followed by a second control study. All studies were performed for 1 week, and although the drug consolidated sleep and increased stage III/IV sleep from 12% to 30% of total sleep time, the apnea index was unchanged with drug (54). Hypopneas were not evaluated.

Zolpidem is a nonbenzodiazepine hypnotic that, like gamma-hydroxybutyrate, increases stage III/IV sleep (55). The effects of this drug on OSDB have been characterized in a randomized, double-blind, crossover study comparing three conditions: a single dose of zolpidem (20 mg) prior to sleep, a single dose of flurazepam (30 mg), and placebo. For the group of 12 patients there were no changes in stage III/IV amount. The AHI was 17 for the placebo group, 21 for flurazepam, and 30 for zolpidem. This did not achieve statistical significance. However, the Sa_{O_2} nadir dropped from 85% for placebo to 81% for flurazepam and 77% for zolpidem. This reached a significance of $p < 0.02$ (56). In summary, myorelaxant hypnotics cannot be recommended to persons with OSDB.

C. Central Nervous System Stimulants

Although these drugs by definition disrupt sleep, several stimulant drugs have been studied for effectiveness in treating OSDB. The results from one study suggest that naloxone, an opioid antagonist, may be of benefit in OSDB (57). In this study, continuous infusion of naloxone was compared to saline infusion in 10 obese subjects with OSDB. Naloxone reduced the frequency of oxyhemoglobin desaturations (by 20%) and the magnitude of desaturation. Interpretation of these results is not straightforward, as the AHI was not measured, and sleep stages were not scored for all subjects, and in the few subjects with sleep scored, REM sleep was suppressed by 80%. A second naloxone study, however, did not find improvement in the AHI in persons with moderate to severe OSDB (58).

Modafinil, a central nervous system stimulant, has been tested in six patients in a pilot study with OSDB using a randomized, crossover, double-blind design (59). The drug appeared to reduce daytime sleepiness but had no impact on AHI or desaturation severity. A more recent study shows that in a larger sample size, also using a crossover design, the effects on sleepiness, although statistically significant, were small, and sleepiness was still clinically evident (60). In the latter study, patients on modafinil used their prescribed CPAP therapy for significantly less time than patients receiving placebo used CPAP (60). In conclusion, modafanil may reduce sleepiness somewhat in persons with OSDB, but the drug has no effect on OSDB and therefore is unlikely to reduce or prevent cardiovascular morbidity from the disease.

D. Noradrenergic Therapies

Prior to the basic science exploration of noradrenergic control of upper airway motoneurons, a noradrenergic reuptake inhibitor, protriptyline, was tested for effectiveness in reducing OSDB events in persons with obstructive sleep apnea (61–66). Protriptyline, a tricyclic antidepressant, is a nonsedating noradrenergic reuptake inhibitor as well as a muscarinic cholinergic antagonist with significant REM sleep–suppressant effects. Because of these characteristics, this drug was studied as a potential therapy for cataplexy and other REM sleep–related phenomena of narcoplepsy (67). Sleep studies before and after protriptyline in narcoleptic patients with OSDB suggested that this agent reduced apneas (67). At the same time, protriptyline administered systemically to paralyzed, ventilated cats increases hypoglossal motoneuronal activity (68). Clinical studies in persons with OSDB followed, specifically addressing the potential for protriptyline in the treatment of sleep apnea. Most of these studies were double-blind randomized trials, with sample sizes being small ranging from 5 to 14 persons. The studies have consistently shown no significant group drug effect on the frequency of NREM or REM OSDB events. Power analyses, however, were not performed for any of these studies, and it is unlikely, given the night-to-night variability, that a sample size of 6–12 subjects would be sufficient to fully evaluate efficacy of this therapy (69). Review of individual subject data shows that none of the subjects ended up with fewer than 5 events per hour on protriptyline. Sleepiness as measured with the multiple sleep latency test did not improve with therapy (61). With chronic therapy, there were group reductions in REM sleep time (by approximately 50%) (62–65). This reduction in REM sleep appears to have contributed in a major way to the overall reductions with drug of oxyhemoglobin desaturations ($Sa_{O_2} < 90\%$) and in the overall number of OSDB events for the night.

A second noradrenergic reuptake inhibitor, imipramine, has also been evaluated for its effects on OSDB (70). Like protriptyline, the effects on OSDB are not significant. In conclusion, it is plausible that noradrenergic reuptake inhibition could reduce SDB, but larger studies are necessary to test this hypothesis, and ideally these should be performed after the active NE receptor subtypes in upper airway motor nuclei have been identified. A larger noradrenergic effect is anticipated from use of α agonists directly activating the relevant motoneurons. Further determination of the noradrenergic α receptor subtypes involved in control of upper airway motoneurons may provide more selective, and therefore more effective and better-tolerated, drugs for OSDB.

E. Serotonergic Agents

The earliest study with a serotonergic drug was a trial of L-tryptophan in 15 patients with sleep apnea (71). Like protriptyline, the concept of L-tryptophan in persons with OSDB developed in a rather indirect manner. L-Tryptophan is a precursor of serotonin (5-HT) and has, at high doses, sedating effects. The drug was tried in persons with idiopathic CNS hypersomnolence in an effort to consolidate sleep (71). It was noted that the drug improved nighttime cardiac arrhythmias. As sleep-related dysrhythmias are a prominent feature of OSDB, the drug was tested for effectiveness on nighttime dysrhythmias in patients with OSDB, and it was found that L-tryptophan improved SDB as well as the dysrhythmias. Patients with apnea indices of ≥5 apneas per hour were then selected to test the effectiveness of L-tryptophan on SDB (70). Fifteen patients were studied in an unblinded non–placebo-controlled study. The doses varied significantly between patients, as did the timing of drug administration and duration of drug treatment (days to weeks). Nevertheless, there were several promising findings. In contrast to the effects of protripytline on REM sleep time, L-tryptophan in this study increased REM sleep time, and despite an increase in REM sleep there were reductions in the individual respiratory disturbance indices for all persons studied. Overall, the index dropped from 46 to 29 events per hour ($p < 0.001$), as did the total duration of such events across the night of study (122 to 79 min, $p < 0.01$). The persons with the greatest improvement with L-tryptophan appeared to be those with apnea indices of <60 per hour. Those with predominantly NREM SDB appeared to show the most profound improvement. However, after cases of pulmonary hypertension and eosinophilic myalgia syndrome were linked to L-tryptophan use (72), this substance was taken off the market. Whether the morbidities relate to impurities within the preparation or directly to L-tryptophan use has never been established. It was nearly a decade later before other serotonin drugs were tested for efficacy in SDB. The newer drugs with serotonergic activity that have been tested in persons with SDB include buspirone, fluoxetine, and paroxetine.

Buspirone is an anxiolytic that acts, in part, as a 5-HT_{1A} agonist. The 5-HT_{1A} receptors are involved in auto-feedback inhibition of brainstem 5-HT neurons, so that this drug would be expected to reduce 5-HT delivery to upper airway motoneurons. The drug has other effects, however, including inhibition at dopaminergic presynaptic receptors involved in inhibiting noradrenaline release, thereby increasing noradrenaline activity (73). The anxiolytic effect of buspirone is unique in that it has no activity at GABA receptors, and it is the only anxiolytic with stimulatory effects on respiration (73). Because of its respiratory stimulant effect, buspirone has been tested for effectiveness in persons with sleep apnea (74). In a preliminary report, the apnea index, in five persons with SDB, improved from 31 ± 9 to 20 ± 10 apneas per hour, but the diffeence was not statistically significant. The apnea index in one person actually worsened from 35 to 59 episodes per hour. Since this initial report, no follow-up studies have been published on the effects of buspirone on OSDB.

After several reports emerged describing the excitatory effects of 5-HT on respiratory motoneurons, a trial of fluoxetine was conducted to compare its effectiveness to that of protriptyline (67). Fluoxetine is classified as a selective 5-HT reuptake inhibitor, although at doses typically used for depression there is some noradrenergic reuptake inhibition as well. The overall effect on 5-HT is far more pronounced after 4–6 weeks of therapy, after the autoreceptors have downregulated (for review, see Ref. 75) and 5-HT neuronal firing rates have returned to baseline. At this time, as a result of both reuptake inhibition of 5-HT and the return of 5-HT neurons to baseline firing activity, 5-HT levels are significantly increased within the brain (75).

The trial of fluoxetine versus protriptyline for OSDB compared effects on both sleep and respiration in 12 patients before and after each of the following conditions. The conditions were: 4 weeks of fluoxetine (20 mg/day), 4 weeks of protriptyline (10 mg/day), and placebo for 4 weeks in a randomized, double-blind, crossover study (67). Importantly, the drug was well tolerated and all patients completed the study. Compliance, however, by determining drug levels or other mechanisms, was not determined. The group AHI improved with fluoxetine from 58 ± 9 to 32 ± 8 ($p < 0.05$). There was tremendous variability in response. One person with a baseline AHI of 46 events per hour had an RDI of 2 on fluoxetine, while in another subject the AHI increased from 18 to 49. There were no significant differences in oxyhemoglobin desaturations or in sleep fragmentation across all subjects. These results suggest that fluoxetine may be effective in some persons with OSDB. Once again, however, it is not clear how much of the variability in response is secondary to simply week-to-week variation in disease severity (69). There was a suggestion that improvement with the drug was more likely in persons with less severe disease. The effectiveness of fluoxetine was comparable to that of protriptyline, with the primary difference being that fluoxetine was better tolerated. Overall, this study suggests that serotonergics warrant further study as pharmacotherapeutics for OSDB. Again, a major obstacle to having sufficient power for studies of drugs for human OSDB may be the night-to-night variability in the AHI. Future studies will need to be designed so that they have sufficient power in view of night-to-night variability.

Fluoxetine, relative to many of the other medications tested for OSDB, appears to have minimal side effects. For this reason, there may be unique circumstances when fluoxetine may be a secondary therapy in persons with mild disease in whom the other therapies cannot be used or tolerated. Because of the variable response to fluoxetine, polysomnography should be repeated on therapy after 4–6 weeks of therapy, and the drug's effect on sleepiness should be determined at that time as well.

There is a report that another serotonin reuptake ihibitor, paroxetine, improves OSDB (76). Paroxetine was studied in a randomized, double-blind, crossover trial of 20 patients with AHIs of 25 ± 13. The drug was administered daily (20 mg) for 6 weeks prior to the on-drug polysomnography, and the washout period was of 4 weeks duration. Paroxetine dropped the apnea index by 10 in NREM sleep ($p < 0.02$) but had no effect on REM sleep events or REM sleep time. Data on the effects of the drug on oxyhemoglobin saturations were not reported. Nevertheless, paroxetine may have a role in persons with very mild NREM OSDB.

Trazodone, a drug that enhances neurotransmitter serotonergic neurotransmission through multiple mechanisms, including reuptake inhibition of 5-HT and a 5-HT agonist metabolite, may improve SDB. In a case report of a person with olivopontocerebellar degeneration and obstructive and central SDB, trazodone markedly reduced both types of SDB events without disrupting sleep architecture (77). The RDI dropped by over 50% without affecting sleep architecture.

To test the hypothesis that administration of serotonergic agents can reduce OSDB, we tested the effectiveness of trazodone and L-tryptophan in our animal model of OSDB, the English bulldog (27). Using a randomized, double-blinded design testing three doses of the two drugs and placebo, each bulldog underwent four sleep studies for each of four conditions. This design allowed adequate power to study five dogs and detect a 20% reduction in the AHI. The combination of L-tryptophan and trazodone significantly reduced NREM SDB events. REM sleep events were reduced as well, with the exception of events coinciding with significant phasic REM phenomena. The drug combination had no apparent effect on the severity of REM sleep onset events.

In summary, it appears that serotonergic drugs may be effective in treating OSDB, particularly 5-HT agonists targeting upper airway motoneuronal excitation (26). However, the effects of 5-HT on respiratory drive are complex, and there are data showing that systemic 5-HT antagonists can *increase* hypoglossal activity (78). The mechanism of 5-HT antagonism increasing respiratory drive may be at the nodose ganglion and involve 5-HT_{2C} or $_3$ (79). It is of interest that central apneas in normal rats may be reduced by a drug with 5-HT_{2C} agonist and 5-HT_3 antagonist effects (80). In contrast, 5-HT_{2C} antagonists result in obstructive breathing in the English bulldog (28) and promote collapsibility in the obese but not the nonobese Zucker rat (81). We believe that these findings are all consistent with different levels of serotonergic drive in animals with obstructive upper airways and animals with normal respiration. Clearly, further work is needed to determine the role of different 5-HT receptor subtypes involved in respiratory control, both centrally and peripherally, and differences in receptor activity must be determined in animal models of OSDB.

IV. Future Directions for Human Trials

Certainly, universally effective and safe pharmacotherapies for OSDB still elude us. We have learned a great deal about the pathogenesis of OSDB, yet we require further insight into the neural mechanisms involved in the waking augmentation of upper airway dilator muscles and the reduction in dilator muscle activity with sleep. Understanding the state-dependent neurochemical control of upper airway motoneurons, and identifying active receptor subtypes for 5-HT and other neurochemicals, should be priorities. Armed with a further refined understanding of the neural mechanisms of OSDB, we will be better poised to direct studies of pharmacotherapeutics for this disorder. This challenge is formidable, in that our endpoint for a successful pharmacotherapy will be identification of drugs that fully alleviate the OSDB and reverse daytime sequelae. By focusing first on neurochemical mechanisms, rather than further human trials, we may identify receptor targets with the greatest potential. Preclinical studies of drugs active at these receptor subtypes in animal models of OSDB should facilitate the identification of promising pharmacotherapies for OSDB. Clinical trials should be reserved for highly selective drugs targeting receptor subtypes and second messenger components important in the pathogenesis of OBSD. It is also clear from the trials described above that these studies must be designed to assure adequate statistical power to detect clinically significant improvements in disease.

Acknowledgment

Original research support by SCOR grant HL-60287.

References

1. Peker Y, Hedner J, Kraiczi H, Loth S. Respiratory Disturbance Index: an independent predictor of mortality in coronary artery disease. Am J Respir Crit Care Med 2000; 162:81–86.
2. Shahar E, Whitney CW, Redline S, Lee ET, Newman AB, Nieto FJ, O'Connor GT, Boland LL, Schwartz JE, Samet JM. Sleep-disordered breathing and cardiovascular disease. Cross-sectional results of the Sleep Heart Health Study. Am J Respir Crit Care Med 2001; 163:19–25.
3. Grunstein RR, Stenlof K, Hedner J, Sjostrom L. Impact of obstructive sleep apnea and sleepiness on metabolic and cardiovascular risk factors in the Swedish Obese Subjects (SOS) study. Int J Obes Rel Met Dis 1995; 19:410–418.
4. Kribbs NB, Pack, AI, Kline LR, Smith PL, Schwartz AR, Schubert NM, Redline S, Henry JN, Getsy JE, Dinges DF. Objective measurement of patterns of nasal CPAP use by patients with obstructive sleep apnea. Am Rev Respir Dis 1993; 147:887–895.
5. Pepin JL, Veale D, Mayer P, Bettega G, Wuyam B, Levy P. Critical analysis of the results of surgery in the treatment of snoring, upper airway resistance syndrome (UARS), and obstructive sleep apnea (OSA). Sleep 1996; 19:S90–S100.
6. Lowe AA, Sjoholm TT, Ryan CF, Fleetham JA, Ferguson KA, Remmers JE. Treatment, airway and compliance effects of a titratable oral appliance. Sleep 2000; 23:S172–S178.
7. Suratt PM, Dee P, Atkinson RL, Armstrong P, Wilhoit SC. Fluoroscopic and computed tomographic features of the pharyngeal airway in obstructive sleep apnea. Am Rev Respir Dis 1983; 127:487–492.
8. Mezzanotte WS, Tangel DJ, White DP. Waking genioglossal electromyogram in sleep apnea patients versus normal controls (a neuromuscular compensatory mechanism). J Clin Invest 1992; 89:1571–1579.
9. Remmers JE, de Groot WJ, Sauerland EK, Anch AM. Pathogenesis of upper airway occlusion during sleep. J Appl Physiol 1978; 44:931–938.

10. Horner RL. Impact of brainstem mechanisms on pharyngeal motor control. Respir Physiol 2000; 119:113–121.
11. Berger AJ. Determinants of respiratory motoneuron output. Respir Physiol 2000; 122: 259–269.
12. Chase MH, Soja PF, Morales FR. Evidence that glycine mediates the postsynaptic potentials that inhibit lumbar motoneurons during the atonia of active sleep. J Neurosci 1989; 9:743–751.
13. Soja PJ, Finch DM, Chase MH. Effect of inhibitory amino acid antagonists on masseteric reflex suppression during active sleep. Exp Neurol 1987; 96:178–193.
14. Si MC, Liu RH, Yamuy J, Morales FR, Chase MH. Electrophysiological properties of lumber motoneurons in the alpha-chloralose-anesthetized cat during carbachol-induced motor inhibition. J Neurophysiol 1997; 78:129–136.
15. Horner RL, Kubin L. Pontine carbachol elicits multiple rapid-eye-movement sleep–like neural events in urethane-anesthetized rats. Neuroscience 1999; 93:215–226.
16. Kubin L, Kimura H, Tojima H, Davies RO, Pack AI. Suppression of hypoglossal motoneurons during the carbachol-induced atonia of REM sleep is not caused by fast synaptic inhibition. Brain Res 1993; 611:300–312.
17. Aghajanian GK. Serotonin-induced inward current in rat facial motoneurons: evidence for mediation by G proteins but not protein kinase C. Brain Res 1990; 524:171–174.
18. Berjer AJ, Bayliss DA, Viana F. Modulation of neonatal rat hypoglossal motoneuron excitability by serotonin. Neurosci Lett 1992; 143:164–168.
19. Al-Zubaidy ZA, Erickson RL, Greer JJ. Serotonergic and noradrenergic effects on respiratory neural discharge in the medullary slice preparation of neonatal rats. Pflug Archiv Eur J Physiol 1996; 431:942–949.
20. Ribeiro-do-valle LE, Metzler CW, Jacobs BL. Facilitation of masseter EMG and masseteric (jaw-closure) reflex by serotonin in behaving cats. Brain Res 1991; 550:197–204.
21. Veasey SC, Fornal CA, Metzler CW, Jacobs BL. Response of serotonergic caudal raphe neurons in relation to specific motor activities in freely moving cats. J Neurosci 1995; 15:5346–5359.
22. Heym J, Steinfels GF, Jacobs BL. Activity of serotonin-containing neurons in the nucleus raphe pallidus of freely-moving cats. Brain Res 1982; 251:259–276.
23. McGinty DJ, Harper RM. Dorsal raphe neurons: depression of firing during sleep in cats. Brain Res 1976; 101:569–575.
24. Kubin L, Reigner C, Tojima H, Taguchi O, Pack AI, Davies RO. Changes in serotonin level in the hypoglossal nucleus region during carbachol induced atonia. Brain Res 1994; 645:291–302.
25. Kubin L, Tojima H, Davies RO, Pack AI. Serotonergic excitatory drive to the hypoglossal motoneurons in the decerebrate cat. Neurosci Lett 1992; 139:243–248.
26. Jelev A, Sood S, Liu H, Nolan P, Horner RL. Microdialysis perfusion of 5-HT into hypoglossal motor nucleus differentially modulates genioglossus activity across natural sleep-wake states in rats. J Physiol 2001; 532:467–481.
27. Veasey SC, Fenik P, Panckeri K, Pack AI, Hendricks JC. The effects of trazodone with L-tryptophan on sleep-disordered breathing in the English bulldog. Am J Respir Crit Care Med 1999; 160:1659–1667.
28. Veasey SC, Panckeri KA, Hoffman EA, Pack AI, Hendricks JC. The effects of serotonin antagonists in an animal model of sleep-disordered breathing. Am J Respir Crit Care Med 1996; 153:776–786.

29. Barnes NM, Sharp T. A review of central 5-HT receptors and their function. Neuropharm 1999; 38:1083–1152.
30. Okabe S, Kubin L. Role of 5-HT1 receptors in the control of hypoglossal motoneurons in vivo. Sleep 1996; 19:S150–S153.
31. Volgin D, Mackiewicz M, Kubin L. Adrenergic receptor mRNA expression profiles in dissociated XII motoneurons; a single cell RT-PCR study. Soc Neurosci 2000; 26:115.
32. Varma DR, Deng XF. Cardiovascular alpha1-adrenoceptor subtypes: functions and signaling. Can J Physiol Pharm 2000; 78:267–292.
33. Weil JV, Kryger MH, Scoggin CH. Sleep and breathing at altitude. In: Sleep Apnea Syndromes. New York: Alan R Liss, 1978:119–136.
34. White DP, Zwillich CW, Pickett CK, Douglas NJ, Findley LJ, Weil JV. Central sleep apnea. Improvement with acetazolamide therapy. Arch Intern Med 1982; 142:1816–1819.
35. DeBacker WA, Verbraecken J, Willemen M, Wittesaele W, DeCock W, Van deHeyning P. Central apnea index decreases after prolonged treatment with acetazolamide. Am J Respir Crit Care Med 1995; 151:87–91.
36. Whyte KF, Gould GA, Airlie MA, Shapiro CM, Douglas NJ. Role of protriptyline and acetazolamide in the sleep apnea/hypopnea syndrome. Sleep 1988; 1:463–472.
37. Skatrud JB, Dempsey JA, Kaiser DG. Ventilatory response to medroxyprogesterone acetate in normal subjects: time course and mechanism. J Appl Physiol 1978; 44:939–944.
38. Cook WR, Benich JJ, Wooten SA. Indices of severity of obstructive sleep apnea syndrome do not change during medroxyprogesterone acetate therapy. Chest 1989; 96: 262–266.
39. Bixler EO, Vgontzas AN, Lin HM, Ten Have T, Rein J, Vela-Bueno A, Kales A. Prevalence of sleep-disordered breathing in women: effects of gender. Am J Respir Crit Care Med 2001; 163:608–613.
40. Collop NA. Medroxyprogesterone acetate and ethanol-induced exacerbation of obstructive sleep apnea. Chest 1994; 106:792–799.
41. Rajagopal KR, Abbrecht PH, Jabbari B. Effects of medroxyprogesterone acetate in obstructive sleep apnea. Chest 1986; 90:815–821.
42. Block JA, Wynne JW, Boysen PG, Lindsey S, Martin C, Cantor B. Menopause, medroxyprogesterone and breathing during sleep. Am J Physiol 1981; 70:506–510.
43. Javaheri S, Parker TJ, Wexler L, Liming JD, Lindover P, Roselle GA. Effect of theophylline on sleep-disordered breathing in heart failure. N Engl J Med 1996; 35:562–566.
44. Dowell AR, Heyman A, Sieker HO, Tripathy K. Effect of aminophylline on respiratory-center sensitivity in Cheyne-Stokes respiration and in pulmonary emphysema. N Engl J Med 1965; 273:1447–1453.
45. Espinoza H, Antic R, Thornton AT, McEvoy RD. The effects of aminophylline on sleep and sleep-disordered breathing in patients with obstructive sleep apnea syndrome. Am Rev Respir Dis 1987; 136:80–84.
46. Berry RB, Desa NM, Braunum JP, Light RW. Effect of theophylline on sleep and sleep-disordered breathing in patients with chronic obstructive pulmonary disease. Am Rev Respir Dis 1991; 143:245–250.
47. Mulloy E, McNicholas WT. Theophylline in obstructive sleep apnea. A double-blind evaluation. Chest 1992; 101:753–757.
48. Haxhiu MA, Van Lunteren E, Van de Graaff WB, Strohl KP, Bruce EN, Mitra J, Cherniack NS. Action of nicotine on the respiratory activity of the diaphragm and genioglossus muscles and the nerves that innervate them. Respir Physiol 1984; 57:153–169.

49. Gothe B, Strohl KP, Levin S, Cherniack NS. Nicotine: a different approach to treatment of obstructive sleep apnea. Chest 1985; 87:11–17.
50. Suratt PM, Wilhoit SC, Brown ED, Findley LJ. Effect of doxapram on obstructive sleep apnea. Bull Eur Physiopathol Respir 1986; 22:127–131.
51. Yamazaki T, Kajiwara M, Itahashi K, Fujimura M. Low-dose doxapram therapy for idiopathic apnea of prematurity. Ped Int 2001; 43:124–127.
52. Hedner J, Grunstein R, Ericksson B, Ejnell H. A double-blind, randomized trial of sabeluzole—a putative glutamate antagonist—in obstructive sleep apnea. Sleep 1996; 19: 287–289.
53. Lapierre O, Montplaisir J, Lamarre M, Bedard MA. The effect of gamma-hydroxybutyrate on nocturnal and diurnal sleep of normal subjects: further considerations on REM sleep-triggering mechanisms. Sleep 1990; 13:24–30.
54. Series F, Series I, Cormier Y. Effects of enhancing slow-wave sleep by gamma-hydroxybutyrate on obstructive sleep apnea. Am Rev Respir Dis 1992; 145:1378–1383.
55. Feinberg I, Maloney T, Campbell IG. Effects of hypnotics on the sleep EEG of healthy young adults: new data and psychopharmacologic implications. J Psych Res 2000; 34: 423–438.
56. Cirignotta F, Mondini S, Zucconi M, Gerardi R, Farolfi A, Lugaresi E. Zolpidem-polysomnographic study of the effect of a new hypnotic drug in sleep apnea syndrome. Pharm Biochem Behav 1988; 29:807–809.
57. Atkinson RL, Suratt PM, Wilhoit SC, Recant L. Naloxone improves sleep apnea in obese humans. Int J Obesity 1985; 9:233–239.
58. Guilleminault C, Hayes B. Naloxone, theophylline, bromocriptive and obstructuve sleep apnea. Negative results. Bull Eur Physiopathol Respir 1983; 19:632–634.
59. Arnulf I, Homeyer P, Garma L, Whitelaw WA, Derenne JP. Modafinil in obstructive sleep apnea-hypopnea syndrome: a pilot study in 6 patients. Respiration 1997; 64:159–161.
60. Kingshott RN, Vennelle M, Coleman EL, Engleman HM, Mackay TW, Douglas NJ. Randomized, double-blind placebo-controlled crossover trial of modafinil in the treatment of residual excessive daytime sleepiness in the sleep apnea-hypopnea syndrome. Am J Respir Crit Care Med 2001; 163:918–923.
61. Clark RW, Schmidt HS, Schaal SF, Boudoulas H, Schuller DE. Sleep apnea: treatment with protriptyline. Neurology 1979; 29:1287–1992.
62. Brownell LG, West P, Sweatman P, Acres JC, Kryger MH. Protriptyline in obstructive sleep apnea: a double-blind trial. N Engl J Med 1982; 307:1037–1042.
63. Smith PL, Haponik EF, Allen RP, Bleecker ER. The effects of protriptyline in sleep-disordered breathing. Am Rev Respir Dis 1983; 127:8–13.
64. Brownell LG, Perez-Padilla R, West P, Kryger MH. The role of protriptyline in ostructive sleep apnea. Bull Eur Physiopathol Respir 1983; 19:621–624.
65. Stepanski EJ, Conway WA, Young DK, Zorick FJ, Wittig RM, Roth T. A double-blind trial of protriptyline in the treatment of sleep apnea syndrome. Henry Ford Hosp Med 1988; 36:5–8.
66. Hanzel DA, Proia NG, Hudgel DW. Response of obstructive sleep apnea to fluoxetine and protriptyline. Chest 1991; 100:416–421.
67. Schmidt HS, Clark RW, Hyman PR. Protriptyline: an effective agent in the treatment of the narcolepsy-cataplexy syndrome and hypersomnia. Am J Psychiatry 1977; 134: 183–185.
68. Bonora M, St. John WM, Bledsoe TA. Differential elevation of protriptyline and depres-

sion by diazepam of upper airway motor activity. Am Rev Respir Dis 1985; 131;41–45.
69. Wittig RM, Romaker A, Zorick FJ, Roehrs TA, Conway WA, Roth T. Night-to-night consistency of apneas during sleep. Am Rev Respir Dis 1984; 129:244–246.
70. Rubin AH, Alroy GG, Peled R, Lavie P. Preliminary clinical experience with imipramine HCl in the treatment of sleep apnea syndrome. Eur Neurol 1986; 25:81–85.
71. Schmidt HS. L-tryptophan in the treatment of impaired respiration in sleep. Bull Eur Physiopathol Respir 1983; 19:625–629.
72. Sack KE, Criswell LA. Eosinophilic-myalgia syndrome: the aftermath. S Med J 1992; 85:878–882.
73. Gobert A, Rivet JM, Cistarelli JM, Milan MJ. Buspirone enhances duloxetine- and fluoxetine-induced increases in dialysate levels of dopamine and noradrenaline, but not serotonin, in the frontal cortex of freely moving rats. J Neurochem 1997; 68:1326–1329.
74. Mendelson WB, Martin JV, Rapoport DM. Effects of buspirone on sleep and respiration. Am Rev Respir Dis 1990; 141;1527–1530.
75. Gardier AM, Malagie I, Trillat AC, Jacquot C, Artigas F. Role of 5-HT_{1A} autoreceptors in the mechanism of action of serotoninergic antidepressant drugs: recent findings from in vivo microdialysis studies. Fund Clin Pharmacol 1996; 10:16–27.
76. Kraiczi H, Hedner J, Dahlof P. Ejnell H. Carlson J. Effect of serotonin uptake inhibition on breathing during sleep and daytime symptoms in obstructive sleep apnea. Sleep 1999; 22:61–67.
77. Salazar-Grueso EF, Rosenberg RS, Roos RP. Sleep apnea in olivopontocerebellar degeneration: treatment with trazodone. Ann Neurol 1988; 23:399–401.
78. Richmonds CR, Hudgel DW. Hypoglossal and phrenic motoneuron responses to serotonergic active agents in rats. Respir Physiol 1996; 106:153–160.
79. Carley DW, Radulovacki M. Role of peripheral serotonin in the regulation of central sleep apnea in rats. Sleep 1998; 21;131–136.
80. Carley DW, Radulovacki M. Mirtazapine, a mixed-profile serotonin in agonist/antagonist, suppresses sleep apnea in rats. Am J Respir Crit Care Med 1999; 160:1824–1829.
81. Nakano H, Magalang UJ, Lee S-D, Krasney JA, Farkas GA. Serotonergic modulation of ventilation and upper airway stability in obese Zucker rats. Am J Respir Crit Care Med 2000; 161:347–352.

AUTHOR INDEX

Italic numbers give the page on which the complete reference is listed.

A

C

E

G

H

K

N

O

P

Q

R

S

U

V

X

Y

Z

SUBJECT INDEX

A

B

C

I

K

L

M

N

P

R

S

T

U

V

W

Z